Current Perspectives in HIV Infection

Current Perspectives in HIV Infection

Editor: Anabella Frost

AMERICAN
MEDICAL PUBLISHERS
www.americanmedicalpublishers.com

AMERICAN
MEDICAL PUBLISHERS
www.americanmedicalpublishers.com

Cataloging-in-Publication Data

Current perspectives in HIV infection / edited by Anabella Frost.
p. cm.
Includes bibliographical references and index.
ISBN 979-8-88740-031-0
1. HIV infections. 2. AIDS (Disease). 3. HIV infections--Treatment. 4. HIV infections--Prevention.
5. AIDS (Disease)--Treatment. 6. AIDS (Disease)--Prevention. I. Frost, Anabella.
RC606.6 .C87 2023
616.979 2--dc23

American Medical Publishers,
41 Flatbush Avenue,
1st Floor, New York,
NY 11217, USA

ISBN 979-8-88740-031-0 (Hardback)

Contents

Preface

The human immunodeficiency virus (HIV) is a retrovirus that causes HIV infection and over time transforms itself into the acquired immunodeficiency syndrome (AIDS). The virus attacks the important immune system cells such as helper T cells (specifically CD4+ T cells), macrophages, and dendritic cells of the human body. HIV gradually damages the immune system, which makes the host susceptible to a range of infections. It is transmitted through the direct transfer of bodily fluids such as blood, semen or breast milk. A major cause of transmission is sexual contact with an infected individual. Preliminary diagnosis of HIV infection is done with the help of enzyme-linked immunosorbent assay (ELISA) test, which tests the blood for the presence of HIV antibodies. Other tests include polymerase chain reaction (PCR) tests, western blot test, and single use diagnostic screening (SUDS) test. The treatment and management of HIV consists of the use of multiple antiretroviral drugs. Preventive measures such as condoms and vaccines can help reduce HIV transmission. Another significant type of prevention strategy is antiretroviral therapy. This book outlines the important aspects of HIV/AIDS infection in a comprehensible and lucid manner. It presents researches and studies performed by experts across the globe. This book will provide comprehensive knowledge to the readers.

After months of intensive research and writing, this book is the end result of all who devoted their time and efforts in the initiation and progress of this book. It will surely be a source of reference in enhancing the required knowledge of the new developments in the area. During the course of developing this book, certain measures such as accuracy, authenticity and research focused analytical studies were given preference in order to produce a comprehensive book in the area of study.

This book would not have been possible without the efforts of the authors and the publisher. I extend my sincere thanks to them. Secondly, I express my gratitude to my family and well-wishers. And most importantly, I thank my students for constantly expressing their willingness and curiosity in enhancing their knowledge in the field, which encourages me to take up further research projects for the advancement of the area.

Editor

1

CXCL13 as a Biomarker of Immune Activation During Early and Chronic HIV Infection

Vikram Mehraj[1,2,3†], Rayoun Ramendra[1,2,4†], Stéphane Isnard[1,2], Franck P. Dupuy[1,2], Bertrand Lebouché[1,2,5], Cecilia Costiniuk[1,2], Réjean Thomas[6], Jason Szabo[1,7], Jean-Guy Baril[7], Benoit Trottier[7], Pierre Coté[7], Roger LeBlanc[8], Madéleine Durand[3], Carl Chartrand-Lefebvre[3], Ido Kema[9], Yonglong Zhang[10], Malcolm Finkelman[10], Cécile Tremblay[3,11] and Jean-Pierre Routy[1,2,12] for the Montreal Primary HIV-infection, Canadian HIV infected Slow Progressors, and Canadian HIV and Aging Cohort Study Groups*

[1] Chronic Viral Illness Service, McGill University Health Centre, Montreal, QC, Canada, [2] Infectious Diseases and Immunity in Global Health Program, Research Institute, McGill University Health Centre, Montreal, QC, Canada, [3] University of Montreal Hospital Health Centre (CRCHUM), Montreal, QC, Canada, [4] Department of Microbiology and Immunology, McGill University, Montreal, QC, Canada, [5] Department of Family Medicine, McGill University, Montreal, QC, Canada, [6] Clinique Médicale l'Actuel, Montreal, QC, Canada, [7] Clinique Médicale Quartier Latin, Montreal, QC, Canada, [8] Clinique Médicale OPUS, Montreal, QC, Canada, [9] Department of Laboratory Medicine, University Medical Center, University of Groningen, Groningen, Netherlands, [10] Associates of CapeCod Inc., Falmouth, MA, United States, [11] Département de Microbiologie, Infectiologie et Immunologie, Université de Montréal, Montreal, QC, Canada, [12] Hematology Clinic, McGill University Health Centre, Montreal, QC, Canada

***Correspondence:**
Jean-Pierre Routy
jean-pierre.routy@mcgill.ca

†These authors have contributed equally to this work*

Background: CXCL13 is preferentially secreted by Follicular Helper T cells (T_{FH}) to attract B cells to germinal centers. Plasma levels of CXCL13 have been reported to be elevated during chronic HIV-infection, however there is limited data on such elevation during early phases of infection and on the effect of ART. Moreover, the contribution of CXCL13 to disease progression and systemic immune activation have been partially defined. Herein, we assessed the relationship between plasma levels of CXCL13 and systemic immune activation.

Methods: Study samples were collected in 114 people living with HIV (PLWH) who were in early (EHI) or chronic (CHI) HIV infection and 35 elite controllers (EC) compared to 17 uninfected controls (UC). A subgroup of 11 EHI who initiated ART and 14 who did not were followed prospectively. Plasma levels of CXCL13 were correlated with CD4 T cell count, CD4/CD8 ratio, plasma viral load (VL), markers of microbial translocation [LPS, sCD14, and (1→3)-β-D-Glucan], markers of B cell activation (total IgG, IgM, IgA, and IgG1-4), and inflammatory/activation markers like IL-6, IL-8, IL-1β, TNF-α, IDO-1 activity, and frequency of $CD38^+HLA\text{-}DR^+$ T cells on $CD4^+$ and $CD8^+$ T cells.

Results: Plasma levels of CXCL13 were elevated in EHI (127.9 ± 64.9 pg/mL) and CHI (229.4 ± 28.5 pg/mL) compared to EC (71.3 ± 20.11 pg/mL), and UC (33.4 ± 14.9 pg/mL). Longitudinal analysis demonstrated that CXCL13 remains significantly elevated after 14 months without ART ($p < 0.001$) and was reduced without normalization after 24 months on ART ($p = 0.002$). Correlations were observed with VL, CD4 T cell count, CD4/CD8 ratio, LPS, sCD14, (1→3)-β-D-Glucan, total IgG, TNF-α, Kynurenine/Tryptophan ratio, and frequency of CD38+HLA-DR+ CD4 and CD8 T cells. In addition, CMV+ PLWH presented with higher levels of plasma CXCL13 than CMV- PLWH ($p = 0.005$).

Conclusion: Plasma CXCL13 levels increased with HIV disease progression. Early initiation of ART reduces plasma CXCL13 and B cell activation without normalization. CXCL13 represents a novel marker of systemic immune activation during early and chronic HIV infection and may be used to predict the development of non-AIDS events.

Keywords: CXCL13, humoral immune response, microbial translocation, inflammation, immune activation, CMV

INTRODUCTION

Despite the success of antiretroviral therapy (ART), people living with HIV (PLWH) still suffer from chronic immune activation and the development of non-AIDS events (1). Progressive CD4 T cell decline, elevated CD8 T cell counts, early damage to the intestinal mucosa, microbial translocation, CMV co-infection, and persistence of HIV in cellular reservoirs all contribute to systemic immune activation (2–6). Chronic immune activation and inflammation among PLWH on ART have been linked with increased risk for mortality and development of non-AIDS events such as cardiovascular dysfunction, renal failure, hepatic steatosis, neurocognitive degeneration, accelerated aging, and cancer (7, 8). Therefore, therapeutic strategies are needed to tackle residual immune activation to improve the quality of life of PLWH.

Apart from the virus itself or its proteins, factors contributing to immune activation among PLWH include elevated circulation of microbial products leaking from the gut and CMV infection (9, 10). It has been reported that epithelial gut damage, leading to microbial translocation, precedes systemic immune activation in a SIV-infected rhesus macaque model of the disease (11). Circulation of gram-negative bacterial cell wall antigen, lipopolysaccharide (LPS), and major component of fungal cell walls, (1→3)-β-D-Glucan (βDG), have been reported to be elevated in the plasma of PLWH (12–16). These markers of microbial translocation have been previously associated with activated CD4 and CD8 T cells, indoleamine 2,3-dioxygenase 1 (IDO-1) activity, and plasma levels of inflammatory cytokines. Thus, the optimal marker of systemic immune activation in PLWH should account for the contribution of circulating microbial products LPS and βDG.

Several cellular and soluble markers of immune activation/inflammation have been identified (17). Frequencies of HLA-DR and CD38 expressing CD4 and CD8 T cells are used to measure lymphoid cell activation (18). Inflammatory myeloid cells including monocytes, macrophages, and dendritic cells (DC) are reported to induce IDO-1 enzyme activity upon antigen stimulation (19). IDO-1 converts essential amino acid tryptophan into immune suppressive kynurenines. Frequency of activated CD4 and CD8 T cells as well as IDO-1 activity of myeloid cells have been associated with the degree of epithelial gut damage, microbial translocation, and size of HIV reservoir (1, 20–22). Plasma level markers of inflammation/immune activation include marker of monocyte activation soluble CD14 (sCD14) as well as inflammatory cytokines such as IL-6, IL-1β, IL-8, and TNF-α which are secreted by activated immune cells (23–25). While there are several validated markers of immune activation/inflammation in PLWH, there is currently no single marker that can account for both lymphoid and myeloid cell activation during early and chronic stages of HIV infection.

B cells play a crucial role in mounting an antiviral humoral immune response. Upon maturation in germinal centers (GCs), they are mainly localized in secondary lymphoid tissues where they present antigens, secrete cytokines, and produce antigen-specific antibodies (26). PLWH have been reported to have humoral immune dysfunction that is regulated by GCs, which have been linked to HIV-associated immune activation (27–29). Both structural and functional impairment of lymph node GCs lead to B cell dysfunction. Subsequent B cell activation results in hypergammaglobulinemia, impaired antibody response, and loss of B cell memory (27). B cell activation and trafficking to lymph node GCs is controlled by secretion of chemokine CXCL13 [(C-X-C motif) ligand 13] that is recognized by leukocytes, which express CXCR5. As such, CXCL13 is considered as a marker of GC activity as it is secreted by follicular DC and helper T (T_{FH}) cells. Furthermore, myeloid cells such as macrophages have also been reported to secrete CXCL13 upon activation (30). It has been previously reported that PLWH have elevated plasma levels of CXCL13 during chronic infection (31). However, plasma levels of CXCL13 during early infection, the effect of ART on CXCL13 secretion, and the contribution of CXCL13 to HIV disease progression and systemic immune activation are poorly understood. Herein, we assessed the validity of plasma levels of CXCL13 as a biomarker of systemic immune activation in a well-defined cohort of early and chronic, untreated and treated PLWH.

METHODS

Study Design and Population

114 adult PLWH were cross-sectionally grouped into those in early HIV-infection (EHI) (n = 37), defined as being within 6 months of the estimated date of infection, and those with chronic HIV-infection (CHI) who were either untreated (n = 13) or ART treated (n = 64). EHI participants were enrolled from the Montreal Primary HIV Infection Study (32); while CHI participants were enrolled from the Chronic Viral Illness Service at the McGill University Health Centre and Canadian HIV and Aging Cohort Study (33). In addition, 35 elite controllers (EC)s, defined as PLWH who control plasma viral loads below 50 copies per mL and maintain CD4 T-cell counts above 500 cells per mm^3 in the absence of ART were included from the Canadian Cohort of HIV-infected Slow Progressors (34). Within the EHI group, 24 participants were prospectively followed-up for about 2 years. During the follow-up, 10 EHI participants were on ART for at

least 1 year while the remaining participants were ART naïve during the time of longitudinal assessment. A group of 17 HIV-uninfected controls (UC) were assessed for comparison with EHI and CHI groups.

Laboratory Measurements

Participants were diagnosed with HIV by measuring plasma HIV-1 p24 antigen/antibody and were further confirmed by Western blot as previously reported (32, 35). HIV viral load (VL) in plasma was quantified by the Abbott RealTime HIV-1 assay (Abbott Laboratories, Abbott Park, Illinois, U.S.A). Assessment of CD4 and CD8 T cell counts was done by 4-color flow cytometry. For further research measurements blood samples of study participants were collected to isolate plasma and peripheral blood mononuclear cells (PBMC) samples and stored at −80°C and in liquid nitrogen, respectively. All participants were fasting at the time of blood collection.

Quantification of Plasma Levels of CXCL13

Plasma CXCL13 levels were measured in duplicate by using the Human CXCL13/BLC/BCA-1 Quantikine ELISA Kit (R&D Systems, Minneapolis, MN), a 4.5-h solid phase enzyme linked immunosorbent assay (ELISA).

Quantification of Markers of B-Cell Activity (Total IgG, IgM, IgA, IgG1-4, BAFF, sCD40L)

Total IgG, IgM, and IgA were measured using the Olympus AU5800 (Beckman Coulter). Further subclasses of IgG (IgG1, IgG2, IgG3, and IgG4) were measured by using ELISA kits (eBiosciences, Saint Laurent, QC, Canada) as per manufacturer's instructions. B cell activating factor (BAFF) and soluble CD40L (sCD40L) were measured in duplicate using an ELISA (R&D Systems, Minneapolis, MN, USA).

Quantification of Markers of Epithelial Gut Damage and Microbial Translocation

Intestinal-fatty acid binding protein (I-FABP) was measured using an ELISA kit (Hycult Biotech, Uden, Netherlands). Soluble suppressor of tumorigenicity 2 (sST2) was measured by ELISA as described before (21). LPS was measured using a human lipopolysaccharide ELISA kit (Cusabio, Wuhan, China). sCD14 was measured by immunoassay (Quantikine, R&D Systems, Minneapolis, MN, USA). (1→3)-β-D-Glucan (βDG) was measured by the Fungitell® Limulus Amebocyte Lysate assay (Associates of Cape Cod, Inc., East Falmouth, MA, USA). All the analytes were measured in duplicate as per manufacturer's instructions.

Multiplex Quantification of Soluble Inflammatory Markers

Plasma levels of IL-1β, Tumor Necrosis Factor α (TNF-α), IL-6, and IL-8 were measured in duplicate using the Meso Scale Discovery (MSD) U-Plex Pro-Inflammatory Combo 4 kit (MSD, Rockville, Maryland, USA).

Measurement of Kynurenine and Tryptophan Plasma Levels

Kynurenine and Tryptophan were measured using an automated on-line solid-phase extraction-liquid chromatographic-tandem mass spectrometric method (36, 37). Ratio of kynurenine to tryptophan was calculated as a measure of IDO-1 enzyme activity.

Flow Cytometry Analyses

Frozen PBMC samples were rapidly thawed and stained for 20 min at 4°C using fluorochrome conjugated antibody panels from BD Biosciences (Mississauga, ON, Canada) or BioLegend (San Diego, CA, USA) using anti-CD56-FITC, anti-CD11c BV711, anti-CD3 PE-Dazzle594, anti-CD4 BUV395, anti-CD8 BUV737, anti-CD38 BV605, anti-HLADR APC-Cy7. Cells were then washed and fixed in 2% paraformaldehyde before acquisition. CD38 and HLA-DR expression were analyzed on CD4 and CD8 T cells. Dead cells were excluded as Live/dead positive (ThermoFisher, Saint Laurent QC, Canada). Fluorescence minus one color controls were used to discriminate auto-fluorescence from positive signals. BD Fortessa X20 flow cytometer was used for FACS and the data was analyzed using FlowJo 10.0.7 (FLOWJO, LLC, Ashland, OR, USA).

In vitro Stimulations

One million PBMC from uninfected donors were stimulated for 18 h in 1 mL complete medium [RPMI (Wisent) + 10% FBS (Wisent) + 1% Penicillin/Streptomycin (ThermoFisher)] with 1 μg/ml of LPS (Sigma), βDG (Sigma) or both. Supernatants were collected and CXCL13 was measured as previously described.

Statistical Analyses

Descriptive and inferential analyses were conducted using SPSS 24.0 (Chicago, IL, USA) and GraphPad Prism 6.0 (La Jolla, CA, USA). Data were summarized using means and standard deviations calculated for the variables with normal distribution and using median with interquartile range (IQR) calculated for variables with a non-normal distribution. Percentages were calculated for categorical variables. Subsequently, both parametric and non-parametric tests including student t, chi-square, Mann-Whitney *U*, χ^2, and ANOVA with LSD test were used for comparisons. Paired *t*-test was used for before-after comparisons. Pearson correlation test was conducted to assess association between two quantitative variables. Statistical significance was determined at $p < 0.05$. Multivariate linear regression analysis was conducted to determine the independent association of CXCL13 with HIV-infection adjusting for the confounding factors such as age, sex, CD4 T cell count and inflammatory markers.

RESULTS

Clinical Characteristics of Study Participants

Eighty one percent of the participating PLWH were male and the median (IQR) age was 47 (37–51). CD4 T-cell count was lower in untreated EHI and CHI vs. controls, which increased amongst

TABLE 1 | Descriptive characteristics of study participants ($n = 166$).

Characteristics	EHI ($n = 37$)	CHI ART− ($n = 13$)	CHI ART+ ($n = 64$)	EC ($n = 35$)	UC ($n = 17$)
Age in years					
Median (IQR)	34 (28–44)	43 (33–51)	50 (55–61)	45 (39–50)	41 (35–49)
Sex					
Male, *n* (%)	36 (97.3)	8 (38.5)	58 (90.6)	21 (60.0)	11 (64.7)
Female, *n* (%)	1 (2.7)	5 (61.5)	6 (9.4)	14 (40.0)	6 (35.3)
CD4 T cells/μL					
Median (IQR)	480 (368–650)	81 (14–319)	605 (412–700)	650 (552–823)	866 (566–1,022)
CD8 T cells/μL					
Median (IQR)	810 (630–1,030)	1,030 (267–1,232)	746 (554–1,001)	690 (409–968)	408 (281–689)
CD4/CD8					
Median (IQR)	0.6 (0.4–0.9)	0.1 (0.1–0.4)	0.8 (0.5–1.1)	1.1 (0.8–1.4)	1.7 (1.2–3.0)
VL (log_{10} copies/mL)					
Median (IQR)	4.4 (3.7–5.0)	5.1 (4.6–5.3)	<1.7	<1.7	NA

EHI, early HIV infection; ART, antiretroviral therapy; CHI, chronic HIV infection; EC, elite controllers; UC, uninfected controls; NA, not applicable.

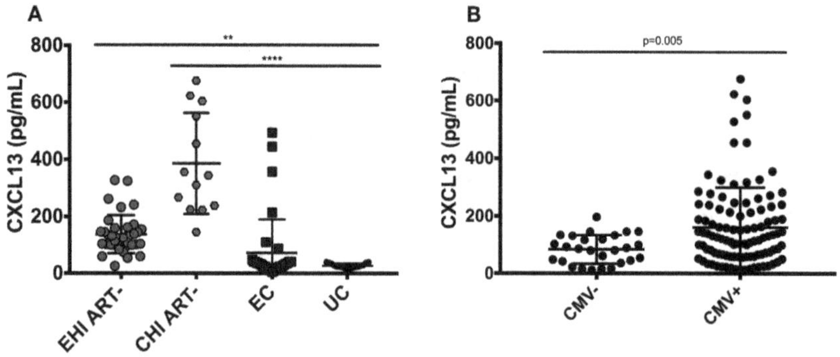

FIGURE 1 | Plasma levels of CXCL13 over the course of HIV-infection. **(A)** Circulating CXCL13 during early and chronic infection compared to elite controllers and uninfected controls. EHI ART− ($n = 37$), CHI ART− ($n = 13$), EC ($n = 35$), UC ($n = 17$). **(B)** Comparison of plasma levels of CXCL13 in CMV+ and CMV− HIV-infected progressors with similar CD4 T cell count. EHI, early HIV infection; CHI, chronic HIV infection; EC, elite controllers; UC, uninfected controls; ART, antiretroviral therapy. $^{**}p < 0.01$; $^{****}p < 0.0001$.

those receiving antiretroviral therapy (ART). In contrast, CD8 T-cell count among untreated PLWH was higher than those receiving ART. Untreated EHI and CHI groups had a median log_{10} plasma viral loads of 4.4 (3.7–5.0) and 5.1 (4.6–5.3) copies per mL, respectively. All the participants on ART and all ECs had plasma viral loads <50 copies/mL (**Table 1**).

Elevation of Plasma CXCL13 Levels During Early and Chronic HIV Infection and Impact of Antiretroviral Therapy

Plasma levels of CXCL13 were significantly elevated in ART-naive EHI (137.3 ± 67.4 pg/mL) and ART-naive CHI (385.91 ± 76.8 pg/mL) compared to EC (71.3119.0 pg/mL) and UC (33.414.9 pg/mL) (**Figure 1A**). EC had lower levels of plasma CXCL13 than EHI and CHI but still had nearly two-fold more CXCL13 than UC. However, this difference was not statistically significant. This is likely because EC are known to have a comparatively preserved immune system compared to progressors (38). We observed PLWH with CMV co-infection to have higher plasma levels of CXCL13 than PLWH without CMV co-infection ($p = 0.005$) (**Figure 1B**). Of note, CMV co-infection has been reported to be linked to HIV-associated immune activation (39). In cross-sectional analysis, both EHI and CHI groups on ART compared to their untreated counterparts showed a significant decrease in their CXCL13 levels without normalization. Longitudinal analysis of the EHI participants that remained without ART for a median of 24 months demonstrated that their plasma CXCL13 levels increased from 133.2 ± 17.3 to 260.5 ± 30.4 pg/mL ($p < 0.001$). On the other hand, EHI participants who received ART for a median of 24 months showed a decrease in their CXCL13 levels without normalization (81.6 ± 10.3 pg/mL, $p = 0.002$) (**Figure 2**). It is important to note that while there is an overall trend of reduced plasma levels of CXCL13 after 24 months of ART, such reduction is pronounced in two participants.

These results suggest that plasma levels of CXCL13 progressively increases with HIV disease progression and is

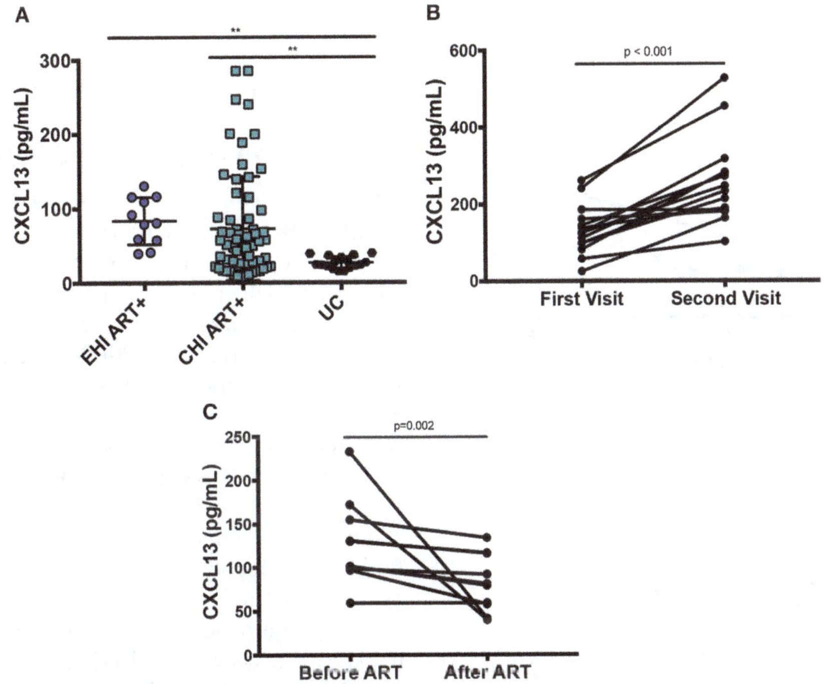

FIGURE 2 | Effect of ART on plasma levels of CXCL13. **(A)** Cross-sectional analysis on the effect of ART on plasma levels of CXCL13 (EHI ART+ $n = 11$; CHI ART+ $n = 64$; UC $n = 17$). **(B)** Longitudinal analysis on the change of plasma levels of CXCL13 over 24 months in PLWH without ART ($n = 14$). **(C)** Longitudinal analysis on the change of plasma levels of CXCL13 in PLWH after 24 months on ART ($n = 10$). EHI, early HIV infection; CHI, chronic HIV infection; UC, uninfected controls; ART, antiretroviral therapy. $^{**}p < 0.01$.

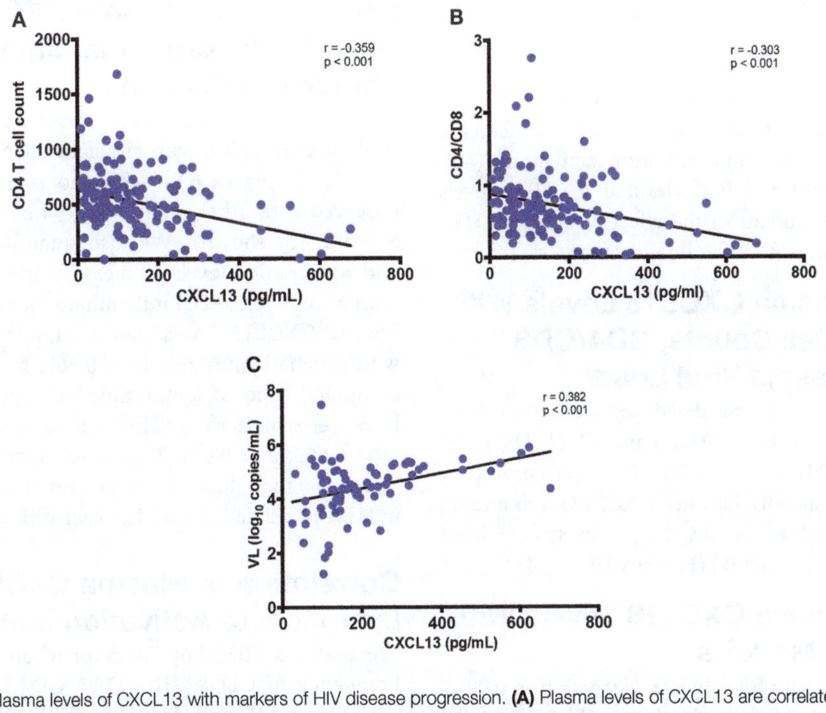

FIGURE 3 | Association of plasma levels of CXCL13 with markers of HIV disease progression. **(A)** Plasma levels of CXCL13 are correlated with CD4 T cell count in HIV-infected progressors ($n = 144$). **(B)** Plasma levels of CXCL13 are correlated with CD4/CD8 T cell ratio in HIV-infected progressors ($n = 144$). **(C)** Plasma levels of CXCL13 are correlated with plasma viral load in untreated PLWH ($n = 72$).

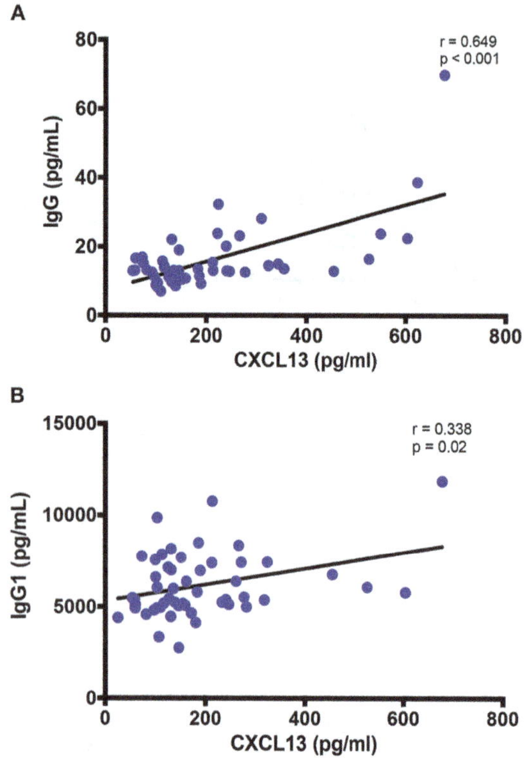

FIGURE 4 | Plasma levels of CXCL13 are associated with immunoglobulin production. **(A)** Plasma levels of CXCL13 are correlated with plasma levels of non-specific IgG in a subset of EHI and CHI PLWH, including participants on and off ART ($n = 49$). **(B)** Plasma levels of CXCL13 are correlated with plasma levels of non-specific IgG1 in a subset of EHI and CHI PLWH, including participants on and off ART ($n = 51$).

decreased without normalization upon initiation of ART. This is in line with previous findings that ART results in a decrease without normalization of systemic immune activation (40). Multivariate analysis confirmed that elevated CXCL13 levels among PLWH were independent of the effect of age, sex, HIV viral load, CD4 T cell count, and inflammatory markers.

Correlation of Plasma CXCL13 Levels With CD4 and CD8 T-Cell Counts, CD4/CD8 T Cell Ratio and Plasma Viral Load

Among PLWH, CXCL13 levels correlated negatively with both CD4 T-cell count ($r = -0.359$; $p < 0.001$) and CD4/CD8 T cell ratio ($r = -0.303$; $p < 0.001$) but not with CD8 T-cell count ($r = 0.107$; $p = 0.232$, data not shown). Elevated CXCL13 levels among untreated participants (both EHI and CHI) positively correlated with viral load ($r = 0.382$; $p < 0.001$) (**Figures 3A–C**) (41).

Correlation of Plasma CXCL13 Levels With B-Cell Activation Markers

CXCL13 levels correlated with total IgG ($r = 0.649$; $p < 0.001$), and IgG1 ($r = 0.338$; $p = 0.02$) in circulation (**Figures 4A,B**), while no correlation was observed with IgG2, IgG3, nor IgG4 (data not shown). Similarly, despite a positive trend, the correlation of plasma CXCL13 was not significant with plasma BAFF and sCD40L levels, two other indicators of B-cell activity (data not shown). These results highlight the distinctive contribution of CXCL13 in B-cell activation and humoral immune response.

Correlation of Plasma CXCL13 Levels With Soluble Markers of Gut Damage and/or Microbial Translocation

Plasma CXCL13 did not correlate with marker of epithelial gut damage, I-FABP (data not shown). We also assessed sST2 as an emerging marker of gut damage (21). CXCL13 levels did not show any correlation with sST2 (data not shown). However, plasma levels of gram-negative bacterial cell wall endotoxin LPS and monocyte activation marker sCD14 positively correlated with systemic CXCL13 levels ($r = 0.332$; $p < 0.001$ and $r = 0.322$; $p = 0.005$, respectively) (**Figures 5A,B**). Both LPS and sCD14 are considered as markers of bacterial translocation. In addition, we also measured fungal translocation using a major fungal cell wall polysaccharide antigen, βDG (42). Plasma levels of βDG correlated significantly with plasma CXCL13 ($r = 0.257$; $p = 0.03$) (**Figure 5C**). Of note, βDG has been used as a diagnostic marker for invasive fungal infections and its role is emerging in HIV-associated fungal translocation as we and others have previously reported (13, 15, 43). *In vitro*, both LPS and βDG induced CXCL13 secretion by PBMC from uninfected donors. Combination of both LPS and βDG did not show an additive effect on CXCL13 secretion compared to LPS or βDG alone (data not shown).

Correlation of Plasma CXCL13 Levels With Soluble Markers of Inflammation and/or Immune Activation

Plasma TNF-α levels were observed to have a significant positive correlation with circulating CXCL13 levels ($r = 0.316$; $p < 0.001$, **Figure 6A**), while no correlation of CXCL13 was observed with other inflammatory markers IL-1β, IL-6, and IL-8 (data not shown). We also quantified plasma Tryptophan and Kynurenine levels to measure IDO-1 enzyme activity as a marker of myeloid cell inflammation and/or immune activation. Plasma CXCL13 levels had a significant positive correlation with plasma kynurenine ($r = 0.569$; $p < 0.001$, **Figure 6B**). We computed ratio of kynurenine to tryptophan as a measure of IDO-1 enzyme activity. This ratio further significantly correlated ($r = 0.653$; $p < 0.001$, **Figure 6C**) with plasma CXCL13 levels. Taken together, these results portray the involvement of CXCL13 in HIV-associated myeloid cell activation and inflammation.

Correlation of Plasma CXCL13 Levels With Lymphocyte Activation Markers

We analyzed PBMC by FACS for whom samples were available. Frequency of $CD38^+HLA\text{-}DR^+$ CD4 T cells ($r = 0.561$; $p = 0.04$, **Figure 6D**) and frequency of $CD38^+HLA\text{-}DR^+$ CD8 T cells ($r = 0.527$; $p = 0.02$, **Figure 6E**) correlated with plasma levels of CXCL13. These findings highlight CXCL13 as a plasma level biomarker of lymphoid cell activation.

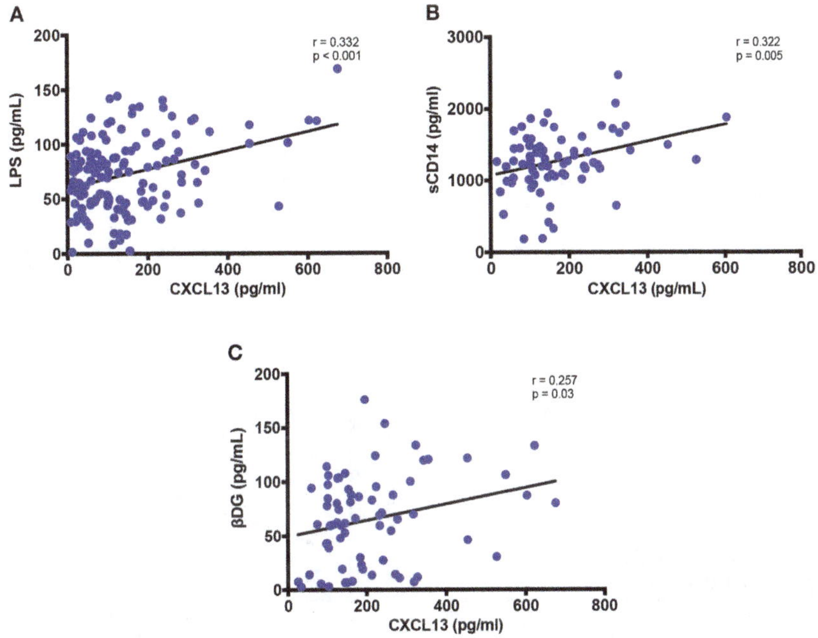

FIGURE 5 | Plasma levels of CXCL13 are associated with markers of microbial translocation. **(A)** Plasma levels of CXCL13 are correlated with plasma levels of LPS ($n = 144$). **(B)** Plasma levels of CXCL13 are correlated with plasma levels of soluble CD14 (sCD14), in a subset of EHI and CHI PLWH, including those on and off ART ($n = 74$). **(C)** Plasma levels of CXCL13 are correlated with plasma levels of (1→3)-β-D-Glucan (βDG), in a subset of EHI and CHI PLWH, including those on and off ART ($n = 68$).

DISCUSSION

We report significant elevation of plasma CXCL13 levels during early and chronic HIV infection that reduced without normalization in PLWH receiving antiretroviral therapy. To our knowledge, this is the first observation reporting a correlation of CXCL13 levels with markers of microbial translocation, inflammatory cytokines, IDO-1 enzyme activity and markers of myeloid and lymphoid cell activation in PLWH. In addition, we also showed a significant correlation of plasma CXCL13 levels with markers of B cell activation in the context of HIV infection. Interestingly, plasma levels of CXCL13 were also associated with CMV co-infection which was reported to be a contributor to HIV-associated systemic inflammation (39). Immune activation is considered as a major factor contributing to the size of HIV reservoirs and development of non-AIDS events despite long-term ART (1, 4, 7). Therefore, therapeutic strategies targeting immune activation remains a priority for curing HIV infection.

Our results are in line with the first report of elevated CXCL13 levels in PLWH. Widney et al. observed a positive correlation of plasma CXCL13 with inflammatory markers and with CD4 T cell count in chronically infected patients (31). In contrast, we observed a negative correlation of CXCL13 with CD4 T cell counts and CD4/CD8 T cell ratio. Progressive decline in the CD4 T cell numbers and CD4/CD8 T cell ratio is a hallmark of HIV-infection (44, 45). Therefore, their negative correlation with CXCL13 levels explains a role of the later in HIV-disease progression via immune activation. Furthermore, in untreated participants, we observed a correlation of plasma CXCL13 with viral load. In untreated participants, the associations of plasma CXCL13 with CD4 T cell count, CD4/CD8 ratio, LPS, sCD14, βDG, and IDO-1 metabolism were independent of HIV viral load.

Moreover, Widney et al. did not observe an association of CXCL13 levels and immunoglobulins. On the other hand, we found a correlation of CXCL13 with IgG and more specifically with its predominant subclass IgG1. This observation shows concordance of plasma CXCL13 levels with B cell activation, which is mediated via CXCR5 expression (46).

Chronic immune activation and inflammation are understood to be the driving factors of HIV disease progression and a significant underlying cause of non-AIDS events in PLWH on long-term ART. As such, it is of clinical interest to validate a biomarker that can monitor myeloid and lymphoid cell activation/inflammation in early and chronic stages of infection in both progressors and non-progressors. In these lines, T_{FH} cells are reported to secrete CXCL13 (47). Cohen et al. have shown that HIV-1 ssRNA induces the production of CXCL13 by DC (48). Furthermore, Carlsen et al. showed that LPS stimulates macrophages to produce CXCL13 *in vitro* (30). We show plasma levels of CXCL13, measured by ELISA, to be a valid marker of HIV disease progression (CD4 T cell count and plasma viral load), microbial translocation (circulation of LPS and βDG), myeloid cell activation (IDO-1 activity and plasma sCD14 levels), lymphoid cell activation (frequency of CD38+ HLA-DR+ CD4 and CD8 T cells), and general inflammation (plasma levels of TNF-α). Thus, we propose plasma levels of CXCL13 as a marker of systemic myeloid and lymphoid cell

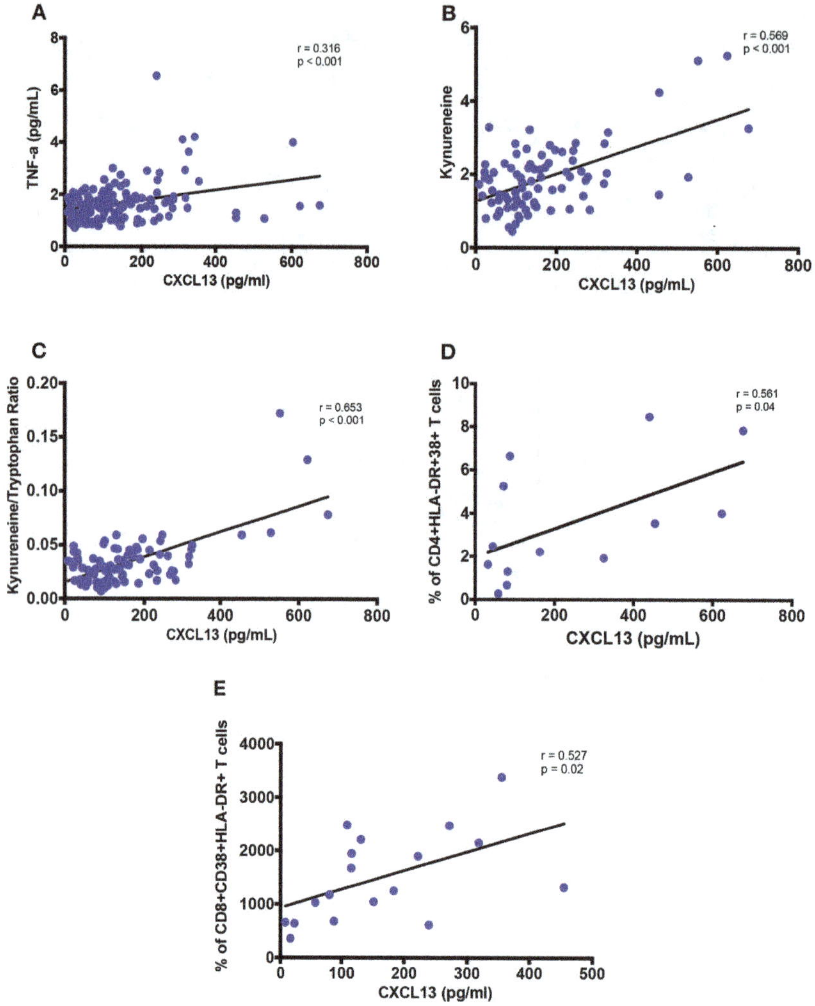

FIGURE 6 | Plasma levels of CXCL13 are associated with markers of myeloid and lymphoid activation. **(A)** Plasma levels of CXCL13 are correlated with plasma levels of TNF-α ($n = 139$). **(B)** Plasma levels of CXCL13 are correlated with plasma levels of Kynurenine, in a subset of PLWH in early and chronic stages of infection, including those on and off ART ($n = 84$). **(C)** Plasma levels of CXCL13 are correlated with IDO-1 metabolism (Kynurenine/Tryptophan), in a subset of EHI and CHI participants including those on and off ART ($n = 84$). **(D)** Plasma levels of CXCL13 are correlated with frequency of HLA-DR$^+$CD38$^+$ CD4 T cells, in a random subset of PLWH from early and chronic HIV-infection ($n = 13$). **(E)** Plasma levels of CXCL13 are correlated with frequency of HLA-DR+CD38+ CD8 T cells, in a random subset of PLWH from early and chronic HIV-infection ($n = 18$).

activation and inflammation in PLWH. Future studies should investigate the contribution of CXCL13 to the development of non-AIDS events and assess if plasma levels of CXCL13 can be used as a prognostic marker for the development of certain non-AIDS events including lymphoma.

T_{FH} cells in GCs and follicular DC in B cell follicles are major producers of CXCL13 owing to their expression of CXCL13 receptor CXCR5 (41, 46, 49). CXCL13 overexpression has been associated with immune activation in chronic conditions such as infection with HIV and systemic sclerosis (31, 50). Havenar-Daughton et al. studied a large longitudinal cohort of PLWH and reported a significant elevation of plasma CXCL13 with the generation of broad neutralizing antibodies (bnAbs) against HIV (41). They further correlated plasma CXCL13 levels with the magnitude of Ab responses and the frequency of T_{FH}-like cells expressing ICOS in the blood of individuals' post-vaccination. Similarly, we observed an association of plasma CXCL13 with Abs such as total IgG and its subtype IgG1 in PLWH. Taken together, such findings display CXCL13 not only as another marker but also as an indicator of GC activity, which is influenced by non-specific and specific stimuli, inflammation, and vaccine response.

Our study has certain limitations that need to be considered while interpreting these findings. Causality cannot be determined as an inherent bias in observational studies like ours despite being conducted on well-defined clinical cohorts. Therefore, this study could not rule out the possibility that the dysfunction caused by chronic immune activation contributes to an increase in plasma CXCL13. Furthermore, limited sample availability did not allow us to assess whether plasma levels of CXCL13 is a marker of immune activation in known HIV reservoirs such as the gut (51). Our multivariate model did not account for potential confounding factors such as risk behaviors, economic status, smoking, alcohol, and drug abuse. Future studies should consider these limitations to further highlight the role of CXCL13 as a biomarker of immune activation among PLWH. Nevertheless, our study represents a novel and comprehensive assessment of plasma CXCL3 in the context of immune activation among PLWH with early HIV infection, before initiation of ART and while being on ART.

CONCLUSION

Globally, our results suggest that elevated plasma levels of CXCL13 in PLWH are partially restored on ART and remains associated with markers of microbial translocation and systemic immune activation. Elevated CXCL13 levels can be used to monitor HIV disease progression and inflammation. Furthermore, it has potential to be used to predict the development of non-AIDS events and residual immune activation after long-term ART.

ETHICS STATEMENT

The study was conducted in accordance with the principles of the declaration of Helsinki and all study participants provided written informed consent for study enrollment. Ethical approval was obtained from the MUHC research ethics board and by each participating medical center.

AUTHOR CONTRIBUTIONS

VM and RR performed the experiments, analyzed the data, wrote the first draft, and revised the final draft of the manuscript. SI, FD, IK, YZ, and MF contributed to the experiments, data analysis, and critical review of the manuscript. J-PR designed the study, contributed to data analysis, and critically reviewed the first and final draft of the manuscript. BL, CC, RT, JS, J-GB, BT, PC, RL, MD, CC-L, CT, and J-PR all contributed to recruitment and follow up of study participants and critically reviewed the manuscript. All authors have read and approved the contents of this manuscript.

FUNDING

This study was financed by the Fonds de la Recherche Québec-Santé (FRQ-S): Réseau SIDA/Maladies infectieuses and Thérapie cellulaire; the Canadian Institutes of Health Research (CIHR; grants MOP 103230 and 154051); the Vaccines & Immunotherapies Core of the CIHR Canadian HIV Trials Network (CTN; grant CTN 257); the Canadian Foundation for AIDS Research (CANFAR; grant 02-512); and the Canadian HIV Cure Enterprise Team Grant (HIG-133050) awarded by the CIHR in partnership with CANFAR. RR is an undergraduate student supported by the H. Grenville Smith Studentship, SI is a post-doctoral fellow supported by the William Turner research fellowship, MD is supported by a salary award from the Fonds de recherche du Québec Santé, J PR is the holder of the Louis Lowenstein Chair in Hematology and Oncology, McGill University and William Turner award holder from the McGill University Health Centre.

ACKNOWLEDGMENTS

We thank Angie Massicotte, Josée Girouard, and Danica Albert for study coordination and assistance as well as Mario Legault and Stéphanie Matte for coordinating the Montreal Primary HIV Infection Study, the Canadian HIV and aging cohort study and the Canadian Cohort of HIV-infected Slow Progressors. We are highly grateful to the study participants for their contribution.

REFERENCES

1. Paiardini M, Muller-Trutwin M. HIV-associated chronic immune activation. *Immunol Rev.* (2013) 254:78–101. doi: 10.1111/imr.12079
2. Sousa AE, Carneiro J, Meier-Schellersheim M, Grossman Z, Victorino RM. CD4 T cell depletion is linked directly to immune activation in the pathogenesis of HIV-1 and HIV-2 but only indirectly to the viral load. *J Immunol.* (2002) 169:3400–6. doi: 10.4049/jimmunol.169.6.3400
3. Cao W, Mehraj V, Kaufmann DE, Li T, Routy JP. Elevation and persistence of CD8 T-cells in HIV infection: the Achilles heel in the ART era. *J Int AIDS Soc.* (2016) 19:20697. doi: 10.7448/IAS.19.1.20697
4. Klatt NR, Chomont N, Douek DC, Deeks SG. Immune activation and HIV persistence: implications for curative approaches to HIV infection. *Immunol Rev.* (2013) 254:326–42. doi: 10.1111/imr.12065
5. Brenchley JM, Price DA, Schacker TW, Asher TE, Silvestri G, Rao S, et al. Microbial translocation is a cause of systemic immune activation in chronic HIV infection. *Nat Med.* (2006) 12:1365–71. doi: 10.1038/nm1511
6. Gianella S, Chaillon A, Mutlu EA, Engen PA, Voigt RM, Keshavarzian A, et al. Effect of cytomegalovirus and Epstein-Barr virus replication on intestinal mucosal gene expression and microbiome composition of HIV-infected and uninfected individuals. *AIDS* (2017) 31:2059–67. doi: 10.1097/QAD.0000000000001579
7. Brites-Alves C, Luz E, Netto EM, Ferreira T, Diaz RS, Pedroso C, et al. Immune activation, proinflammatory cytokines, and conventional risks for cardiovascular disease in HIV patients: a case-control study in Bahia, Brazil. *Front Immunol.* (2018) 9:1469. doi: 10.3389/fimmu.2018.01469
8. Nasi M, De Biasi S, Gibellini L, Bianchini E, Pecorini S, Bacca V, et al. Ageing and inflammation in patients with HIV infection. *Clin Exp Immunol.* (2017) 187:44–52. doi: 10.1111/cei.12814
9. Klatt NR, Funderburg NT, Brenchley JM. Microbial translocation, immune activation, and HIV disease. *Trends Microbiol.* (2013) 21:6–13. doi: 10.1016/j.tim.2012.09.001
10. Maidji E, Somsouk M, Rivera JM, Hunt PW, Stoddart CA. Replication of CMV in the gut of HIV-infected individuals and epithelial barrier dysfunction. *PLoS Pathog.* (2017) 13:e1006202. doi: 10.1371/journal.ppat.1006202
11. Hensley-McBain T, Berard AR, Manuzak JA, Miller CJ, Zevin AS, Polacino P, et al. Intestinal damage precedes mucosal immune dysfunction in SIV infection. *Mucosal Immunol.* (2018) 11:1429–40. doi: 10.1038/s41385-018-0032-5

12. Ancuta P, Kamat A, Kunstman KJ, Kim EY, Autissier P, Wurcel A, et al. Microbial translocation is associated with increased monocyte activation and dementia in AIDS patients. *PLoS ONE* (2008) 3:e2516. doi: 10.1371/journal.pone.0002516
13. Hoenigl M, Perez-Santiago J, Nakazawa M, de Oliveira MF, Zhang Y, Finkelman MA, et al. (1→3)-β-d-Glucan: a biomarker for microbial translocation in individuals with acute or early HIV infection? *Front Immunol.* (2016) 7:404. doi: 10.3389/fimmu.2016.00404
14. Morris A, Hillenbrand M, Finkelman M, George MP, Singh V, Kessinger C, et al. Serum (1→3)-β-D-glucan levels in HIV-infected individuals are associated with immunosuppression, inflammation, and cardiopulmonary function. *J Acquir Immune Defic Syndr.* (2012) 61:462–8. doi: 10.1097/QAI.0b013e318271799b
15. Mehraj V, Ramendra R, Costiniuk C, Lebouché B, Ponte R, Thomas R, et al. Circulating (1→3)-β-d-glucan as a marker of microbial translocation in HIV infection. In: *The Annual Conference on Retroviruses and Opportunistic Infections CROI 2018*, Poster 254. Boston, MA (2018).
16. Hoenigl M, Moser C, Funderburg N, Bosch R, Kantor A, Zhang Y, et al. Soluble Urokinase Plasminogen Activator Receptor (suPAR) is predictive of non-AIDS events during antiretroviral therapy-mediated viral suppression. *Clin Infect Dis.* (2018). doi: 10.1093/cid/ciy966. [Epub ahead of print].
17. Siewe B, Landay A. Cellular and soluble immune activation markers in HIV-infected subjects. In: Hope TJ, Stevenson M, Richman D, editors. *Encyclopedia of AIDS*. New York, NY: Springer (2014). p. 1–8.
18. Kestens L, Vanham G, Vereecken C, Vandenbruaene M, Vercauteren G, Colebunders RL, et al. Selective increase of activation antigens HLA-DR and CD38 on CD4+ CD45RO+ T lymphocytes during HIV-1 infection. *Clin Exp Immunol.* (1994) 95:436–41. doi: 10.1111/j.1365-2249.1994.tb07015.x
19. Mehraj V, Routy JP. Tryptophan catabolism in chronic viral infections: handling uninvited guests. *Int J Tryptophan Res.* (2015) 8:41–8. doi: 10.4137/IJTR.S26862
20. Cockerham LR, Siliciano JD, Sinclair E, O'Doherty U, Palmer S, Yukl SA, et al. CD4+ and CD8+ T cell activation are associated with HIV DNA in resting CD4+ T cells. *PLoS ONE* (2014) 9:e110731. doi: 10.1371/journal.pone.0110731
21. Mehraj V, Jenabian MA, Ponte R, Lebouche B, Costiniuk C, Thomas R, et al. The plasma levels of soluble ST2 as a marker of gut mucosal damage in early HIV infection. *AIDS* (2016) 30:1617–27. doi: 10.1097/QAD.0000000000001105
22. Chen J, Xun J, Yang J, Ji Y, Liu L, Qi T, et al. Plasma indoleamine 2,3-dioxygenase activity is associated with the size of HIV reservoir in patients receiving antiretroviral therapy. *Clin Infect Dis.* (2018) ciy676. doi: 10.1093/cid/ciy676. [Epub ahead of print].
23. Feghali CA, Wright TM. Cytokines in acute and chronic inflammation. *Front Biosci.* (1997) 2:d12–26. doi: 10.2741/A171
24. Esser R, von Briesen H, Brugger M, Ceska M, Glienke W, Muller S, et al. Secretory repertoire of HIV-infected human monocytes/macrophages. *Pathobiology* (1991) 59:219–22. doi: 10.1159/000163649
25. Scherberich JE, Nockher WA. Blood monocyte phenotypes and soluble endotoxin receptor CD14 in systemic inflammatory diseases and patients with chronic renal failure. *Nephrol Dial Transplant.* (2000) 15:574–8. doi: 10.1093/ndt/15.5.574
26. Moir S, Buckner CM, Ho J, Wang W, Chen J, Waldner AJ, et al. B cells in early and chronic HIV infection: evidence for preservation of immune function associated with early initiation of antiretroviral therapy. *Blood* (2010) 116:5571–9. doi: 10.1182/blood-2010-05-285528
27. Moir S, Fauci AS. B cells in HIV infection and disease. *Nat Rev Immunol.* (2009) 9:235–45. doi: 10.1038/nri2524
28. Velu V, Mylvaganam G, Ibegbu C, Amara RR. Tfh1 cells in germinal centers during chronic HIV/SIV infection. *Front Immunol.* (2018) 9:1272. doi: 10.3389/fimmu.2018.01272
29. Pallikkuth S, de Armas L, Rinaldi S, Pahwa S. T follicular helper cells and B cell dysfunction in aging and HIV-1 infection. *Front Immunol.* (2017) 8:1380. doi: 10.3389/fimmu.2017.01380
30. Carlsen HS, Baekkevold ES, Morton HC, Haraldsen G, Brandtzaeg P. Monocyte-like and mature macrophages produce CXCL13 (B cell-attracting chemokine 1) in inflammatory lesions with lymphoid neogenesis. *Blood* (2004) 104:3021–7. doi: 10.1182/blood-2004-02-0701
31. Widney DP, Breen EC, Boscardin WJ, Kitchen SG, Alcantar JM, Smith JB, et al. Serum levels of the homeostatic B cell chemokine, CXCL13, are elevated during HIV infection. *J Interferon Cytokine Res.* (2005) 25:702–6. doi: 10.1089/jir.2005.25.702
32. Mehraj V, Cox J, Lebouche B, Costiniuk C, Cao W, Li T, et al. Socio-economic status and time trends associated with early ART initiation following primary HIV infection in Montreal, Canada: 1996 to 2015. *J Int AIDS Soc.* (2018) 21:e25034. doi: 10.1002/jia2.25034
33. Durand M, Chartrand-Lefebvre C, Baril JG, Trottier S, Trottier B, Harris M, et al. The Canadian HIV and aging cohort study - determinants of increased risk of cardio-vascular diseases in HIV-infected individuals: rationale and study protocol. *BMC Infect Dis.* (2017) 17:611. doi: 10.1186/s12879-017-2692-2
34. El-Far M, Kouassi P, Sylla M, Zhang Y, Fouda A, Fabre T, et al. Proinflammatory isoforms of IL-32 as novel and robust biomarkers for control failure in HIV-infected slow progressors. *Sci Rep.* (2016) 6:22902. doi: 10.1038/srep22902
35. Cao W, Mehraj V, Trottier B, Baril JG, Leblanc R, Lebouche B, et al. Early initiation rather than prolonged duration of antiretroviral therapy in HIV infection contributes to the normalization of CD8 T-cell counts. *Clin Infect Dis.* (2016) 62:250–7. doi: 10.1093/cid/civ809
36. Jenabian MA, El-Far M, Vyboh K, Kema I, Costiniuk CT, Thomas R, et al. Immunosuppressive tryptophan catabolism and gut mucosal dysfunction following early HIV infection. *J Infect Dis.* (2015) 212:355–66. doi: 10.1093/infdis/jiv037
37. Jenabian MA, Patel M, Kema I, Kanagaratham C, Radzioch D, Thebault P, et al. Distinct tryptophan catabolism and Th17/Treg balance in HIV progressors and elite controllers. *PLoS ONE* (2013) 8:e78146. doi: 10.1371/journal.pone.0078146
38. Zaunders J, van Bockel D. Innate and adaptive immunity in long-term non-progression in HIV disease. *Front Immunol.* (2013) 4:95. doi: 10.3389/fimmu.2013.00095
39. Lurain NS, Hanson BA, Hotton AL, Weber KM, Cohen MH, Landay AL. The association of human cytomegalovirus with biomarkers of inflammation and immune activation in HIV-1-infected women. *AIDS Res Hum Retroviruses* (2016) 32:134–43. doi: 10.1089/aid.2015.0169
40. Chen J, Ramendra R, Lu H, Routy JP. The early bird gets the worm: benefits and future directions with early antiretroviral therapy initiation in primary HIV infection. *Fut. Virol.* (2018) 13, 779–786. doi: 10.2217/fvl-2018-0110
41. Havenar-Daughton C, Lindqvist M, Heit A, Wu JE, Reiss SM, Kendric K, et al. CXCL13 is a plasma biomarker of germinal center activity. *Proc Natl Acad Sci USA.* (2016) 113:2702–7. doi: 10.1073/pnas.1520112113
42. Camilli G, Tabouret G, Quintin J. The complexity of fungal beta-Glucan in health and disease: effects on the mononuclear phagocyte system. *Front Immunol.* (2018) 9:673. doi: 10.3389/fimmu.2018.00673
43. Farhour Z, Mehraj V, Chen J, Ramendra R, Lu H, Routy JP. Use of (1→3)-β-d-glucan for diagnosis and management of invasive mycoses in HIV-infected patients. *Mycoses* (2018) 61:718–22. doi: 10.1111/myc.12797
44. Lu W, Mehraj V, Vyboh K, Cao W, Li T, Routy JP. CD4:CD8 ratio as a frontier marker for clinical outcome, immune dysfunction and viral reservoir size in virologically suppressed HIV-positive patients. *J Int AIDS Soc.* (2015) 18:20052. doi: 10.7448/IAS.18.1.20052
45. Vidya Vijayan KK, Karthigeyan KP, Tripathi SP, Hanna LE. Pathophysiology of CD4+ T-cell depletion in HIV-1 and HIV-2 infections. *Front Immunol.* (2017) 8:580. doi: 10.3389/fimmu.2017.00580
46. Rasheed AU, Rahn HP, Sallusto F, Lipp M, Muller G. Follicular B helper T cell activity is confined to CXCR5(hi)ICOS(hi) CD4 T cells and is independent of CD57 expression. *Eur J Immunol.* (2006) 36:1892–903. doi: 10.1002/eji.200636136
47. Gu-Trantien C, Migliori E, Buisseret L, de Wind A, Brohee S, Garaud S, et al. CXCL13-producing TFH cells link immune suppression and

adaptive memory in human breast cancer. *JCI Insight.* (2017) 2:91487. doi: 10.1172/jci.insight.91487
48. Cohen KW, Dugast AS, Alter G, McElrath MJ, Stamatatos L. HIV-1 single-stranded RNA induces CXCL13 secretion in human monocytes via TLR7 activation and plasmacytoid dendritic cell-derived type I IFN. *J Immunol.* (2015) 194:2769–75. doi: 10.4049/jimmunol.1400952
49. Wang X, Cho B, Suzuki K, Xu Y, Green JA, An J, et al. Follicular dendritic cells help establish follicle identity and promote B cell retention in germinal centers. *J Exp Med.* (2011) 208:2497–510. doi: 10.1084/jem.20111449
50. Taniguchi T, Miyagawa T, Toyama S, Yamashita T, Nakamura K, Saigusa R, et al. CXCL13 produced by macrophages due to Fli1 deficiency may contribute to the development of tissue fibrosis, vasculopathy and immune activation in systemic sclerosis. *Exp Dermatol.* (2018) 27:1030–7. doi: 10.1111/exd.13724
51. Mehraj V, Ghali P, Ramendra R, Costiniuk C, Lebouche B, Ponte R, et al. The evaluation of risk-benefit ratio for gut tissue sampling in HIV cure research. *J Virus Erad.* (2017) 3:212–7.

2

A T Cell Receptor Sequencing-Based Assay Identifies Cross-Reactive Recall CD8$^+$ T Cell Clonotypes Against Autologous HIV-1 Epitope Variants

Hok Yee Chan[1,2], Jiajia Zhang[1,2], Caroline C. Garliss[3], Abena K. Kwaa[3], Joel N. Blankson[3,4] and Kellie N. Smith[1,2]**

[1] Bloomberg-Kimmel Institute for Cancer Immunotherapy, Johns Hopkins School of Medicine, Baltimore, MD, United States, [2] Sidney Kimmel Comprehensive Cancer Center, Johns Hopkins School of Medicine, Baltimore, MD, United States, [3] Department of Medicine, Johns Hopkins School of Medicine, Baltimore, MD, United States, [4] Department of Molecular and Comparative Pathobiology, Johns Hopkins School of Medicine, Baltimore, MD, United States

***Correspondence:**
Joel N. Blankson
jblanks@jhmi.edu
Kellie N. Smith
ksmit228@jhmi.edu

HIV-1 positive elite controllers or suppressors control viral replication without antiretroviral therapy, likely via CTL-mediated elimination of infected cells, and therefore represent a model of an HIV-1 functional cure. Efforts to cure HIV-1 accordingly rely on the existence or generation of antigen-specific cytotoxic T lymphocytes (CTL) to eradicate infected cells upon reversal of latency. Detecting and quantifying these HIV-1-specific CTL responses will be crucial for developing vaccine and T cell-based immunotherapies. A recently developed assay, called MANAFEST, uses T cell receptor (TCR) Vβ sequencing of peptide-stimulated cultures followed by a bioinformatic pipeline to identify neoantigen-specific T cells in cancer patients. This assay is more sensitive than conventional immune assays and therefore has the possibility to identify HIV-1 antigenic targets that have not been previously explored for vaccine or T cell immunotherapeutic strategies. Here we show that a modified version of the MANAFEST assay, called ViraFEST, can identify memory CD8$^+$ T cell responses against autologous HIV-1 Gag and Nef epitope variants in an elite suppressor. Nine TCR Vβ clonotypes were identified and 6 of these were cross-reactive for autologous variants or known escape variants. Our findings are a proof of principle that the ViraFEST assay can be used to detect and monitor these responses for downstream use in immunotherapeutic treatment approaches.

Keywords: HIV, cure, elite suppressors, elite controllers, clonotype, CD8 lymphocytes+

INTRODUCTION

Antiretroviral therapy (ART) reduces viral load to undetectable levels in the majority of HIV-1-infected patients. Despite this, a persistent latent viral reservoir in tissues and blood prevents complete viral eradication and results in viral rebound upon ART cessation in the vast majority of patients (1). HIV elite suppressors (ES) are patients who control viral replication without ART (2). These patients may represent a model of a functional cure for HIV-1 since many are infected with replication-competent viruses (3, 4) and are thought to control viral replication through HIV-specific CTL (5–8). Thus it may be possible to control the rebound of viremia following the cessation of ART in patients with progressive disease with immunotherapy. One such strategy is the "shock and kill" approach (9), whereby viral replication is induced from within latent reservoirs and endogenously- or exogenously-generated cytotoxic T lymphocytes (CTL) specific for the patient's own virus (autologous virus) kill infected cells. Several immunotherapeutic approaches have been evaluated to induce CTL killing of infected cells, including dendritic cell-based strategies (10), adoptive transfer of CAR T cells (11), and checkpoint inhibition therapy (12).

Identifying antigenic CTL epitopes and evaluating endogenous memory CTL responses will be crucial for developing these immunotherapies into effective treatments. ELISpot, intracellular cytokine staining, and multimer staining have traditionally been employed when assessing HIV-1-specific T cell responses. However, these assays can underestimate the breadth and magnitude of the response (13) and do not enable identification at the clonotypic level, which will be crucial for engineered T cell-based treatments. The mutation associated neoantigen functional expansion of specific T cells (MANAFEST) assay uses peptide-stimulated T cell cultures coupled with T cell receptor Vβ sequencing and a bioinformatic pipeline to identify neoantigen specific CD8$^+$ T cell clonotypes (13–15). This assay has yet to be utilized to evaluate HIV-1-specific responses. This could be particularly useful given the potential for cross-reactivity of HIV-specific T-cell receptors (16–21).

Our goal was to therefore provide a proof-of-principle demonstrating the utility of the MANAFEST assay in identifying T cell responses at the clonotypic level against closely related autologous HIV-1 epitope variants. Elite suppressors are the ideal model for this analysis, owing to well-documented HIV-specific T cell responses and presumed CTL-mediated viral control in these patients. Here we demonstrate that modified use of the MANAFEST assay, called ViraFEST (viral functional expansion of specific T cells), combined with a novel analytical platform can detect cross-reactive CD8$^+$ T cell responses to autologous epitope variants in an HIV-1$^+$ elite suppressor (ES). This is the first report using this assay to evaluate the cross-reactive nature of T cells specific for autologous HIV-1 epitope variants. Routine use of this assay to detect and monitor T cell responses to HIV-1 antigens could reveal a broad range of immunogenic antigens not previously identified and can identify HIV-1-specific TCRs that could be exploited in vaccine or T cell-based immunotherapies.

METHODS

Study Patient

Blood samples from the study subject were obtained in 2018 and 2019 after written informed consent and subsequently handled in accordance with protocols approved by the Johns Hopkins University IRB.

HIV-1 Sequencing and Epitope Selection

Peptides corresponding to previously described autologous variants found in HLA-B*57 restricted Gag and Nef proviral, plasma, and replication competent clones were synthesized (22–25). Replication-competent isolates from 2018 were obtained as previously described (3, 4). Briefly, unfractionated CD4$^+$ T cells were isolated by negative selection with Miltenyi beads and replicates of 1 million cells were stimulated with PHA (0.5 ug/ml) and 10 million irradiated allogeneic PBMCs. Four million healthy donor lymphoblasts were added on days 2 and 9 to amplify the virus and positive cultures were identified by p24 ELISA (Perkin Elmer). gag and nef were sequenced from 2 isolates as previously described (3, 4).

T Cell Culture

A total of 25 peptides representing autologous Gag and Nef epitope variants were synthesized by GenScript with a purity of > 85% and used to stimulate T cells in a modified version of the MANAFEST assay (13–15, 26), called ViraFEST. On day 0, peripheral blood mononuclear cells (PBMC) were isolated fresh from whole blood. T cells were isolated using the EasySep Human T Cell Enrichment Kit (Stemcell Technologies). The T cell and T cell-negative fraction were washed, counted, and resuspended at 2.5 × 10^6/mL in IMDM supplemented with 50 µg/mL gentamicin (ThermoFisher Scientific). The T cell-negative cells were added to a 96-well plate at 100 µL per well. An equal number of T cells was added to each well. Peptide antigens representing the 25 autologous epitope variants were added to individual wells (10 µg/mL), along with a CMV, EBV, and flu peptide pool (1 µg/mL; Miltenyi), and the Ebola virus AY9 epitope, ATAAATEAY, as a negative control, and a condition without peptide to evaluate non-specific T cell expansion. Each culture condition was evaluated in triplicate, with the exception of the ISPRTLNAW peptide, which was done in duplicate, for a total of 83 T cell cultures. An aliquot of 1M T cells was saved as the uncultured baseline condition. Cells were cultured for a total of 10 days at 37°C in a 5% CO_2 atmosphere. On day 3, half of the culture media was replaced with fresh culture media supplemented with 100 IU/mL IL2, 50 ng/mL IL7, and 50 ng/mL IL15 (for final concentrations of 50 IU/mL IL2, 25 ng/mL IL7, and 25 ng/mL IL15). On day 7, half of the culture media was replaced again with fresh media supplemented with 200 IU/mL IL2, 50 ng/mL IL7, and 50 ng/mL IL15 (for final concentrations of 100 IU/mL IL2, 25 ng/mL IL7, and 25 ng/mL IL15). On day 10, cultured cells were harvested and washed, and CD8+ T cells were isolated using the EasySep Human CD8$^+$ T Cell Enrichment Kit (Stemcell Technologies).

TCR Sequencing, Bioinformatic Processing, and Assessment of Antigen-Specific Expansions

DNA was extracted from each individual cultured CD8$^+$ T cell population, as well as the uncultured baseline CD8$^+$ T cells, using the QIAamp DNA micro kit (Qiagen). TCR Vβ CDR3 sequencing was performed using the survey sequencing ImmunoSEQ platform (Adaptive Biotechnologies). Conditions with less than 5,000 productive reads after TCR sequencing were excluded from further analysis (**Supplementary Table 1**). TCR sequencing. tsv files were exported from the ImmunoSEQ analyzer and were uploaded to our publicly-available MANAFEST analysis web app (http://www.stat-apps.onc.jhmi.edu/FEST/). This package prepares TCR sequencing files for analysis, which includes alignment and trimming of nucleotide sequences to obtain only the CDR3 region and removal of nonproductive CDR3 sequences with premature stops or frame-shifts, sequences with an amino acid length <5, and sequences not starting with "C" or ending with "F/W".

We used a modified version of our statistical criteria to identify antigen-specific T cell clonotypes. To be classified as antigen-specific, a clonotype at the nucleotide level must (1) significantly expand in at least 2 out of 3 replicates relative to the no peptide control well at an FDR of 0.01, (2) only significantly expand in other wells with peptides from the same epitope family using an FDR of 0.01, and (3) have a frequency at least 5 times higher than the frequency of the clone in wells stimulated with peptides from a different epitope family. For visualization, the mean frequency +/- standard deviation of positive and negative expansions was graphed for each well.

RESULTS

Clinical Characteristics and Viral Evolution

ES8 is a previously described elite controller who had undetectable viral loads until 5 years prior to this study when he developed persistent low level viremia. The patient's HLA haplotype is A 02/03, B-57/44.

Autologous HIV-1 *gag* and *nef* was sequenced from provirus and plasma obtained in 2004, 2005, 2007, and 2010 and from replication-competent virus cultured in 2006 and 2018 (3, 21–24) as outlined in **Table 1**. The patient initially had wild type sequence in the HLA-B*57 restricted Gag epitopes TW10 and IW9 in proviral clones and in replication-competent virus (3, 22), but he consistently had variants in both epitopes in plasma clones starting in 2004, the earliest time point studied (22). These plasma variants evolved over time (24) and by 2018, replication-competent virus also contained multiple substitutions in both epitopes. A similar discrepancy between proviral and plasma variants was seen in the non-HLA-B*57 restricted Gag epitope KK15 and in the HLA-B*57 restricted Nef epitope KF9 (22, 23). In contrast there was concordance in sequence between proviral and plasma clones in the HLA-B*57 restricted Nef epitopes HW9 and YT9 (23).

Evaluation of Memory CD8+ T Cell Responses to Autologous Gag and Nef Epitope Variants

We next assessed the memory T cell responses against autologous epitope variants using a modified version of the MANAFEST assay, called ViraFEST (Viral Functional Expansion of Specific T cells). A schema of the general experimental approach is shown in **Figure 1**. Three Gag epitope families were selected for functional validation (**Table 1**). T cells isolated from PBMC were stimulated with individual peptides. When testing mutation associated neoantigens (MANAs), there is customarily only one epitope tested per mutation (there are rarely 2 nonsynonymous passenger mutations in the same codon). However, owing to the possibility of memory T cells existing against closely-related HIV-1 epitope variants (33, 34), we performed each peptide stimulation in triplicate, with the exception of the ISPRTLNAW peptide, which was evaluated in duplicate, to increase the statistical power of identifying true antigen-specific TCRs for a total of 75 HIV-1 peptide-stimulated cultures. TCR sequencing was performed on DNA extracted from each T

TABLE 1 | Characteristics of the autologous and known epitopes evaluated for $CD8^+$ T cell recognition*.

Protein	AA sequence	Description	References
GAG TW10 (240-249)	TSTLQEQIGW	Consensus epitope	
		ES8 provirus, 2005, 2007, 2010	(3, 22, 24, 27)
		ES8 replication-competent virus 2006	(28)
	TSTLTEQVAW	ES8 plasma variant 2004 and 2008	(22, 24)
	TSTLAEQVAW	ES8 plasma variant 2008	(24)
	TSTLVEQIAW	ES8 plasma variant 2008	(24)
	TSTLAEQIAW	ES8 plasma variant 2009	(24)
	TSTLSEQVAW	ES8 plasma variant 2009	(24)
	TSTLSEQIAW	ES8 plasma variant 2009	(24)
	TSTLTEQIAW	ES8 plasma variant 2009	(24)
	TSTLQEQIEW	ES plasma variant 2004	(22)
	TSTLAEQMAW	ES8 replication-competent virus 2018	
	TSNLQEQIGW	Common escape mutant	(29–31)
	TSNLQEQIAW	Common escape mutant	(30)
GAG IW9 (147-155)	ISPRTLNAW	Consensus sequence: ES8 provirus 2005	(22, 24)
		ES8 replication-competent virus 2006	
	MSPRTLNAW	ES8 plasma variant, 2004, 2009. RC virus 2018	(22, 24)
GAG KK15 (17-31)	KIRLRPGGKKKYKLK	Consensus sequence. ES8 provirus 2005	(22, 24)
	KIRLRPGGKKRYKLK	ES8 plasma variant 2004.	(22, 24)
		ES8 replication-competent virus 2006	
NEF KF9 (82-90)	KAAVDLSHF	Consensus sequence	
	KSALDLSHF	ES8 provirus variant 2005	(3, 23, 25)
	TAALDMSHF	ES8 plasma variant 2004 and 2010. RC virus 2018	(23, 25)
	KGALDLSHF	Common variant	
	KAALDLSHF	Common variant	
NEF HW9 (116-124)	HTQGYFPDW	Consensus sequence.	
		ES8 replication-competent virus 2018	
	NTQGYFPDW	Previously described escape mutation	(32)
NEF YT9 (120-128)	YFPDWQNYT	Consensus sequence.	
		ES8 replication-competent virus 2018	
	FFPDWQNYT	ES8 provirus and plasma variant (2004, 2010)	(23, 25)

*All peptides except for Gag KK15 represent HLA-B*57 restricted epitopes. Residues highlighted in red are variants of the consensus sequence.*

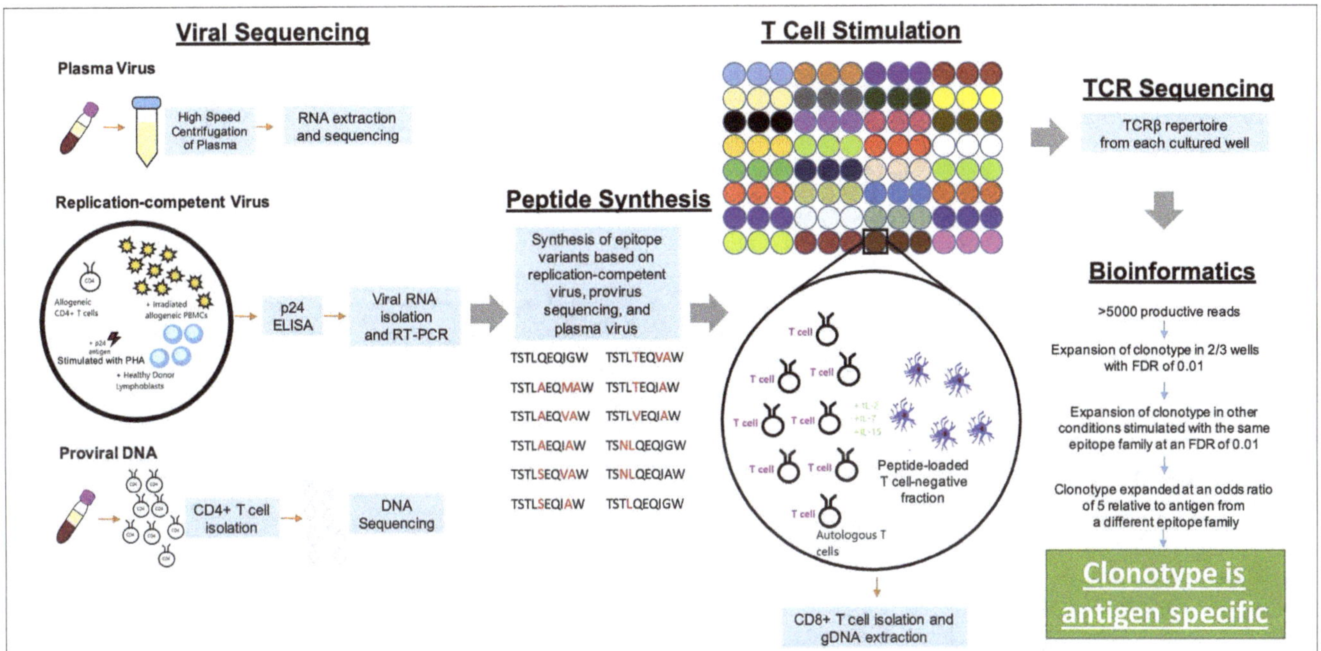

FIGURE 1 | Schematic diagram of the experimental approach. Autologous HIV-1 was sequenced from plasma, replication-competent virus, or proviral DNA. Peptides representing autologous variants of known HLA B57-restricted epitopes were synthesized and used to stimulated T cells in a modified version of the MANAFEST assay. TCR Vβ sequencing was performed on CD8+ T cells from each peptide-stimulated well, as well as uncultured and "no peptide" controls. A bioinformatic pipeline was then used to identify antigen-specific T cell clonotypes.

cell culture. After TCR sequencing, 5 of the 75 samples were removed from further analysis due to an insufficient number of productive reads (**Supplementary Table 1**). TCR sequencing files were run through a pre-processing and statistical analysis pipeline to identify antigen-specific T cell clonotypes. The conventional MANAFEST analytical platform relies on several key requirements to confirm antigen specificity, one of which is that the T cell clone must significantly expand in the relevant well relative to every other peptide-stimulated well. Because we evaluated each peptide in triplicate, and considering the potential for T cell cross-reactivity (16, 17), these criteria were modified to evaluate T cell responses to closely-related viral epitope variants where a given T cell clone could be specific for more than one epitope within an epitope family. Specifically, T cell clones should significantly expand in at least 2 out of 3 culture replicates and satisfy all additional criteria as described in the Methods to be considered antigen specific. Given that there are ~1.4 x 10^6 unique TCR Vβ clonotypes in the memory T cell compartment of a given individual (35), and that we are evaluating responses to 4 different epitope families consisting of 25 unique epitopes, the probability of the same T cell clone expanding in multiple replicates of the same peptide by chance is less than 1.53×10^{-12}.

Three T cell clones specific for the Gag $p24_{235-243}$ TW10 epitope family were identified (**Figure 2**). The first clone, T GTGCCAGCAGCCCAGGGGTGGGGAACACTGAAGCT TTCTTT (CASSPGVGNTEAFF), significantly expanded at an FDR < 0.01 and an odds ratio of at least 5 in all three replicates in the T cell culture of the consensus TW10 epitope, TSTLQEQIGW, and satisfied all additional criteria to be considered antigen-specific. This consensus epitope was the predominant proviral variant seen in 2005, 2007, and 2009 (22, 24) (**Figure 2A**, **Supplementary Data 1**). Interestingly, this T cell clone was cross-reactive for the TSTLAEQIAW and TSTLSEQVAW variants that were both detected in plasma in 2009 (24) and the variant epitope TSTLAEQMAW that was present in replication-competent isolates cultured in 2018. There was no cross-reactivity with epitopes from other Gag or Nef families or the CEF- or ebola AY9-stimulated control wells. The second clone, TGTGCCAGCAGCTTAGATCCGGG GGCGAACACTGAAGCTTTCTTT (CASSLDPGANTEAFF), was also specific for the consensus TW10 epitope and was cross-reactive for the variant TSTLAEQMAW (**Figure 2B**, **Supplementary Data 1**). Although this clone significantly expanded in all three wells stimulated with the TSTLSEQVAW plasma variant from 2009, it only reached the minimum odds ratio threshold in one of the replicates and therefore cannot be considered specific for this antigen. The third clone, TGTGCC AGCAGCCCGAGACAGGCGGGTCTGGTGACCCAGTACT TC (CASSPRQAGLVTQYF) was specific for TSTLAEQMAW (**Figure 2C**; **Supplementary Data 1**) and did not demonstrate any cross-reactivity with other epitope family members.

Five T cell clones specific for the Nef_{81-90} KF9 epitope family and one clone specific for the $Nef_{116-124}$ HW9 epitope family were also identified (**Figure 3**). The first KF9-specific clone, TG TGCCAGCAGCCCTCGATGGGGGACGCCGGGGAGCTG TTTTTT (CASSPRWGDAGELFF), recognized KAALDLSHF, a

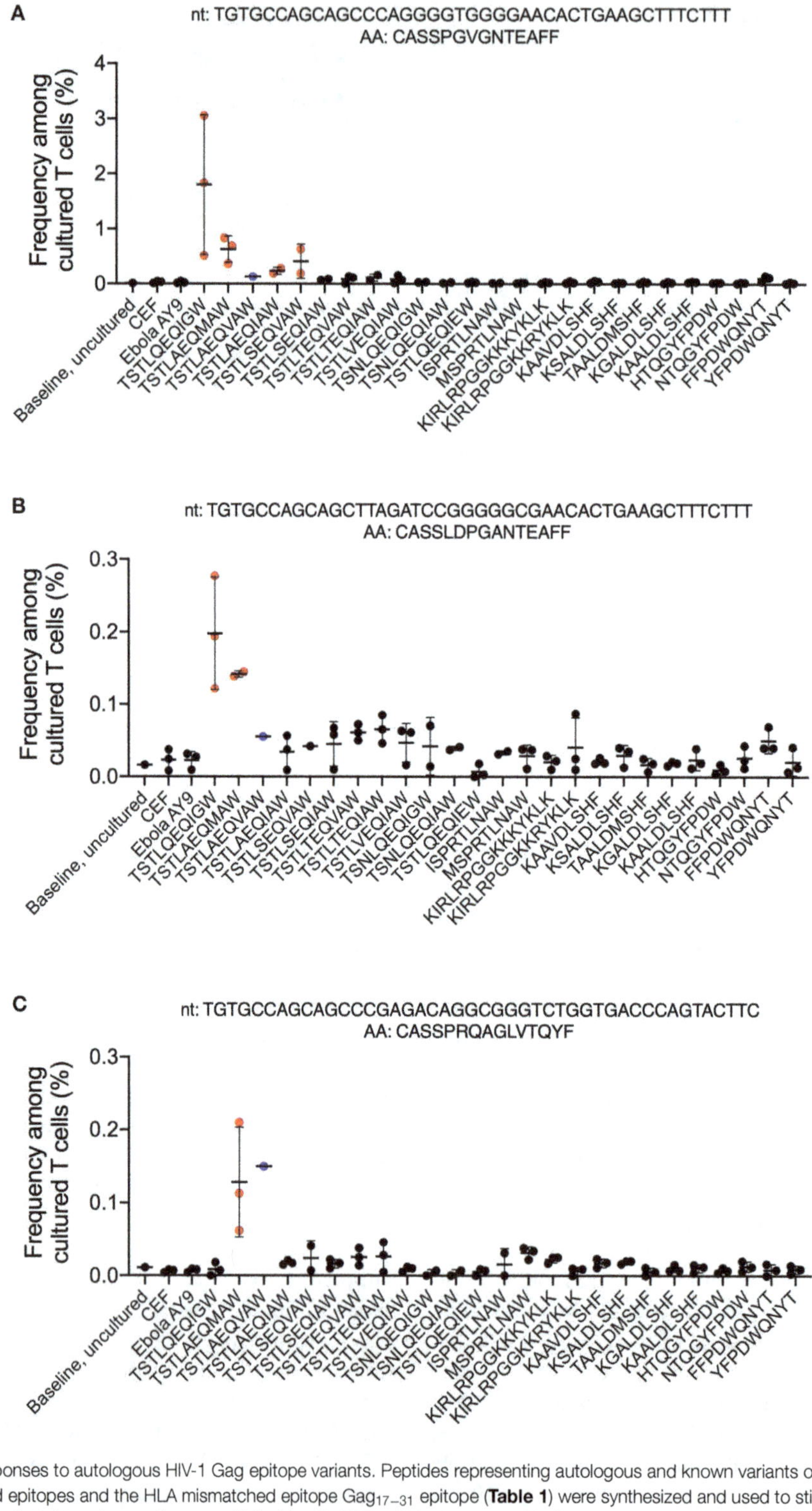

FIGURE 2 | CD8+ T cell responses to autologous HIV-1 Gag epitope variants. Peptides representing autologous and known variants of the HIV-1 $Gag_{240-249}$ and Gag_{17-31} HLA-B57-restricted epitopes and the HLA mismatched epitope Gag_{17-31} epitope (**Table 1**) were synthesized and used to stimulate T cells in the ViraFEST assay. A bioinformatic pipeline that determines antigen specificity identified 3 T cell Vβ clonotypes **(A-C)** that were antigen-specific. The nucleotide (nt) and amino acid (AA) sequence for each clone is shown above their respective graph. The mean frequency (%) after culture +/- standard deviation is shown for each condition where the clonotype contributed to a positive (red) or negative (black) T cell response. In the TSTLAEQIAW-stimulated condition, two of the three triplicates were excluded from analysis, and therefore no determination of a positive or negative response could be determined (blue).

common variant of the consensus epitope and was cross-reactive for the KSALDLSHF variant which was present in proviral clones in 2005 and 2010 (23, 25) (**Figure 3A**, **Supplementary Data 1**). The second clone, TGTGCCTGGGAGACAGGGGTTAGGGA TGGCTACACCTTC (CAWETGVRDGYTF), only recognized KAALDLSHF (**Figure 3B**, **Supplementary Data 1**). The third clone, TGTGCCAGCAGCCTGTTAGCGGGAGGGAGCCTTG ATGAGCAGTTCTTC (CASSLLAGGSLDEQFF), demonstrated the most cross-reactivity, recognizing KAAVDLSHF (the consensus epitope), KAALDLSHF, and KSALDLSHF (**Figure 3C**, **Supplementary Data 1**). The fourth clone, TGCGCCAGCAG CTTGGATTTACGGACCTTTACTTACGAGCAGTACTTC (CASSLDLRTFTYEQYF), was reactive against KAALDLSHF and KSALDLSHF (**Figure 3D**, **Supplementary Data 1**) and the fifth clone, TGCGCCAGCAGCTTGGAGAGGGTGGGC TACAATGAGCAGTTCTTC (CASSLERVGYNEQFF) only recognized KAALDLSHF (**Figure 3E**, **Supplementary Data 1**). There were no T cell responses against the TAALDMSHF variant that was present in plasma in 2005 and 2010 (23, 25) and in replication-competent virus from 2018. The only clone recognizing the HW9 family, TGTGCCATCAGCCTCATGG GCACTGAAGCTTTCTTT (CAISLMGTEAFF), was specific

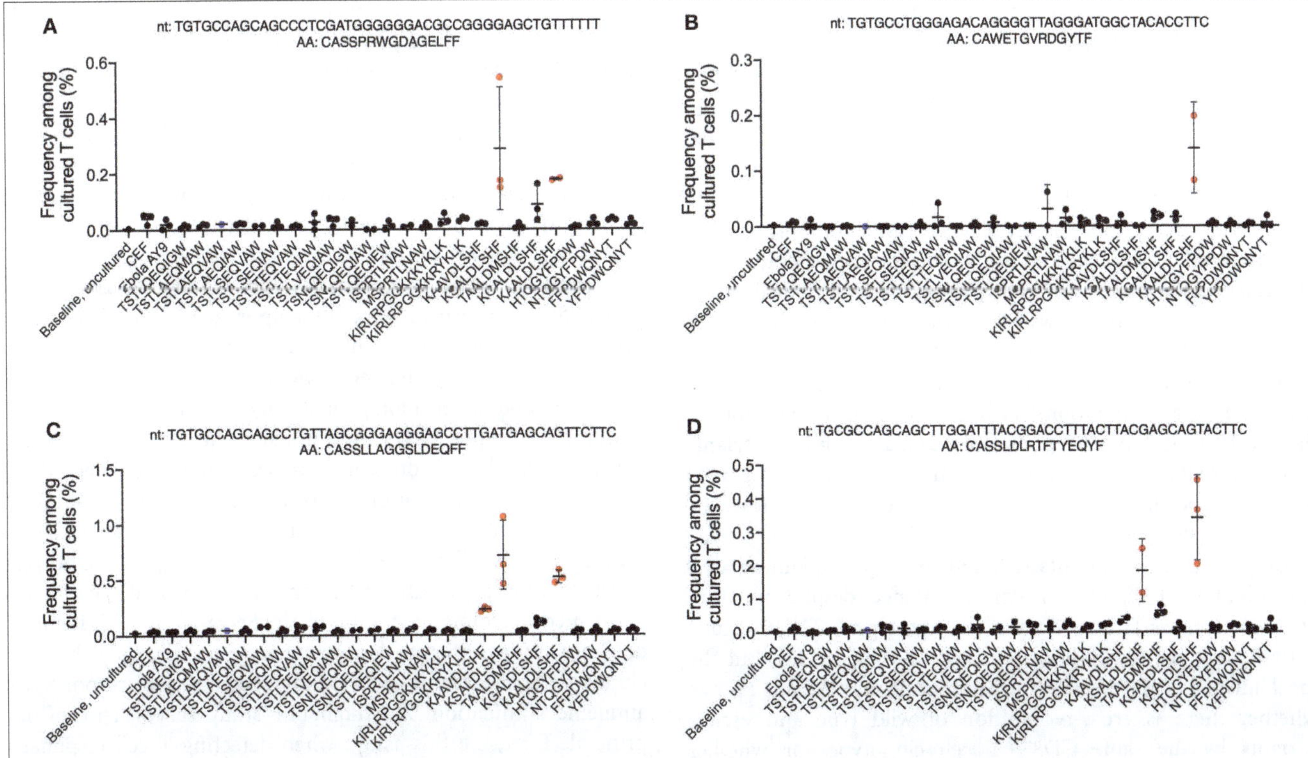

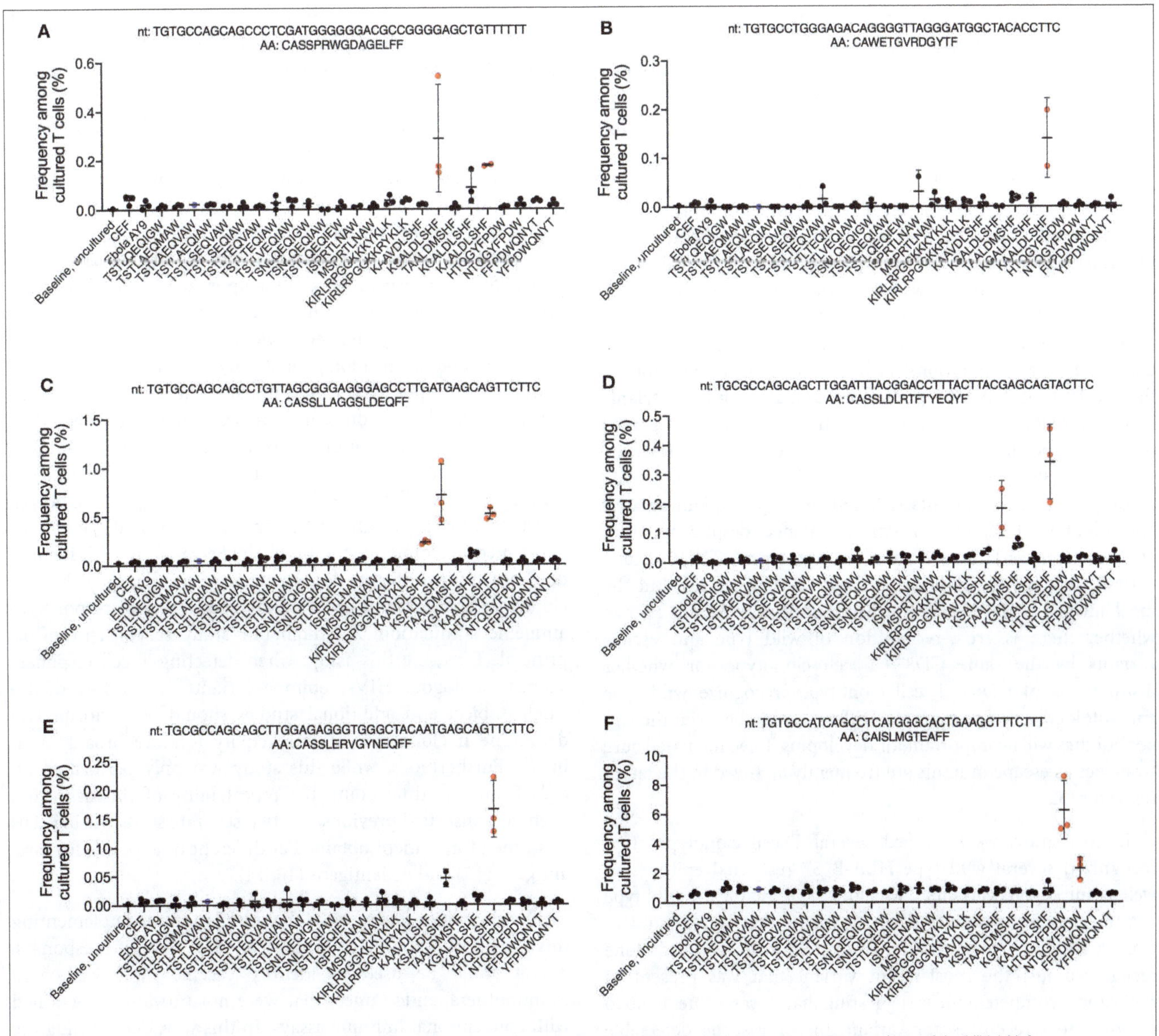

FIGURE 3 | CD8+ T cell responses to autologous HIV-1 Nef epitope variants. Peptides representing autologous and known variants of the HIV-1 Nef$_{82-90}$, Nef$_{116-1204}$, and Nef$_{120-128}$ HLA-B57-restricted epitopes (**Table 1**) were synthesized and used to stimulate T cells in the ViraFEST assay. A bioinformatic pipeline that determines antigen specificity identified 6 T cell Vβ clonotypes **(A–F)** that were antigen-specific. The nucleotide (nt) and amino acid (AA) sequence for each clone is shown above their respective graph. The mean frequency (%) after culture +/- standard deviation is shown for each condition where the clonotype contributed to a positive (red) or negative (black) T cell response. In the TSTLAEQIAW-stimulated condition, two of the three triplicates were excluded from analysis, and therefore no determination of a positive or negative response could be determined (blue).

for the HTQGYFPDW consensus epitope which was present in replication-competent virus from 2018 and the NTQGYFPDW escape variant (**Figure 3F, Supplementary Data 1**).

Taken together, these data demonstrate the feasibility of using a modified ViraFEST analytical platform to identify cross-reactive T cell clonotypes in an ES.

DISCUSSION

This is the first use of the MANAFEST assay to evaluate T cell responses to HIV-1 antigens. This assay, which has been used to identify memory CD8$^+$ T cell responses to tumor-derived neoantigens (13–15, 26), uses TCR Vβ sequencing of peptide-stimulated T cell cultures and a bioinformatic pipeline to identify antigen-specific T cell clonotypes. In this proof of concept study, we chose to evaluate HIV-1-specific responses in ES8. ES serve as a model of a T cell-mediated functional cure of HIV. HLA-B*57 and HLA-B*27 are over-represented in ES (36, 37) and a CTL response that is focused on HLA-B*57 restricted epitopes is associated with elite control (36). In prior studies we analyzed HLA-B*57 restricted epitopes in proviral and plasma clones from ES and found that while wild-type consensus sequences were present in most proviral clones, plasma clones contained multiple substitutions in these epitopes (22). While some of these substitutions were previously well-described escape mutations such as the T242N mutation in the TW10 Gag 240-249 epitope (29–31), ES8 plasma variants had rare mutations in this epitope that were not recognized by TW10-specific CD8$^+$ T cells from other ES. However, CD8$^+$ T cells from ES8 and other ES generally recognized autologous plasma variants (22, 28), perhaps explaining why control of viral replication was maintained despite apparent virologic escape. This recognition of autologous TW10 escape variants has previously been reported (22, 27, 38–40), but the mechanism has not been identified. Specifically it's not known whether there is cross-recognition of wild type and escape variants by the same CD8$^+$ T cell clonotypes or whether distinct sets of CD8$^+$ T cell clonotypes recognize wild type and autologous escape mutants. Differentiating between the two possibilities will be important for developing T cell mediated cure strategies as escape mutants are frequently archived in the latent reservoir (32).

In this study, we identified several T cell clonotypes that recognized several wild type HLA-B*57 restricted epitopes as well as autologous variants. Two clones specific for the wild type TW10 epitope cross-reacted with variants that were found in plasma and later in replication-competent virus. A third clone recognized just the most-recent variant that was present in replication-competent virus suggesting that it was a true de novo response to a recent escape variant. In contrast, no detectable responses were made to some prior plasma variants or to epitopes containing the common T242N mutation that was never detected in ES8.

Five clones were specific for a common variant of the Nef KF9 epitope. Although this variant was never detected in any viral clones from ES8, it could have been present in the initial transmitter/founder clone and/or present at a level below the limit of detection. Three of the five CD8$^+$ T cell clones cross reacted with the proviral variant of this epitope which may represent an early escape mutation that was archived into the reservoir. Finally, the clone specific for the Nef wild type epitope HW9, cross reacted with NW9 a well characterized escape mutation (41) that was not detected in ES8.

While HIV-1-specific cross-reactivity at the clonotype level has been previously described (18), this is the first use of a TCR immunogenomic platform to identify HIV-1-specific T cell responses. As described previously (13), our MANAFEST-based approach is more sensitive than conventional IFNγ ELISpot assays and has the advantage of being able to identify oligo- and polyclonal T cell responses to antigens. Additionally, once HIV-1-specific clonotypes are identified, the TCR can be used as a molecular barcode to track these antigen-specific cells across biological compartments or in serial blood draws. This provides a benefit for immune monitoring of treatment and therapeutic interventions because the functional assay only needs to be performed once. Our approach is novel and has the potential for broad utility within and outside the HIV research community, however we recognize that this assay is costlier and more bioinformatically-intensive compared to traditional ELISpot assays. Additionally, the limitations of this approach should be considered before being implemented in routine monitoring of immune responses. First, the ViraFEST assay only identifies the Vβ chain corresponding to antigen-specific T cells. Therefore, in order to investigate engineered T cell therapy approaches additional assays would have to be performed to enumerate the Vα chain. Second, the TCR identity does not inform on function or cytokine profile, only that the clonotype is capable of proliferating specifically in response to antigenic stimulation. Although our study serves a proof-of-principle for using this assays when detecting T cell responses against autologous HIV-1 epitope variants, we only studied a single subject and additional studies should be performed to determine if clonotypic cross-reactivity is more broadly seen in ES. Furthermore, while this study was only performed on cells from one time point, the repeatability of this assay has been demonstrated previously in two separate studies using cells from the same patient obtained at different time points for viral antigens (13) and neoantigens (13, 14).

Not only does this serve as the foundation for implementing this assay during routine monitoring of HIV-1-specific responses, but it could be used to identify vaccine or T cell-based immunotherapeutic targets that were not previously identified with conventional immune assays. In this way, determining the clonotypic identity of HIV-1-specific T cells paves the way for engineered T cell therapies that could be used across many patients with common epitope variants and HLA alleles.

ETHICS STATEMENT

The studies involving human participants were reviewed and approved by Johns Hopkins IRB. The patients/participants provided their written informed consent to participate in this study. Written informed consent was obtained from the individual(s) for the publication of any potentially identifiable images or data included in this article.

AUTHOR CONTRIBUTIONS

HC and CG performed the experiments described here. JZ analyzed the experimental data. AK analyzed the clinical data. JB and KS conceived of the experiments, analyzed the data and wrote the paper.

REFERENCES

1. Churchill MJ, Deeks SG, Margolis DM, Siliciano RF, Swanstrom R. HIV reservoirs: what, where and how to target them. *Nat Rev Microbiol.* (2016) 14:55–60. doi: 10.1038/nrmicro.2015.5
2. Autran B, Descours B, Avettand-Fenoel V, Rouzioux C. Elite controllers as a model of functional cure. *Curr Opin HIV AIDS.* (2011) 6:181–7. doi: 10.1097/COH.0b013e328345a328
3. Blankson JN, Bailey JR, Thayil S, Yang HC, Lassen K, Lai J, et al. Isolation and characterization of replication-competent human immunodeficiency virus type 1 from a subset of elite suppressors. *J Virol.* (2007) 81:2508–18. doi: 10.1128/JVI.02165-06
4. Salgado M, Swanson MD, Pohlmeyer CW, Buckheit RW, 3rd, Wu J, Archin NM, et al. HLA-B*57 elite suppressor and chronic progressor HIV-1 isolates replicate vigorously and cause CD4+ T cell depletion in humanized BLT mice. *J Virol.* (2014) 88:3340–52. doi: 10.1128/JVI.03380-13
5. Migueles SA, Laborico AC, Shupert WL, Sabbaghian MS, Rabin R, Hallahan CW, et al. HIV-specific CD8+ T cell proliferation is coupled to perforin expression and is maintained in nonprogressors. *Nat Immunol.* (2002) 3:1061–8. doi: 10.1038/ni845
6. Migueles SA, Osborne CM, Royce C, Compton AA, Joshi RP, Weeks KA, et al. Lytic granule loading of CD8+ T cells is required for HIV-infected cell elimination associated with immune control. *Immunity.* (2008) 29:1009–21. doi: 10.1016/j.immuni.2008.10.010
7. Saez-Cirion A, Lacabaratz C, Lambotte O, Versmisse P, Urrutia A, Boufassa F, et al. HIV controllers exhibit potent CD8 T cell capacity to suppress HIV infection *ex vivo* and peculiar cytotoxic T lymphocyte activation phenotype. *Proc Natl Acad Sci USA.* (2007) 104:6776–81. doi: 10.1073/pnas.0611244104
8. Betts MR, Nason MC, West SM, De Rosa SC, Migueles SA, Abraham J, et al. HIV nonprogressors preferentially maintain highly functional HIV-specific CD8+ T cells. *Blood.* (2006) 107:4781–9. doi: 10.1182/blood-2005-12-4818
9. Deeks SG. HIV: shock and kill. *Nature.* (2012) 487:439–40. doi: 10.1038/487439a
10. Martin-Moreno A, Munoz-Fernandez MA. Dendritic cells, the double agent in the war against HIV-1. *Front Immunol.* (2019) 10:2485. doi: 10.3389/fimmu.2019.02485
11. Kim GB, Hege K, Riley JL. CAR talk: how cancer-specific CAR T cells can instruct how to build CAR T cells to cure HIV. *Front Immunol.* (2019) 10:2310. doi: 10.3389/fimmu.2019.02310
12. Sperk M, Domselaar RV, Neogi U. Immune Checkpoints as the Immune System Regulators and Potential Biomarkers in HIV-1 Infection. *Int J Mol Sci.* (2018) 19:7. doi: 10.3390/ijms19072000
13. Danilova L, Anagnostou V, Caushi JX, Sidhom JW, Guo H, Chan HY, et al. The mutation-associated neoantigen functional expansion of specific T cells (MANAFEST) assay: a sensitive platform for monitoring antitumor immunity. *Cancer Immunol Res.* (2018) 6:888–99. doi: 10.1158/2326-6066.CIR-18-0129
14. Forde PM, Chaft JE, Smith KN, Anagnostou V, Cottrell TR, Hellmann MD, et al. Neoadjuvant PD-1 blockade in resectable lung cancer. *N Engl J Med.* (2018) 378:1976–86. doi: 10.1056/NEJMoa1716078
15. Smith KN, Llosa NJ, Cottrell TR, Siegel N, Fan H, Suri P, et al. Persistent mutant oncogene specific T cells in two patients benefitting from anti-PD-1. *J Immunother Cancer.* (2019) 7:40. doi: 10.1186/s40425-019-0547-7
16. Mailliard RB, Smith KN, Fecek RJ, Rappocciolo G, Nascimento EJ, Marques ET, et al. Selective induction of CTL helper rather than killer activity by natural epitope variants promotes dendritic cell-mediated HIV-1 dissemination. *J Immunol.* (2013) 191:2570–80. doi: 10.4049/jimmunol.1300373
17. Smith KN, Mailliard RB, Piazza PA, Fischer W, Korber BT, Fecek RJ, et al. Effective cytotoxic T lymphocyte targeting of persistent HIV-1 during Antiretroviral therapy requires priming of naive CD8+ T cells. *mBio.* (2016) 7:e00473-16. doi: 10.1128/mBio.00473-16
18. Chen H, Ndhlovu ZM, Liu D, Porter LC, Fang JW, Darko S, et al. TCR clonotypes modulate the protective effect of HLA class I molecules in HIV-1 infection. *Nat Immunol.* (2012) 13:691–700. doi: 10.1038/ni.2342
19. Mason D. A very high level of crossreactivity is an essential feature of the T-cell receptor. *Immunol Today.* (1998) 19:395–404. doi: 10.1016/S0167-5699(98)01299-7
20. Wooldridge L, Laugel B, Ekeruche J, Clement M, van den Berg HA, Price DA, et al. CD8 controls T cell cross-reactivity. *J Immunol.* (2010) 185:4625–32. doi: 10.4049/jimmunol.1001480
21. Pohlmeyer CW, Laskey SB, Beck SE, Xu DC, Capoferri AA, Garliss CC, et al. Cross-reactive microbial peptides can modulate HIV-specific CD8+ T cell responses. *PLoS One.* (2018) Feb 21;13(2):e0192098. doi: 10.1371/journal.pone.0192098
22. Bailey JR, Williams TM, Siliciano RF, Blankson JN. Maintenance of viral suppression in HIV-1-infected HLA-B*57+ elite suppressors despite CTL escape mutations. *J Exp Med.* (2006) 203:1357–69. doi: 10.1084/jem.200 52319
23. Bailey JR, Brennan TP, O'Connell KA, Siliciano RF, Blankson JN. Evidence of CD8+ T-cell-mediated selective pressure on human immunodeficiency virus type 1 nef in HLA-B*57+ elite suppressors. *J Virol.* (2009) 83:88–97. doi: 10.1128/JVI.01958-08
24. O'Connell KA, Brennan TP, Bailey JR, Ray SC, Siliciano RF, Blankson JN. Control of HIV-1 in elite suppressors despite ongoing replication and evolution in plasma virus. *J Virol.* (2010) 84:7018–28. doi: 10.1128/JVI.00548-10
25. Salgado M, Brennan TP, O'Connell KA, Bailey JR, Ray SC, Siliciano RF, et al. Evolution of the HIV-1 nef gene in HLA-B*57 positive elite suppressors. *Retrovirology.* (2010) 7:94. doi: 10.1186/1742-46 90-7-94
26. Anagnostou V, Smith KN, Forde PM, Niknafs N, Bhattacharya R, White J, et al. Evolution of Neoantigen Landscape during Immune Checkpoint Blockade in Non-Small Cell Lung Cancer. *Cancer Discov.* (2017) 7:264–76. doi: 10.1158/1538-7445.AM2017-NG01
27. Pohlmeyer CW, Buckheit RW, 3rd, Siliciano RF, Blankson JN. CD8+ T cells from HLA-B*57 elite suppressors effectively suppress replication of HIV-1 escape mutants. *Retrovirology.* (2013) 10:152. doi: 10.1186/1742-4690-10-152
28. O'Connell KA, Hegarty RW, Siliciano RF, Blankson JN. Viral suppression of multiple escape mutants by de novo CD8(+) T cell responses in a human immunodeficiency virus-1 infected elite suppressor. *Retrovirology.* (2011) 8:63. doi: 10.1186/1742-4690-8-63
29. Leslie AJ, Pfafferott KJ, Chetty P, Draenert R, Addo MM, Feeney M, et al. HIV evolution: CTL escape mutation and reversion after transmission. *Nat Med.* (2004) 10:282–9. doi: 10.1038/nm992
30. Brockman MA, Schneidewind A, Lahaie M, Schmidt A, Miura T, Desouza I, et al. Escape and compensation from early HLA-B57-mediated cytotoxic

T-lymphocyte pressure on human immunodeficiency virus type 1 Gag alter capsid interactions with cyclophilin A. *J Virol.* (2007) 81:12608–18. doi: 10.1128/JVI.01369-07
31. Durand CM, O'Connell KA, Apuzzo LG, Langan SJ, Imteyaz H, Ahonkhai AA, et al. HIV-1 Gag evolution in recently infected human leukocyte antigen-B*57 patients with low-level viremia. *AIDS.* (2010) 24:2405–8. doi: 10.1097/QAD.0b013e32833d8a38
32. Deng K, Pertea M, Rongvaux A, Wang L, Durand CM, Ghiaur G, et al. Broad CTL response is required to clear latent HIV-1 due to dominance of escape mutations. *Nature.* (2015) 517:381–5. doi: 10.1038/nature14053
33. Melhem NM, Smith KN, Huang XL, Colleton BA, Jiang W, Mailliard RB, et al. The impact of viral evolution and frequency of variant epitopes on primary and memory human immunodeficiency virus type 1-specific CD8(+) T cell responses. *Virology.* (2014) 450-451:34–48. doi: 10.1016/j.virol.2013.10.015
34. Smith KN, Mailliard RB, Larsen BB, Wong K, Gupta P, Mullins JI, et al. Dendritic cells restore CD8+ T cell reactivity to autologous HIV-1. *J Virol.* (2014) 88:9976–90. doi: 10.1128/JVI.01275-14
35. Robins HS, Campregher PV, Srivastava SK, Wacher A, Turtle CJ, Kahsai O, et al. Comprehensive assessment of T-cell receptor beta-chain diversity in alphabeta T cells. *Blood.* (2009) 114:4099–107. doi: 10.1182/blood-2009-04-217604
36. Migueles SA, Sabbaghian MS, Shupert WL, Bettinotti MP, Marincola FM, Martino L, et al. HLA B*5701 is highly associated with restriction of virus replication in a subgroup of HIV-infected long term nonprogressors. *Proc Natl Acad Sci USA.* (2000) 97:2709–14. doi: 10.1073/pnas.050567397
37. International HIV Controllers Study. The major genetic determinants of HIV-1 control affect HLA class I peptide presentation. *Science.* (2010) 330:1551–7. doi: 10.1126/science.1195271
38. Feeney ME, Tang Y, Pfafferott K, Roosevelt KA, Draenert R, Trocha A, et al. HIV-1 viral escape in infancy followed by emergence of a variant-specific CTL response. *J Immunol.* (2005) 174:7524–30. doi: 10.4049/jimmunol.174.12.7524
39. Navis M, Schellens I, van Baarle D, Borghans J, van Swieten P, Miedema F, et al. Viral replication capacity as a correlate of HLA B57/B5801-associated nonprogressive HIV-1 infection. *J Immunol.* (2007) 179:3133–43. doi: 10.4049/jimmunol.179.5.3133
40. Miura T, Brockman MA, Schneidewind A, Lobritz M, Pereyra F, Rathod A, et al. HLA-B57/B*5801 human immunodeficiency virus type 1 elite controllers select for rare gag variants associated with reduced viral replication capacity and strong cytotoxic T-lymphocyte [corrected] recognition. *J Virol.* (2009) 83:2743–55. doi: 10.1128/JVI.00579-09
41. Navis M, Schellens IM, van Swieten P, Borghans JA, Miedema F, Kootstra NA, et al. A nonprogressive clinical course in HIV-infected individuals expressing human leukocyte antigen B57/5801 is associated with preserved CD8+ T lymphocyte responsiveness to the HW9 epitope in Nef. *J Infect Dis.* (2008) 197:871–9. doi: 10.1086/528695

3

Redirection of Cord Blood T Cells and Natural Killer Cells for Elimination of Autologous HIV-1-Infected Target Cells Using Bispecific DART® Molecules

Justin Pollara[1,2], R. Whitney Edwards[2], Shalini Jha[1,2], Chia-Ying Kao Lam[3], Liqin Liu[3], Gundo Diedrich[3], Jeffrey L. Nordstrom[3], Tori Huffman[1], Joy A. Pickeral[1], Thomas N. Denny[2], Sallie R. Permar[2,4] and Guido Ferrari[1,2]*

[1] *Department of Surgery, Duke University School of Medicine, Durham, NC, United States,* [2] *Human Vaccine Institute, Duke University School of Medicine, Durham, NC, United States,* [3] *Macrogenics, Inc., Rockville, MD, United States,* [4] *Department of Pediatrics, Duke University School of Medicine, Durham, NC, United States*

***Correspondence:**
Justin Pollara
justin.pollara@duke.edu

Mother-to-child transmission of HIV-1 remains a major global health challenge. Currently, HIV-1-infected infants require strict lifelong adherence to antiretroviral therapy to prevent replication of virus from reservoirs of infected cells, and to halt progression of disease. There is a critical need for immune interventions that can be deployed shortly after infection to eliminate HIV-1-infected cells in order to promote long-term remission of viremia, or to potentially cure pediatric HIV-1-infection. Bispecific HIV × CD3 DART® molecules able to co-engage the HIV-1 envelope protein on the surface of infected cells and CD3 on cytolytic T cells have been previously shown to eliminate HIV-1 infected cells *in vitro* and are candidates for passive immunotherapy to reduce the virus reservoir. However, their potential utility as therapy for infant HIV-1 infection is unclear as the ability of these novel antibody-based molecules to work in concert with cells of the infant immune system had not been assessed. Here, we use human umbilical cord blood as a model of the naïve neonatal immune system to evaluate the ability of HIV x CD3 DART molecules to recruit and redirect neonatal effector cells for elimination of autologous CD4$^+$ T cells infected with HIV-1 encoding an envelope gene sequenced from a mother-to-child transmission event. We found that HIV × CD3 DART molecules can redirect T cells present in cord blood for elimination of HIV-infected CD4$^+$ T cells. However, we observed reduced killing by T cells isolated from cord blood when compared to cells isolated from adult peripheral blood—likely due to the absence of the memory and effector CD8$^+$ T cells that are most cytolytic when redirected by bispecific DART molecules. We also found that newly developed HIV × CD16 DART molecules were able to recruit CD16-expressing natural killer cells from cord blood to eliminate HIV-infected cells, and the activity of cord blood natural killer cells could be substantially increased by priming with IL-15. Our results support continued development of HIV-specific DART molecules using relevant preclinical animal models to optimize strategies for effective use of this immune therapy to reduce HIV-1 infection in pediatric populations.

Keywords: pediatric HIV-1, umbilical cord blood, cytotoxic T cells, natural killer cells, redirected cytotoxicity, bispecific DART molecules

INTRODUCTION

Despite the effectiveness of perinatal and postnatal antiretroviral prophylaxis, and the relatively low transmission rates of HIV-1 *in utero*, intrapartum, and during breast-feeding, there remain over 160,000 new pediatric HIV-1 infections annually worldwide (1–4). The overwhelming majority of these infections occur perinatally, via mother-to-child transmission. Treatment is critical as infant HIV-1 peak and set-point viral loads are typically 10-fold above those observed for primary adult infection and are highly predictive of disease outcome (5–12). With proper adherence, antiretroviral therapy (ART) can successfully control viremia in infants, and if initiated shortly after birth, ART may appreciably limit the size of the latently infected cell reservoir (13, 14). However, evidence to date suggests that strict adherence to ART will need to be maintained lifelong to prevent reemergence of virus replication resulting from reactivation of latent infection. Therefore, to provide long-term control or cure of pediatric HIV infection and abrogate the need for lifelong viral suppression, early initiation of ART will need to be combined with additional strategies to eliminate HIV-1-infected cells responsible for persistence of the virus reservoir.

One promising approach to increase elimination of HIV-infected cells is passive immunotherapy with antibody-based molecules capable of recruiting and redirecting endogenous cytolytic effector cells (15, 16). Bispecific HIV × CD3 DART® molecules based on HIV-specific monoclonal antibodies (mAbs) can effectively mediate *in vitro* elimination of HIV-1 infected and reactivated latently infected cells (17, 18). Bispecific HIV × CD3 DART molecules use a monovalent HIV-targeting arm comprised of the antigen-binding region of mAbs specific for highly conserved regions of the HIV envelope protein (Env) to recognize HIV-1-infected target cells, and a monovalent CD3 binding arm for recruitment of cytolytic T cells. Only when both arms are co-engaged will polyclonal T cells be activated and redirected for cytolytic responses against Env-expressing, HIV-1-infected target cells in a major histocompatibility complex-independent manner (18, 19). As a result of these properties, HIV × CD3 DART molecule-mediated activity should be unaffected by mutations among circulating or latent viruses that confer escape from viral-specific T-cell responses, or by the low frequency and functionality of HIV-specific T cells in patients on ART (20, 21). Therefore, passive immunization with HIV × CD3 DART molecules could form the basis of a strategy for cure of HIV by combining early initiation of ART to control viral load and reduce the size of the reservoir with concurrent initiation of HIV × CD3 DART molecule immunotherapy to eliminate infected cells. Once viral load is below detection, ART and DART molecule immunotherapy would be maintained with the addition of compounds that reactivate latent virus-infected cells to generate targets for DART molecule-mediated clearance.

Newborn infant infection resulting from mother-to-child transmission of HIV-1 (MTCT) likely represents the most favorable clinical context for successful passive immunotherapy to eliminate the reservoir of HIV-infected cells. Therapy can be initiated shortly after birth, and therefore near the time of transmission events occurring late *in utero*, during labor and delivery, or via breast milk —likely prior to the establishment of large populations of latently infected cells and the onset of immune dysregulation (22–25). However, neonatal cytolytic immune cells have phenotypic and functional differences compared to the same cell populations in adults (26, 27), and the impact of these differences on the activity of cytotoxic antibody-based immunotherapeutic drugs is not known. Thus, it is crucial to first evaluate infant passive immunotherapies in a model system that recapitulates the effector cells present in newborn infants.

In this study, we used human umbilical cord blood as surrogate for neonatal peripheral blood to test the hypothesis that bispecific DART molecules could redirect neonatal effector cells for elimination of cells infected with HIV-1 encoding an envelope gene sequenced from a mother-to-child transmission event. Our data demonstrate that HIV × CD3 DART molecules can redirect cord blood T cells to kill autologous cord blood $CD4^+$ T cells infected by HIV-1 *in vitro*. However, we observed reduced killing by T cells isolated from cord blood when compared to those isolated from adult peripheral blood. We also found that HIV × CD16 DART molecules can recruit and redirect natural killer (NK) cells from cord blood to eliminate autologous HIV-infected $CD4^+$ T cells; and we determined that the redirected activity of cord blood NK cells can be substantially increased by priming with IL-15. Our data suggest that HIV-specific DART molecules combined with current ART regimens may provide a novel treatment option intended to improve virus control, promote long-term remission, or cure pediatric HIV-1 infection. Our data also indicate that strategies to optimize and enhance the cytotoxic potential of neonatal effector cells, or allowing additional time after birth for the immune system to develop, will likely be needed to maximize the therapeutic potential of HIV-specific DART molecules for use in pediatric populations.

MATERIALS AND METHODS

Study Samples

Blood and Mononuclear Cell Samples

Anonymized human umbilical cord blood donations that failed to meet the volume and/or nucleated cell count criteria required for clinical use were obtained with informed written consent. Human peripheral venous blood was collected by leukapheresis from healthy consenting adult volunteers (28, 29). All samples were collected in accordance with the policies and regulations of the Duke Health Institutional Review Board. Cord blood mononuclear cells (CBMC) and adult peripheral blood mononuclear cells (PBMC) were processed from umbilical cord blood and human peripheral blood, respectively, using density gradient centrifugation with Ficoll-Paque plus (GE Healthcare Life Sciences, Pittsburg, PA), and were cryopreserved in 10% DMSO 90% Fetal Bovine Serum (FBS). All samples were processed within 12 h after collection.

Bispecific HIV × CD3 and HIV × CD16 DART Molecules

HIV × CD3 DART molecules were constructed with anti-HIV-1 envelope specificities based on non-neutralizing mAbs, 7B2 or A32, or an irrelevant control specificity based on the anti-respiratory syncytial virus (RSV) mAb, palivizumab, and with an anti-human CD3ε specificity based on the mAb, hXR32, as described previously (18, 30). These molecules are referred to as 7B2 × CD3, A32 × CD3, and RSV × CD3. HIV × CD16 DART molecules were constructed with anti-human CD16 specificities based on mAb h3G8 as the effector arm, which included 7B2 × CD16 and 4420 × CD16, where 4420 is an anti-fluorescein (control) specificity, and Fc-bearing ones based on mAb h5H2 as the effector arm included 7B2 × CD16, A32 × CD16, and RSV × CD16. The human immunoglobulin G1 (IgG1) Fc domain, which is incorporated to prolong circulating half-life *in vivo*, contains mutations to greatly reduce or eliminate effector function via binding to Fc-gamma receptors (FcγRs) and complement, while retaining binding to the neonatal Fc receptor (FcRn) to take advantage of the IgG salvage pathway mediated by this receptor.

Laboratory Methods

Phenotypic Characterization of T Cells

Immunophenotyping of human T cells was performed using flow cytometry analyses. Cryopreserved PBMC (5 donors) and CBMC (14 donors) were thawed and incubated overnight (18 h) in RPMI 1640 medium supplemented with 10% FBS at 37°C, 5% CO_2. The cells were then washed with buffered saline and stained with a viability marker (Fixable Aqua Dead Cell Stain Kit, Thermo Fisher Scientific, San Diego, CA) prior to surface and intracellular staining with fluorescently conjugated antibodies using standard techniques as described (31). The staining panel used to identify T cell subsets and phenotypes was based on the Optimized Multicolor Immunofluorescence Panel 22 (OMIP-22) described previously (31). Fluorescently conjugated Abs used for cell surface staining were: APC-eFluor780-CD4 (clone RPA-T4, ebioscience, San Diego, CA); Horizon V500-CD14 (clone M5E2, BD Biosciences, San Jose, CA); Horizon V500-CD19 (clone HIB19, BD Biosciences); BV785-CD45RO (clone UCHL1, Biolegend, San Diego, CA); BV605-CCR7 (clone G043H7, Biolegend); and APC-CD366 (clone F38-2E2, Biolegend). Intracellular staining was performed with PE-TR-CD3 (clone UCHT1, Beckman Coulter, Brea, CA); and Ax700-CD8 (clone HIT8a, Biolegend). Data analyses were performed using FlowJo software (v10.5.3) from BD Biosciences.

Phenotypic Characterization of NK Cells and CD16 DART-Molecule NK Cell Binding

Immunophenotyping of human NK cells was performed as previously described (32). Cryopreserved PBMC collected from 15 healthy normal adult donors, and CBMC from 15 umbilical cord blood donors, were thawed and incubated overnight (18 h) in RPMI1640 medium supplemented with 10% FBS, or in RPMI 1640 medium supplemented with 10% FBS and 10 ng/mL recombinant human IL-15 (Miltenyi Biotec, GmbH) at 37°C, 5% CO_2. The cells were then washed with buffered saline and stained with a viability marker (Fixable Aqua Dead Cell Stain Kit, Thermo Fisher Scientific) prior to surface and intracellular staining with fluorescently conjugated Abs using standard techniques as described previously (33). Fluorescently conjugated antibodies used for surface staining were based on OMIP-007 and are as follows: PE-TR-CD3 (clone S4.1, Thermo Fisher Scientific); APC-H7-CD4 (clone SK3, BD Biosciences); PE-Cy5-CD14 (clone Tuk4, Thermo Fisher Scientific); PE-Cy5-CD19 (clone SJ25-C1, Thermo Fisher Scientific); PacificBlue-CD16 (clone 3G8, BD Biosciences); PE-Cy7-CD56 (clone NCAM16.2, BD Biosciences); BV606-CD62L (clone DREG-56, Biolegend); FITC-HLA-DR (clone G46-6, BD Biosciences); APC-CD57 (clone HCD57, Biolegend); and BV785-CD69 (clone FN50, Biolegend). Intracellular staining was performed with BV711-Perforin (clone dG9, Biolegend), and PE-Granzyme B (clone GB11, BD Biosciences). Quantum™ Simply Cellular® beads (Bangs Laboratories, Inc., Fishers, Indiana) were used to determine the antibody binding capacity (ABC) of perforin and granzyme within cells according the manufacturers recommended procedure. Data analyses were performed using FlowJo software (v10.5.3).

To determine if DART molecules with CD16 targeting arms could specifically bind the surface of human NK cells, we incubated purified human NK cells with DART molecules at 1 μg/ml for 40 min at room temperature. Cells were then washed (PBS with 1% FBS) and incubated with 1 μg/ml mouse anti-EK antibody (recognizes the E/K heterodimerization region of DART molecules, MacroGenics) for 20 min at 4°C in wash buffer. Cells were then washed and incubated with PE rat-anti mouse IgG1 (BD Biosciences), at the manufactures recommended concentration, in wash buffer, for 25 min at 4°C. Finally, cells were washed, fixed, and analyzed by flow cytometry. Data are reported as mean fluorescent intensity (MFI) of PE.

Redirected T Cell Cytotoxicity Assay Against Autologous HIV-1 Env-Expressing CD4+ T Cells

Redirected T cell cytotoxicity assays were performed with methods similar to those previously described (18). Cryopreserved resting CBMC and PBMC from normal healthy donors were activated for 72 h with anti-human CD3 antibody (clone OKT3, eBioscience), anti-human CD28 antibody (clone 28.2, BD Biosciences) each at 150 ng/mL, and recombinant human IL-2 (30 U/mL, Proleukin, Prometheus Therapeutics and Diagnostics) in RPMI 1640 media supplemented with 20% FBS. Next, $CD8^+$ T cells were depleted using magnetic beads (Miltenyi Biotec), leaving a $CD4^+$ T cell-enriched population that was then infected with HIV-1 infectious molecular clone virus

(HIV-1 4403bmC5) encoding a subtype C infant postnatally-transmitted/founder envelope protein (34) and Tat-inducible *Renilla* luciferase reporter gene (35), by spinoculation as described (36). Where indicated, cells were alternatively infected with an infectious molecular clone virus representing HIV-1 subtype B isolate BaL. After 48 h of infection, the $CD4^+$ T cells were incubated with $CD8^+$ T cells purified from autologous PBMC or CBMC using negative selection with magnetic beads (human $CD8^+$ T cell isolation kit, Miltenyi Biotec) at a $CD8^+$ T cell to target cell ratio of 30:1 in ½ area opaque flat bottom plates (Corning Life Sciences, Corning, NY). HIV × CD3 DART molecules were added, in duplicate, using 10-fold serial dilutions starting at 1 μg/mL, and the plates were incubated for an additional 24 h at 37°C, 5% CO_2. Control plates included only infected $CD4^+$ target cells and DART molecules without autologous $CD8^+$ T effector cells. Percent of specific killing was calculated based on the change in Relative Light Units (RLU) (ViviRen luciferase assay; Promega, Fithchburg, WI) resulting from the loss of live, intact target cells in test wells containing effector cells, target cells, and DART molecules relative to RLU in control wells containing target cells and effector cells alone (without DART molecules) according to the following formula: percent of specific killing = [(number of RLU of control well - number of RLU of test well)/number of RLU of control well] ×100. Positive responses were defined as specific killing >20%. Data were fit to a sigmoidal dose-response function for graphing and for determination of 50% effective concentrations (EC_{50}). In most cases, data are reported as positive area under the curve (pAUC), defined as the area under the log-transformed dilution curve that is above the threshold for positivity (20% specific killing), calculated with the trapezoidal method using SAS software (SAS Institute Inc., Cary, NC).

In vitro Evaluation of Strategies to Improve Redirected T Cell Cytotoxicity

Exogenous cytokines and T-cell co-stimulators were incorporated into the redirected T cell cytotoxicity assay to test their ability to improve the cytolytic activity of T cells present in CBMC and PBMC. The impact of exogenous IL-12 was evaluated by overnight incubation of the CBMC and PBMC with exogenous recombinant human IL-12 (10 ng/mL, Miltenyi Biotec), before isolation of $CD8^+$ T cells used as effector cells in the redirected cytotoxicity assay. IL-12 was maintained in the assay plates at 10 ng/mL throughout the 24-h killing assay. The impact of coreceptor signaling was assessed by incubating the CBMC and PBMC overnight with anti-CD28 (150 ng/mL, clone 28.2, BD Biosciences) or anti-CD137 (150 ng/mL, clone 4B4-1, BioLegend), prior to isolation of $CD8^+$ T cells, and maintaining the presence of the anti-coreceptor antibodies throughout the killing assay. Experiments were also performed using exogenous IL-12, anti-CD28, and anti-CD137 together, or with cells stimulated for 48 h by incubation with 150 ng/mL anti-human CD3 antibody (clone OKT3, eBioscience), anti-human CD28 antibody, and 30 U/mL recombinant human IL-2 in RPMI 1640 media supplemented with 20% FBS prior to isolation of $CD8^+$ T cells. In one set of experiments, T cells in CBMC and PBMC were activated for 72 h with anti-CD3, anti-CD28, and IL-2, before isolation of $CD8^+$ T cells, which were then allowed to rest for 72 h in absence of any stimulation before use as effector cells according to the methods described above.

Redirected NK Cell Cytotoxicity Assay Against Autologous HIV-1 Env-Expressing $CD4^+$ T Cells

Cryopreserved CBMC and PBMC samples were thawed and rested overnight (18 h) at 37°C 5% CO_2 in RPMI 1640 media supplemented with 10% FBS, or media supplemented with 10 ng/mL recombinant human IL-15 (Miltenyi Biotec), as previously described (32). Subsequently, NK cells were purified by negative selection with magnetic beads (human NK cell isolation kit, Miltenyi Biotec) and used as effector cells (NK cell to target cell ratio of 5:1) in redirected cytotoxicity assays using HIV × CD16 DART molecules, performed as described above. Positive responses were defined as specific killing >20%, and data were not fit to a dose-response function for graphing due to the presence of a prozone (37).

CD107a Degranulation Assay

Cell-surface expression of CD107a was used as a marker for T cell degranulation (38). Redirected cytotoxicity assays were performed as described above, with the following modification [as previously described in (18)]. After plating the target cells, effector cells, and DART molecules, the plate was incubated for 18 h and then FITC- or APC-Cy7-CD107a antibody (clone H4A3, BD Biosciences), brefeldin A (GolgiPlug, 1 μL/mL, BD Biosciences), and monensin (GolgiStop, 4 μL/6mL, BD Biosciences) were added to each well and the plates were incubated for an additional 6 h. Plates were then washed and stained with a viability marker and fluorescently conjugated antibodies as described above (phenotypic characterization of T cells), or with a truncated staining panel that included only antibodies specific for CD3, CD4, and CD8, using standard techniques. Data analyses were performed using FlowJo software (v10.5.3).

Statistical Methods

Kruskal Wallis tests were used to compare response magnitudes across groups. In order to assess if two groups have different response magnitudes, pairwise comparisons between groups were conducted using Wilcoxon rank sum test. Two-tailed $p < 0.05$ were considered significant. Statistical analysis was performed using SAS software (SAS Institute Inc.).

RESULTS

Cord Blood T Cells Have Modest Ability to Eliminate Autologous HIV-Infected CD4 T Cells Directed by HIV x CD3 DART Molecules *in vitro*

We and others have demonstrated that bispecific DART molecules able to co-engage HIV-1 Env on infected cells, and CD3 antigen on cytolytic T cells, can be used to eradicate acutely infected and reactivated latently-infected cells *in vitro* (17, 18). However, these initial studies were performed using immune cells from adults —the ability of these novel antibody-based molecules to work in concert with cells present in the neonatal immune system cells had not been explored. To address this limitation, we performed redirected T cell cytotoxicity assays using CBMC as a source of neonatal CD8$^+$ T cells for use as effectors, and autologous cord blood CD4$^+$ T cells for use as targets after infection with HIV-1 *in vitro*. Target cells were infected with a subtype C HIV-1 infectious molecular clone virus that encodes the *env* gene from HIV-1 4403bmC5, a postnatally-transmitted founder virus isolated from infant plasma, and identical to a virus isolate present in matched maternal breast milk (34). Thus, this isolate is expected to be a representative of those present in the early active and latent virus reservoirs of infected infants. Assays were also performed using adult PBMC as a source of effector cells and autologous HIV-1 4403bmC5-infected target cells for comparison. We observed minimal background activity (specific killing <20%) by the negative control DART molecule, RSV × CD3, in assays performed with CD8$^+$ T cells and autologous 4403bmC5-infected CD4$^+$ cells isolated from adult PBMC (black lines and open squares, **Figure 1A**) or CBMC (blue lines and circles, **Figure 1A**). In contrast, HIV-specific DART molecules, 7B2 × CD3 and A32 × CD3, mediated specific killing activity with cells isolated from most donors (80% of CBMC samples, and 89% of PBMC samples with 7B2 × CD3; 17% of CBMC and 100% of PBMC samples with A32 × CD3) as shown in **Figures 1B,C**, respectively. However, we observed that the specific killing activity of cells from cord blood is reduced when compared to those from adult PBMC for the majority of samples, both in terms of maximum observed killing activity (**Figures 1B,C**), and EC_{50} (mean ~100 ng/mL for 7B2 × CD3 with CBMC samples that were positive for killing, and ~4 ng/mL with positive PBMC samples). To better compare the killing activities, we calculated the positive area under the dilution curves (**Figure 1D**), and confirmed that specific killing of HIV-1 4403bmC5-infected cells was significantly lower in assays performed with cells isolated from CBMC compared to adult PBMC ($p \leq 0.001$, Wilcoxon rank sum tests). These data demonstrate that HIV-specific DART molecules can redirect cord blood T cells to kill HIV-1 infected, Env-expressing, autologous cord blood CD4$^+$ T cells, however with activity subordinate to that mediated by adult peripheral blood T cells. Therefore, we next sought to identify characteristics of cord blood T cells that may limit their functionality when redirected by HIV-specific DART molecules.

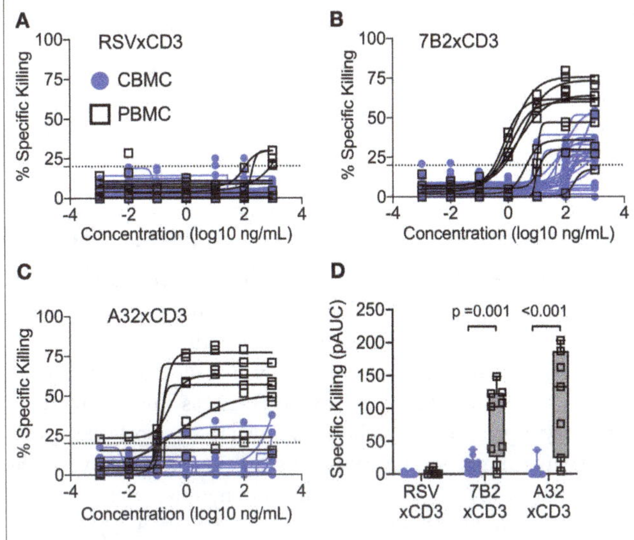

FIGURE 1 | Redirection of cytolytic T cells to autologous HIV-infected CD4$^+$ T cells by HIV × CD3 DART molecules. The ability of T cells isolated from cord blood mononuclear cells (CBMC, blue lines, and symbols) and adult peripheral blood mononuclear cells (PBMC, black lines, and open symbols) to eliminate autologous CD4$^+$ T cells infected with an HIV-1 molecular clone virus representing an infant postnatally-transmitted founder isolate (HIV-1 4403bmC5) after being redirected by **(A)** RSV × CD3 control DART molecules ($n = 25$ CBMC samples, $n = 9$ PBMC samples), **(B)** 7B2 × CD3 DART molecules ($n = 25$ CBMC samples, $n = 9$ PBMC samples), and **(C)** A32 × CD3 DART molecules ($n = 18$ CBMC samples, $n = 7$ PBMC samples). Dashed line indicates the threshold for positivity. The positive areas under the dilution curves (pAUC) are presented in **(D)** with blue circles and bars representing assays performed with cells from CBMC and black/gray squares and bars representing assays performed with cells from adult PBMC. Box plots represent the interquartile ranges, horizontal lines indicate the medians, and error bars extend to the minimum and maximum observed values. Data are from 24 h killing assays with a CD8$^+$ effector to HIV-infected autologous CD4$^+$ target cell ratio of 30:1.

Comparison of Effector and Memory T Cell Subsets in Cord Blood and Adult Peripheral Blood

We used flow cytometry immunophenotyping to compare T cell subsets present in CBMC to those present in adult PBMC. Comparisons were made using cells isolated from 14 cord blood and 5 adult peripheral blood samples. The gating strategy used to identify total T cells, and T cell subsets —naïve, effector, effector memory (T_{EM}), and central memory (T_{CM})— is indicated in **Figure 2A**. Flow plots showing representative examples of CD4$^+$ and CD8$^+$ T cell subsets among PBMC and CBMC are shown in **Figures 2B,C**, respectively. Consistent with prior observations (39, 40), we found that although CBMC contained similar frequencies of CD4$^+$ and CD8$^+$ T cells as adult PBMC, there were marked differences in the distribution of functional subsets with cord blood CD4$^+$ (**Figure 2D**) and CD8$^+$ T cells (**Figure 2E**) being predominantly naïve (naïve CD4: median 95%, interquartile range 92–97%; naïve CD8: median 89%, interquartile range 84–94%), and therefore deficient in memory and effector subsets. We hypothesized that although DART molecules are able to redirect resting T cells for killing of HIV-infected cells without need for pre-activation (17, 18), they may be more effective when redirecting effector or memory subsets. To test this, we assessed CD107a degranulation concomitant with redirected killing activity with PBMC from two healthy adult donors as a source of effector cells, and HIV-1 subtype B BaL IMC virus-infected cells as targets. We previously demonstrated high levels of HIV × CD3 DART molecule-induced CD8$^+$ T cell degranulation in the presence of CD4$^+$ cells infected by this HIV-1 isolate (18). We found that although HIV-specific DART molecules induced degranulation in all subsets of CD8$^+$ T cells during redirected cytotoxicity assays, the majority of degranulated cells were CCR7$^-$ and therefore expressed phenotypes consistent with T_{EM} and effector cells (**Figure 2F**).

These data suggest that the reduced DART molecule-mediated cytotoxicity observed in assays performed using CBMC-derived T cells is likely due in part to the predominance of naïve cells in cord blood, and the absence of memory and effector CD8$^+$ T cells, which are preferentially redirected by the HIV × CD3 DART molecules.

Evaluation of Strategies to Increase the Cytolytic Potential of T Cells in Cord Blood

We explored strategies to increase the activity of cord blood cytolytic T cells for HIV DART molecule-redirected elimination of HIV-infected cells. We first evaluated the impact of priming CBMC-derived T cells with IL-12, as this cytotoxic-T-lymphocyte-promoting cytokine is known to be poorly expressed by the naïve infant immune system (41). We found that overnight incubation with exogenous IL-12, and maintenance of IL-12 treatment throughout the redirected cytotoxicity assay, did not improve cytotoxic activity of cord blood CD8$^+$ T cells when used in combination with HIV × CD3 DART molecules (**Figure 3A**), nor was there any impact on activity of CD8$^+$ T cells from adult PBMC. Next, reasoning that the naïve CD8$^+$ T cells present in cord blood cells may require a more substantial activation signal compared to CD8$^+$ T cells present in adult PBMC, we explored if killing activity could be improved by providing additional co-stimulatory signaling via co-engagement of CD28 or CD137 receptors (42). However, the results of experiments performed using T cells isolated from CBMC and adult PBMC demonstrated that exogenous anti-CD28 or anti-CD137 co-stimulation did not significantly improve killing mediated by HIV × CD3 DART molecules (**Figure 3B**). Moreover, we found that treatment of CBMC with IL-12 combined with anti-CD28 and anti-CD137 co-stimulation also had no impact on the cytolytic activity of T cells from CBMC when used with HIV × CD3 DART molecules, but did increase activity in assays performed with adult PBMC (**Figure 3C**), although the increase did not reach statistical significance ($p = 0.064$, Wilcoxon rank sum test). We next assessed if pre-activation of cord blood T cells would increase their cytotoxic activity. Interestingly, we found that pre-activation of cord blood T cells via T cell receptor (TCR) cross linking using anti-CD3 and anti-CD28 monoclonal antibodies in combination with exogenous recombinant human IL-2 (30 U/mL) improved the ability of T cells from 5 of 5 tested cord blood samples to eliminate HIV-infected cells upon redirection by 7B2 × CD3 DART molecules, and 4 of 5 tested samples upon redirection by A32 × CD3 DART molecules (**Figure 3D**). This observation indicates that CD8$^+$ T cells present in cord blood are capable of improved cytotoxic activity when given sufficient stimulation.

We next determined if cord blood-derived CD8$^+$ cells, which had experienced prior activation and subsequently transitioned back to a resting state, were able to maintain higher cytolytic activity. To test this, we activated cord blood CD8$^+$ T cells for 72 h via TCR stimulation as described above, then allowed the cells to rest for an additional 72 h before use in the redirected killing assay. Flow cytometry analysis was used to define cell phenotypes during activation, and the return to resting state as shown in **Figures 4A–C**. As previously described, the preponderance of resting cord blood CD8$^+$ T cell presented a naïve (CD45RO$^-$, CCR7$^+$) cell surface phenotype (**Figure 4A**). CD45RO expression increased along with expression of the activation markers CD69 and HLA-DR after TCR stimulation (**Figure 4B**). Upon returning to a resting state, cell-surface expression of activation markers CD69 and HLA-DR were reduced, but the vast majority of cells maintained a cell-surface phenotype consistent with that of T_{CM} cells (CD45RO$^+$, CCR7$^+$, **Figure 4C**). Despite these changes to cell-surface phenotypes, induced during activation and maintained after returning to rest, we observed similarly low levels of cytolytic activity for resting cord blood CD8$^+$ T cells (**Figure 4D**), and CD8$^+$ T cells that were transitioned from an active to resting state *in vitro* (**Figure 4E**). Collectively, these results demonstrated that redirected killing activity of cord blood T cells mediated by HIV × CD3 DART molecules was not affected by providing exogenous IL-12 or costimulatory signals, but could be improved when given sufficient stimulation leading to activation. However, the improved cytolytic activity was not maintained when activation waned.

Cord Blood CD4$^+$ T Cells Are Recruited by HIV × CD3 DART Molecules

In parallel to the assays performed using CBMC-derived CD8$^+$ T cells as effector cells, we also evaluated whether HIV × CD3 DART molecules had anti-HIV activity when incubated with infected cord blood CD4$^+$ T cells alone. As the epitope recognized by the 7B2 × CD3 DART molecules is non-neutralizing (43) we expected minimal anti-HIV activity in absence of CD8$^+$ effector cells. In contrast, we observed 7B2 × CD3 DART molecule-dependent specific killing of HIV-infected cells at similar levels for assays performed with and without CD8$^+$ T cells from CBMC (**Figure 5A**, filled and open blue circles, respectively). We also observed 7B2 × CD3 DART molecule-dependent specific killing in assays performed without CD8$^+$ T cells from PBMC (**Figure 5A**, open black squares), however killing was higher in the presence of PBMC-derived CD8$^+$ T cells (**Figure 5A**, filled black squares). To determine if HIV × CD3 DART molecules were capable of activating effector responses from the cord blood CD4$^+$ T cells themselves, we assessed CD107a degranulation during redirected cytotoxicity assays as described previously. The gating strategy for identification of cord blood-derived CD4$^+$ T cells in this assay is shown in **Figure 5B**, with representative flow cytometry plots depicting detection of CD107a on CD4$^+$ T cells in presence of control or HIV × CD3 DART molecules. These data demonstrate that CD4$^+$ T cells from CBMC are capable of being induced to degranulate by DART molecules in redirected cytotoxicity assays. The specific killing activity observed using cord blood CD4$^+$ T cells as effectors to eliminate HIV-1 BaL-infected autologous T cells from two cord blood donations is shown in **Figure 5C**. The frequency of CD107a$^+$ CD4$^+$ T cells detected in these assays is shown in **Figure 5D**. The specific killing and concomitant degranulation responses observed across the tested HIV × CD3 DART molecule concentrations show comparable

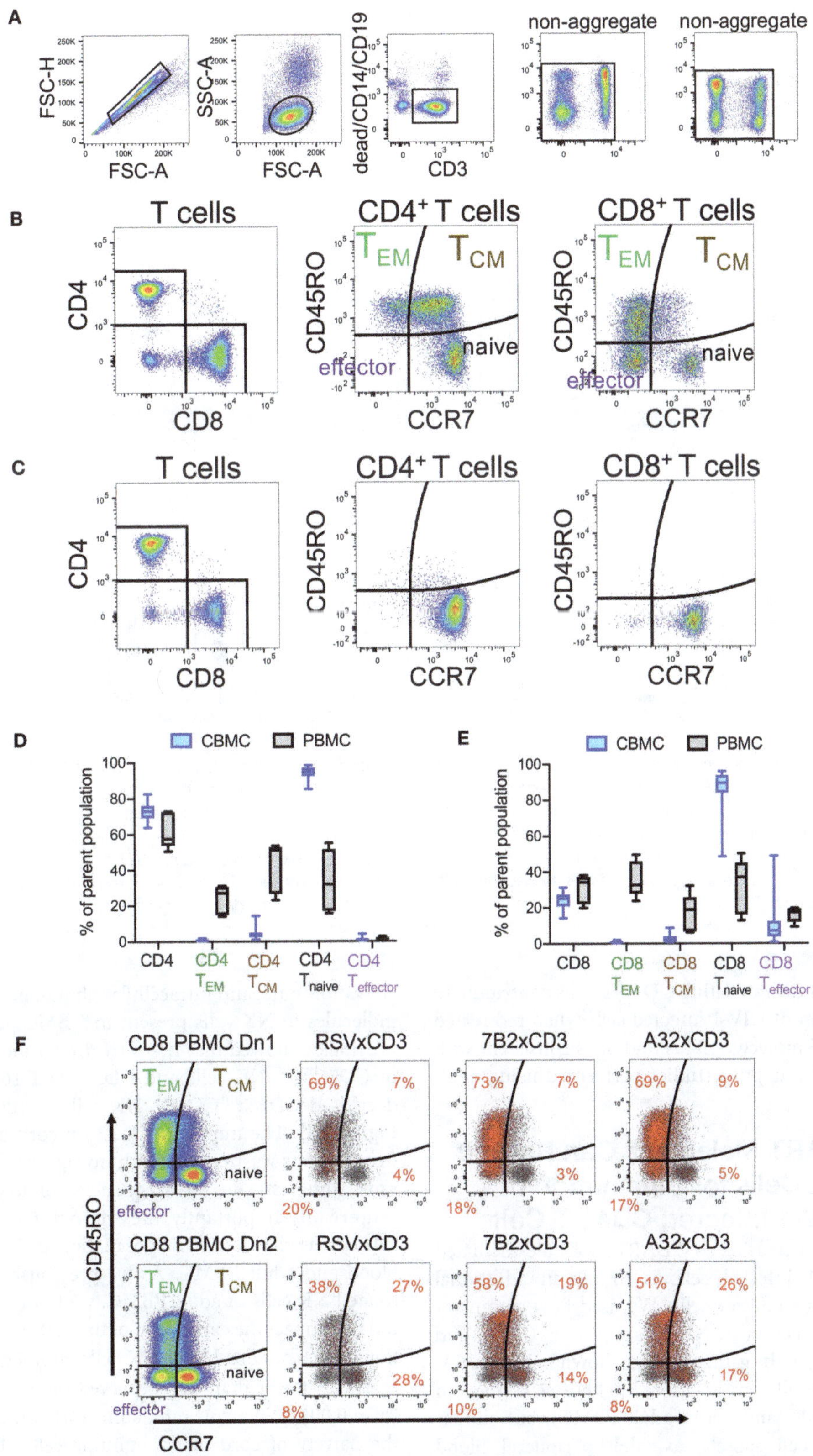

FIGURE 2 | Comparison of T cell subsets in adult peripheral blood mononuclear cells (PBMC) and cord blood mononuclear cells (CBMC) **(A)** Gating strategy. **(B)** Flow cytometry plots showing representative example of CD4+ and CD8+ T cell subsets among adult PBMC or **(C)** CBMC. Comparison of frequencies of **(D)** total CD4+ T

(Continued)

FIGURE 2 | Cells and CD4$^+$ T cell subsets or **(E)** CD8$^+$ T cells and CD8$^+$ T cell subsets in CBMC ($n = 14$) and adult PBMC ($n = 5$). In **(D,E)**, box plots represent the interquartile ranges, horizontal lines indicate the medians, and error bars extend to the minimum and maximum observed values. **(F)** CD8$^+$ T cells subsets that degranulate concomitant with HIV × CD3 or control (RSV × CD3) DART molecule mediated cytolytic activity. Rows represent assay results using PBMC from two different adult donors, Dn1 and Dn2. Distribution of CD8$^+$ T cell subsets is shown in the first column. Red dots in the remaining columns represent CD8 T cells that have degranulated (CD107a+) in response to the indicated DART molecules (frequencies within each quadrant indicated with red text), overlaid on the total CD8$^+$ T cells (gray dots) acquired for each condition. 24 h killing assay with a CD8$^+$ effector to Bal-infected autologous CD4$^+$ target cell ratio of 30:1 and DART molecule concentration of 100 ng/mL.

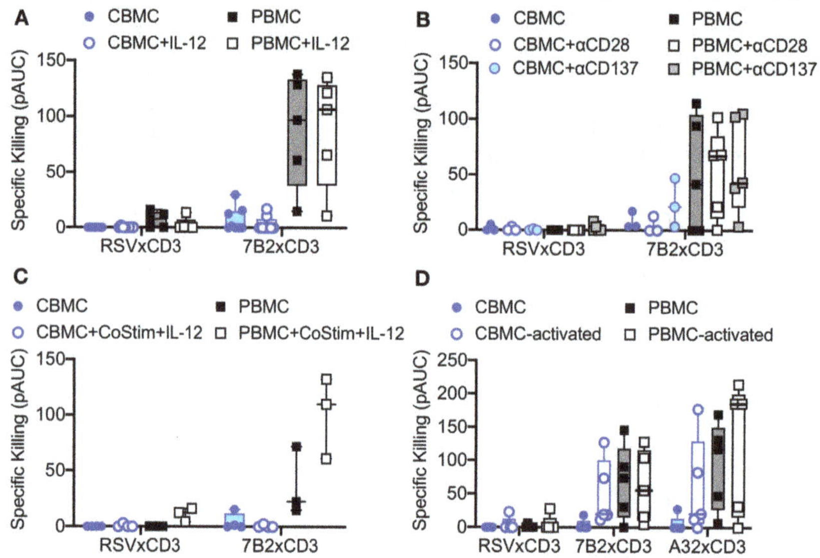

FIGURE 3 | Redirection of cord blood mononuclear cell (CBMC)-derived cytolytic T cells for elimination of autologous HIV-1 infected CD4 T cells by HIV × CD3 DART molecules is not improved by incubation with **(A)** 10 ng/mL exogenous IL-12 (CBMC $n = 8$, PBMC $n = 5$), **(B)** costimulation with anti-CD28 or anti-CD137 antibodies (CBMC $n = 3$, PBMC $n = 5$), or **(C)** a combination of costimulation with anti-CD28 and anti-CD137 (CoStim) and exogenous IL-12 (CBMC $n = 4$, PBMC $n = 3$). **(D)** HIV × CD3 DART molecule-mediated elimination of autologous HIV-1-infected CD4$^+$ T cells is improved when CD8$^+$ T cells used as effectors are activated by T cell receptor stimulation (anti-CD28, anti-CD3, and IL-2) for 48 h prior to use in the cell killing assays (CBMC and PBMC $n = 5$). Box plots represent the interquartile ranges, horizontal lines indicate the medians, and error bars extend to the minimum and maximum observed values. 24 h killing assays with a CD8$^+$ effector to HIV-1 4403bmC5-infected autologous CD4$^+$ target cell ratio of 30:1. All data reported as positive area under the dilution curve (pAUC).

trends, suggesting that degranulating CD4$^+$ T cells contribute to the *in vitro* elimination of HIV-1 infected cells when redirected by HIV × CD3 DART molecules. This finding is consistent with observations made in our prior studies performed using adult PBMC (18).

HIV x CD16 DART Molecules Can Recruit Cord Blood NK Cells for Elimination of Autologous HIV-1 Infected CD4$^+$ T Cells

Another approach for increasing HIV DART-molecule-mediated elimination of HIV-1 infected cells is to recruit additional populations of cytotoxic effector cells. We used flow cytometry immunophenotyping to compare NK cells present in CBMC and adult PBMC according to the gating strategy shown in **Figure 6A**. We found that cord blood contains more total NK cells (median 11% total NK in CBMC and 5% in adult PBMC), but similar distributions of NK cell subsets, as adult peripheral blood (**Figure 6B**). As we, and others, have previously demonstrated that pretreatment with IL-15 augments the cytotoxic potential of NK cells (32, 44–46) we compared the impact of overnight incubation with IL-15 (10 ng/mL) on the subset distribution, activation state, and intracellular abundance of cytotoxic effector molecules in NK cells present in CBMC and adult PBMC. We previously showed that IL-15 treatment increased the frequency of CD56^{bright} NK cells and CD56^{dim}CD16$^{-/dim}$ NK cells, and decreased CD56^{dim}CD16$^+$ NK cells in adult PBMC [(32) and **Figure 6B**]. The impact of IL-15 on cord blood NK cell subset distributions was modest, with no significant change (Wilcoxon rank sum tests) in the frequencies of major NK cell subsets (**Figure 6B**). Importantly, the cytotoxic CD56^{dim}CD16$^+$ NK cell subset was the dominant population of NK cells in both cord blood and adult PBMC. As we previously described for IL-15 treated NK cells in adult PBMC, we found that IL-15 treatment did not impact the expression of the maturation marker CD57 on the surface of cord blood NK cells, although its expression was markedly lower than that observed on NK cells in adult PBMC ($p < 0.001$, Wilcoxon rank sum test), which is consistent with the naivety of cord blood immune cells (**Figure 6C**). We also found that fewer cord blood NK cells expressed the secondary lymphoid homing marker CD62L when compared to NK cells in adult PBMC ($p < 0.001$, Wilcoxon rank sum test), and treatment of cord blood with IL-15 further reduced the percentage of

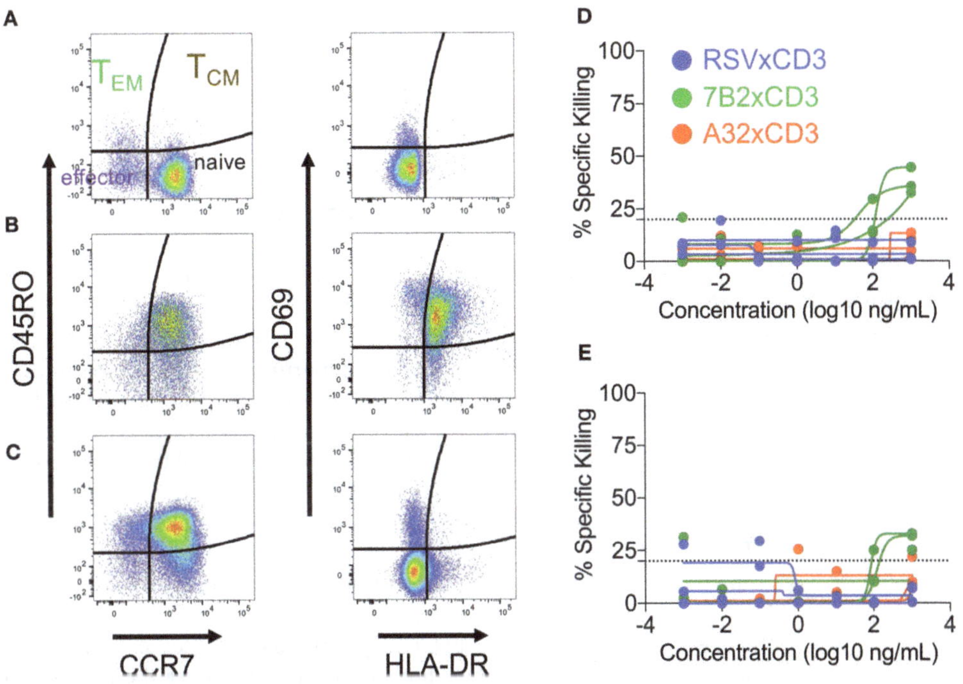

FIGURE 4 | Cord blood mononuclear cell (CBMC) CD8$^+$ T cells subset distribution (left panels) and activation state (right panels) after **(A)** overnight rest, **(B)** 3 days of T cell receptor stimulation (anti-CD3, anti-CD28, and IL-2), or **(C)** 3 day transition from activated cells back to the resting state. Representative example shown. Similar levels of DART molecule-redirected killing of autologous HIV-1 4403bmC5-infeced CD4$^+$ T cells were observed in assays performed with **(D)** CD8$^+$ T cell effectors after overnight rest, and **(E)** as they returned back to a resting state following 3 days of T cell receptor stimulation. **(D,E)** represent data from 24 h killing assays with a CD8$^+$ effector to HIV-1 4403bmC5-infected autologous CD4$^+$ target cell ratio of 30:1, performed using three different CBMC donors, each represented by individual lines.

NK cells expressing CD62L (**Figure 6D**). Moreover, and as expected, cord blood NK cells incubated with IL-15 presented a more active phenotype than untreated NK cells as evident by cell surface expression of HLA-DR (**Figure 6E**) and CD69 (**Figure 6F**), although overall, the frequency of activated NK cells was lower in CBMC compared to adult PBMC following IL-15 treatment ($p < 0.001$ for both CD69 and HLA-DR, Wilcoxon rank sum tests). Finally, using fluorescent quantitation beads to measure the intracellular content of perforin and granzyme B, we found that cord blood NK cells contained more perforin (**Figure 6G**) but less granzyme B (**Figure 6H**) than NK cells in adult PBMC, whether untreated (perforin, $p = 0.001$; granzyme B, $p < 0.001$, Wilcoxon rank sum tests) or treated with IL-15 (granzyme B, $p < 0.001$, Wilcoxon rank sum test). Collectively, these data suggest that cord blood contains similar distributions of NK cell subsets as adult peripheral blood, however the NK cells present in cord blood are less mature, less lymphoid homing, less active, and contain less of the cytotoxic effector molecule granzyme B when compared to NK cells in adult PBMC.

To recruit and redirect NK cells, DART-molecules comprised of our previously characterized HIV-1 targeting arms (18) linked to CD16 targeting arms were developed. We used flow cytometry staining to confirm that DART-molecules with CD16-targeting arms were capable of binding to the surface of human NK cells (**Figure 7A**). We next evaluated the ability of cord blood NK cells to eliminate autologous CD4$^+$ T cells infected with HIV-1 4403bmC5 virus when redirected by HIV × CD16 (clone hG38) DART molecules based on the 7B2 mAb. Similar to the data observed for cord blood CD8$^+$ T cells, we found that resting cord blood NK cells had modest ability to eliminate autologous HIV-1 infected T cells when redirected by the 7B2 × CD16 DART molecule (**Figure 7B**, filled symbols). However, overnight treatment with IL-15 significantly increased ($p = 0.007$, Wilcoxon rank sum test) the cytotoxic activity of cord blood NK cells when redirected by the HIV-specific DART molecule (**Figure 7B**, open symbols). The 7B2 × CD16 DART molecule redirected cytolytic activity of IL-15 treated CBMC NK cells was similar to that observed in assays performed with NK cells from adult PBMC (**Figure 7B**, black squares). These data demonstrate that NK cells in cord blood have potential to be effective mediators of DART molecule-redirected killing after priming with IL-15. We next explored whether combinations of HIV × CD16 DART molecules specific for different epitopes improved elimination of HIV-infected cells. For these experiments, we used HIV × CD16 DART molecules (A32 × CD16 and 7B2 × CD16) and a control molecule (RSV × CD16) that were generated using a different anti-CD16 arm (clone h5H2, **Figure 7A**). Assays were performed using NK cells from three cord blood samples that we identified as having cytolytic activity in previous assays. Using equivalent concentrations of the A32 × CD16 and 7B2 × CD16 molecules we found that activity of the combination was similar to that of the A32 × CD16 molecule alone (**Figure 7C**). Thus, there was no

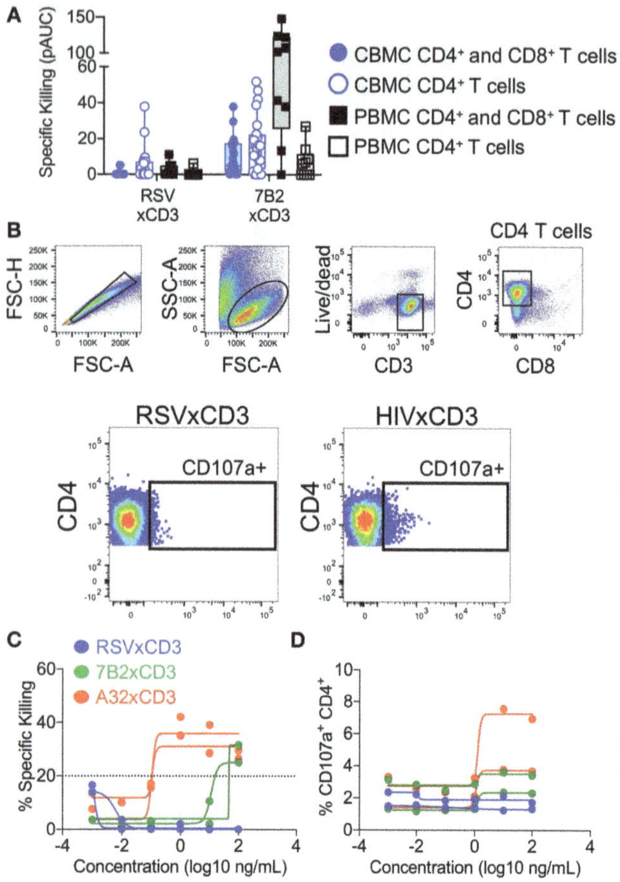

FIGURE 5 | Redirection of cord blood mononuclear cell (CBMC)-derived CD4+ T cells for elimination of HIV-infected cells by HIV × CD3 or control (RSV × CD3) DART molecules. **(A)** Similar levels of HIV-1 4403bmC5 infected CBMC-derived CD4+ T cell killing were observed in assays performed with autologous CD8+ T cell effectors (filled blue circles and box, $n = 23$ CBMC samples) or with CD4+ T cells alone, no additional effector cells (open blue circles and box). HIV-1 4403bmC5 infected PBMC-derived CD4+ T cell killing observed in assays performed with autologous CD8+ T cell effectors (filled black squares and box, $n = 9$ PBMC samples) or with CD4+ T cells alone, no additional effector cells (open black squares and box). **(B)** Gating strategy used to identify cord blood CD4+ T cells that degranulated concomitant with DART molecule mediated cytolytic activity. Redirection of CBMC-derived CD4+ T cells for elimination of HIV-1 Bal-infected autologous CD4+ T cells as measured by **(C)** luciferase cell killing assay, and **(D)** CD107a degranulation assay. Data are from 24 h killing assays performed using two different CBMC donors, each represented by individual lines.

evidence in these assays of an additive effect, nor of interference, when using these two HIV × CD16 DART molecules to mediate redirected killing with cord blood NK cells.

Finally, we investigated whether combinations of HIV × CD3 and HIV × CD16 DART molecules could work cooperatively for improved killing. To test this, we utilized IL-15 treated CBMC from two donors which we identified as having T cells and NK cells that supported redirected killing of autologous HIV-infected CD4+ T cells. 7B2 × CD3 and 7B2 × CD16 DART-molecules were used either alone, or in combination at equivalent concentrations. RSV × CD3 and 4420 × CD16 DART molecules in equivalent combination were used as a negative control. As shown in **Figure 7D**, combinations of 7B2 × CD3 and 7B2 × CD16 DART molecules did not improve the killing of HIV-1-infected autologous CD4+ T cells by cord blood cells in these assays.

DISCUSSION

Mother-to-child transmission is the principal cause of the approximate 400 new pediatric HIV-1 infections that occur each day, mostly in resource limited countries (4). Infants born into these unfortunate circumstances must strictly adhere to a lifetime of ART to control virus replication and prevent disease progression. Thus, there is a critical need for innovative therapeutic approaches enabling long-term remission or cure of infant HIV-1 infection in order to offer these children the chance to lead normal, healthy lives. One potential strategy is the use of antibody-based immunotherapy in combination with ART and latency reversing agents as a "shock and kill" approach to eliminate the virus reservoir (15, 16, 47, 48). Infants are potentially ideal candidates for immunotherapy due to the ability to initiate therapy soon after the perinatal transmission event and prior to establishment of a large virus reservoir (49, 50), and proven history of safe administration of passive antibody therapy against another infectious disease, respiratory syncytial virus (51). Here, we used human umbilical cord blood as a surrogate model of neonatal peripheral blood to test the hypothesis that HIV × CD3 DART molecules based on HIV-specific mAbs could redirect neonatal effector cells for elimination of cells infected with HIV-1. Importantly, our *in vitro* assays used autologous cord blood-derived CD4+ T cells as target cells, after infecting with an HIV IMC molecular clone virus encoding an HIV-1 subtype C *env* gene sequenced from plasma of a postnatally-infected infant, and identical to an isolate found in the matched maternal breast milk (34). Thus, these assays attempt to recapitulate the effector cells and HIV-1 Env-expressing target cells expected to be present in perinatally infected infants. Our results demonstrated that T cells present in cord blood can be recruited and redirected by HIV × CD3 DART molecules to eliminate HIV-1 infected target cells. This key finding supports the continued development of HIV-specific DART molecules as immunotherapies to combat pediatric HIV infection. However, we also found that the DART molecule-dependent killing activity by T cells from cord blood is significantly lessened as compared to that by T cells from adult PBMC. We therefore explored approaches to improve the cytotoxicity of cord blood effector cells with the goal of identifying strategies to maximize the potential effectiveness of DART molecule-based immunotherapy for use in early life.

We found that cord blood T cells were largely refractory to *in vitro* cytokine treatment and co-stimulatory receptor engagement intended to increase their cytolytic activity. We observed no impact of exogenous IL-12 (41), CD28 and CD137 co-stimulatory receptor engagement via specific antibodies, nor of combined use of IL-12 and co-stimulatory receptor engagement on the ability of cord blood T cells to eliminate HIV-1 infected cells when redirected by HIV × CD3 DART

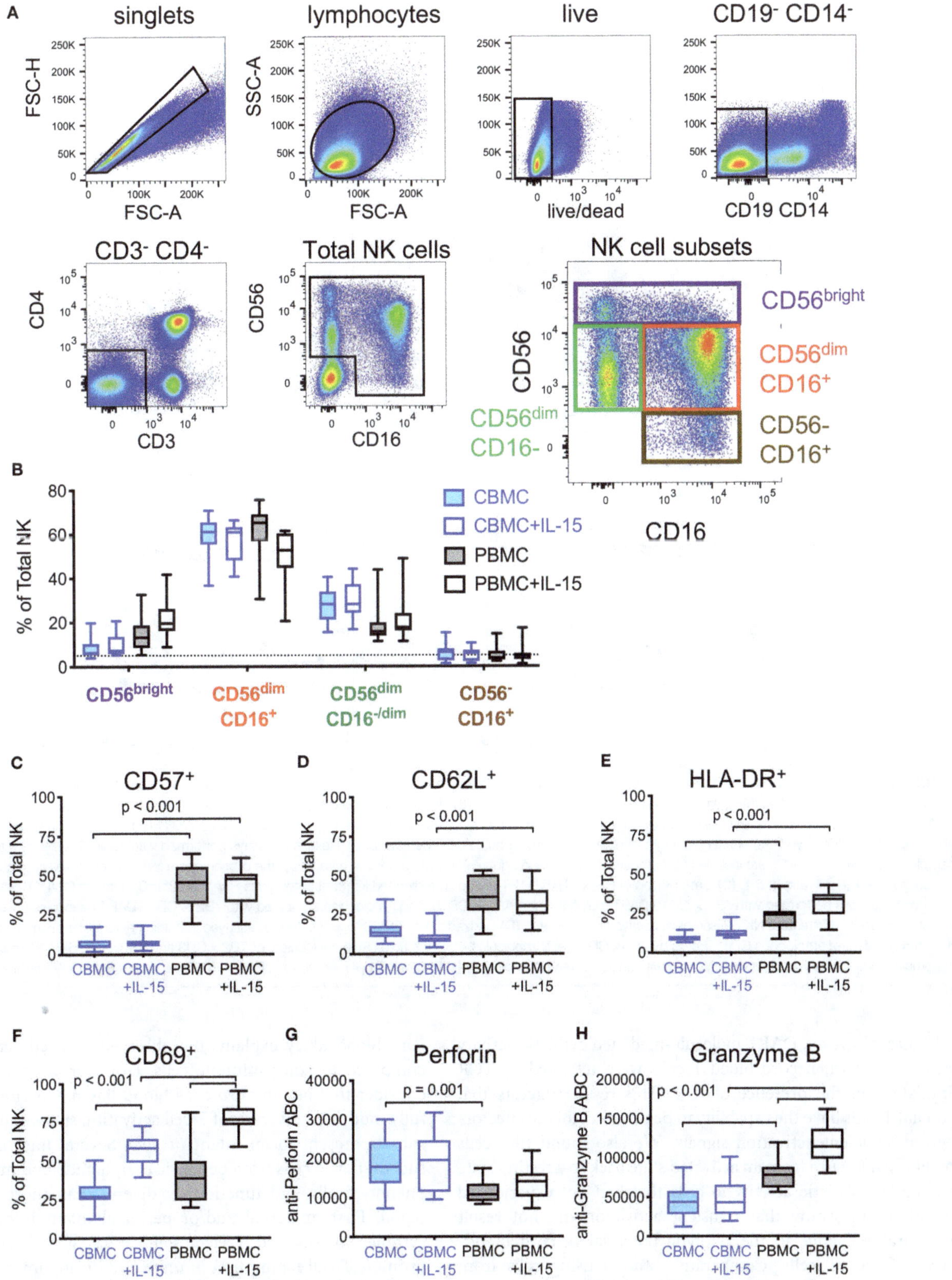

FIGURE 6 | Effect of exogenous IL-15 treatment on phenotypes of natural killer (NK) cells present in cord blood mononuclear cells (CBMC) with comparison to adult peripheral blood (PBMC). **(A)** Gating strategy used to identify total and subsets of NK cells. Data representing all CBMC samples ($n = 30$, 15 CBMC donors +/- IL-15)

(Continued)

FIGURE 6 | were combined and included in the flow cytometry plots shown. **(B)** Comparison of NK cell subset frequencies between untreated, and after overnight treatment with 10 ng/mL IL-15 ($n = 15$ CBMC and $n = 15$ PBMC samples per condition). Frequencies of total NK cells expressing **(C)** CD57, **(D)** CD62L, **(E)**, HLA-DR, and **(F)** CD69 in cells left untreated or treated overnight with 10 ng/mL IL-15. Amount of intracellular **(G)** Perforin and **(H)** Granzyme B in NK cells left untreated or after overnight treatment with 10 ng/mL IL-15, measured by antibody binding capacity (see Methods). In **(B–H)**, box plots represent the interquartile ranges, horizontal lines indicate the medians, and error bars extend to the minimum and maximum observed values.

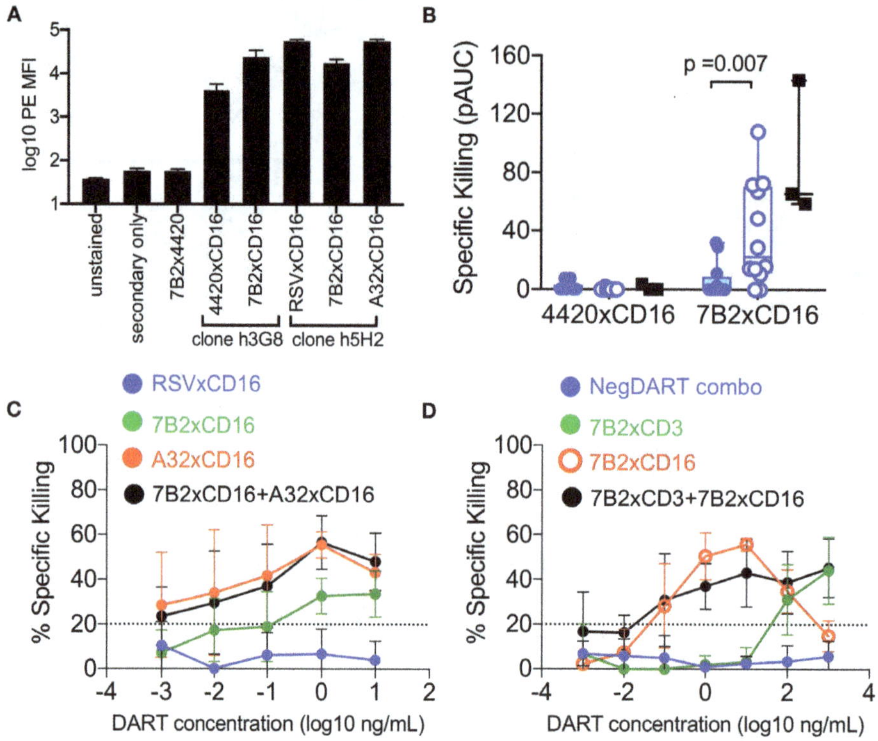

FIGURE 7 | (A) DART-molecules with CD16-targeting arms bind to the surface of human NK cells (from $n = 4$ donors) by flow cytometry analysis. Data are reported as mean fluorescent intensities (MFI), error bars represent standard deviation. **(B)** Redirection of cord blood mononuclear cell (CBMC)-derived NK cells (from $n = 12$ CBMC samples, blue circles) for elimination of HIV-1 4403bmC5-infected autologous $CD4^+$ T cells by 7B2 × CD16 or control (4420 × CD16) DART molecules in the absence of IL-15 (filled symbols) or after overnight incubation with 10 ng/mL IL-15 (open symbols). Results of assays performed with adult NK cells from three PBMC samples, in absence of IL-15, are included for comparison (black filled squares). Data are positive area under the dilution curve (pAUC) from 24 h killing assays with a NK cell to $CD4^+$ T cell ratio of 5:1. **(C)** Similar levels of HIV x CD16 DART molecule-redirected killing of autologous HIV-1 4403bmC5-infeced $CD4^+$ T cells were observed in assays performed with A32 × CD16 DART molecules and A32 × CD16 DART molecules combined with 7B2 × CD16 DART molecules ($n = 3$ CBMC-derived, IL-15 treated, NK cell samples, assayed in duplicate). **(D)** Redirection of CBMC ($n = 2$ samples, assayed in duplicate) for elimination of HIV-1 4403bmC5-infected autologous $CD4^+$ T cells by 7B2 x CD3 DART molecules, 7B2 × CD16 DART molecules, or 7B2 x CD3 and 7B2 x CD16 DART molecules used in combination. Twenty four hours killing assay with an IL-15 treated whole CBMC to $CD4^+$ T cell ratio of 30:1. Data in **(C,D)** represent mean +/− standard deviation.

molecules. However, DART molecule-mediated cytolytic activity was increased when cord blood T cells were activated by TCR stimulation in the presence of IL-2. This result suggests that neonatal T cells have the capability to be potent cytolytic effectors if given sufficient activation signals. We also found that cells transitioned *in vitro* from an activated state back to a resting state had similar cytolytic activity to cells that had not experienced activation, suggesting that transient activation did not result in a durable change in the cytolytic potential of cord blood-derived $CD8^+$ T cells. Comparative studies using cells from adult peripheral blood demonstrated that HIV × CD3 DART molecules effectively recruit and redirect memory and effector T cells —populations of cells that are poorly represented in cord blood. Thus, the limited maturation of T cell subsets in cord blood likely explains the observed reduced activity when compared to adult immune cells. However, it is important to consider that our *in vitro* cord blood-based experiments fail to fully model the diversity of T cell activation states and functional subsets present in an infant *in vivo*. Several lines of evidence suggest that T cells from pediatric peripheral blood may be more phenotypically and functionally diverse than those from cord blood. First, maternal and/or perinatal infant infections with cytomegalovirus and *Trypanosoma cruzi*, have been found to promote T cell maturation *in utero* and during infancy (52, 53). As cytomegalovirus, *T. cruzi*, and a myriad of other infectious agents and parasites are endemic in regions of high HIV-1 prevalence (54), it is likely that infants infected with HIV-1 via mother-to-child transmission have circulating T cells that differ in maturation, activation, and functionality when compared to those in cord blood from healthy United States-based mothers, as utilized in this study. It also has been shown that there are differences between pediatric circulating T cells, as modeled by cord blood in this study, and T cells present in pediatric tissues. Seminal work by Thome and collaborators using tissues obtained from pediatric organ donors from 2 months to 2 years of age demonstrated that, although naïve cells constitute the majority of T cells in pediatric peripheral blood, spleen, and lymph nodes, T_{EM} cells comprise a large portion of the T cells in intestinal mucosal tissues (40). Moreover, they demonstrated that memory T cells from the intestine were capable of rapid secretion of the effector cytokine IFNγ in response to stimulation. Because we found that T_{EM} cells are preferentially recruited by HIV × CD3 DART molecules, the cytolytic activity of these molecules mediated by tissue-derived T cells at mucosal sites may be higher than that observed by cord blood-derived T cells *in vitro*. It is important to note that Thome and collaborators also identified higher frequencies of T regulatory cells in pediatric blood and tissues relative to adults (40). The $CD4^+$ T regulatory cells may act to either limit the cytolytic activity of infant T cell responses, or may themselves serve as effector cells for CD3 DART molecule mediated lysis of target cells as has been previously shown (55). Thus, accurate characterization of the cytolytic activity of pediatric tissue-resident T cells when recruited by HIV × CD3 DARTs will likely require *in vivo* testing using a biologically relevant model, such as infant rhesus macaques. Finally, immune system development during early life will likely also affect the therapeutic potential of HIV × CD3 DART molecules. In fact, $CD8^+$ T cell responses may mature rather quickly, as young children (2–3 years of age) have been shown to have $CD8^+$ T cells with potent antiviral activity (56, 57). These observations suggest that the ability of HIV × CD3 DART molecules to mediate elimination of HIV-1-infected cells may improve over the first few years of life. Interestingly, we also found that cord blood $CD4^+$ T cells contributed to elimination of infected cells *in vitro*. Whether these cells would contribute to HIV × CD3 DART molecule-dependent elimination of infected cells *in vivo* is not yet known. Additional studies using blood samples collected longitudinally from HIV-infected infants and age-appropriate non-human primate models would likely help to identify relevant populations of effector cells, and to determine the optimal timing post birth for usage of HIV × CD3 DART molecules to eliminate the HIV-1 infected cell reservoir during early life. However, the presence of higher birth levels of memory T cells, and rapid expansion of T cell memory in rhesus macaques may complicate human translation of such studies (58).

Effective control and/or cure of pediatric HIV will likely require early and aggressive interventions. Thus, the likelihood of success with the HIV-specific DART molecule-based approach might be increased by recruitment of additional populations of cytolytic effector cells to further promote eradication of infected cells, and to potentially reach additional tissues and anatomical compartments. NK cells are abundant in cord blood and pediatric peripheral blood, with cytotoxic $CD56^{dim}CD16^+$ NK cells representing the dominant subset (39, 45, 59). We found that HIV × CD16 DART molecules were able to recruit and redirect neonatal NK cells present in cord blood for elimination of HIV-1 infected cells and killing activity could be substantially increased by treatment with IL-15. The ability of IL-15 to augment the cytolytic activity of cord blood derived NK cells is consistent with previously reported results from assays measuring cord blood NK cell natural cytotoxicity against sensitive target cells (45). Currently, the mechanisms by which IL-15 improves NK cell cytotoxicity are incompletely defined. We previously demonstrated that IL-15 treatment of NK cells from adult peripheral blood increases the levels of cytolytic effector molecules, perforin and granzyme B (32). By contrast, we found that cord blood NK cells contained more perforin, but less granzyme B, than NK cells in adult PBMC —and the levels of neither were impacted by IL-15 treatment. Thus, intracellular abundance of perforin and granzyme B does not explain how cord blood NK cells become more cytolytic after incubation with IL-15, which suggests involvement of other activatory or regulatory processes. Exogenous IL-15 was previously shown to increase cord blood NK cell expression of intracellular adhesion molecule 1 (ICAM-1) —a cell surface protein involved in cell-to-cell interactions including formation of NK cell immunologic synapses (60). However, this effect was only seen after extended culture for 7 days (61), not after a short overnight incubation as in our study. It has also been proposed that the higher frequency of cord blood NK cells expressing cell-surface inhibitory receptor NKG2A compared to NK cells from adult peripheral blood may contribute to the reduced activity of cord blood derived NK cells (62). In contrast, we have previously demonstrated that IL-15 promotes expression of the activating receptors NKG2D and NKp30 (46). Additional research will be required to define the impact of IL-15 on the multitude of cord blood NK inhibitory and activating receptors, and to determine how these signals may integrate with the CD16-mediated signaling that occurs when NK cells interact with HIV x CD16 DART molecules.

Having found that IL-15 stimulation is able to maximize the functionality of cord blood NK cells for DART molecule-redirected killing has generated another important question: are neonatal NK cells naturally primed by IL-15 *in vivo* during HIV-1 infection? IL-15 was transiently detected in the plasma during acute HIV-1 infection of adults, with a median time of first detection being 6 days after viremia reached detectable levels in peripheral blood plasma (63). Although a similar inflammatory cytokine response is expected in neonates, it has also been demonstrated that stimulated CBMC produce less IL-15 than adult peripheral blood (64). Whether or not sufficient levels of IL-15 to activate neonatal NK cells would be present at sites of infection will require additional research. If an absence of natural IL-15 is identified, alternative strategies including the administration of recombinant human IL-15, or engineered forms of IL-15 (65, 66), in combination with the HIV × CD16 DART molecules could be tested in the infant rhesus macaque model.

Although we found that combinations of 7B2 × CD3 and A32 × CD3 DART molecules did not result in improved cytolytic activity, it is important to note that these studies were intended to explore the cytolytic potential of neonatal effector cells, not to identify optimal combinations of DART molecules. We used 7B2 and A32 DART molecules as an extension of our original study (18), but additional DART molecules targeting other Env epitopes have been described (17). It is probable that combinations of DART molecules targeting both broad-binding neutralizing and non-neutralizing epitopes, could be the most effective in recognizing the HIV Env diversity that results from the genetic diversity of HIV-1, and the variety of Env conformations that may be found on the surface of infected cells *in vivo* (43, 67, 68). Research aimed at identifying optimal combinations of anti-HIV antibodies using diverse HIV isolates, and patient-derived latent reservoir virus (Tuyishime et al., submitted) will likely help identify optimal combinations of DART molecules.

At present, blinatumomab, a CD19 × CD3 antibody-based bispecific molecule, is the only example of an immune cell-engaging bispecific drug that has FDA approval for the treatment of disease—B cell acute lymphoblastic leukemia (69, 70). However, there are dozens of bispecific antibody-based molecules in various stages of development, and clinical testing, against multiple types of cancers (71, 72). This includes several DART molecules being evaluated for potential use in treatment of leukemias and lymphomas (73, 74), colorectal cancer (55), and solid tumors (75). The majority of bispecifics in development are intended to recruit T cells via an anti-CD3 arm, however NK cell recruitment by anti-CD16 targeting is also being explored (76, 77). The continued development and clinical testing of DART molecules, and other antibody-based bispecifics, for use against human cancers will provide important safety, durability, and efficacy data that will help inform the best strategies for use of these types of therapies against other diseases, including HIV-1 infection.

In summary, we demonstrated that HIV × CD3 and HIV × CD16 DART molecules can recruit and redirect cytolytic immune cells present in cord blood to eliminate autologous T cells infected with HIV-1, albeit less effectively than cells present in adult peripheral blood. Our work supports the continued development of these antibody-based molecules as components of passive immunization strategies aimed at treatment and cure of pediatric HIV. However, future studies using early life blood and tissue samples, and infant or juvenile preclinical animal models, will be required to identify tenable strategies to optimize their efficacy.

ETHICS STATEMENT

Anonymized human umbilical cord blood donations that failed to meet the criteria required for clinical use were obtained with informed written consent. Human peripheral venous blood was collected by leukapheresis from healthy consenting adult volunteers (28, 29). All samples were collected in accordance with the policies and regulations of the Duke Health Institutional Review Board.

AUTHOR CONTRIBUTIONS

JP conceived the study, performed experiments, analyzed and interpreted data, and wrote the manuscript. RE performed experiments and analyzed data. SJ performed statistical analyses. TH and JAP performed experiments and analyzed data. C-YL, LL, GD, and JN led the design, development, and production of the bispecific dart molecules. SP isolated and characterized the breast milk transmitted/founder HIV-1 virus. TD collected and characterized the adult leukapheresis samples. SP and GF interpreted data and contributed to design of the study. All authors commented on the manuscript and approved the final version.

ACKNOWLEDGMENTS

We thank Dr. Joanne Kurtzberg and the staff of the Carolinas Cord Blood Bank for assistance in acquiring human umbilical cord blood samples used for this study.

REFERENCES

1. Nduati R, John G, Mbori-Ngacha D, Richardson B, Overbaugh J, Mwatha A, et al. Effect of breastfeeding and formula feeding on transmission of HIV-1: a randomized clinical trial. *JAMA*. (2000) 283:1167–74. doi: 10.1001/jama.283.9.1167
2. Chasela CS, Hudgens MG, Jamieson DJ, Kayira D, Hosseinipour MC, Kourtis AP, et al. Maternal or infant antiretroviral drugs to reduce HIV-1 transmission. *N Engl J Med*. (2010) 362:2271–81. doi: 10.1056/NEJMoa0911486
3. Tobin NH, Aldrovandi GM. Immunology of pediatric HIV infection. *Immunol Rev*. (2013) 254:143–69. doi: 10.1111/imr.12074
4. UNAIDS. *Communities at the Centre - Global AIDS Update 2019*. (2019) Geneva: WHO Library.
5. De Rossi A, Masiero S, Giaquinto C, Ruga E, Comar M, Giacca M, et al. Dynamics of viral replication in infants with vertically acquired human immunodeficiency virus type 1 infection. *J Clin Invest*. (1996) 97:323–30. doi: 10.1172/JCI118419
6. Rouzioux C, Burgard M, Chaix ML, Delamare C, Cirau N, Bouiller B, et al. Human immunodeficiency virus-1 infection in neonates: correlation of plasma and cellular viremia and clinical outcome. French pediatric cohort study group. *Acta Paediatr Suppl*. (1997) 421:17–21. doi: 10.1111/j.1651-2227.1997.tb18314.x
7. Shearer WT, Quinn TC, Larussa P, Lew JF, Mofenson L, Almy S, et al. Viral load and disease progression in infants infected with human immunodeficiency virus type 1. Women and infants transmission study group. *N Engl J Med*. (1997) 336:1337–42. doi: 10.1056/NEJM199705083361901
8. Abrams EJ, Weedon J, Steketee RW, Lambert G, Bamji M, Brown T, et al. Association of human immunodeficiency virus (HIV) load early in life with disease progression among HIV-infected infants. New York city perinatal HIV transmission collaborative study group. *J Infect Dis*. (1998) 178:101–8. doi: 10.1086/515596
9. Dickover RE, Dillon M, Leung KM, Krogstad P, Plaeger S, Kwok S, et al. Early prognostic indicators in primary perinatal human immunodeficiency virus type 1 infection: importance of viral RNA and the timing of transmission on long-term outcome. *J Infect Dis*. (1998) 178:375–87. doi: 10.1086/515637
10. Palumbo PE, Raskino C, Fiscus S, Pahwa S, Fowler MG, Spector SA, et al. Predictive value of quantitative plasma HIV RNA and CD4+ lymphocyte count in HIV-infected infants and children. *JAMA*. (1998) 279:756–61. doi: 10.1001/jama.279.10.756

11. Rich KC, Fowler MG, Mofenson LM, Abboud R, Pitt J, Diaz C, et al. Maternal and infant factors predicting disease progression in human immunodeficiency virus type 1-infected infants. Women and infants transmission study group. *Pediatrics.* (2000) 105:e8. doi: 10.1542/peds.105.1.e8
12. Richardson BA, Mbori-Ngacha D, Lavreys L, John-Stewart GC, Nduati R, Panteleeff DD, et al. Comparison of human immunodeficiency virus type 1 viral loads in Kenyan women, men, and infants during primary and early infection. *J Virol.* (2003) 77:7120–3. doi: 10.1128/JVI.77.12.7120-7123.2003
13. Persaud D, Gay H, Ziemniak C, Chen YH, Piatak M Jr, Chun TW, et al. Absence of detectable HIV-1 viremia after treatment cessation in an infant. *N Engl J Med.* (2013) 369:1828–35. doi: 10.1056/NEJMoa1302976
14. Luzuriaga K, Gay H, Ziemniak C, Sanborn KB, Somasundaran M, Rainwater-Lovett K, et al. Viremic relapse after HIV-1 remission in a perinatally infected child. *N Engl J Med.* (2015) 372:786–8. doi: 10.1056/NEJMc1413931
15. Richman DD. HIV: cure by killing. *Nature.* (2015) 528:198–9. doi: 10.1038/nature16321
16. Ferrari G, Haynes BF, Koenig S, Nordstrom JL, Margolis DM, Tomaras GD, et al. Envelope-specific antibodies and antibody-derived molecules for treating and curing HIV infection. *Nat Rev Drug Discov.* (2016) 15:823–34. doi: 10.1038/nrd.2016.173
17. Sloan DD, Lam CY, Irrinki A, Liu L, Tsai A, Pace CS, et al. Targeting HIV reservoir in infected CD4 T cells by dual-affinity re-targeting molecules (DARTs) that bind HIV envelope and recruit cytotoxic T cells. *PLoS Pathog.* (2015) 11:e1005233. doi: 10.1371/journal.ppat.1005233
18. Sung JA, Pickeral J, Liu L, Stanfield-Oakley SA, Lam CY, Garrido C, et al. Dual-affinity re-targeting proteins direct T cell-mediated cytolysis of latently HIV-infected cells. *J Clin Invest.* (2015) 125:4077–90. doi: 10.1172/JCI82314
19. Moore PA, Zhang W, Rainey GJ, Burke S, Li H, Huang L, et al. Application of dual affinity retargeting molecules to achieve optimal redirected T-cell killing of B-cell lymphoma. *Blood.* (2011) 117:4542–51. doi: 10.1182/blood-2010-09-306449
20. Shan L, Deng K, Shroff NS, Durand CM, Rabi SA, Yang HC, et al. Stimulation of HIV-1-specific cytolytic T lymphocytes facilitates elimination of latent viral reservoir after virus reactivation. *Immunity.* (2012) 36:491–501. doi: 10.1016/j.immuni.2012.01.014
21. Deng K, Pertea M, Rongvaux A, Wang L, Durand CM, Ghiaur G, et al. Broad CTL response is required to clear latent HIV-1 due to dominance of escape mutations. *Nature.* (2015) 517:381–5. doi: 10.1038/nature14053
22. Strain MC, Little SJ, Daar ES, Havlir DV, Gunthard HF, Lam RY, et al. Effect of treatment, during primary infection, on establishment and clearance of cellular reservoirs of HIV-1. *J Infect Dis.* (2005) 191:1410–8. doi: 10.1086/428777
23. Chun TW, Nickle DC, Justement JS, Meyers JH, Roby G, Hallahan CW, et al. Persistence of HIV in gut-associated lymphoid tissue despite long-term antiretroviral therapy. *J Infect Dis.* (2008) 197:714–20. doi: 10.1086/527324
24. Boasso A, Shearer GM, Chougnet C. Immune dysregulation in human immunodeficiency virus infection: know it, fix it, prevent it?. *J Intern Med.* (2009) 265:78–96. doi: 10.1111/j.1365-2796.2008.02043.x
25. Martinez-Bonet M, Puertas MC, Fortuny C, Ouchi D, Mellado MJ, Rojo P, et al. Establishment and replenishment of the viral reservoir in perinatally HIV-1-infected children initiating very early antiretroviral therapy. *Clin Infect Dis.* (2015) 61:1169–78. doi: 10.1093/cid/civ456
26. Strauss-Albee DM, Liang EC, Ranganath T, Aziz N, Blish CA. The newborn human NK cell repertoire is phenotypically formed but functionally reduced. *Cytometry B Clin Cytom.* (2017) 92:33–41. doi: 10.1002/cyto.b.21485
27. Fike AJ, Kumova OK, Carey AJ. Dissecting the defects in the neonatal CD8(+) T-cell response. *J Leukoc Biol.* (2019) 106:1051–61. doi: 10.1002/JLB.5RU0319-105R
28. Garcia A, Keinonen S, Sanchez AM, Ferrari G, Denny TN, Moody MA. Leukopak PBMC sample processing for preparing quality control material to support proficiency testing programs. *J Immunol Methods.* (2014) 409:99–106. doi: 10.1016/j.jim.2014.05.019
29. Sambor A, Garcia A, Berrong M, Pickeral J, Brown S, Rountree W, et al. Establishment and maintenance of a PBMC repository for functional cellular studies in support of clinical vaccine trials. *J Immunol Methods.* (2014) 409:107–16. doi: 10.1016/j.jim.2014.04.005
30. Johnson S, Burke S, Huang L, Gorlatov S, Li H, Wang W, et al. Effector cell recruitment with novel Fv-based dual-affinity re-targeting protein leads to potent tumor cytolysis and *in vivo* B-cell depletion. *J Mol Biol.* (2010) 399:436–49. doi: 10.1016/j.jmb.2010.04.001
31. Graves AJ, Padilla MG, Hokey DA. OMIP-022: comprehensive assessment of antigen-specific human T-cell functionality and memory. *Cytometry A.* (2014) 85:576–9. doi: 10.1002/cyto.a.22478
32. Fisher L, Zinter M, Stanfield-Oakley S, Carpp LN, Edwards RW, Denny T, et al. Vaccine-induced antibodies mediate higher antibody-dependent cellular cytotoxicity after interleukin-15 pretreatment of natural killer effector cells. *Front Immunol.* (2019) 10:2741. doi: 10.3389/fimmu.2019.02741
33. Eller MA, Currier JR. OMIP-007: phenotypic analysis of human natural killer cells. *Cytometry A.* (2012) 81:447–9. doi: 10.1002/cyto.a.22033
34. Fouda GG, Mahlokozera T, Salazar-Gonzalez JF, Salazar MG, Learn G, Kumar SB, et al. Postnatally-transmitted HIV-1 envelope variants have similar neutralization-sensitivity and function to that of non-transmitted breast milk variants. *Retrovirology.* (2013) 10:3. doi: 10.1186/1742-4690-10-3
35. Edmonds TG, Ding H, Yuan X, Wei Q, Smith KS, Conway JA, et al. Replication competent molecular clones of HIV-1 expressing *Renilla* luciferase facilitate the analysis of antibody inhibition in PBMC. *Virology.* (2010) 408:1–13. doi: 10.1016/j.virol.2010.08.028
36. O'doherty U, Swiggard WJ, Malim MH. Human immunodeficiency virus type 1 spinoculation enhances infection through virus binding. *J Virol.* (2000) 74:10074–80. doi: 10.1128/JVI.74.21.10074-10080.2000
37. Lewis GK. Qualitative and quantitative variables that affect the potency of Fc- mediated effector function *in vitro* and *in vivo*: considerations for passive immunization using non-neutralizing antibodies. *Curr HIV Res.* (2013) 11:354–64. doi: 10.2174/1570162X113116660060
38. Betts MR, Brenchley JM, Price DA, De Rosa SC, Douek DC, Roederer M, et al. Sensitive and viable identification of antigen-specific CD8+ T cells by a flow cytometric assay for degranulation. *J Immunol Methods.* (2003) 281:65–78. doi: 10.1016/S0022-1759(03)00265-5
39. D'arena G, Musto P, Cascavilla N, Di Giorgio G, Fusilli S, Zendoli F, et al. Flow cytometric characterization of human umbilical cord blood lymphocytes: immunophenotypic features. *Haematologica.* (1998) 83:197–203.
40. Thome JJ, Bickham KL, Ohmura Y, Kubota M, Matsuoka N, Gordon C, et al. Early-life compartmentalization of human T cell differentiation and regulatory function in mucosal and lymphoid tissues. *Nat Med.* (2016) 22:72–7. doi: 10.1038/nm.4008
41. Mccarron MJ, Reen DJ. Neonatal CD8+ T-cell differentiation is dependent on interleukin-12. *Hum Immunol.* (2010) 71:1172–9. doi: 10.1016/j.humimm.2010.09.004
42. Chen L, Flies DB. Molecular mechanisms of T cell co-stimulation and co-inhibition. *Nat Rev Immunol.* (2013) 13:227–42. doi: 10.1038/nri3405
43. Moore PL, Crooks ET, Porter L, Zhu P, Cayanan CS, Grise H, et al. Nature of nonfunctional envelope proteins on the surface of human immunodeficiency virus type 1. *J Virol.* (2006) 80:2515–28. doi: 10.1128/JVI.80.5.2515-2528.2006
44. Carson WE, Giri JG, Lindemann MJ, Linett ML, Ahdieh M, Paxton R, et al. Interleukin (IL) 15 is a novel cytokine that activates human natural killer cells via components of the IL-2 receptor. *J Exp Med.* (1994) 180:1395–403. doi: 10.1084/jem.180.4.1395
45. Dalle JH, Menezes J, Wagner E, Blagdon M, Champagne J, Champagne MA, et al. Characterization of cord blood natural killer cells: implications for transplantation and neonatal infections. *Pediatr Res.* (2005) 57:649–55. doi: 10.1203/01.PDR.0000156501.55431.20
46. Garrido C, Abad-Fernandez M, Tuyishime M, Pollara JJ, Ferrari G, Soriano-Sarabia N, et al. Interleukin-15-stimulated natural killer cells clear HIV-1-infected cells following latency reversal *ex vivo*. *J Virol.* (2018) 92:e00235–18. doi: 10.1128/JVI.00235-18

47. Ferrari G, Pollara J, Tomaras GD, Haynes BF. Humoral and innate antiviral immunity as tools to clear persistent HIV infection. *J Infect Dis.* (2017) 215:S152–9. doi: 10.1093/infdis/jiw555
48. Kim Y, Anderson JL, Lewin SR. Getting the "kill" into "shock and kill:" strategies to eliminate latent HIV. *Cell Host Microbe.* (2018) 23:14–26. doi: 10.1016/j.chom.2017.12.004
49. Rainwater-Lovett K, Luzuriaga K, Persaud D. Very early combination antiretroviral therapy in infants: prospects for cure. *Curr Opin HIV AIDS.* (2015) 10:4–11. doi: 10.1097/COH.0000000000000127
50. Luzuriaga K. Early combination antiretroviral therapy limits HIV-1 persistence in children. *Annu Rev Med.* (2016) 67:201–13. doi: 10.1146/annurev-med-091114-111159
51. Sandritter T. Palivizumab for respiratory syncytial virus prophylaxis. *J Pediatr Health Care.* (1999) 13:191–5. doi: 10.1016/S0891-5245(99)90039-1
52. Hermann E, Truyens C, Alonso-Vega C, Even J, Rodriguez P, Berthe A, et al. Human fetuses are able to mount an adultlike CD8 T-cell response. *Blood.* (2002) 100:2153–8. doi: 10.1182/blood.V100.6.2153
53. Marchant A, Appay V, Van Der Sande M, Dulphy N, Liesnard C, Kidd M, et al. Mature CD8(+) T lymphocyte response to viral infection during fetal life. *J Clin Invest.* (2003) 111:1747–55. doi: 10.1172/JCI200317470
54. Dauby N, Goetghebuer T, Kollmann TR, Levy J, Marchant A. Uninfected but not unaffected: chronic maternal infections during pregnancy, fetal immunity, and susceptibility to postnatal infections. *Lancet Infect Dis.* (2012) 12:330–40. doi: 10.1016/S1473-3099(11)70341-3
55. Moore PA, Shah K, Yang Y, Alderson R, Roberts P, Long V, et al. Development of MGD007, a gpA33 x CD3-bispecific DART protein for T-cell immunotherapy of metastatic colorectal cancer. *Mol Cancer Ther.* (2018) 17:1761–72. doi: 10.1158/1535-7163.MCT-17-1086
56. Sandberg JK, Fast NM, Jordan KA, Furlan SN, Barbour JD, Fennelly G, et al. HIV-specific CD8+ T cell function in children with vertically acquired HIV-1 infection is critically influenced by age and the state of the CD4+ T cell compartment. *J Immunol.* (2003) 170:4403–10. doi: 10.4049/jimmunol.170.8.4403
57. Chen SF, Tu WW, Sharp MA, Tongson EC, He XS, Greenberg HB, et al. Antiviral CD8 T cells in the control of primary human cytomegalovirus infection in early childhood. *J Infect Dis.* (2004) 189:1619–27. doi: 10.1086/383249
58. Pitcher CJ, Hagen SI, Walker JM, Lum R, Mitchell BL, Maino VC, et al. Development and homeostasis of T cell memory in rhesus macaque. *J Immunol.* (2002) 168:29–43. doi: 10.4049/jimmunol.168.1.29
59. Verneris MR, Miller JS. The phenotypic and functional characteristics of umbilical cord blood and peripheral blood natural killer cells. *Br J Haematol.* (2009) 147:185–91. doi: 10.1111/j.1365-2141.2009.07768.x
60. Liu D, Bryceson YT, Meckel T, Vasiliver-Shamis G, Dustin ML, Long EO. Integrin-dependent organization and bidirectional vesicular traffic at cytotoxic immune synapses. *Immunity.* (2009) 31:99–109. doi: 10.1016/j.immuni.2009.05.009
61. Lin SJ, Yan DC. ICAM-1 (CD54) expression on T lymphocytes and natural killer cells from umbilical cord blood: regulation with interleukin-12 and interleukin-15. *Cytokines Cell Mol Ther.* (2000) 6:161–4. doi: 10.1080/mccm.6.4.161.164
62. Wang Y, Xu H, Zheng X, Wei H, Sun R, Tian Z. High expression of NKG2A/CD94 and low expression of granzyme B are associated with reduced cord blood NK cell activity. *Cell Mol Immunol.* (2007) 4:377–82.
63. Stacey AR, Norris PJ, Qin L, Haygreen EA, Taylor E, Heitman J, et al. Induction of a striking systemic cytokine cascade prior to peak viremia in acute human immunodeficiency virus type 1 infection, in contrast to more modest and delayed responses in acute hepatitis B and C virus infections. *J Virol.* (2009) 83:3719–33. doi: 10.1128/JVI.01844-08
64. Qian JX, Lee SM, Suen Y, Knoppel E, Van De Ven C, Cairo MS. Decreased interleukin-15 from activated cord versus adult peripheral blood mononuclear cells and the effect of interleukin-15 in upregulating antitumor immune activity and cytokine production in cord blood. *Blood.* (1997) 90:3106–17. doi: 10.1182/blood.V90.8.3106
65. Xu W, Jones M, Liu B, Zhu X, Johnson CB, Edwards AC, et al. Efficacy and mechanism-of-action of a novel superagonist interleukin-15: interleukin-15 receptor αSu/Fc fusion complex in syngeneic murine models of multiple myeloma. *Cancer Res.* (2013) 73:3075–86. doi: 10.1158/0008-5472.CAN-12-2357
66. Thaysen-Andersen M, Chertova E, Bergamaschi C, Moh ES, Chertov O, Roser J, et al. Recombinant human heterodimeric IL-15 complex displays extensive and reproducible N- and O-linked glycosylation. *Glycoconj J.* (2016) 33:417–33. doi: 10.1007/s10719-015-9627-1
67. Alsahafi N, Bakouche N, Kazemi M, Richard J, Ding S, Bhattacharyya S, et al. An asymmetric opening of HIV-1 envelope mediates antibody-dependent cellular cytotoxicity. *Cell Host Microbe.* (2019) 25:578 e575. doi: 10.1016/j.chom.2019.03.002
68. Lu M, Ma X, Castillo-Menendez LR, Gorman J, Alsahafi N, Ermel U, et al. Associating HIV-1 envelope glycoprotein structures with states on the virus observed by smFRET. *Nature.* (2019) 568:415–9. doi: 10.1038/s41586-019-1101-y
69. Nagorsen D, Kufer P, Baeuerle PA, Bargou R. Blinatumomab: a historical perspective. *Pharmacol Ther.* (2012) 136:334–42. doi: 10.1016/j.pharmthera.2012.07.013
70. Przepiorka D, Ko CW, Deisseroth A, Yancey CL, Candau-Chacon R, Chiu HJ, et al. FDA approval: blinatumomab. *Clin Cancer Res.* (2015) 21:4035–9. doi: 10.1158/1078-0432.CCR-15-0612
71. Clynes RA, Desjarlais JR. Redirected T cell cytotoxicity in cancer therapy. *Annu Rev Med.* (2019) 70:437–50. doi: 10.1146/annurev-med-062617-035821
72. Suurs FV, Lub-De Hooge MN, De Vries EGE, De Groot DJA. A review of bispecific antibodies and antibody constructs in oncology and clinical challenges. *Pharmacol Ther.* (2019) 201:103–19. doi: 10.1016/j.pharmthera.2019.04.006
73. Chichili GR, Huang L, Li H, Burke S, He L, Tang Q, et al. XA CD3xCD123 bispecific DART for redirecting host T cells to myelogenous leukemia: preclinical activity and safety in non-human primates. *Sci. Transl. Med.* Blinatumoma 7:289ra282. doi: 10.1126/scitranslmed.aaa5693
74. Liu L, Lam CK, Long V, Widjaja L, Yang Y, Li H, et al. MGD011, A CD19 x CD3 dual-affinity retargeting bi-specific molecule incorporating extended circulating half-life for the treatment of B-cell malignancies. *Clin Cancer Res.* (2017) 23:1506–18. doi: 10.1158/1078-0432.CCR-16-0666
75. Spira A, Goldberg S, Strauss J, Bendell J, Cote G, Rahma E, et al. A phase 1, open label, dose escalation study of MGD009, a B7-H3 x CD3 DART® protein, in combination with MGA012, an anti-PD-1 antibody, in patients with relapsed or refractory B7-H3-expressing tumors. *J Immuno Ther Cancer.* (2018) 6:P305. doi: 10.1200/JCO.2018.36.15_suppl.TPS2601
76. Rothe A, Sasse S, Topp MS, Eichenauer DA, Hummel H, Reiners KS, et al. A phase 1 study of the bispecific anti-CD30/CD16A antibody construct AFM13 in patients with relapsed or refractory Hodgkin lymphoma. *Blood.* (2015) 125:4024–31. doi: 10.1182/blood-2014-12-614636
77. Vallera DA, Felices M, Mcelmurry R, Mccullar V, Zhou X, Schmohl JU, et al. IL15 trispecific killer engagers (TriKE) make natural killer cells specific to CD33+ targets while also inducing persistence, *in vivo* expansion, and enhanced function. *Clin Cancer Res.* (2016) 22:3440–50. doi: 10.1158/1078-0432.CCR-15-2710

4

Elevated Expression of miR-19b Enhances CD8$^+$ T Cell Function by Targeting PTEN in HIV Infected Long Term Non-progressors With Sustained Viral Suppression

Lin-Bo Yin[1,2,3,4], Cheng-Bo Song[1,2,3,4], Jie-Fu Zheng[1,2,3,4], Ya-Jing Fu[1,2,3,4], Shi Qian[1,2,3,4], Yong-Jun Jiang[1,2,3,4], Jun-Jie Xu[1,2,3,4], Hai-Bo Ding[1,2,3,4], Hong Shang[1,2,3,4] and Zi-Ning Zhang[1,2,3,4]**

[1] NHC Key Laboratory of AIDS Immunology (China Medical University), Department of Laboratory Medicine, The First Affiliated Hospital of China Medical University, Shenyang, China, [2] Key Laboratory of AIDS Immunology of Liaoning Province, The First Affiliated Hospital of China Medical University, Shenyang, China, [3] Key Laboratory of AIDS Immunology, Chinese Academy of Medical Sciences, Shenyang, China, [4] Collaborative Innovation Center for Diagnosis and Treatment of Infectious Diseases, Hangzhou, China

***Correspondence:**
Hong Shang
hongshang100@hotmail.com
Zi-Ning Zhang
zi_ning101@hotmail.com

Human immunodeficiency virus (HIV)-infected long-term non-progressors (LTNPs) are of particular importance because of their unique disease progression characteristics. Defined by the maintenance of normal CD4$^+$T cells after more than 8 years of infection, these LTNPs are heterogeneous. Some LTNPs exhibit ongoing viral production, while others do not and are able to control viral production. The underlying basis for this heterogeneity has not been clearly elucidated. In this study, the miRNA expression profiles of LTNPs were assessed. The levels of microRNA-19b (miR-19b) were found to be significantly increased in peripheral blood mononuclear cells of LTNPs with lower rather than higher viral load. We made clear that miR-19b may regulate CD8$^+$T cell functions in HIV infection, which has not been addressed before. Overexpression of miR-19b promoted CD8$^+$T cell proliferation, as well as interferon-γ and granzyme B expression, while inhibiting CD8$^+$T cells apoptosis induced by anti-CD3/CD28 stimulation. The target of miR-19b was found to be the "phosphatase and tensin homolog", which regulates CD8$^+$T cells function during HIV infections. Furthermore, we found that miR-19b can directly inhibit viral production in *in-vitro* HIV infected T cells. These results highlight the importance of miR-19b to control viral levels, which facilitate an understanding of human immunodeficiency virus pathogenesis and provide potential targets for improved immune intervention.

Keywords: CD8$^+$T cells, long-term non-progressors, microRNA-19b, phosphatase and tensin homolog, HIV

INTRODUCTION

Human immunodeficiency virus (HIV) infected patients with atypical disease progression are of particular importance because they can provide important information regarding HIV pathogenesis and therapy. The first evidence of long-term non-progressors (LTNPs) was reported in 1993, showing that 15% of individuals infected with HIV maintain a CD4 count >500 cells/μl (1, 2).

In 2005, study showed that ~1/300 HIV-infected patients had undetectable plasma HIV RNA loads without antiretroviral therapy (ART) (3). Described as "Elite Controllers" (ECs) in 2007, these patients maintained HIV RNA levels below 50 copies/ml for at least 1 year in the absence of ART (4–8). Although there is overlap between LTNPs and ECs, they are not identical. Most ECs exhibit minimal reductions in CD4$^+$ T cells over time, although reductions are observed in some ECs. Furthermore, some LTNPs have ongoing viral production, while others do not (3, 5, 7, 9–11). Transcriptomic analysis showed that ECs with higher CD4$^+$T cell numbers were indistinguishable from HIV-1-negative individuals. In contrast, ECs with lower CD4$^+$ T cell numbers were similar to ART-treated patients, but different from HIV-1-negative individuals (12). Alterations in T cell homeostasis predict the loss of immunological control in ECs (13)4. However, viral control differs among LTNPs and the reason for this difference is currently unknown. LTNPs maintaining high viral loads are prone to long-term disease progression, with reduced life expectancy compared to HIV negative individuals (14, 15). Analysis of the underlying reason for the differing levels of viral control in LTNPs may facilitate an understanding of HIV pathogenesis and may provide for new approaches to immune intervention.

The level of virus control is affected by immunologic and virologic factors. MicroRNAs (miRNAs) may be a potential mechanistic factor involved in this process. It has been shown that miRNAs play important roles in the regulation of immune responses and viral production. In HIV infection, miRNAs can directly modulate viral production by targeting the HIV-1 genome or by indirectly modulating cellular genes that influence viral propagation (16–20). Dramatic advances have been made in understanding how miRNAs regulate the development and function of immune cells (21, 22), including CD8$^+$T cells which are key players in the antiviral immune response (23, 24). It is established that miRNAs modulate the expression of numerous regulatory proteins required for the development, differentiation, and function of CD8$^+$T cells (25). Studies have shown that, in HIV infection, miRNAs modulate the expression of key markers associated with T cell exhaustion or dysfunction, such as interleukin 10 and B lymphocyte-induced maturation protein-1 (26). We postulated that differential miRNA profiles may contribute to the divergent control of viral load in LTNPs by affecting viral production and/or CD8$^+$T cell function. Although previous studies have identified miRNA profiles in HIV-infected ECs and LTNPs (16, 27–30), the role of miRNAs in the differential control of viral load in LTNPs has not been addressed.

In this study, miRNA expression profiles of LTNPs were assessed. The expression of miR-19b was found to be significantly increased in the peripheral blood mononuclear cells (PBMCs) of LTNPs with low (LTNP-Ls) compared to high levels (LTNP-Hs) of virus production. In addition, miR-19b promoted proliferation, and expression of interferon gamma (IFN-γ) and granzyme B, while inhibiting CD8$^+$T apoptosis induced by anti-CD3/CD28 stimulation. The phosphatase and tensin homolog (PTEN) is a target of miR-19b regulating CD8$^+$T cell function in HIV infection. Furthermore, we found that miR-19b directly inhibits viral production in HIV-infected T cells *in vitro*. Our results revealed a previously unknown mechanism of sustained viral control by miR-19b in a subtype of LTNPs, suggesting that miR-19b may be a novel target for immune intervention in HIV infection.

MATERIALS AND METHODS

Study Population

In total, samples obtained from 27 LTNPs, six typical progressors (TPs), and four healthy controls (HCs) were analyzed. The LTNPs were HIV positive patients who maintained normal CD4$^+$ T cell counts (CD4 >500 cells/μl) for >10 years (mean ± SD: 14.72 ± 1.79 years at the time of sample collection) without receiving ART (**Supplemental Table 1**). The TPs were ART naive HIV positive patients who progressed to CD4 counts <500 cells/μl at 2.53 ± 0.95 years (**Supplemental Table 2**). The initial 347-miRNA array was performed in a training cohort, including nine LTNPs (age, mean ± SD: 41 ± 6 years; gender, eight males and one female), six TPs (age, mean ± SD: 30 ± 15 years; gender, six males) and four HCs (age, mean ± SD: 37 ± 6 years; gender, four males). From the training cohort, miRNAs differentially expressed in LTNPs with differing viral loads were detected in a subsequent validation group that included 18 LTNPs. Ethical approval was obtained from the First Hospital of China Medical University, Shenyang, China and written informed consent was provided by all participants.

miRNA Array Analysis

Quantitative real-time polymerase chain reaction (qRT-PCR)-based high-throughput miRNA profiling was performed at QuantoBio Biotechnology Co. Ltd. (Beijing, China). Briefly, total RNA extracted from peripheral blood mononuclear cells (PBMCs) was isolated using TRIzol® (Invitrogen, Carlsbad, USA). *Escherichia coli* poly (A) polymerase was used to add adenines to the 3′ end of RNA molecules lacking a poly (A) tail. After oligo dT annealing, a universal tag was attached to the 3′ end of cDNAs during cDNA synthesis using retrotranscriptase Superscript III (Invitrogen). With this universal tag, a SYBR®-based qRT-PCR was performed using miRNA-specific forward primers and a reverse universal primer mix. Of note, U1 and U6 were used in the training cohort for normalization. The variation of change in the threshold cycle (CT, target-CT, and control) was evaluated and used as a relative qualitative value.

RT-PCR Quantification of miRNA and mRNA

We extracted miRNAs from cells using the miRNeasy Micro kit (Qiagen, Hilden, Germany). The RNA was reverse transcribed using a Primpscript® RT reagent kit (TAKARA, Dalian, China) according to the instructions provided by the manufacturer. Subsequently, RT-PCR was performed using a SYBR® Premix Ex Taq™ II (TAKARA). The levels of miRNA were normalized to the U6 small nucleolar RNA and quantified through the relative quantification method ($2^{-\Delta\Delta Ct}$), as previously described (31). Cellular total mRNA was isolated using the RNeasy Micro kit (Qiagen). The cDNA was generated using the Primpscript® RT reagent kit (TAKARA). The levels of mRNA were quantified through the SYBR® Premix Ex Taq™ II (TAKARA), normalized to GAPDH transcripts, and expressed using the relative quantification method ($2^{-\Delta\Delta Ct}$). All primer sequences for the quantification of miRNA and mRNA are listed in **Supplemental Table 3**.

Isolation of Cells

PBMCs were obtained by Ficoll–Hypaque density gradient centrifugation. If indicated, $CD8^+$ or $CD4^+$ T cells were further purified from isolated PBMCs by negative selection with magnetic beads using a $CD8^+$ or $CD4^+$ T cell Enrichment Kit (Cell purity >95%, Stem Cell Technologies, Vancouver, Canada). The following antibodies were used for immunostaining to isolate cell subtypes: FITC-CD3, APC-cy7-CD8, APC-CD4, PE-cy7-CD14 and 7-AAD (Biolegend, San Diego, CA, USA). $CD4^+$ T cells ($CD3^+CD4^+$), $CD8^+$ T cells ($CD3^+CD8^+$), and monocytes ($CD3^-CD14^+$) were selected from 7-AAD-negative live PBMCs using a FACSAria™ flow cytometer (BD Biosciences, Franklin Lake, NJ, USA).

Cell Culture

The Jurkat human leukemia T cells, Clone-X cells, and primary cells were maintained in RPMI1640 media (HyClone, Logan, UT, USA) supplemented with 10% fetal bovine serum and 1% penicillin-streptomycin. The 293T cells were maintained in DMEM media (HyClone) supplemented with 10% fetal bovine serum and 1% penicillin-streptomycin.

Transfection

Transfection of miRNAs to cell lines was achieved using Lipofectamine® 2000 (Invitrogen). Briefly, 20 μM miR-19b mimics or controls (GenePharma, Shanghai, China) were transfected to 293T cells, Jurkat cells, or Clone-X cells according to the protocol provided by the manufacturer. In primary cells, Lipofectamine® RNAiMAX (Invitrogen) was used for the transfection according to the protocol provided by the manufacturer. Briefly, 20 μM miR-19b mimics, inhibitors (GenePharma), or controls were transfected to isolated $CD8^+$T or $CD4^+$T cell-depleted PBMCs. In addition, isolated primary $CD4^+$ T cells from healthy controls were transfected with 20 μM miR-19b mimics or controls. The forced reduction of phosphatase and tensin homolog (PTEN) was achieved by introducing 20 μM PTEN siRNA (Invitrogen) to isolated $CD8^+$T cells. The siRNA control used in this experiment was non-specific Stealth RNAi® Negative Control Duplexes. The sequences of the mimics and inhibitors are listed in **Supplemental Table 3**.

Proliferation Assays

After transfection (24 h), Jurkat cells and primary $CD8^+$T cells were labeled with Cell Trace™ Violet (Thermo Fisher Scientific, Waltham, USA) for 15 min at 37°C according to the instructions provided by the manufacturer, washed with complete medium, and cultured (1×10^6 cells/ml). Primary $CD8^+$T cells were cultured in the presence of anti-CD3/CD28 (3 μg/ml; Gibco, New York, NY, USA). After incubation for 5 days, the dividing cells were analyzed using a BD LSR II flow cytometer and the FlowJo software.

Detection of Apoptosis

After transfection (72 h), Jurkat cells were stained with PE-conjugated anti-Annexin V and 7-AAD (Biolegend). After transfection (24 h), primary $CD8^+$T cells were stimulated using anti-CD3/CD28 (3 μg/ml). After stimulation (48 h), $CD8^+$T cells were stained with PE-cy7-conjugated anti-CD3, APC-cy7-conjugated anti-CD8, PE-conjugated anti-Annexin V, and 7-AAD (Biolegend). The cells were analyzed using a BD LSR II flow cytometer and the FlowJo software.

Cell Cycle Assay

Cell cycle phases were determined using the BD Cycletest™ Plus DNA Reagent Kit (BD Biosciences) according to the instructions provided by the manufacturer. In brief, Jurkat cells were cultured for 72 h after transfection. After transfection (24 h), primary $CD8^+$T cells were cultured for 48 h under stimulation using anti-CD3/CD28 (3 μg/ml). The distribution of DNA content was determined using a BD LSR II flow cytometer and analyzed using the FlowJo software.

Intracellular Staining of IFN-γ and Granzyme B

After transfection (24 h), primary $CD8^+$T cells were stimulated using anti-CD3/CD28 (3 μg/ml) for 24 h. The protein transport inhibitor (GolgiStop; 1 μl/ml, BD Biosciences) was added to the culture for the last 6 h. The cells were stained with PE-cy7-conjugated anti-CD3 and APC-cy7-conjugated anti-CD8 (Biolegend). Subsequently, intracellular staining was performed by incubating the cells in 1X Perm/Wash Buffer for 15 min in the dark, followed by incubation with APC-conjugated anti-IFN-γ and FITC-conjugated anti-granzyme B for 30 min at 4°C. After staining, the cells were fixed in 1% formaldehyde. The intracellular expression of IFN-γ and granzyme B was determined using a BD LSR II flow cytometer and data were analyzed using the FlowJo software.

IFN-γ ELISpot Assay

$CD4^+$ T cells were depleted from PBMCs using anti-CD4 MAb-coated magnetic beads (Biolegend) as described in the instructions provided by the manufacturer. The Human IFN-γ ELISpot Kit (Mabtech, Nacka, Sweden) was used to detect the secretion of IFN-γ according to the instruction manual. After transfection (24 h), 2×10^5 $CD4^+$ T cell-depleted PBMCs were added per well (in duplicates) in a volume of 200 μl. The HIV-1 gag peptide pools (10 μg/ml, Sigma) were added for 20 h. Anti-CD3/CD28 (3 μg/ml) were used as a positive control, and negative controls consisted of cells without stimuli. The number of IFN-γ-secreting cells was calculated by subtracting the negative control (medium only) values. A positive response was defined as >50 spot-forming units/10^6 PBMC.

In-vitro Infection

Viral particles were produced by transfecting 293T cells with HIV-1 pNL4-3 plasmids and vesicular stomatitis virus glycoprotein (VSV-G) plasmids. Transfection of miR-19b mimics, pNL4-3 plasmids, and VSV-G plasmids into 293T cells was performed to detect the effects of miR-19 on HIV production. The levels of p24 in the supernatants were measured by ELISA (Biomedical Engineering Center of Hebei Medical University, Hebei, China) 2 days later. For the infection of Clone-X cells, the cells were transfected with miR-19b mimics for 24 h and subsequently infected with VSV-G pseudotyped HIV-1 (NL4-3) virus. GFP^{+} cells were detected by flow cytometry 48 h after infection.

Replication-competent HIV-1 isolate was used to test the effects of miR-19b in primary $CD4^{+}$ T cells. Isolated primary $CD4^{+}$ T cells from healthy controls were transfected with miR-19b mimics or controls. After transfection (24 h), the cells were stimulated using anti-CD3/CD28 (3 μg/ml). A cryopreserved primary HIV-1 isolate—obtained by a co-culture using mixed PBMCs from an HIV-1-infected patient and a healthy donor—was thawed and added to the cells. The supernatant was collected after 3 days of infection and the levels of p24 in the supernatants were measured by ELISA.

Statistical Analysis

Principal component analysis (PCA) was used (Origin 9.1 software) to analyze the distribution of miRNAs in HIV-infected patients with differing disease progression. The non-parametric Mann–Whitney test was used to determine differences between LTNPs with a relatively high viral load (>1,000 copies/ml) (LTNP-Hs) and LTNPs with relative control of viral load (<1,000 copies/ml) (LTNP-Ls). A paired *t*-test was used to analyze differences in $CD8^{+}$T cell function between groups. Data analysis was performed using the SPSS 21.0 and GraphPad Prism Version 5.0 software packages. A $P < 0.05$ was considered statistically significant.

RESULTS

miRNA Profiles Distinguish LTNPs With Different Virus Levels

A training cohort was formed including nine LTNPs, six TPs, and four HCs to identify the miRNA profiles of LTNPs. Using qRT-PCR-based arrays, the expression levels of 347 miRNAs were quantified. Based on an unsupervised PCA of all array data, the six TPs, nine LTNPs and four HCs were segregated into two groups (**Figure 1A**). All the HCs were clustered in one group. Most of the TPs were clustered in the other group, except one TP with a relatively low viral load (<1,000 copies/ml), indicating that HIV infection alters miRNAs. This finding was consistent with those reported in previous studies (30, 32, 33). Interestingly, the nine LTNPs were divided into two groups, one of which was very close to the TPs (Group A, $n = 6$) and another that was intertwined with the HCs (Group B, $n = 3$) (**Figure 1A**). We subsequently sought to identify differences between the two groups of LTNPs. By comparison of clinical characteristics (i.e., age, number of $CD4^{+}$T cells, and viral loads), we found that viral load was the only significantly different parameter between the two groups of LTNPs ($P = 0.024$, **Figure 1B**). Six LTNPs in Group A, whose miRNA profiles were similar to those of TPs, had a relatively high level of viral load (>1,000 copies/ml, hereinafter referred to as "LTNP-Hs"). Three LTNPs in Group B, whose miRNA profiles were similar to those of HCs, had relative control of viral load (VL < 1,000 copies/ml, hereinafter referred to as "LTNP-Ls," **Supplemental Table 1**). The results of the unsupervised PCA suggest that the expression of miRNAs can distinguish LTNP-Hs and LTNP-Ls, and may account for the differing viral loads observed in LTNPs.

Expression of miR-19b Is High in LTNP-Ls in Comparison With That in LTNP-Hs

Subsequently, the differential expression of miRNAs in LTNP-Hs and LTNP-Ls was assessed. The miRNAs were determined to be significantly differentially expressed in LTNP-Hs and LTNP-Ls with a Benjamini–Hochberg false discovery rate-adjusted $P < 0.05$. We found that 78 miRNAs were differentially expressed with >2-fold change between the three LTNP-Ls and six LTNP-Hs in the training cohort (adj. $P < 0.05$, **Supplemental Table 4**). Among those, 55 miRNAs were upregulated and 23 were downregulated in LTNP-Ls compared with that in LTNP-Hs. Using an unsupervised clustering method, 78 miRNAs accurately distinguished and clustered LTNP-Hs and LTNP-Ls (**Figure 2A**). A total of 75 miRNAs with differential expression levels between LTNP-Hs or LTNP-Ls and HCs or TPs ($P < 0.05$) were excluded to identify miRNAs that can uniquely differentiate LTNP-Hs from LTNP-Ls (**Figure 2B; Supplemental Table 4**). This exclusion was carried out because these miRNAs may reflect differences caused by HIV infection or the stages of infection. Only three miRNAs which were differentially expressed between LTNP-Hs and LTNP-Ls in the training cohort were selected, including miR-15a ($P = 0.024$), miR-19b ($P = 0.048$), and miR-33 ($P = 0.024$, **Figure 2C**).

The expression levels of these three miRNAs were assessed in a subsequent validation group, including ten LTNP-Hs and eight LTNP-Ls (**Supplemental Table 1**). In the validation cohort, only miR-19b was verified to be highly expressed in LTNP-Ls compared with LTNP-Hs ($P = 0.034$, **Figures 2D–F**). Subsequently, $CD8^{+}$, $CD4^{+}$ T cells, and monocytes from LTNPs were sorted to identify the cell subtypes in which the expression of miR-19b was altered. We found that the expression of miR-19b decreased in $CD4^{+}$T cells and $CD8^{+}$ T cells in LTNP-Hs ($n = 10$) compared with that observed in LTNP-Ls ($n = 9$) ($P = 0.041$, **Figure 2G**; $P = 0.028$, **Figure 2H**). There were no differences observed in the expression of miR-19b in monocytes between the two groups (data not shown).

miR-19b Promotes Proliferation and Expression IFN-γ, and Inhibits the Apoptosis of Primary $CD8^{+}$T Cells

As the most important immune effector cell population, $CD8^{+}$T cells play a key role in anti-HIV immune responses. We hypothesized that miR-19b may contribute to the control of the virus in LTNP-Ls by regulating $CD8^{+}$T cell function. This was the first study addressing this question. Initially, we overexpressed miR-19b in Jurkat cells by transfection with miRNA mimics to investigate the effect of miR-19b on lymphocyte proliferation and apoptosis. After transfection (48 h), miR-19b was highly expressed (**Supplemental Figure 1**). After 5 days, the proliferation of miR-19b-overexpressing cells

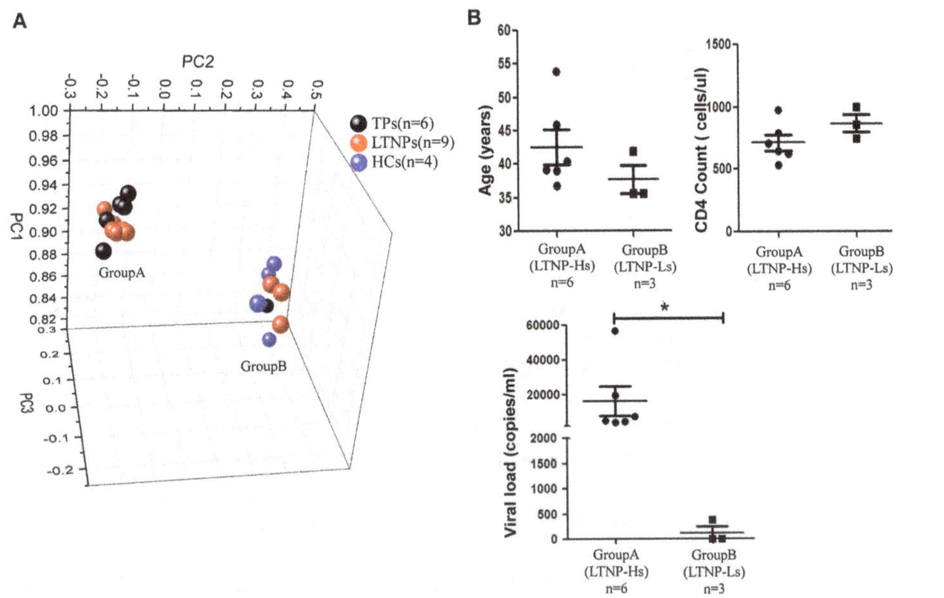

FIGURE 1 | miRNA profiles distinguish LTNPs with different levels of virus. **(A)** Principal component analysis (PCA) plot of miRNA expression data from LTNPs, TPs, and HCs in the training cohort. Nine LTNPs were divided into two groups, one of which was very close to the TPs (Group A, $n = 6$) and another that was intertwined with the HCs (Group B, $n = 3$). **(B)** Comparison of age, CD4 counts, and viral load between Group A and Group B of LTNPs. $^{*}P < 0.05$.

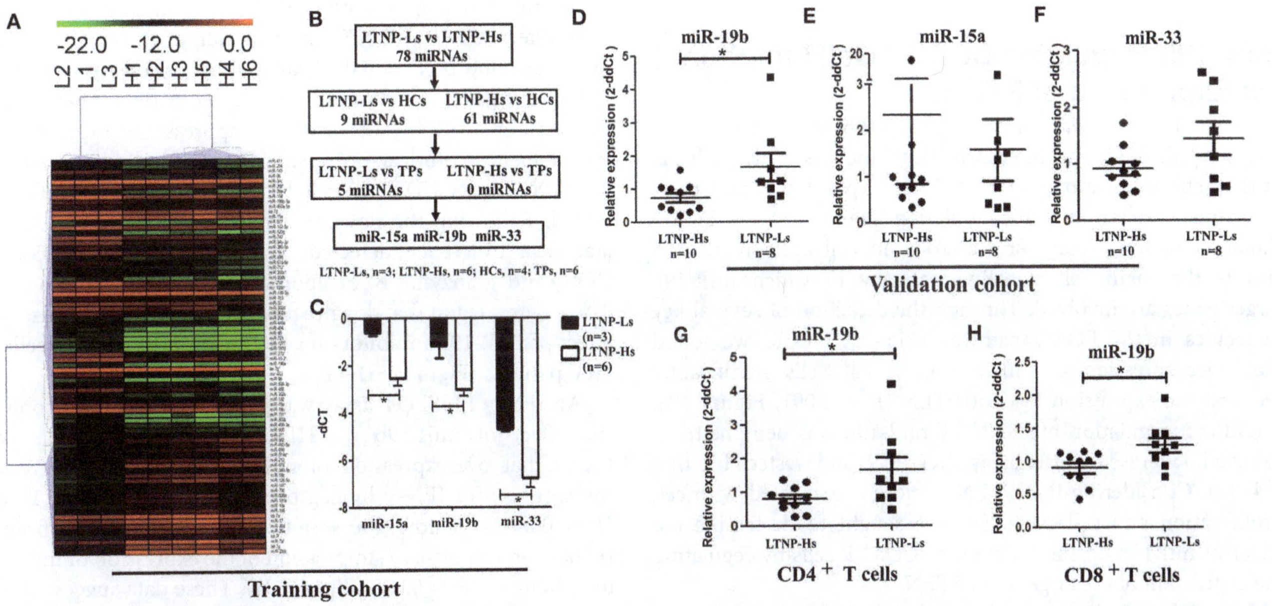

FIGURE 2 | Expression of miR-19b is high in LTNP-Ls compared with that observed in LTNP-Hs. **(A)** Heatmap demonstrating 78 miRNAs differentially expressed between LTNP-Hs ($n = 6$) and LTNP-Ls ($n = 3$) in the training cohort (Benjamini–Hochberg false discovery rate-adjusted $P < 0.05$ and fold change >2). Hierarchical clustering of change in the threshold cycle (ΔCT) was performed using the complete linkage method and Pearson correlation coefficient. **(B)** The protocol for the selection of candidate miRNA from the training cohort. Among the 78 miRNAs differentially expressed between LTNP-Hs ($n = 6$) and LTNP-Ls ($n = 3$), 70 miRNAs differentially expressed between LTNPs and HCs ($P < 0.05$) were excluded. Subsequently, five differentially expressed miRNAs between LTNPs and TPs were excluded. Three candidate miRNAs, namely miR-15a, miR-19b, and miR-33 were selected. **(C)** Comparison of the three candidate miRNAs between LTNP-Ls ($n = 3$) and LTNP-Hs ($n = 6$) in the training cohort. **(D,F)** Relative expression of miR-19b **(D)**, miR-15a **(E)** and miR-33 **(F)** in PBMCs obtained from LTNP-Ls ($n = 8$) and LTNP-Hs ($n = 10$) in the subsequent validation group. **(G,H)** $CD4^{+}$ and $CD8^{+}$T cells from LTNPs were sorted through flow cytometry. The expression of miR19b in $CD4^{+}$ **(G)** and $CD8^{+}$ T **(H)** cells was compared between LTNP-Ls ($n = 9$, one from training cohort, eight from validation cohort) and LTNP-Hs ($n = 10$, two from training cohort, eight from validation cohort) using qRT-PCR. $^{*}P < 0.05$.

was significantly increased compared with that observed in the control group, suggesting that miR-19b promotes cell proliferation ($P = 0.013$, **Figure 3A**). Overexpression of miR-19b significantly accelerated the cell cycle ($P = 0.033$, **Figure 3B**). Furthermore, the percentage of Annexin V^+ 7-AAD^- apoptotic cells was lower following the overexpression of miR-19b ($P = 0.005$, **Figure 3C**). These data indicate that miR-19b promotes proliferation and inhibits apoptosis of T cell lines.

We subsequently assessed the role of miR-19b in regulating the function of primary $CD8^+$T cells by transfection of miR-19b mimics into $CD8^+$T cells obtained from HCs. We found that overexpression of miR-19b significantly promoted the proliferation of $CD8^+$T cells after anti-CD3/CD28 stimulation ($P = 0.010$, **Figure 3D**). Similarly, forced expression of miR-19b significantly inhibited apoptosis of $CD8^+$T cells after stimulation of the anti-CD3/CD28 ($P = 0.009$, **Figure 3E**). $CD8^+$T cells were sorted using magnetic beads to study the effect of miR-19b on the cytotoxic function of $CD8^+$T cells. Overexpression of miR-19b in $CD8^+$T cells significantly increased the intracellular levels of IFN-γ and granzyme B after stimulation of the anti-CD3/CD28 ($P = 0.006$, **Figure 3F**; $P = 0.002$, **Figure 3G**, respectively). These results demonstrate that miR-19b promotes cell proliferation, and the expression of IFN-γ and granzyme B in $CD8^+$T cells. Moreover, it inhibits the apoptosis of $CD8^+$T cells after stimulation of the anti-CD3/CD28.

miR-19b Regulates $CD8^+$ T Cell Function via Expression of PTEN

Cell signaling pathways involving miR-19b target genes were assessed through a bioinformatics analysis (http://diana.imis.athena-innovation.gr/) to further explore the molecular mechanistic basis of miR-19b regulation (**Figure 4A**). The FOXO signaling pathway plays critical roles in cell cycle regulation and is the main cell signaling pathway in which miR-19b target genes are involved. Through the detection of several key molecules in the FOXO pathway using qRT-PCR, we found that overexpression of miR-19b in Jurkat cells significantly reduced the expression level of PTEN ($P < 0.001$, **Figure 4B**). The direct regulation of PTEN by miR-19b was demonstrated using a Luciferase reporter assay, qRT-PCR, and western blotting (34–38). Considering that PTEN is closely associated with cell proliferation and cell cycle (39), we sought to determine the effect of miR19b on the function of $CD8^+$T cells by regulating the expression of the target gene PTEN.

We reduced the expression of PTEN in primary HCs $CD8^+$T cells using specific siRNAs (**Supplemental Figure 1**). Cell proliferation was promoted and apoptosis was inhibited via the knockdown of PTEN in comparison with the negative control group ($P = 0.040$ **Figure 4C**; $P = 0.047$, **Figure 4D**, respectively). Moreover, the secretion of granzyme B by $CD8^+$ T cells was significantly increased ($P = 0.006$, **Figure 4E**) and that of IFN-γ showed an increasing trend ($P = 0.094$, **Figure 4F**) after stimulation of the anti-CD3/CD28, in response to the suppression of PTEN. These findings demonstrate that inhibition of PTEN, which is a potential target of miR-19b, exerts similar effects on $CD8^+$T cell function to those observed following the overexpression of miR-19b.

miR-19b Regulates the Function of $CD8^+$ T Cells From HIV-Infected Patients

The function of miR-19b in $CD8^+$T cells from 7 HIV-infected patients (**Supplemental Table 5**) was also studied. Primary $CD8^+$T cells from HIV-infected patients were sorted. Following the overexpression of miR-19b (**Supplemental Figure 1**), $CD8^+$T cells showed a significant increase in proliferation ($P = 0.010$), and secretion of IFN-γ ($P = 0.010$) and granzyme B ($P = 0.003$) after stimulation of the anti-CD3/CD28 (**Figure 5A**). Apoptosis of $CD8^+$T cells was significantly reduced in comparison with the controls ($P = 0.040$, **Figure 5A**). Furthermore, the expression of miR-19b was inhibited by transfection of miR-19b inhibitors into $CD8^+$ T cells from HIV patients (**Supplemental Figure 1**). Contrary to the miRNA overexpression results, the proliferation of $CD8^+$ T cells was reduced ($P = 0.043$, **Figure 5B**), the secretions of IFN-γ ($P = 0.023$) and granzyme B ($P = 0.049$) were reduced, and the apoptosis of $CD8^+$T cells was increased ($P = 0.035$, **Figure 5B**).

Subsequently, the expression of PTEN in primary $CD8^+$T cells was inhibited using siRNA to verify that PTEN was a miR-19b target gene involved in the regulation of $CD8^+$T cell function in HIV infection. Consistent with the findings reported in healthy patients, inhibition of PTEN resulted in an increase in proliferation ($P = 0.005$) and secretion of IFN-γ ($P < 0.001$) and granzyme B ($P = 0.012$), as well as a decrease in $CD8^+$T cell apoptosis ($P = 0.006$) in HIV-infected patients (**Figure 5C**). Furthermore, siRNA was used to suppress the expression of PTEN in miR-19b-low-expressing $CD8^+$ T cells to verify that miR-19b affects $CD8^+$ T cell function through regulation of PTEN. Following the downregulation of PTEN, there was no statistical difference detected in proliferation, expression of IFN-γ and granzyme B, or apoptosis compared with controls. These data suggest that downregulation of PTEN antagonizes the effect of miR-19b inhibitors on the function of $CD8^+$T cells in HIV patients (**Figures 5D–G**).

An IFN-γ ELISPOT assay was performed to further confirm the effect of miR-19b on HIV specific $CD8^+$T cells. We found that overexpression of miR-19b significantly increased the secretion of IFN-γ by gag peptide-stimulated $CD8^+$T cells ($P = 0.041$). Of note, the secretion of IFN-γ was significantly reduced in response to suppression of the expression of miR-19b by inhibitors ($P = 0.020$, **Figure 5H**). These data suggested that miR-19b augments the function of HIV specific $CD8^+$T cells.

miR-19b Inhibits Viral Replication in *in-vitro* HIV-Infected T Cells

Lastly, we hypothesized that miR-19b may play a role in the direct inhibition of HIV replication, besides its regulation of $CD8^+$T cells. The levels of miR-19b in the plasma have been reported to be associated with $CD4^+$ T cell counts, indicating that miR-19b may be a biomarker for the monitoring of the HIV immune status (40). However, its direct effects on HIV viral production

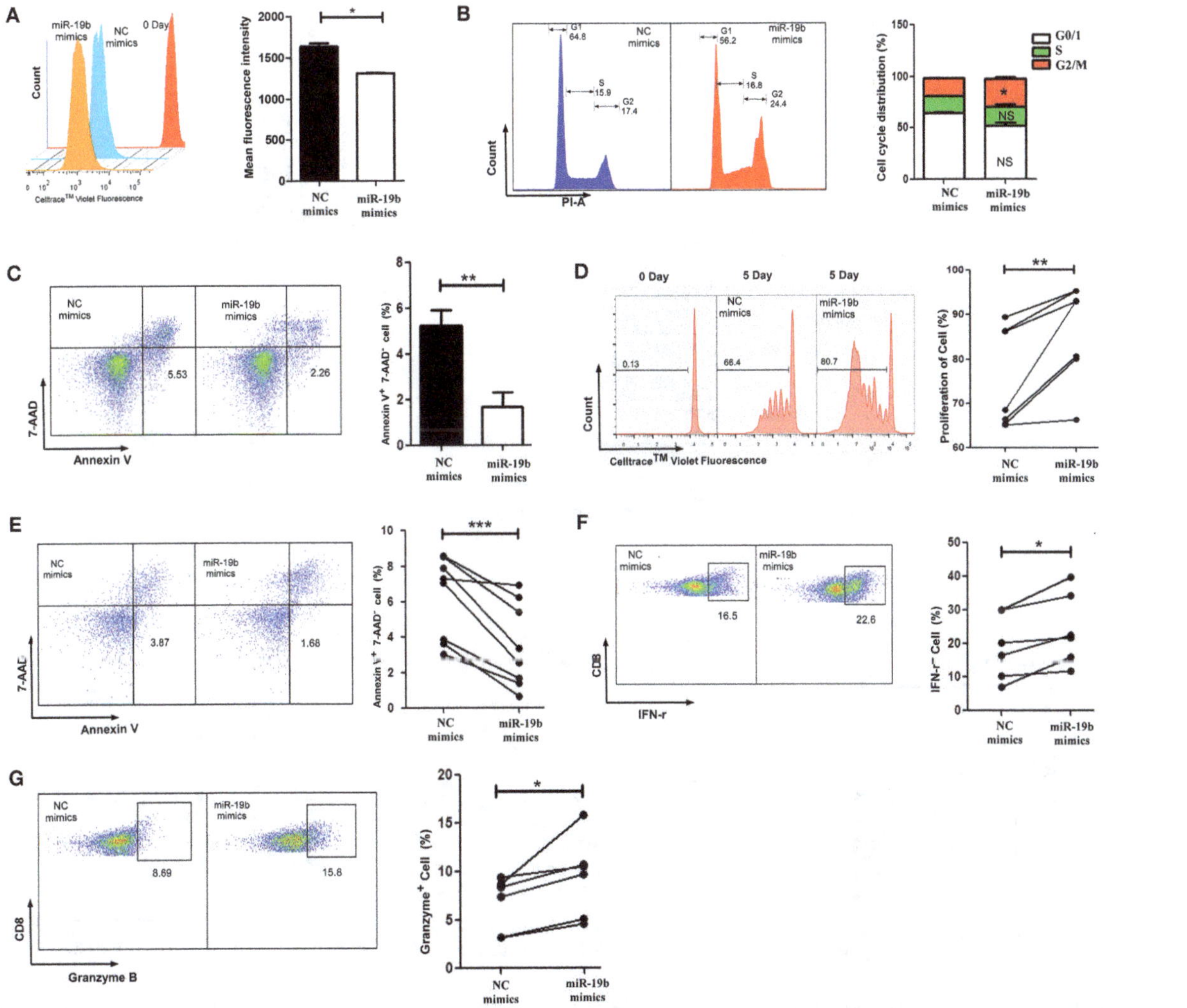

FIGURE 3 | Overexpression of miR-19b regulates the function of $CD8^+$ T cells from healthy controls. Jurkat cells were transfected with miR-19b mimics using Lipofectamine® 2000. **(A)** After transfection (24 h), Jurkat cells were labeled with Cell Trace^{TM} Violet. After incubation for 5 days, the dividing cells were analyzed. **(B)** After transfection (72 h), the cell cycle of Jurkat cells was determined. **(C)** After transfection (72 h), Jurkat cells were stained with Annexin V and 7-AAD and the apoptosis of the cells was determined. **(D–G)** $CD8^+$ T cells from healthy controls were sorted and transfected with miR-19b mimics or controls using Lipofectamine® RNAiMAX. **(D)** After transfection (24 h), $CD8^+$T cells were labeled with Cell Trace^{TM} Violet and stimulated with anti-CD3/CD28 (3 μg/ml) for 5 days, the proliferation of $CD8^+$T cells was determined. **(E)** After transfection (24 h), $CD8^+$T cells were stimulated using anti-CD3/CD28 (3 μg/ml) for 48 h and the rate of apoptosis were determined. **(F,G)** After transfection (24 h), $CD8^+$ T cells were stimulated using anti-CD3/CD28 (3 μg/ml) for 24 h and expression of intracellular IFN-γ **(F)** and granzyme B **(G)** was determined. In each part, representative flow cytometry data and comparisons of the parameters between miR-19b-overexpressing cells and controls are shown. $n = 7$ for each group in **(D)**, $n = 8$ for each group in **(E)**, $n = 6$ for each group in **(F,G)**. $^*P < 0.05$. $^{**}P < 0.01$, $^{***}P < 0.001$, respectively.

have not been reported. We found that overexpression of miR-19b by mimics reduced the production of HIV. Following the co-transfection of miR-19b mimics and the pNL4-3 plasmid into 293T cells, the expression level of P24 in supernatants was lower than that in the control group after 48 h of culture ($P = 0.040$, **Figure 6A**). Furthermore, Clone-X cells were infected with the same titer of HIV pseudovirus, the percentage of HIV-positive cells overexpressing miR-19b was lower compared with that in the control group ($P = 0.007$, **Figure 6B**). Finally, we infected primary $CD4^+$ T cells from normal controls using replication-competent HIV-1 virus isolates and found that overexpression of miR-19b inhibited the production of HIV ($P = 0.001$, **Figure 6C**). These data demonstrated that, besides its role in the regulation of $CD8^+$T cells, miR-19b inhibits viral production, leading to lower viral levels.

DISCUSSION

LTNPs are defined by the maintenance of normal $CD4^+$T cells counts for more than 8 years after infection. However, LTNPs exhibit heterogeneity in their viral loads. LTNPs maintaining high viral loads are prone to long-term progression, with reduced overall life expectancy vs. healthy individuals. However, the factors involved in the differential control of viral levels in LTNPs

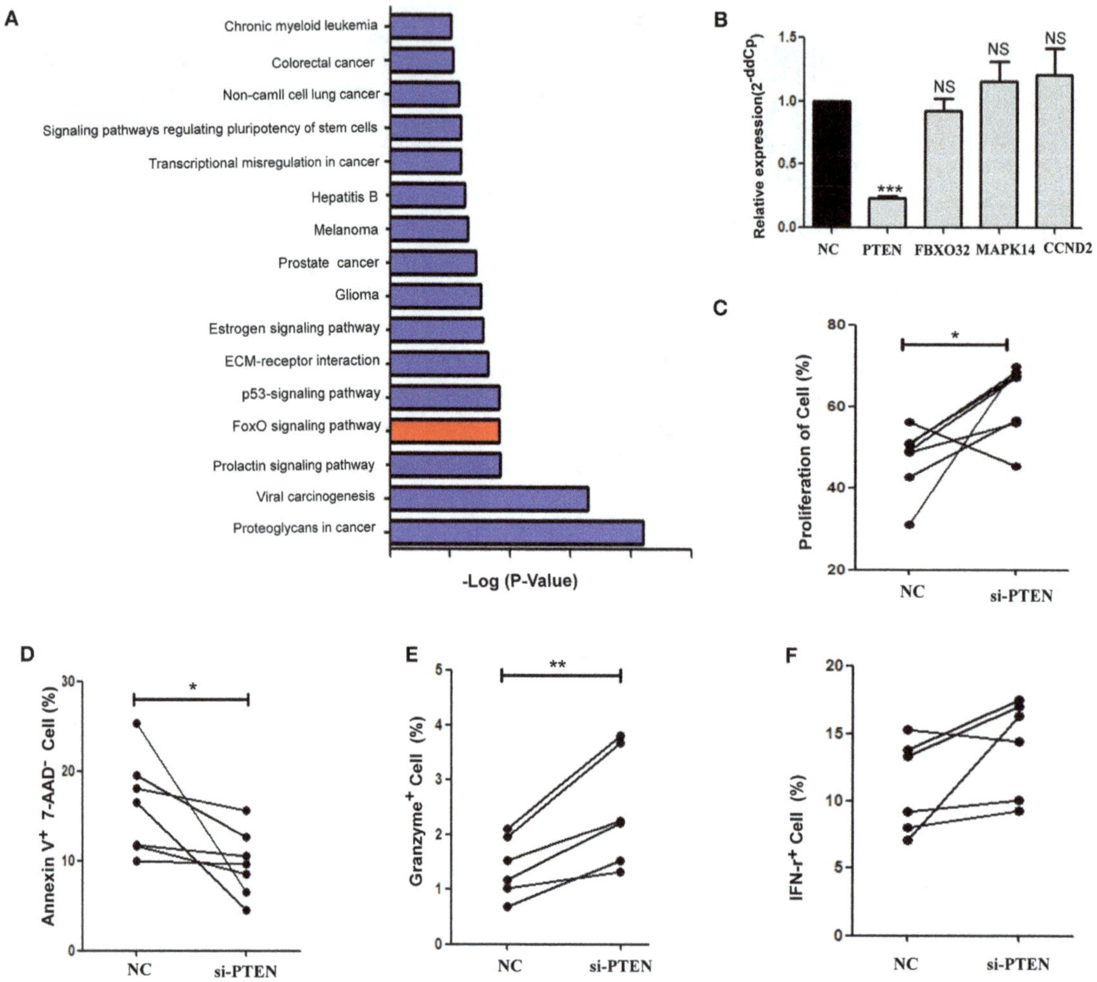

FIGURE 4 | PTEN is a potential target of miR-19b. **(A)** Cell signaling pathways involving miR-19b target genes were assessed through a bioinformatics analysis (http://diana.imis.athena-innovation.gr/). The FOXO signaling pathway (Red) is a major cellular signaling pathway playing a key role in cell cycle regulation. **(B)** The expression of miR-19b was enhanced by mimics in Jurkat cells. Four genes in the FOXO pathway were detected through qRT-PCR. **(C–F)** The expression of PTEN was inhibited by introducing 20 μM PTEN siRNA to isolated CD8$^+$T cells. **(C)** After transfection (24 h), CD8$^+$T cells were labeled with Cell Trace^{TM} Violet and stimulated using anti-CD3/CD28 (3 μg/ml) for 5 days. The proliferation of CD8$^+$T cells was determined. **(D)** After transfection (24 h), CD8$^+$ T cells were stimulated using anti-CD3/CD28 (3 μg/ml) for 48 h and the rate of apoptosis of CD8$^+$ T cells was determined. **(E,F)** After transfection (24 h), CD8$^+$ T cells were stimulated using anti-CD3/CD28 (3 μg/ml) for 24 h and the intracellular expression of IFN-γ **(E)** and granzyme B **(F)** was determined. $n = 6$ for each group in **(C)**, $n = 7$ for each group in **(D)**, $n = 6$ for each group in **(E,F)**. $^*P < 0.05$. $^{**}P < 0.01$. $^{***}P < 0.001$, respectively.

have not been identified. In this study, we found that miR-19b is highly expressed in LTNP-Ls vs. LTNP-Hs. It was shown that miR-19b influences the low viral load of LTNP-Ls by promoting the function of CD8$^+$T cells in HIV infection and directly inhibiting viral production of HIV.

Factors contributing to the different levels of CD4$^+$T cells in ECs have already been studied (12, 13). However, thus far, the underlying mechanistic basis for the differing levels of viral control in LTNPs has not been investigated. Considering the important role of miRNAs in regulating immune responses and viral replication, we performed a miRNA profiling analysis of HIV-infected individuals. The miRNA profiles distinguished LTNPs with differing viral loads. LTNPs whose miRNA profiles were similar to those of TPs exhibited a relatively high viral load. In contrast, LTNPs with miRNA profiles similar to those of HCs showed relatively well-controlled viral loads. Based on the results of the miRNA array analysis and subsequent validation, miR-19b was verified to be highly expressed in LTNP-Ls compared with LTNP-Hs. In HIV infection, plasma miR-19b was associated with CD4$^+$ T cell counts and may be a useful biomarker for monitoring the HIV immune status (40). Our study showed that the expression of miR-19b is significantly different between LTNP-Hs and LTNP-Ls. We speculated that miR-19b contributes to the control of viral load in LTNP-Ls by affecting viral production and/or regulating immune cell function.

CD8$^+$T cells play a crucial role in the control of HIV replication by direct cytolysis of infected cells and production

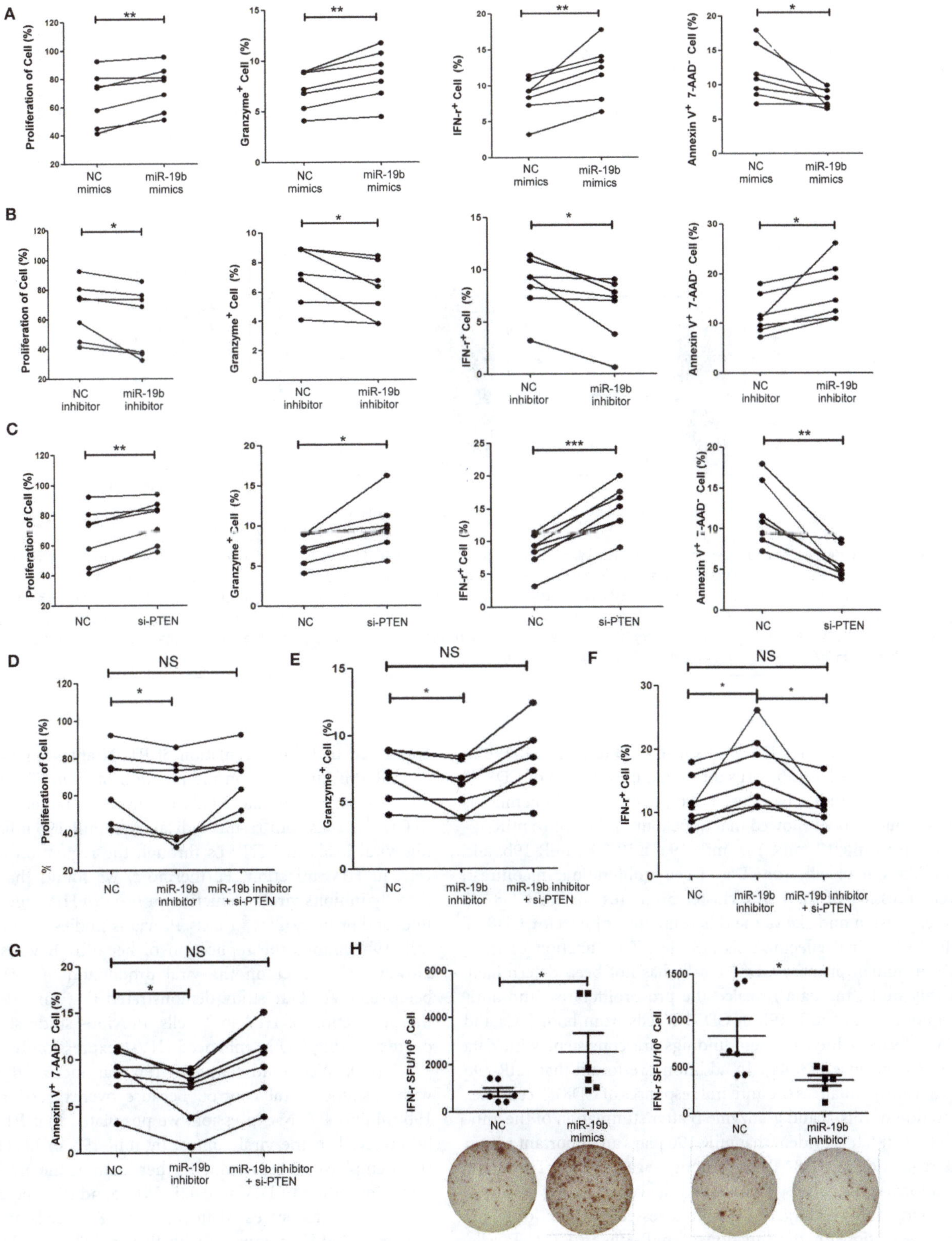

FIGURE 5 | miR-19b regulates CD8$^+$T cell function in HIV-infected patients. CD8$^+$ T cells from HIV-infected treatment-naive patients were sorted. **(A)** CD8$^+$ T cells were transfected with miR-19b mimics using Lipofectamine® RNAiMAX. After transfection (24 h), CD8$^+$ T cells were stimulated using anti-CD3/CD28 (3 μg/ml). Proliferation (day 5), intracellular expression of IFN-γ and granzyme B (day 1), and apoptosis (day 2) were compared between miR-19b-overexpressing CD8$^+$ T

(Continued)

FIGURE 5 | cells and controls. **(B)** $CD8^+$ T cells were transfected with miR-19b inhibitors using Lipofectamine® RNAiMAX. After transfection (24 h), $CD8^+$ T cells were stimulated using anti-CD3/CD28 (3 μg/ml). Proliferation (day 5), intracellular expression of IFN-γ and granzyme B (day 1), and apoptosis (day 2) were compared between miR-19b-overexpressing $CD8^+$T cells and controls. **(C)** The expression of PTEN was inhibited by introducing 20 μM PTEN siRNA to isolated $CD8^+$ T cells. Proliferation (day 5), intracellular expression of IFN-γ and granzyme B (day 1), and apoptosis (day 2) were compared between PTEN-inhibited $CD8^+$ T cells and controls. **(D–G)** $CD8^+$ T cells were transfected with a miR-19b inhibitor and PTEN siRNAs simultaneously. After transfection (24 h), $CD8^+$ T cells were stimulated using anti-CD3/CD28 (3 μg/ml). Proliferation **(D)**, apoptosis **(G)**, and intracellular expression of granzyme B **(E)** and IFN-γ **(F)** were compared. **(H)** $CD4^+$ T cells were depleted from PBMCs and transfected with miR-19b mimics or inhibitors. An IFN-γ ELISPOT assay was performed 24 h after transfection. Spot-forming units were compared between miR-19b-overexpressing/inhibited cells and controls. $n = 7$ for each group in **(A–G)**, $n = 6$ for each group in **(H)**. $^*P < 0.05$. $^{**}P < 0.01$. $^{***}P < 0.001$, respectively.

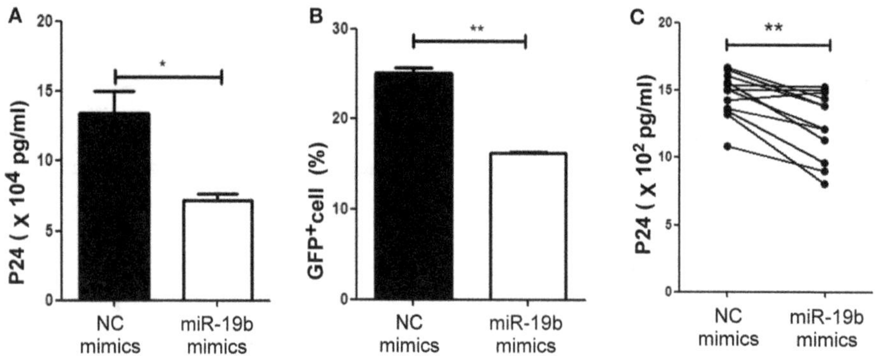

FIGURE 6 | miR-19b inhibits viral replication in *in-vitro* HIV-infected T cells. **(A)** Mimics of miR-19b and the pseudoviral plasmid NL4-3 were co-transfected into 293T cells and the level of P24 in the supernatants was measured through ELISA. **(B)** Clone-X cells were transfected with miR-19b mimics for 24 h and subsequently infected with vesicular stomatitis virus glycoprotein (VSV-G) pseudotyped HIV-1 (NL4-3) virus. GFP^+ cells were detected through flow cytometry 48 h after infection. **(C)** Primary $CD4^+$ T cells isolated from healthy controls were transfected with miR-19b mimics or controls. After transfection (24 h), the cells were stimulated using anti-CD3/CD28 (3 μg/ml). A cryopreserved primary HIV-1 isolate was added to the cells and the levels of p24 in the supernatants were measured after 3 days of infection through ELISA. $n = 12$ for each group in **(C)** $^*P < 0.05$. $^{**}P < 0.01$.

of secreted factors (41, 42). We assessed the role of miR-19b in maintaining low levels of virus through the regulation of $CD8^+$T cell function. Studies based on a lymphocytic choriomeningitis virus mouse model showed that knockout of the entire miR-17-92 cluster (miR-17, miR-18a, miR-19a, miR-20a, miR-19b, and miR-92a) impairs effector $CD8^+$ T cell proliferation. In contrast, overexpression of the entire cluster promotes effector $CD8^+$ T cell expansion and skews the differentiation of effector $CD8^+$T cells to terminal effector cells (43, 44). The function of miR-19b in human primary $CD8^+$T cells has not been determined. In this study, the data revealed the pro-proliferative and anti-apoptotic role of miR-19b in $CD8^+$T cells from both HCs and HIV-infected patients. These findings are consistent with data reported in mice (43, 44). In addition, we found that miR-19b significantly enhances the antiviral responses of $CD8^+$T cells (i.e., secretion of IFN-γ and granzyme B after stimulation of the anti-CD3/CD28). It is evident that miR-19b plays an important role in the regulation of $CD8^+$T cell responses against HIV. Through a bioinformatics analysis, we analyzed the cell signaling pathways involving miR-19b target genes and assessed the effect of PTEN downregulation on the function of miR-19b in $CD8^+$T cells. Previous studies have shown that miR-19b downregulates the expression of the target gene PTEN. However, the involvement of PTEN in the regulation of $CD8^+$T cell functions by miR-19b in HIV infection had not been investigated. This study confirmed that downregulation of PTEN antagonizes the effect of miR-19b inhibition on the function of $CD8^+$T cells in HIV patients, suggesting that PTEN is one of the targets of miR-19b in $CD8^+$T cells. Our results indicate that miR-19b influences the low viral loads in LTNP-Ls through the regulation of $CD8^+$T cells in HIV infection. Furthermore, we found that miR-19b directly inhibits viral production in *in-vitro* HIV-infected T cell lines and primary $CD4^+$T cells. Previous studies have shown that miR-19b inhibits the replication of hepatitis B virus (45, 46). However, its effect on the viral production of HIV has not been reported. Our study demonstrated that miR-19b inhibits the production of HIV in T cells. Previous study showed that overexpressing PTEN enhanced HIV-1 expression by inhibiting PI3K (47). We found that miR-19b was increased in LTNPs with sustained viral control. Because overexpression of miR-19b inhibits PTEN expression, we postulated that PTEN might be involved in the viral control by miR-19b in LNTP-Ls. Our study emphasized the need to further examine the mechanism of direct inhibition of HIV in detail. We found that the expression of miR-19b was decreased in sorted $CD8^+$T cells and $CD4^+$T cells in LTNP-Hs compared with that in LTNP-Ls. The current data highlighted the importance of miR-19b in HIV infection, promoting $CD8^+$T cell function and inhibiting viral production. These results provide potential targets for improved immune intervention.

In summary, this study provided the first comprehensive overview of the expression of miRNA in LTNP-Hs and LTNP-Ls. The investigation identified miR-19b as a highly expressed miRNA in LTNP-Ls, contributing to low viral load in LTNPs through promotion of $CD8^{+}$T cell function and inhibition of viral production. This study provides useful information for the exploration of new intervention paths in HIV infection.

AUTHOR CONTRIBUTIONS

HS, Z-NZ, and L-BY conceived and designed the experiments. L-BY performed the experiments. L-BY analyzed the data. C-BS, J-FZ, Y-JF, SQ, Y-JJ, J-JX, and H-BD contributed reagents, materials, and analysis tools. L-BY and Z-NZ wrote the article.

REFERENCES

1. Sheppard HW, Lang W, Ascher MS, Vittinghoff E, Winkelstein W. The characterization of non-progressors: long-term HIV-1 infection with stable $CD4^{+}$ T-cell levels. *Aids* (1993) 7:1159–66.
2. Pantaleo G, Fauci AS. New concepts in the immunopathogenesis of HIV infection. *Annu Rev Immunol.* (1995) 13:487–512. doi: 10.1146/annurev.iy.13.040195.002415
3. Lambotte O, Boufassa F, Madec Y, Nguyen A, Goujard C, Meyer L, et al. HIV controllers: a homogeneous group of HIV-1-infected patients with spontaneous control of viral replication. *Clin Infect Dis.* (2005) 41:1053–6. doi: 10.1086/433188
4. Grabar S, Selinger-Leneman H, Abgrall S, Pialoux G, Weiss L, Costagliola D. Prevalence and comparative characteristics of long-term nonprogressors and HIV controller patients in the French Hospital Database on HIV. *Aids* (2009) 23:1163–9. doi: 10.1097/QAD.0b013e32832b44c8
5. Lambotte O, Delfraissy JF. HIV controllers: a homogeneous group of HIV-1 infected patients with a spontaneous control of viral replication. *Pathol Biol (Paris)* (2006) 54:566–71. doi: 10.1016/j.patbio.2006.07.035
6. O'Connell KA, Bailey JR, Blankson JN. Elucidating the elite: mechanisms of control in HIV-1 infection. *Trends Pharmacol Sci.* (2009) 30:631–7. doi: 10.1016/j.tips.2009.09.005
7. Deeks SG, Walker BD. Human immunodeficiency virus controllers: mechanisms of durable virus control in the absence of antiretroviral therapy. *Immunity* (2007) 27:406–16. doi: 10.1016/j.immuni.2007.08.010
8. Okulicz JF, Lambotte O. Epidemiology and clinical characteristics of elite controllers. *Curr Opin HIV AIDS* (2011) 6:163–8. doi: 10.1097/COH.0b013e328344f35e
9. Walker BD. Elite control of HIV Infection: implications for vaccines and treatment. *Top HIV Med.* (2007)15:134–6.
10. Saez-Cirion A, Pancino G, Sinet M, Venet A, Lambotte O. HIV controllers: how do they tame the virus? *Trends Immunol.* (2007) 28:532–40. doi: 10.1016/j.it.2007.09.002
11. Autran B, Descours B, Avettand-Fenoel V, Rouzioux C. Elite controllers as a model of functional cure. *Curr Opin HIV AIDS* (2011) 6:181–7. doi: 10.1097/COH.0b013e328345a328
12. Vigneault F, Woods M, Buzon MJ, Li C, Pereyra F, Crosby SD, et al. Transcriptional profiling of CD4 T cells identifies distinct subgroups of HIV-1 elite controllers. *J Virol.* (2011) 85:3015–9. doi: 10.1128/JVI.01846-10
13. Benito JM, Ortiz MC, Leon A, Sarabia LA, Ligos JM, Montoya M, et al. Class-modeling analysis reveals T-cell homeostasis disturbances involved in loss of immune control in elite controllers. *BMC Med.* (2018) 16:30. doi: 10.1186/s12916-018-1026-6
14. Grabar S, Selinger-Leneman H, Abgrall S, Pialoux G, Weiss L, Costagliola D. Loss of long-term non-progressor and HIV controller status over time in the French Hospital Database on HIV–ANRS CO4. *PLoS ONE* (2017) 12:e0184441. doi: 10.1371/journal.pone.0184441
15. van der Helm JJ, Geskus R, Lodi S, Meyer L, Schuitemaker H, Gunsenheimer-Bartmeyer B, et al. Characterisation of long-term non-progression of HIV-1 infection after seroconversion: a cohort study. *Lancet HIV* (2014) 1:e41–8. doi: 10.1016/s2352-3018(14)70016-5
16. Witwer KW, Watson AK, Blankson JN, Clements JE. Relationships of PBMC microRNA expression, plasma viral load, and $CD4^{+}$ T-cell count in HIV-1-infected elite suppressors and viremic patients. *Retrovirology* (2012) 9:5. doi: 10.1186/1742-4690-9-5
17. Huang J, Wang F, Argyris E, Chen K, Liang Z, Tian H, et al. Cellular microRNAs contribute to HIV-1 latency in resting primary $CD4^{+}$ T lymphocytes. *Nat Med.* (2007) 13:1241–7. doi: 10.1038/nm1639
18. Wang X, Ye L, Hou W, Zhou Y, Wang YJ, Metzger DS, et al. Cellular microRNA expression correlates with susceptibility of monocytes/macrophages to HIV-1 infection. *Blood* (2009) 113:671–4. doi: 10.1182/blood-2008-09-175000
19. Ahluwalia JK, Khan SZ, Soni K, Rawat P, Gupta A, Hariharan M, et al. Human cellular microRNA hsa-miR-29a interferes with viral nef protein expression and HIV-1 replication. *Retrovirology* (2008) 5:117. doi: 10.1186/1742-4690-5-117
20. Triboulet R, Mari B, Lin YL, Chable-Bessia C, Bennasser Y, Lebrigand K, et al. Suppression of microRNA-silencing pathway by HIV-1 during virus replication. *Science* (2007) 315:1579–82. doi: 10.1126/science.1136319
21. Mehta A, Baltimore D. MicroRNAs as regulatory elements in immune system logic. *Nat Rev Immunol.* (2016) 16:279–94. doi: 10.1038/nri.2016.40
22. O'Connell RM, Rao DS, Chaudhuri AA, Baltimore D. Physiological and pathological roles for microRNAs in the immune system. *Nat Rev Immunol.* (2010) 10:111–22. doi: 10.1038/nri2708
23. Kuerten S, Nowacki TM, Kleen TO, Asaad RJ, Lehmann PV, Tary-Lehmann M. Dissociated production of perforin, granzyme B, and IFN-gamma by HIV-specific CD8(+) cells in HIV infection. *AIDS Res Hum Retroviruses* (2008) 24:62–71. doi: 10.1089/aid.2007.0125
24. Nasi A, Chiodi F. Mechanisms regulating expansion of $CD8^{+}$ T cells during HIV-1 infection. *J Intern Med.* (2018) 283:257–67. doi: 10.1111/joim.12722
25. Liang Y, Pan HF, Ye DQ. microRNAs function in $CD8^{+}$T cell biology. *J Leukoc Biol.* (2015) 97:487–97. doi: 10.1189/jlb.1RU0814-369R
26. Swaminathan S, Kelleher AD. microRNA modulation of key targets associated with T cell exhaustion in HIV-1 infection. *Curr Opin HIV AIDS* (2014) 9:464–71. doi: 10.1097/COH.0000000000000089
27. Zwolińska K. Host genetic factors associated with susceptibility to HIV infection and progression of infection. *Postepy Hig Med Dosw.* (2009) 63:73–91.
28. Dey R, Soni K, Saravanan S, Balakrishnan P, Kumar V, Boobalan J, et al. Anti-HIV microRNA expression in a novel Indian cohort. *Sci Rep.* (2016) 6:28279. doi: 10.1038/srep28279
29. Reynoso R, Laufer N, Hackl M, Skalicky S, Monteforte R, Turk G, et al. MicroRNAs differentially present in the plasma of HIV elite controllers reduce HIV infection *in vitro*. *Sci Rep.* (2014) 4:05915. doi: 10.1038/srep05915
30. Egaña-Gorroño L, Escribà T, Boulanger N, Guardo AC, León A, Bargalló ME, et al. Differential MicroRNA expression profile between stimulated PBMCs from HIV-1 infected elite controllers and viremic progressors. *PLoS ONE* (2014) 9:e0106360. doi: 10.1371/journal.pone.0106360
31. Schmittgen TD, Livak KJ. Analyzing real-time PCR data by the comparative CT method. *Nat Protoc.* (2008) 3:1101–8. doi: 10.1038/nprot.2008.73
32. Zhu LY, Qiu C, Lv JX, Xu JQ. HIV-1 infection changes miRNA expression profile in the whole blood. *Bing Du Xue Bao* (2013) 29:323–9. doi: 10.13242/j.cnki.bingduxuebao.002394
33. Gupta A, Nagilla P, Le HS, Bunney C, Zych C, Thalamuthu A, et al. Comparative expression profile of miRNA and mRNA in primary peripheral blood mononuclear cells infected with human immunodeficiency virus (HIV-1). *PLoS ONE* (2011) 6:e22730. doi: 10.1371/journal.pone.0022730

34. Jia Z, Wang K, Zhang A, Wang G, Kang C, Han L, et al. miR-19a and miR-19b overexpression in gliomas. *Pathol Oncol Res.* (2013) 19:847–53. doi: 10.1007/s12253-013-9653-x
35. Wang F, Li T, Zhang B, Li H, Wu Q, Yang L, et al. MicroRNA-19a/b regulates multidrug resistance in human gastric cancer cells by targeting PTEN. *Biochem Biophys Res Commun.* (2013) 434:688–94. doi: 10.1016/j.bbrc.2013.04.010
36. Ventura W, Koide K, Hori K, Yotsumoto J, Sekizawa A, Saito H, et al. Placental expression of microRNA-17 and−19b is down-regulated in early pregnancy loss. *Eur J Obstet Gynecol Reprod Biol.* (2013) 169:28–32. doi: 10.1016/j.ejogrb.2013.01.025
37. Riley KJ, Rabinowitz GS, Yario TA, Luna JM, Darnell RB, Steitz JA. EBV and human microRNAs co-target oncogenic and apoptotic viral and human genes during latency. *EMBO J.* (2012) 31:2207–21. doi: 10.1038/emboj.2012.63
38. Mavrakis KJ, Wolfe AL, Oricchio E, Palomero T, de Keersmaecker K, McJunkin K, et al. Genome-wide RNA-mediated interference screen identifies miR-19 targets in Notch-induced T-cell acute lymphoblastic leukaemia. *Nat Cell Biol.* (2010) 12:372–9. doi: 10.1038/ncb2037
39. Groszer M, Erickson R, Scripture-Adams DD, Lesche R, Trumpp A, Zack JA, et al. Negative regulation of neural stem/progenitor cell proliferation by the Pten tumor suppressor gene *in vivo. Science* (2001) 294:2186–9. doi: 10.1126/science.1065518
40. Qi Y, Hu H, Guo H, Xu P, Shi Z, Huan X, et al. MicroRNA profiling in plasma of HIV-1 infected patients: potential markers of infection and immune status. *J Pub Health Emerg.* (2017) 1:65. doi: 10.21037/jphe.2017.05.11
41. Walker BD, Chakrabarti S, Moss B, Paradis TJ, Flynn T, Durno AG, et al. HIV-specific cytotoxic T lymphocytes in seropositive individuals. *Nature* (1987) 328:345–8. doi: 10.1038/328345a0
42. Levy JA. The search for the $CD8^+$ cell anti-HIV factor (CAF). *Trends Immunol.* (2003) 24:628–32. doi: 10.1016/j.it.2003.10.005
43. Wu T, Wieland A, Araki K, Davis CW, Ye L, Hale JS, et al. Temporal expression of microRNA cluster miR-17-92 regulates effector and memory $CD8^+$ T-cell differentiation. *Proc Natl Acad Sci USA.* (2012) 109:9965–70. doi: 10.1073/pnas.1207327109
44. Khan AA, Penny LA, Yuzefpolskiy Y, Sarkar S, Kalia V. MicroRNA-17–92 regulates effector and memory CD8 T-cell fates by modulating proliferation in response to infections. *Blood* (2013) 121:4473–83. doi: 10.1182/blood-2012-06-435412
45. Jung YJ, Kim JW, Park SJ, Min BY, Jang ES, Kim NY, et al. c-Myc-mediated overexpression of miR-17-92 suppresses replication of hepatitis B virus in human hepatoma cells. *J Med Virol.* (2013) 85:969–78. doi: 10.1002/jmv.23534
46. Ji F, Yang B, Peng X, Ding H, You H, Tien P. Circulating microRNAs in hepatitis B virus-infected patients. *J Viral Hepat.* (2011) 18:e242–51. doi: 10.1111/j.1365-2893.2011.01443.x
47. Cook JA, August A, Henderson AJ. Recruitment of phosphatidylinositol 3-kinase to CD28 inhibits HIV transcription by a Tat-dependent mechanism. *J Immunol.* (2002) 169:254–60. doi: 10.4049/jimmunol.169.1.254

5

Nanoparticle-Based Immunoengineered Approaches for Combating HIV

Allan Bowen[1], *Elizabeth E. Sweeney*[1] *and Rohan Fernandes*[1,2*]

[1] *The George Washington Cancer Center, The George Washington University, Washington, DC, United States,*

[2] *Department of Medicine, The George Washington University, Washington, DC, United States*

Correspondence:
Rohan Fernandes
rfernandes@gwu.edu

Highly active antiretroviral therapy (HAART) serves as an effective strategy to combat HIV infections by suppressing viral replication in patients with HIV/AIDS. However, HAART does not provide HIV/AIDS patients with a sterilizing or functional cure, and introduces several deleterious comorbidities. Moreover, the virus is able to persist within latent reservoirs, both undetected by the immune system and unaffected by HAART, increasing the risk of a viral rebound. The field of immunoengineering, which utilizes varied bioengineering approaches to interact with the immune system and potentiate its therapeutic effects against HIV, is being increasingly investigated in HIV cure research. In particular, nanoparticle-based immunoengineered approaches are especially attractive because they offer advantages including the improved delivery and functionality of classical HIV drugs such as antiretrovirals and experimental drugs such as latency-reversing agents (LRAs), among others. Here, we present and discuss the current state of the field in nanoparticle-based immunoengineering approaches for an HIV cure. Specifically, we discuss nanoparticle-based methods for improving HAART as well as latency reversal, developing vaccines, targeting viral fusion, enhancing gene editing approaches, improving adoptively transferred immune-cell mediated reservoir clearance, and other therapeutic and prevention approaches. Although nanoparticle-based immunoengineered approaches are currently at the stage of preclinical testing, the promising findings obtained in these studies demonstrate the potential of this emerging field for developing an HIV cure.

Keywords: HIV cure strategies, immunoengineering, nanoparticles, immune activation, HAART (highly active antiretroviral therapy), combination therapy for HIV, latency reversing agents

INTRODUCTION

Approximately 37 million people worldwide are living with HIV for which there is no practical cure (1). There are two main types of the virus: HIV-1 and HIV-2. HIV-1, which is the focus of cure strategies discussed in this paper, is more prevalent and pathogenic, and primarily infects $CD4^+$ T helper cells (2). Other cell populations susceptible to HIV-1 include dendritic cells, macrophages, microglia, and astrocytes although the mechanisms of infection for these cell types are not yet fully understood (3–8). HAART is an effective treatment regimen for HIV-1 (9), however, it allows the virus to remain viable and does not provide a sterilizing or functional cure in patients. Further HAART causes several deleterious comorbidities (10, 11). Since HAART targets the HIV-1 replication cycle, HIV-1 evades targeting by undergoing latency (12, 13). Latent HIV-1 reservoirs are also able to go undetected by the immune system, which increases the risk of a viral rebound. Another confounding factor is the lack of unique surface markers on latently infected cells, which has hindered the development of strategies to generate total viral clearance or permanent latency (14–16). This challenge is supported by the fact that there have been only two well-documented cases wherein patients have experienced total HIV-1 viral clearance. This suggests that it is extremely rare for individuals to adequately control HIV-1 without a sustained antiretroviral treatment regimen (17, 18). Hence, there is an urgent need for novel HIV cure strategies.

The field of immunoengineering encompasses a broad variety of bioengineering approaches and technologies to manipulate the immune system. A notable component of these approaches involves engineered biomaterials including nanoparticles, polymeric scaffolds, and hydrogels to engage the immune system to fight disease, and represents an attractive strategy for developing a cure for HIV-1 (19–21). While numerous nanoparticle-based immunoengineered approaches have been successfully applied in the field of cancer immunotherapy (22–26), fewer studies have utilized these promising benefits for an HIV cure. The goal of this mini-review is to familiarize the reader with the field of nanoparticle-based immunoengineering approaches for an HIV cure. In particular, we focus on the use of nanoparticles to enhance HAART, latency reversal, vaccination strategies, gene editing, cell therapies, among others (**Figure 1**). We highlight both immune-mediated strategies (e.g., nanoparticles in conjunction with adoptive cell transfer) and those targeting endogenous immune cells involved in HIV (e.g., nanovaccines). For a comprehensive discussion on the use of nanoparticles for treating HIV/AIDS in the context of nanoparticles classes, formulation, and their use in drug delivery, we direct the readers to several published reviews in the literature (27–29).

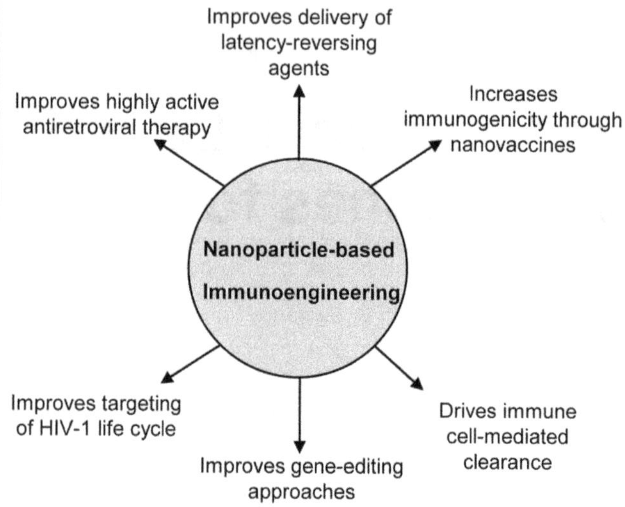

FIGURE 1 | Overview of the applications of nanoparticle-based immunoengineering approaches for combating HIV-1.

NANOPARTICLES EXHIBIT BENEFICIAL PROPERTIES FOR IMMUNOENGINEERING CURES FOR HIV-1

Nanoparticle sizes range from ~1 to 100 nm (30). On account of their sizes, nanoparticle-based therapies can easily be administered by varied techniques (i.e., intravenously, subcutaneously, intraperitoneally) and penetrate body barriers (31). Related to their sizes and pertinent to HIV cure strategies, nanoparticles accumulate in lymphoid tissue and lymphatic organs (32), the sites of anatomical HIV reservoirs (33, 34) when parenterally injected (especially when injected intradermally, subcutaneously, and/or intramuscularly). Additionally, because nanoparticles have a large surface area-to-volume ratio, diverse molecules such as drug payloads, immunological adjuvants, and targeting ligands can be bioconjugated to their surface (35), which can then be trafficked to sites of latent HIV reservoirs. Nanoparticles can also be synthesized in the form of depots/reservoirs that encapsulate and release therapeutic drugs or immunomodulatory agents (36), allowing for their improved bioavailability and sustained release kinetics in an HIV cure setting. In the following sections, we review various examples of nanoparticles used for immunoengineering HIV cures.

Nanoparticles for Improving HAART

HAART can successfully inactivate HIV-1, however the virus is able to persist within latent lymphoid, gut, and CNS reservoirs (5–8). This requires patients to remain adherent to the HAART regimen for the duration of their lifetime to prevent viral rebound (9). Since nanoparticles facilitate the sustained release of drugs, a group of researchers have developed a long-acting slow-effective release antiretroviral therapy (termed "LASER ART"), which utilizes nanoparticles for controlled release of HAART agents, thereby improving regimen adherence (37, 38). In a recent study, the same group of researchers demonstrated that a nanocrystallized product of lamivudine, a nucleoside reverse transcriptase inhibitor (NM23TC), maintained antiretroviral activity in HIV-1-infected monocyte-derived macrophages after viral challenge for up to 30 days. NM23TC was taken up by HIV-1-infected monocyte-derived macrophages and remained in high prodrug concentration in whole blood for 30 days after a single dose. In addition, at day 28, M23TC, a metabolized version of lamivudine, was detected at high levels in the liver, lymph nodes, and spleen (39), suggesting that this nanoplatform may improve delivery of the drug to HIV-1 niches. Other groups have also developed nanoparticles for improving HAART (40–43) (**Table 1**).

Nanoparticles for Improving Latency Reversal

Latency-reversing agents (LRAs) are able to reactivate viral replication. LRAs are used in "shock and kill" treatment approaches, wherein the LRA-elicited viral replication is coupled

TABLE 1 | Nanoparticle-based immunoengineering approaches for HIV/AIDS.

Nanoparticle class	Key findings	References
NANOPARTICLES FOR IMPROVING HAART		
Poloxamer-based nanoparticles	LASER ART (also known as nanoART) nanoparticles for controlled release of HAART agents	(37–40)
Lipid nanoparticle	Lipid-drug nanoparticles exhibited 5-fold increased bioavailability of HAART drugs in lymph nodes, and markedly increased sustained release over the course of 7 days	(41)
PLGA/pluronic nanoparticle	Nanoformulation of HAART drugs demonstrate greater bioavailability in plasma and absorption in various tissues over the course of 14 days	(42)
Lactoferrin nanoparticle	First-line nanoformulated HAART drugs exhibited 4-fold increase in bioavailability and an increase in anti-HIV activity compared to soluble agents	(43)
NANOPARTICLES FOR IMPROVING LATENCY REVERSAL		
Lipid nanoparticle	LRA and protease inhibitor encapsulated within nanoparticle reversed latency and prevented HIV-1 viral spread	(44)
Lipid-coated PLGA nanoparticle	Co-administration of LRAs-individually encapsulated within nanoparticles exhibited synergistic induction of HIV-1 mRNA levels at low cytotoxicity	(45)
Iron oxide nanoparticle	LRA and vorinostat-loaded nanoparticle penetrated BBB, reversed HIV-1 latency and exhibited antiviral efficacy in astrocytes.	(46)
PLG/PEG nanoparticle	LRA and protease inhibitor encapsulated within PLGA-PEG nanoparticles reversed latency and inhibited viral spread	(47)
NANOVACCINES		
PLGA nanoparticle	Encapsulating TLR-agonist improved HIV-1 vaccine immunogenicity and decrease required dose for immunogenic effect	(48)
Lumazine synthase- and ferritin-based nanoparticles	Antigens encapsulated within nanoparticles were trafficked within germinal centers promoting a potent immunogenic response	(49)
Polyethylenimine mannose/DNA/ glucose nanoparticle	DermaVir nanoformulation delivered HIV-1 antigen to Langerhans cells, which matured into Dendritic cells, mounting an immune response	(50)
eOD-GT8 nanoparticle	Engineered outer domain (eOD)-60 mer nanoparticle exhibited sufficient precursor naïve B cell binding for bnAb production	(51)
Liposome nanoparticle	Clade C-derived trimers decorated on liposomal surface induced enhanced germinal center and bnAb responses compared to soluble trimers	(52)
Ferritin nanoparticle	Consensus-derived Env trimers conjugated to nanoparticles induced greater bnAb targeting of apex trimers of *in vivo* models	(53)
Protein nanoparticle	Nanomaterial presenting SOSIP trimer increased B-cell activation and induced greater bnAb titers against Tier-1A viral strains	(54)
Liposome nanoparticle	Vaccination with liposomes formulated with HIV envelope protein elicits bnAb targeting and neutralization	(55)
Ferritin nanoparticle	HIV antigens are presented on nanoparticles in native trimeric structure as a tool for vaccine development	(56)
NANOPARTICLES TARGETING HIV VIRAL FUSION TO IMMUNE CELLS		
Silver nanoparticle	Silver nanoparticles exert anti-HIV activity through gp120 binding in various viral strains	(57)
Poly (acrylate)-based nanoparticle	Hydrophobic nanoparticle impedes amyloid fiber structure, thereby disrupting HIV-1 trafficking to its target cell	(58)
PLGA nanoparticle	Nanoparticles coated with a T-cell membrane were able to serve as a "decoy" for HIV-1 binding, resulting in viral suppression	(59)
Extracellular vesicles	Extracellular vesicles (EVs) released by *Lactobacillus* inhibited HIV-1 viral attachment and entry to target cells	(60)
Extracellular vesicles	EVs isolated from semen inhibited HIV-1 regardless of donor infection status; EVs from ART-treated subjects inhibited HIV-1 *in vivo*	(61)
NANOPARTICLES TO ENHANCE GENE EDITING APPROACHES		
Gold nanoparticles	Au-nanoparticles can mediate CRISPR-Cas9 components to target cells with higher efficiency and lower cytotoxicity	(62)
Poloxamer-based nanoparticles	LASER ART combined with CRISPR/Cas9 eliminated HIV-1 in a small subset of mice	(63)
NANOPARTICLES TO ENHANCE CLEARANCE BY ADOPTIVELY TRANSFERRED IMMUNE CELLS		
PLGA nanoparticles	Nanoparticles encapsulating neutralizing antibody and LRA improved NK cell effector function toward J-Lat cells compared to free agents	(64)
Lipid nanoparticle	IL-15-loaded nanocapsules conjugated to HIV-1-specific CTLs improved elimination of infected cells	(65)
OTHER THERAPIES		
PEG-*b*-PR co-polymer nanoparticles	STING agonist nanoformulation reversed HIV-1 immune evasion mechanism	(66)
Quantum dots	Graphene quantum dots mediated HIV-1 viral suppression	(67)
Nanodiamonds	Efavirenz-nanodiamond conjugation improved bioavailability and blood brain barrier penetration	(68)
Gold nanoparticles	Gold conjugated with HIV integrase inhibitors could penetrate the BBB and exert antiviral efficacy in targeted HIV-1-infected microglial cells	(69)
PLGA nanoparticles	FTC-loaded nanoparticles exhibited greater bioavailability and lower IC_{50} compared to soluble agents	(70)
PLGA nanoparticles	TDF-loaded nanoparticles in thermosensitive gel conferred 100% protection from HIV-1 strains within 24 h time period and had no detectable viral levels in plasma throughout 4 weeks period	(71)
Cellulose acetate phthalate nanoparticles	DTG-loaded nanoparticles in thermosensitive gel were uptaken into vaginal epithelial cells with low cytotoxicity	(72)

(Continued)

to the actions of HIV-1 cell-specific cytotoxic agents or immune-mediated clearance (73). Several classes of molecules and macromolecules have been used as LRAs including protein kinase C (PKC) agonists, histone deacetylase inhibitors, and cytokines, and their mechanisms of latency reversal are well-described. For example, PKC agonists function via the NF-KB pathway. Activated PKC isoforms downregulate the inhibitor IKB, thereby releasing the transcription factor NF-KB, which translocates into the nucleus, and binds to the HIV-1 proviral long terminal repeats, thereby mediating viral transcription (74). Similar to HAART, nanoparticles have been utilized to improve the delivery of LRAs (**Table 1**). In one study, Kovochich et al. encapsulated bryostatin, a potent PKC agonist (75) and nelfinavir, an HIV-1 protease inhibitor, into nanoparticles. Their nanoplatform targeted $CD4^+$ cells in a peripheral blood mononuclear cells (PBMC) culture, activated latent virus, and inhibited viral spread (76). In a more recent study, Cao et al. synthesized hybrid lipid-coated PLGA nanocarriers that incorporated diverse LRAs. These lipid-coated nanoparticles could selectively activate $CD4^+$ T cells in nonhuman primate PBMCs as well as in murine lymph nodes with substantially reduced toxicity (44). Despite the fact that it is currently impossible to identify and target every HIV-1-infected cell in the latent reservoir (45), the ability of nanoparticles and nanocarriers to traffic and deliver LRAs to sites of latent HIV reservoirs can maximize their therapeutic benefit, and serve as an important component of successful shock and kill cure regimens. Other examples of nanoparticles for improving latency reversal appear in **Table 1** (46, 47).

Nanovaccines

Traditional vaccines for HIV-1 have been difficult to develop, and clinical trials using HIV-1 vaccines have demonstrated poor efficacy (77, 78). Vaccines fail for several reasons including poor delivery to dendritic cells, reversion of a live attenuated virus to its virulent form, or if the vaccine is too weak to facilitate an immune response (68). Consequently, an ideal vaccine should be clinically safe, stable, and capable of inducing a potent immune response (79). Nanoparticles have been shown to overcome these limitations (80) by protecting antigens from proteolytic enzymes, promoting antigen uptake and processing by antigen-presenting cells (APCs), in addition to being biocompatible and biodegradable (81). Several groups have leveraged favorable properties of nanoparticles to develop nanovaccines for HIV-1 (**Table 1**).

One effective strategy is utilizing nanovaccines to activate dendritic cells (DCs), which in turn cause T cell activation (82). To this end, Rostami et al. decorated antigens onto the surface of nanoparticles to facilitate greater interaction with the APCs due to the high surface area to volume ratio of the nanoparticles (48). Specifically, a flagellin molecule sequence derived from *Pseudomonas aeruginosa* (FLiC), a toll-like receptor 5 agonist, was conjugated to an HIV-1 p24-NeF peptide, and encapsulated within PLGA nanoparticles. The FLiC-p24-NeF-encapsulated nanoparticle elicited higher levels of lymphocyte proliferation and cytotoxic T cell activity compared to controls (48), suggesting its potential use in an HIV-1 vaccination strategy. In a more recently study by Tokatlian et al., nanoparticles encapsulating HIV-1 antigens were observe to localize to the lymph nodes more than corresponding soluble antigen counterparts, and remained localized there for up to 4 weeks (49). In another study, Lori et al. showed that their nanoplatform "DermaVir" could administer HIV-1 antigens to Langerhans cells, which resulted in a potent immunogenic response (50). DermaVir is currently undergoing a phase 3 clinical trial evaluation based on excellent responses observed in Phase I/II clinical trials (83). Together, these studies along with others summarized in **Table 1** (51–56), clearly suggest the importance of nanovaccines for treating HIV-1.

Nanoparticles Targeting HIV Viral Fusion to Immune Cells

Targeting the HIV replication cycle by inhibiting the ability of HIV-1 to fuse and/or enter a target cell has been the focus of several published studies (**Table 1**). Fusion or entry inhibition leads to inhibition of viral activity and viral cytotoxicity. In one approach, Lara et al. showed that silver nanoparticles are antiviral and prophylactic against HIV-1 fusion to target cells (57). Silver nanoparticles exert anti-HIV activity at an early stage of viral replication, likely as a virucidal agent or as an inhibitor of viral entry. Silver nanoparticles bind to gp120 in a manner that prevents CD4-dependent virion binding, fusion, and infectivity, acting as an effective virucidal agent against cell-free and cell-associated virus. Further, silver nanoparticles inhibit post-entry stages of the HIV-1 life cycle (57).

Another approach utilized semen-derived enhancer of viral infection (SEVI), which is a type of amyloid fibril present in human semen that enhances HIV-1 infection of target cells by capturing HIV-1 virions, resulting in increased viral fusion (84). SEVI serves as a mediator for HIV-1 viral attachment due to its highly cationic nature (84, 85). In their study, Sheik et al., synthesized a hydrophobic polymeric nanoparticle to reduce SEVI fibril-mediated infection (58). The hydrophobicity of the nanoparticle interferes with Aβ amyloid structure, forming amorphous aggregates, thereby disrupting the amyloid HIV-1 trafficking protein to target cells (86–88). Thus, the hydrophobic nanoparticles were able to reduce HIV-1 virion binding affinity toward their target cells (58).

Biomimicry approaches, such as plasma membrane-coated nanoparticles, represent a unique strategy to target a variety of human pathologies (89). A pivotal study showed the efficacy of coating a nanoparticle with a cell membrane to imitate and model endogenous cell activity. HIV-1 infection begins when an exposed HIV-1 surface protein, gp120, interacts with CD4 receptor and chemokine receptor type 5 (CCR5) co-receptor on target cells (90). Wei et al. coated polymeric nanoparticles with a $CD4^+$ T cell membrane, causing the modified membrane-coated nanoparticle to preferentially interact with HIV-1. This preferential binding ultimately neutralized HIV-1 viral activity in PBMCs *in vitro* (59), illustrating the potential of biomimicking nanoparticle approaches to reduce HIV-1 viral spread by blocking viral fusion to T cells.

Unlike synthetic nanoparticles, extracellular vesicles (EVs) are naturally occurring nanoscale structures that carry cargo (e.g., proteins, lipids, nucleic acids) and can be released from both healthy and apoptotic cells (91). Recently, Palomino et al. discovered that EVs released by Lactobacillus in the healthy vaginal microbiota prevented HIV-1 attachment to target cells and thereby inhibited HIV-1 infection (60). In a recent study by Welch et al., EVs extracted from semen inhibited HIV-1 *in vitro* regardless of HIV infection status of the donor, while EVs extracted from the blood and semen of ART-treated subjected inhibited HIV-1 *in vivo* (61). These studies suggest a potential avenue for bacterial and/or EV-based treatment strategies in preventing HIV-1 viral spread.

Nanoparticles to Enhance Gene Editing Approaches

Gene therapy technologies have been explored for HIV-1 cure strategies (**Table 1**). Clustered regularly interspaced short palindromic repeats and CRISPR-associated protein 9 (CRISPR-Cas9) is a gene editing platform wherein genes can be added, removed, or altered at given genetic loci (92). CRISPR-Cas9 is a faster and more efficient technique than other genetic editing platforms using other viral vectors or the Cre-Lox system, although current CRISPR-Cas9 delivery techniques use electroporation to facilitate DNA entry into living cells, which is difficult to control and can generate cytotoxicity (92, 93). Previously, gene-editing tools have knocked out CCR5 in $CD4^+$ T cells to block HIV-1 viral entry (94, 95). However, gold nanoparticles (AuNPs) have a unique ability to safely deliver CRISPR-Cas9 components to their targets (96). AuNPs have large surface area to volume ratios and are biocompatible with low toxicity (5). Shahbazi et al. developed AuNPs with layer-by-layer surface conjugation of CRISPR components (AuNP/CRISPR), targeting two locations within the hematopoietic stem and progenitor cell (HSPC) genome, CCR5 and the gamma-globin gene promoter. Genetic deficiency in CCR5 is linked to HIV-1 resistance through the elimination of viral anchoring and entry through its CCR5 co-receptor (62, 97). AuNP/CRISPR was able to penetrate into $CD34^+$ hematopoietic cell line, which is difficult to transfect. At micromolar concentrations, AuNP/CRISPR exhibited an overall low amount of gene editing and homologous directed repair (HDR) at the CCR5 and the gamma-globin promoter locus. This demonstrates that AuNP/CRISPR functioned with low efficacy. However, genetic editing and HDR via AuNP/CRISPR was higher than the electroporation-driven process. This suggests that AuNP/CRISPR could be effective in delivering gene editing for HIV-1 therapy (62).

With the promising innovations of LASER ART and CRISPR-Cas9, Dash et al. combined the two methodologies to evaluate a potentially synergistic functionality. Two of seven HIV-1-infected mice that received LASER ART followed by subsequent AAV_9-CRISPR-Cas9 treatment targeting a fragment of the HIV-1 genome were cured of viral rebound and experienced a restoration of their $CD4^+$ T cells, suggesting HIV-1 regression/elimination (63). Additionally, HIV-1 RNA levels diminished to undetectable levels in the plasma, spleen, liver, gut, and brain in the cured mice. Further, naïve humanized mice that were challenged with adoptively transferred cells isolated from the cured mice showed no detectable HIV-1 viral loads. This study demonstrates the possibility of eliminating HIV-1 in plasma and infectious tissues through this novel combination approach (63).

Nanoparticles to Enhance Clearance by Adoptively Transferred Immune Cells

Recent studies show promising effects of cell therapies for treating HIV-1 (98–100). Here, autologous or allogenic immune cells are transferred to the patient after *ex vivo* expansion and/or modification to clear HIV-1 infected cells. Nanoparticles may offer the ability to enhance the ability of immune cells to target and kill target cells in the context of HIV-1. In their study, Sweeney et al. generated a PLGA nanoplatform that co-encapsulated an LRA and a target cell-specific antibody to improve NK cell effector function in an *in vitro* cell model of latent HIV-1 (64). The nanoplatform was able to increase NK cell cytotoxicity of the target cells, thereby illustrating an example of nanoparticles enhancing immune cell function in the context of latent HIV-1 (64). In another studies, Jones et al. demonstrated that cytotoxic T lymphocytes (CTLs) were made more potent by conjugating drug-loaded lipid nanoparticles to their surface (65). HIV-1-specific CTLs were able to specifically target HIV-1-infected cells and deliver the nanoparticle-encapsulated payload (65).

Other Focus Areas

Nanoparticles to Boost Innate Immunity

HIV-1, like many other viruses, has evolved mechanisms to evade or disrupt immune surveillance. Therefore, one strategy to eliminate HIV-1 viral load is to reverse immune evasion. HIV-1 typically inhibits the cGAS-STING pathway that normally functions via cGAMP binding to STING on the endoplasmic reticulum resulting in an IFN-1-mediated antiviral response (66, 101, 102). pH-sensitive polymeric nanoparticles were engineered to deliver a STING agonist to counteract HIV-1 immune evasion via the cGAS-STING pathway. These STING agonist-nanoparticles demonstrated potent antiretroviral activity for up to 12 days (66).

Nanoparticles to Inhibit HIV-1 Reverse Transcriptase Activity

Quantum dots are biocompatible semiconductor crystal nanoparticles with low toxicity that have been used for biosensing, image contrast, and drug delivery (103, 104). These nanomaterials are attractive due to their intrinsic antiviral activity and thus, their potential as inhibitors of HIV-1. In a proof-of-concept study by Iannazzo et al., a reverse transcriptase inhibitor (RTI; CHI499) was readily conjugated onto the surface of the graphene quantum dots (GQDs) via intrinsic functional groups (67). The conjugated GQD product (GQD-CHI499) achieved remarkable anti-reverse transcriptase and cellular anti-HIV-1 activities compared to the free drug alone. This additive improvement may be the result of the GQDs' intrinsic structure, where the polycarboxylation group could mediate the inhibition of HIV-1 reverse transcriptase through viral fusion (67), suggesting the potential of GQDs in treatment for HIV-1.

Nanoparticles to Enhance Blood Brain Barrier Penetration

Aside from persistent HIV-1 in $CD4^+$ helper T cells, HIV-1 may also persist in microglial cells, which are the resident macrophages of the CNS (6). These cells may confer HAART resistance, perpetuate HIV-1 infection in peripheral tissues, and are critical in the development of HIV-1 associated neurocognitive diseases (105). The brain poses an anatomical barrier, where there is low drug penetration by virtue of the blood brain barrier (BBB). Therefore, there is a need to develop ways to penetrate the BBB to target persistent HIV-1 in microglial cells (6, 105). Nanodiamonds are ~10 nm diamonds which are known for their inexpensive production, surface modifications, and low cytotoxic profile. In the context of HIV-1, Roy et al. complexed efavirenz (EFV), an effective non-nucleoside RTI, to a nanodiamond to effectively improve the poor bioavailability of EFV (ND-EFV) (68). ND-EFV allowed for sustained release of EFV in a BBB model *in vitro*. In addition, ND-EFV was effective in controlling HIV-1 replication for 7 days, where the EFV alone drug was able to inhibit HIV-1 for 5 days (68). Similarly, gold nanoparticles have also been used entry through the BBB. Garrido et al. showed that gold nanoparticles conjugated with HIV integrase inhibitors could penetrate the BBB with antiviral efficacy, providing another nanoplatform for targeting HIV-1-infected microglial cells (69).

Nanoparticles for Prophylactic HIV-1 Prevention

Another application of nanoparticles is in improving pre-exposure prophylaxis (PrEP), which provides a >90% effective approach to prevent HIV-1 infection but requires daily oral administration (106). PrEP comprises tenofovir disoproxil fumarate (TDF) and emtricitabine (FTC), two nucleoside RTIs that have low half-lives and require high dosing, thereby increasing the risk of adverse effects (107). Mandal et al. encapsulated FTC within PLGA nanoparticles (FTC-NPs), and demonstrated improved bioavailability of FTC with significantly lower inhibitory concentration (IC_{50}) than free FTC *in vitro* (70). Alternatively, Destache et al. loaded TDF into PLGA nanoparticles (TDF-NPs), and subsequently incorporated them within a thermosensitive vaginal gel (71). Mice challenged with two strains of HIV-1 and treated with the TDF-NP gel were 100% protected against the virus with no detectable viral plasma load (71), suggesting the efficacy of sustained release of TDF by nanoparticles via vaginal administration to prevent HIV-1 infection. In another study, Mandal et al. encapsulated dolutegravir (DTG), an integrase strand transfer inhibitor, within nanoparticles made from cellulose acetate phthalate, a pH-sensitive polymer that intrinsically inhibits HIV-1 entry into its target cells (DTG-CAP-NPs) (72). Similarly to above, DTG-CAP-NPs were incorporated into a thermosensitive vaginal gel. Vaginal epithelial cells were able to take up DTG-CAP-NPs, where they persisted for up to 7 days with low cytotoxicity (72). These studies demonstrate the potential of nanoparticles for use in HIV-1 preventative strategies, including enhancing PrEP.

CONCLUSION

Here, we have reviewed the field of nanoparticle-based immunoengineered approaches toward an HIV-1 cure. We highlighted the potential and use of nanoparticles to facilitate and improve the delivery, bioavailability, and/or functionality of HAART, LRAs, vaccines, gene-editing approaches, and other therapeutic or preventative strategies. The innovative advances described herein demonstrate the potential of the field of nanoparticle-based immunoengineering in treating and preventing HIV-1.

AUTHOR CONTRIBUTIONS

AB, ES, and RF all participated in the writing and the preparation of the manuscript, and approved it for publication.

REFERENCES

1. Jordan A, Bisgrove D, Verdin E. HIV reproducibly establishes a latent infection after acute infection of T cells *in vitro*. *EMBO J.* (2003) 22:1868–77. doi: 10.1093/emboj/cdg188
2. Martinez Rivas CJ, Tarhini M, Badri W, Miladi K, Greige-Gerges H, Nazari QA, et al. Nanoprecipitation process: from encapsulation to drug delivery. *Int J Pharm.* (2017) 532:66–81. doi: 10.1016/j.ijpharm.2017.08.064
3. Fredenberg S, Wahlgren M, Reslow M, Axelsson A. The mechanisms of drug release in poly(lactic-co-glycolic acid)-based drug delivery systems–a review. *Int J Pharm.* (2011) 415:34–52. doi: 10.1016/j.ijpharm.2011.05.049
4. Wiemann B, Starnes CO. Coley's toxins, tumor necrosis factor and cancer research: a historical perspective. *Pharmacol Ther.* (1994) 64:529–64. doi: 10.1016/0163-7258(94)90023-X
5. Murphy CJ, Gole AM, Stone JW, Sisco PN, Alkilany AM, Goldsmith EC, et al. Gold nanoparticles in biology: beyond toxicity to cellular imaging. *Acc Chem Res.* (2008) 41:1721–30. doi: 10.1021/ar800035u
6. Wallet C, De Rovere M, Van Assche J, Daouad F, De Wit S, Gautier V, et al. Microglial cells: the main HIV-1 reservoir in the brain. *Front Cell Infect Microbiol.* (2019) 9:362. doi: 10.3389/fcimb.2019.00362
7. Chauveau L, Donahue DA, Monel B, Porrot F, Bruel T, Richard L, et al. HIV fusion in dendritic cells occurs mainly at the surface and is limited by low CD4 levels. *J Virol.* (2017) 91:e01248-17. doi: 10.1128/JVI.01248-17
8. Wu L, KewalRamani VN. Dendritic-cell interactions with HIV: infection and viral dissemination. *Nat Rev Immunol.* (2006) 6:859–68. doi: 10.1038/nri1960
9. Chesney M. Adherence to HAART regimens. *Aids Patient Care St.* (2003) 17:169–77. doi: 10.1089/108729103321619773
10. Sension MG. Long-Term suppression of HIV infection: benefits and limitations of current treatment options. *J Assoc Nurses AIDS Care.* (2007) 18(1 Suppl.):S2–10. doi: 10.1016/j.jana.2006.11.012
11. Margolis AM, Heverling H, Pham PA, Stolbach A. A review of the toxicity of HIV medications. *J Med Toxicol.* (2014) 10:26–39. doi: 10.1007/s13181-013-0325-8

12. Reeves DB, Duke ER, Wagner TA, Palmer SE, Spivak AM, Schiffer JT. A majority of HIV persistence during antiretroviral therapy is due to infected cell proliferation. *Nat Commun.* (2018) 9:4811. doi: 10.1038/s41467-018-06843-5
13. Richman DD, Margolis DM, Delaney M, Greene WC, Hazuda D, Pomerantz RJ. The challenge of finding a cure for HIV infection. *Science.* (2009) 323:1304–7. doi: 10.1126/science.1165706
14. Siliciano RF, Greene WC. HIV latency. *Cold Spring Harb Perspect Med.* (2011) 1:a007096. doi: 10.1101/cshperspect.a007096
15. Williams SA, Chen LF, Kwon H, Ruiz-Jarabo CM, Verdin E, Greene WC. NF-kappaB p50 promotes HIV latency through HDAC recruitment and repression of transcriptional initiation. *EMBO J.* (2006) 25:139–49. doi: 10.1038/sj.emboj.7600900
16. Dahabieh MS, Battivelli E, Verdin E. Understanding HIV latency: the road to an HIV cure. *Annu Rev Med.* (2015) 66:407–21. doi: 10.1146/annurev-med-092112-152941
17. Gupta RK, Abdul-Jawad S, McCoy LE, Mok HP, Peppa D, Salgado M, et al. HIV-1 remission following CCR5Delta32/Delta32 haematopoietic stem-cell transplantation. *Nature.* (2019) 568:244–8. doi: 10.1038/s41586-019-1027-4
18. Hutter G, Nowak D, Mossner M, Ganepola S, Mussig A, Allers K, et al. Long-term control of HIV by CCR5 Delta32/Delta32 stem-cell transplantation. *N Engl J Med.* (2009) 360:692–8. doi: 10.1056/NEJMoa0802905
19. Goldberg MS. Immunoengineering: how nanotechnology can enhance cancer immunotherapy. *Cell.* (2015) 161:201–4. doi: 10.1016/j.cell.2015.03.037
20. Delcassian D, Sattler S, Dunlop IE. T cell immunoengineering with advanced biomaterials. *Integr Biol (Camb).* (2017) 9:211–22. doi: 10.1039/c6ib00233a
21. Xie YQ, Wei L, Tang L. Immunoengineering with biomaterials for enhanced cancer immunotherapy. *Wiley Interdiscip Rev Nanomed Nanobiotechnol.* (2018) 10:e1506. doi: 10.1002/wnan.1506
22. Wang C, Xu L, Liang C, Xiang J, Peng R, Liu Z. Immunological responses triggered by photothermal therapy with carbon nanotubes in combination with anti-CTLA-4 therapy to inhibit cancer metastasis. *Adv Mater.* (2014) 26:8154–62. doi: 10.1002/adma.201402996
23. Chen Q, Xu L, Liang C, Wang C, Peng R, Liu Z. Photothermal therapy with immune-adjuvant nanoparticles together with checkpoint blockade for effective cancer immunotherapy. *Nat Commun.* (2016) 7:13193. doi: 10.1038/ncomms13193
24. Nam J, Son S, Ochyl LJ, Kuai R, Schwendeman A, Moon JJ. Chemo-photothermal therapy combination elicits anti-tumor immunity against advanced metastatic cancer. *Nat Commun.* (2018) 9:1074. doi: 10.1038/s41467-018-03473-9
25. Sweeney EE, Cano-Mejia J, Fernandes R. Photothermal therapy generates a thermal window of immunogenic cell death in neuroblastoma. *Small.* (2018) 14:e1800678. doi: 10.1002/smll.201800678
26. Cano-Mejia J, Bookstaver ML, Sweeney EE, Jewell CM, Fernandes R. Prussian blue nanoparticle-based antigenicity and adjuvanticity trigger robust antitumor immune responses against neuroblastoma. *Biomater Sci.* (2019) 7:1875–87. doi: 10.1039/C8BM01553H
27. Mamo T, Moseman EA, Kolishetti N, Salvador-Morales C, Shi J, Kuritzkes DR, et al. Emerging nanotechnology approaches for HIV/AIDS treatment and prevention. *Nanomedicine (Lond).* (2010) 5:269–85. doi: 10.2217/nnm.10.1
28. Victor OB. Nanoparticles and its implications in HIV/AIDS therapy. *Curr Drug Discov Technol.* (2019) 16:1. doi: 10.2174/1570163816666190620111652
29. Cao S, Woodrow KA. Nanotechnology approaches to eradicating HIV reservoirs. *Eur J Pharm Biopharm.* (2019) 138:48–63. doi: 10.1016/j.ejpb.2018.06.002
30. International Organization for Standardization (ISO). *Nanotechnologies — Vocabulary — Part 2: Nano-objects.* ISO/TS 80004-2:2015 (2015).
31. Blanco E, Shen H, Ferrari M. Principles of nanoparticle design for overcoming biological barriers to drug delivery. *Nat Biotechnol.* (2015) 33:941–51. doi: 10.1038/nbt.3330
32. Rao DA, Forrest ML, Alani AW, Kwon GS, Robinson JR. Biodegradable PLGA based nanoparticles for sustained regional lymphatic drug delivery. *J Pharm Sci.* (2010) 99:2018–31. doi: 10.1002/jps.21970
33. Vanhamel J, Bruggemans A, Debyser Z. Establishment of latent HIV-1 reservoirs: what do we really know? *J Virus Erad.* (2019) 5:3–9.
34. Pantaleo G, Graziosi C, Butini L, Pizzo PA, Schnittman SM, Kotler DP, et al. Lymphoid organs function as major reservoirs for human immunodeficiency virus. *Proc Natl Acad Sci USA.* (1991) 88:9838–42. doi: 10.1073/pnas.88.21.9838
35. Sinha R, Kim GJ, Nie S, Shin DM. Nanotechnology in cancer therapeutics: bioconjugated nanoparticles for drug delivery. *Mol Cancer Ther.* (2006) 5:1909–17. doi: 10.1158/1535-7163.MCT-06-0141
36. Reis CP, Neufeld RJ, Ribeiro AJ, Veiga F. Nanoencapsulation I. Methods for preparation of drug-loaded polymeric nanoparticles. *Nanomedicine.* (2006) 2:8–21. doi: 10.1016/j.nano.2005.12.003
37. Edagwa B, McMillan J, Sillman B, Gendelman HE. Long-acting slow effective release antiretroviral therapy. *Expert Opin Drug Deliv.* (2017) 14:1281–91. doi: 10.1080/17425247.2017.1288212
38. Gnanadhas DP, Dash PK, Sillman B, Bade AN, Lin Z, Palandri DL, et al. Autophagy facilitates macrophage depots of sustained-release nanoformulated antiretroviral drugs. *J Clin Invest.* (2017) 127:857–73. doi: 10.1172/JCI90025
39. Smith N, Bade AN, Soni D, Gautam N, Alnouti Y, Herskovitz J, et al. A long acting nanoformulated lamivudine ProTide. *Biomaterials.* (2019) 223:119476. doi: 10.1016/j.biomaterials.2019.119476
40. Guo D, Zhou T, Arainga M, Palandri D, Gautam N, Bronich T, et al. Creation of a long-acting nanoformulated 2',3'-dideoxy-3'-thiacytidine. *J Acquir Immune Defic Syndr.* (2017) 74:e75–e83. doi: 10.1097/QAI.0000000000001170
41. Freeling JP, Koehn J, Shu C, Sun J, Ho RJ. Long-acting three-drug combination anti-HIV nanoparticles enhance drug exposure in primate plasma and cells within lymph nodes and blood. *Aids.* (2014) 28:2625–7. doi: 10.1097/QAD.0000000000000421
42. Prathipati PK, Mandal S, Pon G, Vivekanandan R, Destache CJ. Pharmacokinetic and tissue distribution profile of long acting tenofovir alafenamide and elvitegravir loaded nanoparticles in humanized mice model. *Pharm Res.* (2017) 34:2749–55. doi: 10.1007/s11095-017-2255-7
43. Kumar P, Lakshmi YS, Kondapi AK. Triple drug combination of zidovudine, efavirenz and lamivudine loaded lactoferrin nanoparticles: an effective nano first-line regimen for HIV therapy. *Pharm Res.* (2017) 34:257–68. doi: 10.1007/s11095-016-2048-4
44. Cao S, Slack SD, Levy CN, Hughes SM, Jiang Y, Yogodzinski C, et al. Hybrid nanocarriers incorporating mechanistically distinct drugs for lymphatic $CD4^+$ T cell activation and HIV-1 latency reversal. *Sci Adv.* (2019) 5:eaav6322. doi: 10.1126/sciadv.aav6322
45. Battivelli E, Dahabieh MS, Abdel-Mohsen M, Svensson JP, Da Silva IT, Cohn LB, et al. Distinct chromatin functional states correlate with HIV latency reactivation in infected primary $CD4^+$ T cells. *Elife.* (2018) 7:e34655. doi: 10.7554/eLife.34655
46. Jayant RD, Atluri VS, Agudelo M, Sagar V, Kaushik A, Nair M. Sustained-release nanoART formulation for the treatment of neuroAIDS. *Int J Nanomed.* (2015) 10:1077–93. doi: 10.2147/IJN.S76517
47. Tang X, Liang Y, Liu X, Zhou S, Liu L, Zhang F, et al. PLGA-PEG nanoparticles coated with anti-CD45RO and loaded with HDAC plus protease inhibitors activate latent HIV and inhibit viral spread. *Nanoscale Res Lett.* (2015) 10:413. doi: 10.1186/s11671-015-1112-z
48. Rostami H, Ebtekar M, Ardestani MS, Yazdi MH, Mahdavi M. Co-utilization of a TLR5 agonist and nano-formulation of HIV-1 vaccine candidate leads to increased vaccine immunogenicity and decreased immunogenic dose: a preliminary study. *Immunol Lett.* (2017) 187:19–26. doi: 10.1016/j.imlet.2017.05.002
49. Tokatlian T, Read BJ, Jones CA, Kulp DW, Menis S, Chang JYH, et al. Innate immune recognition of glycans targets HIV nanoparticle immunogens to germinal centers. *Science.* (2019) 363:649–54. doi: 10.1126/science.aat9120
50. Lori F, Calarota SA, Lisziewicz J. Nanochemistry-based immunotherapy for HIV-1. *Curr Med Chem.* (2007) 14:1911–9. doi: 10.2174/092986707781368513

51. Jardine JG, Kulp DW, Havenar-Daughton C, Sarkar A, Briney B, Sok D, et al. HIV-1 broadly neutralizing antibody precursor B cells revealed by germline-targeting immunogen. *Science.* (2016) 351:1458–63. doi: 10.1126/science.aad9195
52. Martinez-Murillo P, Tran K, Guenaga J, Lindgren G, Adori M, Feng Y, et al. Particulate array of well-ordered HIV clade C env trimers elicits neutralizing antibodies that display a unique V2 cap approach. *Immunity.* (2017) 46:804–17.e7. doi: 10.1016/j.immuni.2017.04.021
53. Sliepen K, Han BW, Bontjer I, Mooij P, Garces F, Behrens AJ, et al. Structure and immunogenicity of a stabilized HIV-1 envelope trimer based on a group-M consensus sequence. *Nat Commun.* (2019) 10:2355. doi: 10.1038/s41467-019-10262-5
54. Brouwer PJM, Antanasijevic A, Berndsen Z, Yasmeen A, Fiala B, Bijl TPL, et al. Enhancing and shaping the immunogenicity of native-like HIV-1 envelope trimers with a two-component protein nanoparticle. *Nat Commun.* (2019) 10:4272. doi: 10.1038/s41467-019-12080-1
55. Dubrovskaya V, Tran K, Ozorowski G, Guenaga J, Wilson R, Bale S, et al. Vaccination with glycan-modified HIV NFL envelope trimer-liposomes elicits broadly neutralizing antibodies to multiple sites of vulnerability. *Immunity.* (2019) 51:915–29.e7. doi: 10.1016/j.immuni.2019.10.008
56. He L, de Val N, Morris CD, Vora N, Thinnes TC, Kong L, et al. Presenting native-like trimeric HIV-1 antigens with self-assembling nanoparticles. *Nat Commun.* (2016) 7:12041. doi: 10.1038/ncomms12041
57. Lara HH, Ayala-Nunez NV, Ixtepan-Turrent L, Rodriguez-Padilla C. Mode of antiviral action of silver nanoparticles against HIV-1. *J Nanobiotechnology.* (2010) 8:1. doi: 10.1186/1477-3155-8-1
58. Sheik DA, Chamberlain JM, Brooks L, Clark M, Kim YH, Leriche G, et al. Hydrophobic nanoparticles reduce the β-sheet content of SEVI amyloid fibrils and inhibit SEVI-enhanced HIV infectivity. *Langmuir.* (2017) 33:2596–602. doi: 10.1021/acs.langmuir.6b04295
59. Wei X, Zhang G, Ran D, Krishnan N, Fang RH, Gao W, et al. T-cell-mimicking nanoparticles can neutralize HIV infectivity. *Adv Mater.* (2018) 30:e1802233. doi: 10.1002/adma.201802233
60. Nahui Palomino RA, Vanpouille C, Laghi L, Parolin C, Melikov K, Backlund P, et al. Extracellular vesicles from symbiotic vaginal lactobacilli inhibit HIV-1 infection of human tissues. *Nat Commun.* (2019) 10:5656. doi: 10.1038/s41467-019-13468-9
61. Welch JL, Kaddour H, Winchester L, Fletcher CV, Stapleton JT, Okeoma CM. Semen extracellular vesicles from HIV-1-infected individuals inhibit HIV-1 replication *in vitro*, and extracellular vesicles carry antiretroviral drugs *in vivo*. *J Acquir Immune Defic Syndr.* (2020) 83:90–8. doi: 10.1097/QAI.0000000000002233
62. Shahbazi R, Sghia-Hughes G, Reid JL, Kubek S, Haworth KG, Humbert O, et al. Targeted homology-directed repair in blood stem and progenitor cells with CRISPR nanoformulations. *Nat Mater.* (2019) 18:1124–32. doi: 10.1038/s41563-019-0385-5
63. Dash PK, Kaminski R, Bella R, Su H, Mathews S, Ahooyi TM, et al. Sequential LASER ART and CRISPR treatments eliminate HIV-1 in a subset of infected humanized mice. *Nat Commun.* (2019) 10:2753. doi: 10.1038/s41467-019-10366-y
64. Sweeney EEBP, Balakrishnan PB, Powell AB, Bowen A, Sarabia I, Burga RA, et al. PLGA nanodepots co-encapsulating prostratin and anti-CD25 enhance primary natural killer cell antiviral and antitumor function. *Nano Res.* (2020) 13:736–44. doi: 10.1007/s12274-020-2684-1
65. Jones RB, Mueller S, Kumari S, Vrbanac V, Genel S, Tager AM, et al. Antigen recognition-triggered drug delivery mediated by nanocapsule-functionalized cytotoxic T-cells. *Biomaterials.* (2017) 117:44–53. doi: 10.1016/j.biomaterials.2016.11.048
66. Aroh C, Wang ZH, Dobbs N, Luo M, Chen ZJ, Gao JM, et al. Innate immune activation by cGMP-AMP nanoparticles leads to potent and long-acting antiretroviral response against HIV-1. *J Immunol.* (2017) 199:3840–8. doi: 10.4049/jimmunol.1700972
67. Iannazzo D, Pistone A, Ferro S, De Luca L, Monforte AM, Romeo R, et al. Graphene quantum dots based systems as HIV inhibitors. *Bioconjugate Chem.* (2018) 29:3084–93. doi: 10.1021/acs.bioconjchem.8b00448
68. Roy U, Drozd V, Durygin A, Rodriguez J, Barber P, Atluri V, et al. Characterization of nanodiamond-based anti-HIV drug delivery to the brain. *Sci Rep.* (2018) 8:1063. doi: 10.1038/s41598-017-16703-9
69. Garrido C, Simpson CA, Dahl NP, Bresee J, Whitehead DC, Lindsey EA, et al. Gold nanoparticles to improve HIV drug delivery. *Future Med Chem.* (2015) 7:1097–107. doi: 10.4155/fmc.15.57
70. Mandal S, Belshan M, Holec A, Zhou Y, Destache CJ. An enhanced emtricitabine-loaded long-acting nanoformulation for prevention or treatment of HIV infection. *Antimicrob Agents Chemother.* (2017) 61:e01475-16. doi: 10.1128/AAC.01475-16
71. Destache CJ, Mandal S, Yuan Z, Kang GB, Date AA, Lu WX, et al. Topical tenofovir disoproxil fumarate nanoparticles prevent HIV-1 vaginal transmission in a humanized mouse model. *Antimicrob Agents Chemother.* (2016) 60:3633–9. doi: 10.1128/AAC.00450-16
72. Mandal S, Khandalavala K, Pham R, Bruck P, Varghese M, Kochvar A, et al. Cellulose acetate phthalate and antiretroviral nanoparticle fabrications for HIV pre-exposure prophylaxis. *Polymers-Basel.* (2017) 9:423–40. doi: 10.3390/polym9090423
73. Deeks SG. HIV: shock and kill. *Nature.* (2012) 487:439–40. doi: 10.1038/487439a
74. Spivak AM, Planelles V. Novel latency reversal agents for HIV-1 cure. *Annu Rev Med.* (2018) 69:421–36. doi: 10.1146/annurev-med-052716-031710
75. Qatsha KA, Rudolph C, Marme D, Schachtele C, May WS. Go-6976, a selective inhibitor of protein-kinase-C, is a potent antagonist of human immunodeficiency virus-1 induction from latent low-level-producing reservoir cells-*in vitro*. *Proc Natl Acad Sci USA.* (1993) 90:4674–8. doi: 10.1073/pnas.90.10.4674
76. Kovochich M, Marsden MD, Zack JA. Activation of latent HIV using drug-loaded nanoparticles. *PLoS ONE.* (2011) 6:e18270. doi: 10.1371/journal.pone.0018270
77. Buchbinder SP, Mehrotra DV, Duerr A, Fitzgerald DW, Mogg R, Li D, et al. Efficacy assessment of a cell-mediated immunity HIV-1 vaccine (the step study): a double-blind, randomised, placebo-controlled, test-of-concept trial. *Lancet.* (2008) 372:1881–93. doi: 10.1016/S0140-6736(08)61591-3
78. Haynes BF, Gilbert PB, McElrath MJ, Zolla-Pazner S, Tomaras GD, Alam SM, et al. Immune-correlates analysis of an HIV-1 vaccine efficacy trial. *N Engl J Med.* (2012) 366:1275–86.
79. Ada GL. The ideal vaccine. *World J Microb Biot.* (1991) 7:105–9. doi: 10.1007/BF00328978
80. Zaman M, Good MF, Toth I. Nanovaccines and their mode of action. *Methods.* (2013) 60:226–31. doi: 10.1016/j.ymeth.2013.04.014
81. Lopez-Sagaseta J, Malito E, Rappuoli R, Bottomley MJ. Self-assembling protein nanoparticles in the design of vaccines. *Comput Struct Biotec.* (2016) 14:58–68. doi: 10.1016/j.csbj.2015.11.001
82. Huleatt JW, Jacobs AR, Tang J, Desai P, Kopp EB, Huang Y, et al. Vaccination with recombinant fusion proteins incorporating toll-like receptor ligands induces rapid cellular and humoral immunity. *Vaccine.* (2007) 25:763–75. doi: 10.1016/j.vaccine.2006.08.013
83. Rodriguez B, Asmuth DM, Matining RM, Spritzler J, Jacobson JM, Mailliard RB, et al. Safety, tolerability, and immunogenicity of repeated doses of dermavir, a candidate therapeutic HIV vaccine, in HIV-infected patients receiving combination antiretroviral therapy: results of the ACTG 5176 trial. *J Acquir Immune Defic Syndr.* (2013) 64:351–9. doi: 10.1097/QAI.0b013e3182a99590
84. Ren RX, Yin SW, Lai BL, Ma LZ, Wen JY, Zhang XX, et al. Myricetin antagonizes semen-derived enhancer of viral infection (SEVI) formation and influences its infection-enhancing activity. *Retrovirology.* (2018) 15:49. doi: 10.1186/s12977-018-0432-3
85. Roan NR, Munch J, Arhel N, Mothes W, Neidleman J, Kobayashi A, et al. The cationic properties of SEVI underlie its ability to enhance human immunodeficiency virus infection. *J Virol.* (2009) 83:73–80. doi: 10.1128/JVI.01366-08
86. Capule CC, Yang J. Enzyme-linked immunosorbent assay-based method to quantify the association of small molecules with aggregated amyloid peptides. *Anal Chem.* (2012) 84:1786–91. doi: 10.1021/ac2030859
87. Giacomelli CE, Norde W. Conformational changes of the amyloid β-peptide (1-40) adsorbed on solid surfaces. *Macromol Biosci.* (2005) 5:401–7. doi: 10.1002/mabi.200400189
88. Moores B, Drolle E, Attwood SJ, Simons J, Leonenko Z. Effect of surfaces on amyloid fibril formation. *PLoS ONE.* (2011) 6:e25954. doi: 10.1371/journal.pone.0025954

89. Hu CM, Zhang L, Aryal S, Cheung C, Fang RH, Zhang L. Erythrocyte membrane-camouflaged polymeric nanoparticles as a biomimetic delivery platform. *Proc Natl Acad Sci USA*. (2011) 108:10980–5. doi: 10.1073/pnas.1106634108
90. Campbell EM, Hope TJ. HIV-1 capsid: the multifaceted key player in HIV-1 infection. *Nat Rev Microbiol.* (2015) 13:471–83. doi: 10.1038/nrmicro3503
91. Yanez-Mo M, Siljander PR, Andreu Z, Zavec AB, Borras FE, Buzas EI, et al. Biological properties of extracellular vesicles and their physiological functions. *J Extracell Vesicles.* (2015) 4:27066. doi: 10.3402/jev.v4.27066
92. Ma Y, Zhang L, Huang X. Genome modification by CRISPR/Cas9. *FEBS J.* (2014) 281:5186–93. doi: 10.1111/febs.13110
93. Lino CA, Harper JC, Carney JP, Timlin JA. Delivering CRISPR: a review of the challenges and approaches. *Drug Deliv.* (2018) 25:1234–57. doi: 10.1080/10717544.2018.1474964
94. Li C, Guan X, Du T, Jin W, Wu B, Liu Y, et al. Inhibition of HIV-1 infection of primary $CD4^+$ T-cells by gene editing of CCR5 using adenovirus-delivered CRISPR/Cas9. *J Gen Virol.* (2015) 96:2381–93. doi: 10.1099/vir.0.000139
95. Xu L, Yang H, Gao Y, Chen Z, Xie L, Liu Y, et al. CRISPR/Cas9-mediated CCR5 ablation in human hematopoietic stem/progenitor cells confers HIV-1 resistance *in vivo. Mol Ther.* (2017) 25:1782–9. doi: 10.1016/j.ymthe.2017.04.027
96. Lee B, Lee K, Panda S, Gonzales-Rojas R, Chong A, Bugay V, et al. Nanoparticle delivery of CRISPR into the brain rescues a mouse model of fragile X syndrome from exaggerated repetitive behaviours. *Nat Biomed Eng.* (2018) 2:497–507. doi: 10.1038/s41551-018-0252-8
97. Lopalco L. CCR5: from natural resistance to a new anti-HIV strategy. *Viruses.* (2010) 2:574–600. doi: 10.3390/v2020574
98. Lam S, Bollard C. T-cell therapies for HIV. *Immunotherapy.* (2013) 5:407–14. doi: 10.2217/imt.13.23
99. Patel S, Jones RB, Nixon DF, Bollard CM. T-cell therapies for HIV: preclinical successes and current clinical strategies. *Cytotherapy.* (2016) 18:931–42. doi: 10.1016/j.jcyt.2016.04.007
100. Sung JA, Patel S, Clohosey ML, Roesch L, Tripic T, Kuruc JD, et al. HIV-Specific, ex vivo expanded T cell therapy: feasibility, safety, and efficacy in ART-suppressed HIV-infected individuals. *Mol Ther.* (2018) 26:2496–506. doi: 10.1016/j.ymthe.2018.08.015
101. Yan N, Regalado-Magdos AD, Stiggelbout B, Lee-Kirsch MA, Lieberman J. The cytosolic exonuclease TREX1 inhibits the innate immune response to human immunodeficiency virus type 1. *Nat Immunol.* (2010) 11:1005–U53. doi: 10.1038/ni.1941
102. Gao DX, Wu JX, Wu YT, Du FH, Aroh C, Yan N, et al. Cyclic GMP-AMP synthase is an innate immune sensor of HIV and other retroviruses. *Science.* (2013) 341:903–6. doi: 10.1126/science.1240933
103. Mansur HS. Quantum dots and nanocomposites. *Wires Nanomed Nanobi.* (2010) 2:113–29. doi: 10.1002/wnan.78
104. Matea CT, Mocan T, Tabaran F, Pop T, Mosteanu O, Puia C, et al. Quantum dots in imaging, drug delivery and sensor applications. *Int J Nanomed.* (2017) 12:5421–31. doi: 10.2147/IJN.S138624
105. Garrido C, Margolis DM. Translational challenges in targeting latent HIV infection and the CNS reservoir problem. *J Neurovirol.* (2015) 21:222–6. doi: 10.1007/s13365-014-0269-z
106. Anderson PL, Glidden DV, Liu A, Buchbinder S, Lama JR, Guanira JV, et al. Emtricitabine-tenofovir concentrations and pre-exposure prophylaxis efficacy in men who have sex with men. *Sci Trans Med.* (2012) 4:151ra125. doi: 10.1126/scitranslmed.3004006
107. Valade E, Treluyer JM, Bouazza N, Ghosn J, Foissac F, Benaboud S, et al. Population pharmacokinetics of emtricitabine in HIV-1-infected adult patients. *Antimicrob Agents Chemother.* (2014) 58:2256–61. doi: 10.1128/AAC.02058-13

6

Modeling the Function of TATA Box Binding Protein in Transcriptional Changes Induced by HIV-1 Tat in Innate Immune Cells and the Effect of Methamphetamine Exposure

*Ryan Tjitro[1], Lee A. Campbell[2], Liana Basova[1,3], Jessica Johnson[1], Julia A. Najera[1], Alexander Lindsey[3] and Maria Cecilia Garibaldi Marcondes[1,3]**

[1] Department of Neurosciences, The Scripps Research Institute, La Jolla, CA, United States, [2] LAC Intramural Research Program, National Institute on Drug Abuse, Baltimore, MD, United States, [3] San Diego Biomedical Research Institute, San Diego, CA, United States

Correspondence:
Maria Cecilia Garibaldi Marcondes
cmarcondes@SDBRI.org

Innate immune cells are targets of HIV-1 infection in the Central Nervous System (CNS), generating neurological deficits. Infected individuals with substance use disorders as co-morbidities, are more likely to have aggravated neurological disorders, higher CNS viral load and inflammation. Methamphetamine (Meth) is an addictive stimulant drug, commonly among HIV+ individuals. The molecular basis of HIV direct effects and its interactions with Meth in host response, at the gene promoter level, are not well understood. The main HIV-1 peptide acting on transcription is the transactivator of transcription (Tat), which promotes replication by recruiting a Tata-box binding protein (TBP) to the virus long-terminal repeat (LTR). We tested the hypothesis that Tat can stimulate host gene expression through its ability to increase TBP, and thus promoting its binding to promoters that bear Tata-box binding motifs. Genes with Tata-box domains are mainly inducible, early response, and involved in inflammation, regulation and metabolism, relevant in HIV pathogenesis. We also tested whether Tat and Meth interact to trigger the expression of Tata-box bearing genes. The THP1 macrophage cell line is a well characterized innate immune cell system for studying signal transduction in inflammation. These cells are responsive to Tat, as well as to Meth, by recruiting RNA Polymerase (RNA Pol) to inflammatory gene promoters, within 15 min of stimulation (1). THP-1 cells, including their genetically engineered derivatives, represent valuable tools for investigating monocyte structure and function in both health and disease, as a consistent system (2). When differentiated, they mimic several aspects of the response of macrophages, and innate immune cells that are the main HIV-1 targets within the Central Nervous System (CNS). THP1 cells have been used to characterize the impact of Meth and resulting neurotransmitters on HIV entry (1), mimicking the CNS micro-environment. Integrative consensus sequence analysis in genes with enriched RNA Pol, revealed that TBP was a major transcription factor in Tat stimulation, while the co-incubation with Meth shifted usage to a distinct and diversified pattern. For validating these findings, we engineered a THP1 clone to be deficient in the expression of all major

TBP splice variants, and tested its response to Tat stimulation, in the presence or absence of Meth. Transcriptional patterns in TBP-sufficient and deficient clones confirmed TBP as a dominant transcription factor in Tat stimulation, capable of inducing genes with no constitutive expression. However, in the presence of Meth, TBP was no longer necessary to activate the same genes, suggesting promoter plasticity. These findings demonstrate TBP as mechanism of host-response activation by HIV-1 Tat, and suggest that promoter plasticity is a challenge imposed by co-morbid factors such as stimulant drug addiction. This may be one mechanism responsible for limited efficacy of therapeutic approaches in HIV+ Meth abusers.

Keywords: HIV, Tat, Methamphetamine, TATA-box, TATA-box binding peptide, Crispr/Cas9, macrophages, inflammation

INTRODUCTION

The infection with the Human Immunodeficiency Virus (HIV) triggers inflammatory pathogeneses in several tissues (3), including in the Central Nervous System (CNS) (4). Inflammation in the brain and cognitive deficits can be significantly aggravated upon the co-morbid use of addictive substances, such as Methamphetamine (Meth), which impair the success of antiretroviral therapies and increase viral load specifically in the brain (5, 6). The Meth-induced aggravation of HIV—induced CNS deficits, inflammatory response, and brain viral load, have been replicated in non-human primate models of neuroHIV (5, 7, 8). Of the HIV-1 peptides, the trans-activator of transcription (Tat) is the only one that is secreted across the plasma membrane (9–12), affecting neighboring cell types. *In vivo*, HIV-Tat is linked to impaired learning and memory, and gray matter deficits (13, 14), suggesting its involvement in HIV-associated neurological disorders (HAND). In a mouse model of neuroHIV, the induction of Tat in CNS glial cells enhances behaviors associated with Meth exposure, while contributing to changes in microglial activation and in the expression of neurotransmitter receptors (15).

In the brain, innate immune cells, microglia and macrophages, are targets of HIV infection. The main role of the HIV Tat peptide is maintaining viral transcription by activating the viral promoter, located within the 5′ long terminal repeat (LTR) of the integrated viral genome. In that process, the virus gains the ability to hijack the host cell RNA polymerase II (RNA Pol II) machinery for initiating viral transcription. In previous experiments, we observed that the SIV infection in rhesus macaques, which is a model of neuroHIV, causes a strong upregulation of TATA-box binding peptide (TBP) and components of the transcription initiation complex in brain microglia, suggesting that a mechanism of gene transcription that involves TATA box may be stimulated by the infection.

HIV-1 proviral transcription starts with the binding of cellular factors, such as NF-κB and Sp1, as well as the TATA box binding protein (TBP), which is a key component for recruiting RNA Pol II to the LTR. This complex allows the production of viral transcripts, which are then spliced and translated. Epigenetic and other limiting host factors, as well as the level of cellular activation, can potentially regulate such process. Tat binds to the trans-activator response (TAR) element hairpin at the 5′ end of viral RNA transcripts (16–19), and to the apical loop, to which the transcriptional elongation factor pTEFb binds in a Tat-dependent manner (20, 21). Upon TAR binding, the kinase component of pTEFb, cyclin-dependent kinase 9 (CDK9), can phosphorylate the C-terminal domain of RNA Pol II (21, 22). The pTEFb also directs the recruitment of TATA box binding protein (TBP) to the LTR, stimulating the assembly of new transcription complexes (23). Core promoter elements participate in the initiation factor TFIID complex, where TBP works as an anchor for TBP-associated factors (TAFs) 4–12 (24). The TFIID complex then makes contact with acidic activator proteins such as Sp1 and the initiator, while TBP recognizes the TATA box. Thus, TBP is a key element in the ability of Tat to recruit the host transcriptional machinery in favor of viral transcription.

The activation of the LTR-directed gene expression by Tat has been observed in CNS-derived cells, and in astrocytic glial cell lines (25). Importantly, it has been demonstrated that this can happen in the absence of a TAR element (25), suggesting that alternative mechanisms may exist. Importantly, HIV Tat can strongly upregulate inflammatory cytokines in the brain, *per se* mimicking aspects of the inflammatory outcomes observed in HIV infection (26, 27). In addition, it has been demonstrated that the ability of Tat to initiate transcription of heterologous genes through the TATA-box element can happen in the absence of any HIV-1 sequence, through mechanisms that are similar to DNA sequence-specific transcription factors (28, 29). This suggests that HIV-1 Tat may have the ability to enhance genes that present a TATA-box promoter element. While the HIV Tat peptide *per se* has the ability to stimulate a diversity of genes, both *in vivo* (15, 26, 27, 30), and *in vitro* (31–37), the contribution of the TATA-box promoter element to upregulated heterologous transcripts has not been examined.

The TATA box is the most well-studied core promoter element. The canonical TATA-box sequence, TATAAA, may be variable in natural promoters (38, 39). Methodologies to estimate the frequency of TATA box-containing promoters also vary. As a result, there is a wide-range of estimates of how many genes have a Tata-box promoter motif [revised by (40)]. It is most accepted that the TATA-containing promoters make up only 10–16% of the genes read by RNA Pol II, of which only 30% contain the canonical TATA box (41). Systematic analysis of genes that bear this promoter element has pointed to specific biological processes, associated to organogenesis and morphogenesis, with an impact in early development, but also has found a second largest contribution to responses to stimulus and to stress, as well as to defense, supporting the role of TATA-box mediated transcription in the elevation of early-response, immune and inflammatory genes. TATA-less promoters, on the other hand, tend to be involved in basic biological maintenance processes, or be constitutively expressed (40, 42).

Here, we have examined the hypothesis that the HIV-1 Tat protein has the property of increasing inflammatory cytokines in innate immune cells through favoring a TATA box-supported mechanism, and that this mechanism may be enhanced by Meth exposure. Using the THP1 innate immune cell line system, we show evidence that the TATA box-binding transcription factor TBP is increased by HIV-1 Tat, along with the recruitment of RNA PolII to promoters of genes that bear the TATA-box promoter. We also show that this effect is enhanced when HIV-1 Tat is combined with Meth.

The lack of TAR in host gene promoters argues against a direct interaction between TBP and Tat. Yet, binding of HIV Tat to the host chromatin has been described in T cells (43), where it functions through master transcriptional regulators bound at promoters and enhancers, rather than through cellular "TAR-like" motifs, to both activate and repress gene sets sharing common functional annotations (44). The functional interaction between HIV-1 Tat and TBP has been proposed in different models (29, 45, 46). In our system, we have not tested whether Tat plays a role at bridging TBP and its binding motifs, or whether Tat just activates TBP as major transcription factor in the innate immune environment. However, we have found evidence that Tat is able to translocate to the nucleus soon after cell exposure.

We have developed a strategy to test the hypothesis of TBP as a major transcription factor in the activation of TATA-box-bearing inflammatory genes by HIV Tat *in vitro*, by engineering a THP1 cell line with impaired transcription of TBP dominant splice variants. As a result, we produced a human innate immune cell line with a deficient expression of TBP protein. In that cell line, we have found that TBP was critical for the upregulation of genes stimulated by HIV Tat, including inflammatory molecules. Yet, in the presence of Meth, alternative transcriptional factors positively enhanced a significant fraction of genes with TATA box motifs, bypassing the TBP disruption.

Our findings demonstrate that TBP is indeed a critical transcription factor in Tat-induced host responses that can result in pathogenesis, but co-morbidities such as the stimulant drug Meth, can increase the transcriptional complexity and promoter plasticity, downgrading the central role of TBP in inflammation.

MATERIALS AND METHODS

THP1 Cell Culture

THP-1 cells were obtained from ATCC (TIB-202). They were maintained in RPMI 1640 containing 2 mM glutamine; 10 mM HEPES; 1 mM sodium pyruvate; 4.5 g/L glucose; 1.5 g/L sodium bicarbonate; 0.05 mM beta2 mercaptoethanol, as well as 10% heat inactivated fetal bovine serum (Hyclone), and 100 ug/ml Pen/Strep.

In vitro Treatments With HIV-1 Tat and With Meth

For treatments, the THP1 cells were plated at 2×10^6 cells/well in 12 well plates, containing 2 ml per well. The HIV-1 IIIB Tat Recombinant Protein (MW: 14,000) was obtained from the NIH AIDS Reagent Program. The doses used were 1–100 ng/ml for Western Blots, and 10 ng/ml for all the other assays. Meth was used at 60 μM, following previously optimized protocols, and for mimicking abuse concentrations in plasma (47). The cells were treated with either Vehicle, HIV-1 Tat, Meth, or HIV-1 Tat and Meth. The concentrations of Tat in culture were 1, 10, and 100 ng/ml. The concentrations of Meth were 30 μM, 60 μM (shown in Figures), and 120 μM, which produced similar results regarding the lack of TBP induction. The cells were then harvested 15 min after exposure for ChIP assays, and 2 h for Western blots, RNA-seq and validations. These time points were selected following a time-course that demonstrated that epigenetic events that result directly from Tat and/or Meth, and not from factors produced by the cells as a result from the stimulation, are detectable in 15 min. Yet, a 2 h period is necessary for confirming productive events at the transcriptional and protein level. All experiments were performed at least 3 times, in triplicate, otherwise stated in the figure legend.

Western Blots

The cells treated as described were centrifuged at 2,500 g for 5 min, and the pellets were washed twice in PBS, and in 0.5% Triton X buffer, for isolation of nuclear fraction, before being resuspended in RIPA buffer (Thermofisher), added 1 mini tablet Complete (Roche protease inhibitors) for protein extraction. Western blots for detection of TBP and TAF9 were performed by loading 20 μg of whole cell lysates and 5 μl of PageRuler Plus Prestained Protein Ladder (Thermofisher) per well, onto a Mini-Protean TGX 4–20% pre-cast gel (Biorad). Proteins were transferred to a nitrocellulose membrane using a G2 Blotter, and blocked with 5% Casein in TBST for 1 h at room temperature. The N-terminus of the TATA binding protein (TBP) was detected at 36–38 kD using a TBP monoclonal antibody (1TBP18/ MA1-189) at a dilution of 1:1,000. TATA box associated factor 9 (TAF9) was detected at ~20 kD using a polyclonal antibody (PA5-40919), at 1:1,000. Both antibodies were incubated overnight at 4oC on a rocking platform, followed by a Goat anti-Mouse IgG (H+L) HRP conjugate (Cell Signaling) for 1 h at room temperature. Chemiluminescent detection was performed using SuperSignal Pico substrate (Thermofisher).

TBP and Tat Nuclear Translocation

The THP1 cells were brought to the concentration of 10^6/ml and stimulated with 50 nM of phorbol-12-myristate-13-acetate (PMA) for 24 h for differentiation, prior to the stimulation with Meth (30 or 60 μM), and/or HIV Tat (10 ng/ml). The cells were fixed with 4% paraformaldehyde, 5, 15, 30, and 60 min following stimulation, and then were washed with PBS. The wells were then treated with PBS containing 0.1% Triton

X-100 for 20 min at room temperature, rinsed 3 times with PBS, and then blocked with 5 g/l Casein (Sigma Aldrich) in PBS, containing 0.5 g/l Thimerosal (Sigma Aldrich) for 1 h at room temperature. The primary antibody against TBP was a rabbit polyclonal (HPA049805, Sigma Aldrich), and the antibody anti-Tat peptide was obtained through the NIH AIDS Reagent Program, Division of AIDS, NIAID, NIH: Anti-HIV-1 Tat Monoclonal (15.1) from NIAID, DAIDS (cat# 1974). Both antibodies were diluted in blocking solution, and then placed overnight, at 4°C, with gentle rotation. Then cells were rinsed 3 times for 10 min with 1% blocking solution in PBS, containing 0.1% Triton-X, followed by incubation with a secondary AlexaFluor 647-labeled anti-rabbit or anti-mouse IgG (Thermo Fisher Scientific), for 2 h at room temperature, in the dark. After rinsing, 4′, 6-Diamidino-2-Phenylindole, Dihydrochloride (DAPI) was diluted to 300 ng/ml in 1% blocking solution for 2 min, in the dark. Cells were rinsed and maintained in PBS, and observed in a Nikon A1R laser-scanning confocal mounted onto a Nikon inverted Ti-E scope (Nikon, Melville, NY), and with a 20x PlanApo objective, 0.8NA (Nikon) and Images were acquired using a NIS-Elements C software (Nikon). Fluorescence intensity was normalized against background (secondary antibody only). Image analysis was performed in Fiji/ImageJ (National Institute of Health, USA). For that, tiff image files from separate channels were opened, transformed into 32-bit images, and manually thresholded to identify DAPI nuclei, and stained cells. A binary mask was obtained from the negative thresholded DAPI image and subtrated from the total transcription factor stained area. The translocation index was calculated as percentage of the total transcription factor stained measurement values that is co-localized within the nuclear area, and derived from the difference between total and nuclear staining. The colocalization was further confirmed in calculated images where 32-bit thresholded channels were averaged.

Fixation for Chromatin Immunoprecipitation

The cells were fixed with a 1.1% Formaldehyde (Sigma Aldrich F-8775), and molecular grade 0.01 M NaCl, 0.1 mM EDTA pH 8, 50 mM HEPES pH 7.9, in H_2O. The plate was then agitated on a titer plate shaker for exactly 15 min at room temperature. The fixation was then interrupted with 125 mM Glycine (Sigma Aldrich G-7403). The samples were let set at room temperature for 5 min. After the glycine incubation, the cells were transferred to conical 15 ml tubes and kept on ice for the remainder of the procedure. The tubes were centrifuge at 800 × g at 4°C for 10 min, the supernatants were removed and the cells were resuspended in 10 ml ice-cold PBS-Igepal (PBS containing 0.5% Igepal CA-630 (Sigma Aldrich I-8896) per tube, by pipetting up and down. The tubes were centrifuged again as before, and pellets were again resuspended in 10 ml PBS-Igepal. Then, 100 μl from a PMSF stock (100 mM in ethanol) was added to each tube for a final concentration of 1 mM. The tubes were centrifuged a third time to pellet the cells, and the supernatant was completely removed from cell pellets. The pellets were snap-frozen on dry ice and store at −80°C, until further procedures. The pellets were sonicated and the DNA sheared to an average length of 300–500 bp. Genomic DNA (input) was prepared by treating aliquots of chromatin with RNase, proteinase K, and heat (65°C) to reverse cross-linking, followed by phenol and chloroform extractions and ethanol precipitation. Pellets were resuspended in 10 mM Tris, 1 mM EDTA, and the resulting DNA was quantified on a Nanodrop spectrophotometer (Thermo Fisher Scientific, Chicago, IL). Results were used to calculate the total chromatin yield.

Chromatin Immunoprecipitation (ChIP) of RNA Pol II

RNA Pol II ChIP reactions were performed using 30 μg of human THP1 cell chromatin and 4 μg of antibody anti-RNA Pol II (Abcam, ab5095). Positive control primers (b-Actin and GAPDH) as well as negative control primer pairs were used to amplify regions in a gene desert on chromosome 12 and 4 (Untr12, Untr4) by qRT-PCR. Signals for RNA Pol II were strong, with enrichments of the best positive control signal over background up to 99-fold. For the library generation and sequencing, 50-nt sequence reads identified using Illumina's Hi-Seq, were mapped to the genome using the BWA algorithm with default settings. Alignment information to Human Hg19 for each read was stored in BAM format. Only reads that passed the purity filter, aligned with no more than 2 mismatches, and mapped uniquely to the genome were used in the subsequent analysis. Duplicate reads were removed. Since the 5′-ends of the aligned reads (= "tags") represent the end of ChIP/IP-fragments, the tags were extended *in silico* (using Active Motif software) at their 3′- ends to a length of 150–250 bp. To estimate the density, the genome was divided into 32-nt bins and the number of fragments in each bin was determined, to provide a "signal map"; histograms of fragment densities were stored in both a BAR file, for viewing in Integrated Genome Browser (IGB), and bigWig file, uploaded to the UCSC Genome Browser. BAR/bigWig files also provide the peak metrics in the Active Motif analysis program as described below. Intervals, describing genomic regions with local enrichments in tag numbers, were defined by the chromosome number, a start and end coordinates. SICER (48) was used to study RNA polymerase II binding to extended regions in the genome, by looking for significant enrichments in the ChIP/IP data file when compared to the Input data file (random background), and also for examining transcription factor binding sites using TRANSFAC Match weight matrix (49, 50). Peaks and false positives were estimated by thresholding of the BAR files. In the default analysis, the tag number of all samples is reduced (by random sampling) to the number of tags present in the smallest sample. Only Input/IgG control peaks that overlapped with Intervals in the ChIP/IP data were used in the analysis. After defining the Intervals and Active Regions, their genomic locations, their proximities to gene annotations, and other genomic features, were determined.

ChIP Analysis

Genes with RNA Pol II peaks found within 10 kb of start/end were compared in the ChIP samples. Overlap between the samples was high (70–90% in pairwise comparisons), reflecting the fact that the majority of gene transcription does not change. There were 4,865 active genomic regions that presented overlapping intervals from all conditions. Active regions were identified for the comparison of all samples, and the peak metrics was used in combination with the present/absent peak call information to find genomic regions with RNA Pol II occupancy patterns of interest. Ratios of treated samples compared to their respective controls were used to average signal values (>1.5-fold change) and to perform transcription factor and pathway analysis using TRANSFAC, iRegulon and Genemania in Cytoscape, and iPathwayGuide. Regions of Pol II enrichment in ChIP-Seq data often did not correlate perfectly with the gene annotations. Typically, a stronger peak was seen at the transcription start site (TSS/promoter), and high enrichments were often seen extending into downstream regions. Therefore, the average fragment densities for 25,143 human genes (from TSS to termination site) and the corresponding promoters (from −1,000 to +1,000 nt relative to TSS) were determined. The values between different gene promoters were comparable because they were based on a 2,000 bp segment. Peak values that were found in gene bodies were corrected by length. **Table 1** shows the total number of reads sequenced and their alignment to the human genome (hg19). For the analysis, the data files were normalized to the same number of unique alignments without duplicate reads, which was 16 million. Intervals were determined using the SICER algorithm at a cutoff of FDR1E-10 and a Gap parameter of 600 bp (which merges peaks located within 600 bp of each other). Gene intervals (peaks) were determined using the SICER algorithm at a cutoff of FDR1E-10 and a Gap parameter of 600 bp (which merges peaks located within 600 bp of each other into a single "island"). The number of intervals identified ranged from 9,775 in Meth-treated cells to 14,124 in cells treated with both Meth and Tat, within 10 kb of start/end. The overlap between the samples was high (70–90% in pairwise comparisons), reflecting the fact that the majority of gene transcription does not change. At 4,865 genomic regions, all conditions showed overlapping intervals. Because RNA Pol II- enriched regions are not typical bell- shaped, symmetrical peaks, average signal values were used in the analysis, and for estimating the ratios between each treatment condition and controls, and in additional pairwise comparisons. Regions of RNA Pol II enrichment in ChIP-Seq data did not correlate perfectly with the gene annotations, but as expected, stronger peaks were typically seen at the transcription start site (TSS/promoter), and high enrichments are often seen extending into the downstream region. Thus, the tag densities/signal metrics relative to the known gene annotation were examined. In this analysis, the average fragment densities for 25,143 human genes (from TSS to termination site) and the corresponding 25,143 human promoters (from −1,000 to +1,000, relative to TSS) were determined. The values between different gene promoters were comparable since they were based on a 2,000 bp segment.

Production of TBP-Knock Out THP1 Clone by CRISPR/Cas9

A template for disruption of the TBP gene (ENST00000412512, NM001172085) was established following described methods (51–54), and based on the conserved protein coding sequence in 8 detected splice variants (ENST00000423353.1, 703 bp). Primers for detection of human TBP and GAPDH by SyBrGreen qRT-PCR were purchased from Qiagen (Germantown, MD). A guide sequence was designed in http://crispr.mit.edu/guides, by introducing the FASTA sequence of the TBP coding region onto the target human genome (h19). Twenty-six high score guide sequences targeting exon 1 coding region mapped to the correct transcript, from which one was selected for oligo synthesis (sgTBP#1.1 AGCCTGCCACCTTACGCTCA), by Integrated DNA Technologies (San Diego, CA). For nickase Cas9, gRNA left GATAGGGATTCCGGGAGTCA, and gRNA right CCAATGATGCCTTATGGCAC were selected. Using the protein coding sequence data from ENSEMBLE and the designed gRNAs from the CRISPR database, the guide binding pattern was mapped out, identifying 5 out of 7 total wild-type gRNA targets transcripts, and 6 out of 7 nickase gRNA targets, with 0 off targets. The gRNAs and the Cas 9 protein were put into a plasmid for expression, using a GFP tag for assessing efficiency and selecting positively transfected cells by flow cytometry. For that, we used the CRISPR/Cas9 gesicle technology (55), with Guide-It CRISPR/Cas9 gesicle system (Clontech, Mountain View, CA). First, the oligos were annealed and cloned into pGuide-it-sgRNA1 vector, following manufacturer's protocols. Positive colonies were picked and expanded in LB, and plasmid DNA was isoladed using NucleoBond Xtra Midi (Clontech), and sequencing analysis was performed by Eton Bioscience Inc (San Diego, CA), using provided Guide-it sequencing primer 1. The gesicle-producing 293T cell line (Clontech) was expanded in DMEM with high glucose (4.5 g/l) (Genesee, San Diego, CA), 4 mM L-glutamine, and sodium bicarbonate, 10% fetal bovine serum Hyclone (GE Healthcare Lifesciences, Pittsburgh, PA), and 1% Penicilin/Streptomycin (Genesee), and split using Trypsine-EDTA (Sigma-Aldrich). These cells were seeded in 10-cm tissue culture dishes treated with poly-L-Lysine (Corning).

TABLE 1 | Number of sequenced reads and their alignment to the human genome (hg19).

	Control	Meth	Tat	Meth + Tat	Pooled Input
Total number of reads	35,582,719	36,449,122	23,742,921	40,019,315	35,838,803
Total number of alignments	32,594,991	34,255,959	21,211,764	36,906,854	34,240,934
Unique alignments (-q 25)	27,536,469	28,943,392	17,774,903	31,197,538	28,385,207
Unique alignments (without duplicate reads)	22,337,553	24,631,143	15,956,453	27,319,946	25,642,285
Normalized	15,956,453	15,956,453	15,956,453	15,956,453	15,956,453

Then 10 μg of plasmids encoding for sgRNA mixed to a plasmid containing Cherry picker red fluorescence, and the Cas9 enzyme were applied to the 293T cells, following manufacture's protocols. The A/C heterodimerizer ligand was added to the cultures for driving active loading of the Cas9/sgRNA complex into gesicles. A similar procedure, using Cas9 without the sgRNA was performed for producing "empty" gesicles, used for control conditions. Seventy-two hours after that, transfected cells were visualized due to Cherry picker red fluorescence. The cell media was harvested, and centrifuged overnight at 8,000 × g in a Beckman J2-HS centrifuge, with a JS 7.5 swinging rotor, and the pellet was concentrated to ~100 μl final volume in PBS. The gesicles were placed at 4°C on a rocking platform for 2 h, and stored in aliquots at −80°C until ready for treating THP1 cells. The cells were resuspended in protamine medium (containing 8 μg/ml protamine sulfate, Sigma), plated at 2 × 10^5 cells/ well in 500 μl, in 24 well plates, and 30 μl of gesicles were added. The plates were centrifuged at 1,150 × g for 30 min at room temperature. The plates were incubated at 37°C overnight, and then positively transfected cells were visualized under a fluorescence-microscope for detection of intracellular red fluorescence signal originated from the Cherry Picker reporter on the gesicle surface. The Cherry Picker positive cells from each positive well were washed in HBSS without phenol red, containing 10% fetal bovine serum, 1% penicillin/streptomycin, and resuspended in this buffer for sorting using a BD FACSJazz (BD Biosciences, San Diego, CA). Sorted positive cells were expanded into clones (1A, 1B, 2A, 2B, 2C, and 8), for at least 7 days before testing the TBP mutation. The detection of the TBP mutation was tested using DNA hybridization with Guide-It Resolvase (Clontech), on the gel-purified TBP band, amplified from QIAmp-extracted genomic DNA (Qiagen), and following manufacturers' protocols. The TBP gene was amplified with primers 5′ GAGTTCCAGCGCAAGGGTT forward, and 5′ TTTTGCAGCTGCGGTACAAT, using Phusion High Fidelity DNA Polymerase (New England Biolabs, Ipswich, MA), following manufacture's protocol, to generate two fragments, one 63 bp and one 465 bp, visualized on 2% agarose gel. Clone 2A presented efficient TBP mutagenesis and was used for the comparison with control clone C, which was generated as above, but with empty gesicles. Clone 1A had poor mutagenesis, and was used in some experiments as a control in addition to clone C. The TBP gene disruption was further tested at the mRNA level, which was extracted from cell pellets using RNeasy Mini kit (Qiagen), and reverse-transcribed with Superscript II (Thermo Fisher). The presence or absence of the TBP transcript confirmed the efficacy of CRISPR/Cas9 to disrupt the TBP gene (**Figure 4**).

Treatment of TBP-Mutant Clone 2A and TBP-Sufficient Clone C

The TBP-deficient clone 2A and control clone C were expanded in RMPI 1640, containing 10% fetal bovine serum (Hyclone), 1% penicillin/streptomycin, and 25 mM HEPES (Invitrogen). The cells were plated in 24-well plates at 2 × 10^6 cell/ml, and then stimulated with 10 ng/ml of HIV-1 IIIB Tat Recombinant Protein (NIH AIDS Reagent Program), 30 or 60 μM of Meth, or both HIV-1 Tat and Meth together. The cells were then harvested 2 h after stimulation, and RNA-seq was performed.

RNA-Seq Protocol

RNA was isolated from TBP-deficient THP1 clone 2A, and TBP-sufficient control clone C using the RNeasy Mini Kit (Qiagen) with on-column DNAse I treatment. quantified using Qubit 2.0 Fluorometer (Life Technologies, Carlsbad, CA, USA). The eluted RNA had a 260/280 of greater than 1.8. RNA integrity was checked with Agilent TapeStation (Agilent Technologies, Palo Alto, CA, USA). RNA samples were quantified using Qubit 2.0 Fluorometer (Life Technologies, Carlsbad, CA, USA) and RNA integrity was checked with Agilent TapeStation (Agilent Technologies, Palo Alto, CA, USA). RNA library preparation, sequencing reaction, and bioinformatics analysis were conducted at GENEWIZ, LLC. (South Plainfield, NJ, USA). RNA sequencing library preparations used the NEBNext Ultra RNA Library Prep Kit for Illumina by following manufacturer's recommendations (NEB, Ipswich, MA, USA). Briefly, mRNA was first enriched with Oligod(T) beads. Enriched mRNAs were fragmented for 15 min at 94°C. First strand and second strand cDNA were subsequently synthesized. cDNA fragments were end repaired and adenylated at 3′ends, and universal adapter was ligated to cDNA fragments, followed by index addition and library enrichment with limited cycle PCR. The sequencing libraries were validated on the Agilent TapeStation (Agilent Technologies, Palo Alto, CA, USA), and quantified by using Qubit 2.0 Fluorometer (Invitrogen, Carlsbad, CA) as well as by quantitative PCR (Applied Biosystems, Carlsbad, CA, USA). The sequencing libraries were clustered on one lane of a flowcell. After clustering, the flow-cell was loaded on the Illumina HiSeq instrument according to manufacturer's instructions. The samples were sequenced using a 2 × 150 Paired End (PE) configuration. Image analysis and base calling were conducted by the HiSeq Control Software (HCS). Raw sequence data (.bcl files) generated from Illumina HiSeq was converted into fastq files and de-multiplexed using Illumina's bcl2fastq 2.17 software. One mis-match was allowed for index sequence identification. After investigating the quality of the raw data, sequence reads were trimmed to remove possible adapter sequences and nucleotides with poor quality using Trim Sequences Module in CLC Genomics Workbench 9.0.1. The trimmed reads were mapped to the Homo sapiens GRCh38 reference genome available on ENSEMBL using the RNA-Seq Analysis Module in CLC Genomics Workbench 9.0.1. BAM files, Unique gene hit counts and Unique transcript hit counts were generated as a result of this step. After extraction of gene and transcript hit counts, the hit counts tables were used for downstream differential expression analysis. Using Kal's test, a comparison of gene expression between the groups of samples was performed. The Kal's test was used to generate *p*-values and Log2 fold changes. Genes and transcripts with adjusted p-values < 0.05 and absolute log2 fold changes > 1 were called as differentially expressed genes and transcripts, respectively, for each comparison. A gene ontology analysis was performed on the statistically significant set of genes by implementing the Hyoergeometric tests in CLC Genomics Workbench 9.0.1. The goa human GO list was used to cluster the set of genes based on their biological process and determine their statistical significance. Sequencing performance was assessed for total number of aligned reads, total number of uniquely aligned reads, and genes detected. All gene counts were then imported into the R/Bioconductor package EdgeR and TMM normalization size factors were calculated to adjust for samples for differences in library size, and then imported into R/Bioconductor package Limma. Performance of the samples was assessed with a Spearman correlation matrix. Weighted likelihoods based on the observed mean-variance relationship of every gene and sample were calculated with the voom WithQualityWeights function and gene performance was assessed with plots of residual standard deviation of every gene to their average log-count with a robustly fitted trend line of the residuals. Generalized linear models were created to test for gene level differential expression, and the results were displayed with FDR p-values $\leq$ 0.05 and log 2-fold-changes greater than an absolute value of 2, in each given comparison.

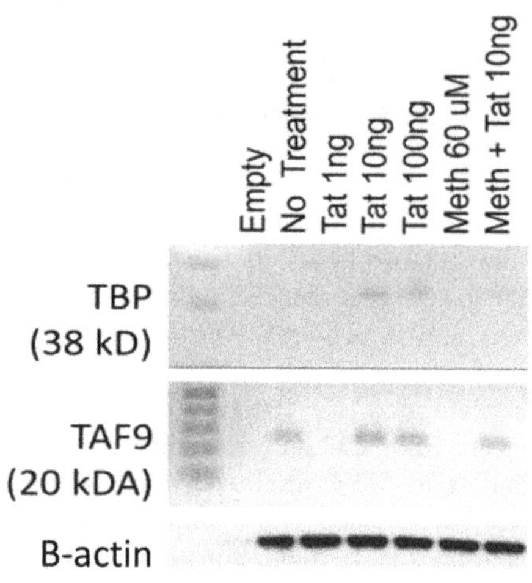

FIGURE 1 | Levels of TBP and TAF9 in the nuclear fraction of THP1 cells stimulated with HIV-1 Tat and with Meth. THP1 cells were incubated with different concentrations of HIV-1 Tat peptide (1, 10, and 100 ng/ml), and with Meth (60 μM). Protein was extracted from nuclear pellets 2 h after stimulation.

Expression Data Analysis

Using the Cytoscape interface platform, Mentha and Biogrid were used for building a network, using transformed fold change and FDR corrected p-values as attributes to visualize the effects of TBP deficiency in changes caused by 2 h of stimulation with HIV Tat, in the presence or absence of Meth. BinGO was used to estimate pathways affected in cells that were engineered to lack TBP expression, following stimulation.

RESULTS

TBP Is Activated and Translocated by HIV-1 Tat in Human THP1 Macrophages

In order to test the hypothesis that the HIV-1 Tat may utilize a TATA-box mediated mechanism, which may be involved in the ability of that protein to activate transcription of inflammatory genes that have a TATA-box promoter domain, we used a human macrophage cell line, THP1. These cells can activate the TBP protein when treated with 10 and 100 ng of the HIV-1 Tat peptide for 2 h, but not with 1 ng (**Figure 1**). Meth alone did not activate TBP at any concentration, but when combined with Tat, there was a detectable increase (**Figure 1**). The optimal concentration of Tat for activation of TBP was 10 ng/ml, which was the concentration maintained throughout the experiments. Other components of the TFIID complex, such as TAF9, were increased by Tat, with or without Meth, but not by Meth alone (**Figure 1**).

We tested the ability of Tat and Meth to translocate TBP by immunocytochemistry, using image analysis strategies illustrated in **Figures 2A,B**, and described in Methods. Representative original images are in of **Supplementary Figure 1**. The treatment of THP1 cells with Tat was able to translocate TBP into the nucleus, detectable since 5 min following the exposure (**Figure 2C**), and maintained TBP translocation throughout the analysis period, with a peak at 15 min (**Figure 2D**). On the other hand, Tat together with Meth induced a stronger translocation at 5 min, but that was gradually decreased. Meth alone also induced TBP translocation at 5 min, but this was quickly decreased and returned to baseline levels at 60 min (**Figures 2E,F**).

We have also tested whether Tat is able to translocate to the nucleus. **Figure 3A** shows that Tat enters the cellular nucleus soon after exposure and over time. The acute translocation of Tat was enhanced by Meth at 5 min, but this was followed by a gradual extinction effect. **Figures 3B,C** show the channel average overlap confirming the entry of Tat (black) into the nuclear structure (gray).

RNA Pol II Recruitment to Promoters Containing the TATA-Box Element Is Increased by HIV-1 Tat, and Further Enhanced by Meth

In order to examine the effects of Tat, and of the interactions with Meth on early transcriptional modifications in innate immune cells, we have used ChIP-seq to estimate changes in RNA Pol II recruitment to gene promoter regions, and to determine commonalities in transcription factor regulation. For that, THP1 macrophages were stimulated with 10 ng/ml of HIV Tat and/or 60 μM of Meth. The cell pellets were examined 15 min after stimulation, for identification of changes that are immediately due, and specific to, the provided stimuli, rather than due to secondary autocrine cytokine stimulation.

The examination of active promoter regions revealed that the majority of the differences in RNA Pol II signal enrichment between conditions were not above 2-fold, except for cells treated with Meth, which showed strongest signals (**Supplementary Materials**—Active Regions).

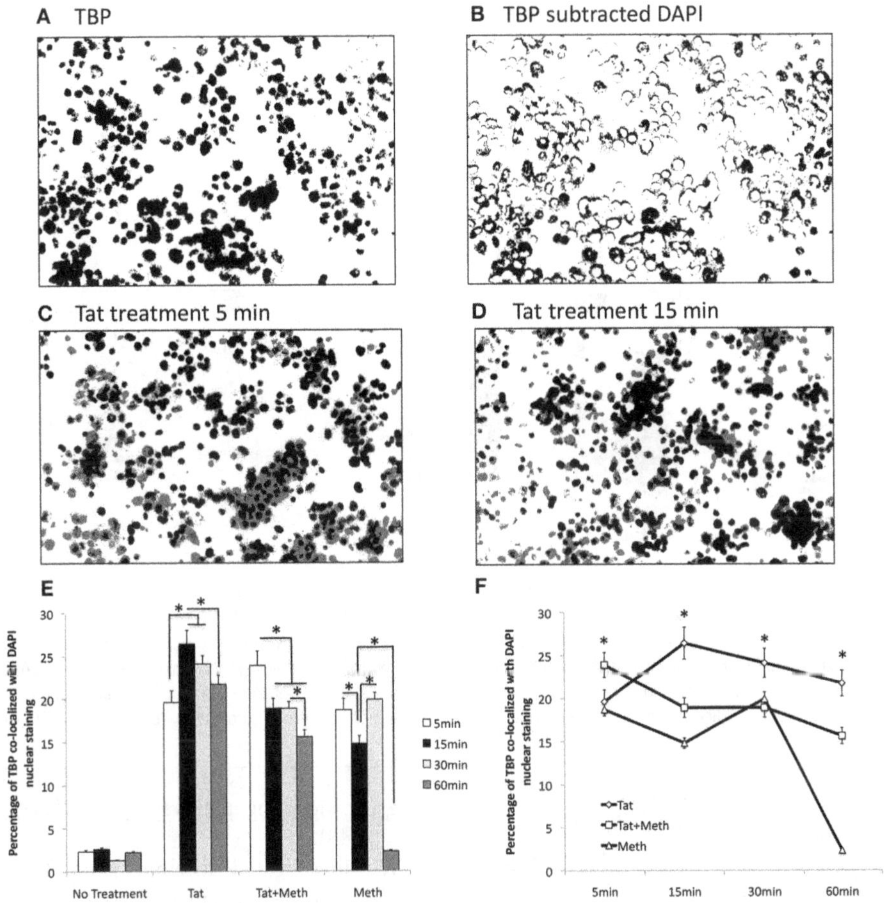

FIGURE 2 | TBP translocation patterns by Tat and by Meth. Translocation was estimated by immunocytochemistry on differentiated THP1 cells that were treated with HIV-1 Tat (10 ng/ml), and/or Meth (60 μM), over 5, 15, 30, and 60 min. Acquired images of cells stained with anti-TBP (rabbit polyclonal), and anti-rabbit AlexaFluor 647, and counterstained with DAPI are in **Supplementary Materials**. The images were digitalized as described in Methods. DAPI staining was converted into a binary mask and subtracted from the total TBP staining **(A)**, to produce an image of cytoplasmatic staining **(B)**. The average of overlapped binary masks confirmed the co-localization of TBP and DAPI upon Tat stimulation at 5 min **(C)**, and with a peak at 15 min **(D)**. After measurements, the translocation index was calculated as the percentage of the total staining that was co-localized with DAPI. **(E)** Bar graph showing translocation indexes for baseline untreated cells, and cells treated with all stimulants over time. **(F)** Line graph for visualization of the effect of time on TBP translocation with the different stimuli. The assays were performed in triplicate, and in three independent experiments. Results represent the average and standard deviation of 3 experiments performed in duplicate. *$p < 0.05$ in two-way ANOVA, followed by Bonferroni's test.

Visualization of Changes in RNA Pol II Recruitment Patterns

Using Cytoscape interface platform, Mentha and Biogrid interactomes were imported from the Proteomics Standard Initiative Common QUery InterfaCe (PSICQUIC) (www.bioconductor.org). These two databases were used for building a network from RNA Pol II recruitment data, ratio between experimental and controls' peaks signal average, and FDR-corrected p-values as node attributes, for visualizing changes.

The network was filtered for eliminating genes that were not represented in our data set. Gene networks were 63.73% due to co-expression, followed by 15.84% due to physical interactions. The organic layouts were restricted to selected default pathway database attributes (combined Wu-Stein-2010, PathwayCommons NCI Nature, IMID, Reactome and Cell_Map), which connected 5.27% of the genes (**Figure 4**). The application of attributes and visualization in Cytoscape suggested that Meth had a stronger effect on RNA Pol II recruitment when compared to HIV-1 Tat (**Figure 4**). Pathway perturbation and over-representation analysis by iPathwayGuide, showed that RNA Pol II recruitment was disturbed by Tat, mainly on genes involved in metabolism, activation and response to stimulus, such as cell adhesion molecules ($p = 0.023$), fatty acid elongation ($p = 0.024$), sulfur-relay system ($p = 0.026$), hematopoietic lineage ($p = 0.034$), Notch-signaling pathway ($p = 0.04$), purine metabolism ($p = 0.043$), systemic lupus erythematous ($p = 0.046$), and tryptophan metabolism ($p = 0.049$). Meth promoted RNA Pol recruitment to genes involved in metabolic pathways, such as fatty acid elongation ($p = 0.007$), glycan degradation ($p = 0.007$), DNA replication ($p = 0.022$), endocrine and other factor-regulated calcium reabsorption ($p = 0.028$), ribosome biogenesis ($p = 0.039$), NOD-like

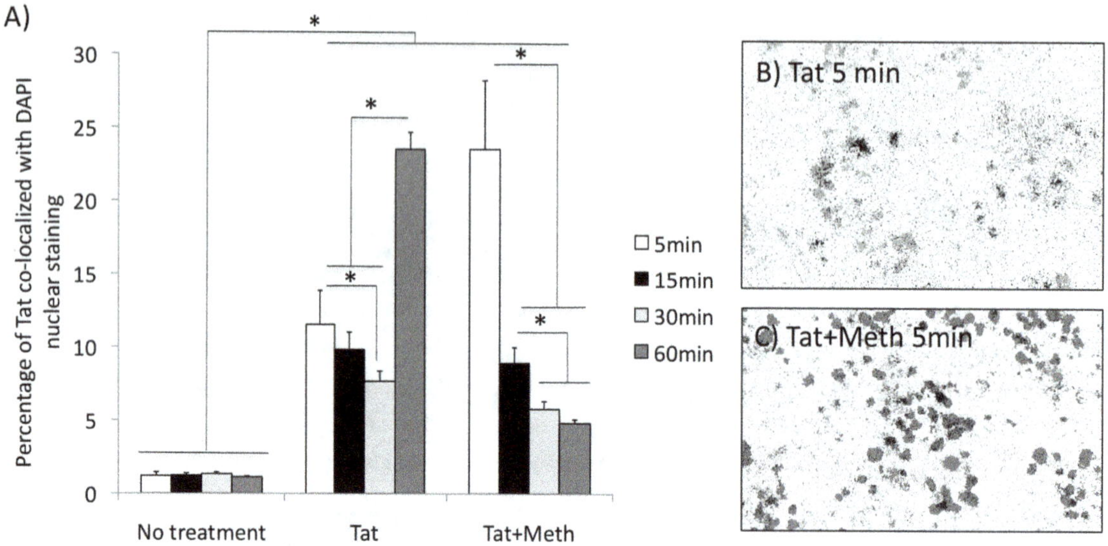

FIGURE 3 | Tat translocation patterns in the presence of Meth. Translocation was estimated by immunocytochemistry on differentiated THP1 cells that were treated with HIV-1 Tat (10 ng/ml), or Tat together with Meth (60 μM), over 5, 15, 30, and 60 min. The cells were stained with anti-Tat (Monoclonal 15.1), and anti-mouse AlexaFluor 647, and counterstained with DAPI. The images were digitalized as described in Methods. DAPI staining was converted into a binary mask and subtracted from the total Tat staining. **(A)** Measurements were used for calculating the percentage of the total Tat staining that was co-localized to DAPI. Results represent the average standard deviation of 3 experiments performed in duplicate. **(B)** Representative image of the averaged overlapped binary masks, which confirmed the co-localization of Tat and DAPI upon Tat stimulation at 5 min), and **(C)** enhancement by Meth simultaneous stimulation. $^{*}p < 0.05$ 2-way ANOVA, followed by Bonferroni's *post hoc* test.

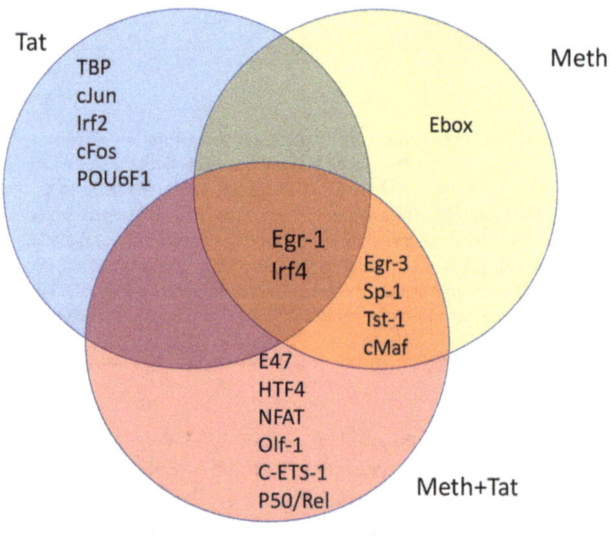

FIGURE 4 | Venn's diagram showing transcription factors with frequent binding motifs among genes with significant changes in RNA Pol II recruitment, immediately following the stimulation of THP1 cells with HIV-1 Tat, Meth, or both together. Matrices for transcription factor binding motifs were generated from ChIP-seq data. For that, SICER raw data in BED format was loaded into TRANSFAC, and the Match-algorithm, was applied as binding factor identifier. Transcription factors with highest frequency of binding motifs in gene promoters affected by HIV-1 Tat, Meth, or both together were estimated. The transcription factors listed in each segment of the Venn's diagram are all significantly increased in comparison to control conditions, and are ranked in order according to frequency matrices, from highest on top to lowest at the bottom of the segregated lists.

receptor signaling pathway ($p = 0.048$) and synaptic vesicle ($p = 0.048$).

We investigated whether promoters where RNA Pol II recruitment was changed by HIV-1 Tat, or Meth, or by both factors together, displayed critical promoter sequence commonalities, based on alignment and frequency of transcription factor binding motifs. This was examined using a combination of strategies, aiming at identifying common transcription master regulators potentially orchestrating the observed effects. First, SICER BED files were analyzed using MATCH tool algorithm (50) with h19 genome as a template, and using a library of mononucleotide weight matrices from TRANSFAC database (Wolfenbuttel, Germany). This tool created nucleotide matrices that calculated frequency of promoter binding motifs among genes exhibiting significant changes in RNA Pol II recruitment. **Figure 4** shows the identified condition-specific transcription factors, in order of importance, in a Venn diagram. The attributed matrix score identified TBP (V$TATA_01, V$TATA_C, VTBP_Q6, VTBP_01, V$TBP_06), as the main transcription factor regulating changes upon HIV-1 Tat exposure, as determined by a consensus sequence matrix (**Table 2**). TBP was followed by other exclusive factors, cJun, Irf2, cFos and POU6F1, which were also statistically significant, but occurred at lower frequency when compared to TBP. Meth stimulation drastically shifted RNA Pol recruitment patterns to genes with high frequency of Egr-3, Sp-1, Tst-1, cMaf, and Ebox binding motifs. Of these, the Ebox (CACGTG/CAGCTG) binding motif aligned exclusively in Meth alone, while the other factors were common to Meth+Tat stimulation. E47, HTF4,

TABLE 2 | TATA box promoter element matrices obtained from THP1 cells stimulated with Tat or with Meth+Tat.

Reverse Consensus	A	C	G	T	Complement Consensus	A	C	G	T
(A) Tat stimulation									
T	4	9	2	29	N	15	10	15	4
T	3	11	1	29	G	8	6	27	3
T	11	2	1	30	N	8	7	21	8
T	2	4	0	38	N	6	13	18	7
A	25	8	0	11	T	5	4	11	24
T	1	5	0	38	A	38	0	5	1
A	24	11	4	5	T	11	0	8	25
N	7	18	13	6	A	38	0	4	2
N	8	21	7	8	A	30	1	2	11
C	3	27	6	8	A	29	1	11	3
N	4	15	10	15	A	29	2	9	4
(B) Meth+Tat stimulation									
T	1	1	1	20	N	5	5	8	2
T	0	0	0	20	T	3	2	3	12
T	0	0	0	20	A	18	0	0	2
A	15	2	1	2	T	2	1	2	15
T	2	0	0	18	A	20	0	0	0
A	12	3	2	3	A	20	0	0	0
N	2	8	5	5	A	17	1	1	1

The frequency of nucleotides matching the TATA box promoter element was calculated on complementary and reverse genomic sequences, using TRANSFAC.

NFAT, Olf-1, cETS-1, and p50/Rel were the transcription factors exclusively associated to Meth+Tat stimulation.

The finding that TBP binding motifs were the most frequent in genes affected by Tat alone is in agreement with the initial finding of increase of TBP at the protein level. It suggests a key role for the TATA-box promoter element in innate immune responses to HIV. **Table 2** shows the frequency of nucleotides comprising the TATA box element matrix compiled from individual genomic sites upon HIV-1 Tat stimulation, in the absence or presence of Meth. The matrices estimating the frequency of nucleotides at the correct positions, suggest that upon Tat stimulation 31.5% of the genes showing enriched RNA Pol recruitment have the TATA box promoter element sequence. In contrast, in Meth+Tat stimulated cells, the average was decreased to 12%. In those cells stimulated with both Meth and Tat, the predominant transcription factor sequence domain (30.6%) identified by TRANSFAC was Egr-1 (GCGCATGCG), followed by Egr-3 (GTGGGT/C), and Sp-1 (GGGGCGGGG), all classified as C2H2 zink finger proteins.

Interestingly, many genes affected by Tat alone and by Meth+Tat were the same. Yet, estimated master regulators differed in those conditions, with Egr-1 and Irf4 in common. These two factors were also identified in genes affected by Meth alone, in addition to Egr-3, Sp-1, Tst-1, and cMaf, which were shared with Meth+Tat. On the other hand, Tat alone and Meth+Tat had no common regulators (**Figure 4**).

The prediction of TBP as a master regulator of changes caused by Tat stimulation was further examined in iRegulon within the Cytoscape platform, using a targeted approach. This method identified all the genes displaying a TATA box element within ± 500 bp from the transcription starting site within the dataset. A table with predicted TBP-controlled genes and attributes was generated, and then utilized to produce a network in Genemania, for comparative analysis and visualization of critical differences between Tat and Meth stimulation (**Figure 5**). Overall, in Tat – stimulated THP1 cells there was a significantly higher number of genes with decreased RNA Pol II recruitment, while in Meth-stimulated cells, more genes were increased. However, upon the generation of a sub-network through targeting TBP and its first neighbors linked through physical interactions, most genes associated with that transcription factor had increased recruitment of RNA Pol II with all treatments (**Figure 6**).

The predicted significance of TBP as a transcription factor in Tat stimulated cells but not in Meth, or Meth+Tat, was challenged by the similarities in RNA Pol II recruitment found in all three conditions. Thus, we developed a strategy to test whether TBP is indeed important for the changes caused by HIV Tat, as well as by Meth, and their interactions. Our strategy consisted on impairing the expression of the TBP gene, using CRISPR/Cas9 guides delivered into THP1 cells by using exosomic gesicles. The efficient transfection of guide sequences was monitored using mCherryPicker reporter (**Figure 7A**). One representative high efficiency clone (2A), was compared to a low efficiency clone (1A) and to a control clone (C) that was treated with empty gesicles. Cells that were positive to mCherryPicker, indicating efficient delivery of guide sequences were sorted using flow cytometry procedures, and placed in culture for expansion and testings (**Figure 7B**). The disruption of the TBP gene was confirmed using Resolvase and visualized in a 2% gel (**Figure 7C**). The significantly decreased baseline expression of the TBP gene was confirmed using qRT-PCR (**Figure 7D**).

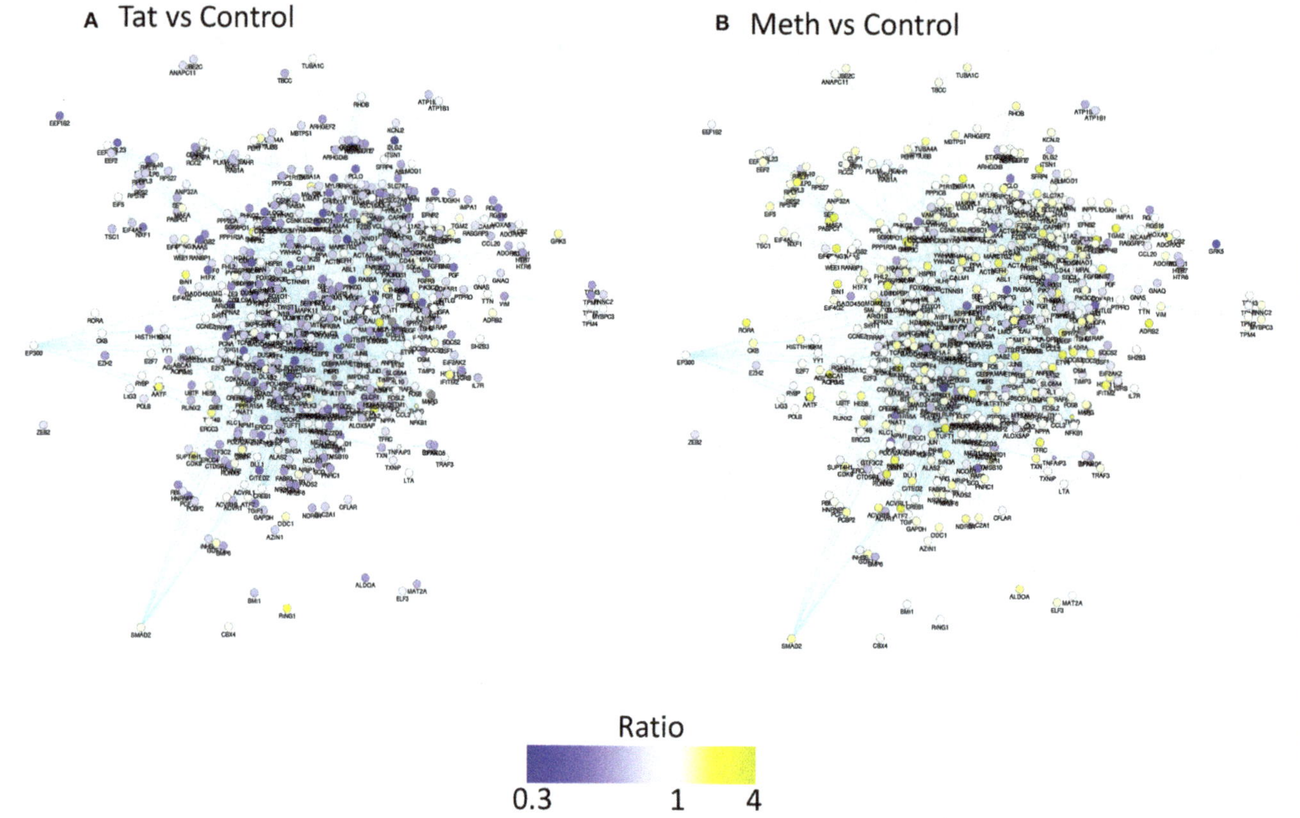

FIGURE 5 | Pathway-based network association of genes with promoter activity changes due to HIV-1 Tat or Meth, compared to vehicle treatment. Ratio between RNA Pol normalized peak values between treated conditions and controls were used for designing a color-coded visualization. Genes were filtered to display only significantly decreased (blue), and increased (yellow) RNA Pol II recruitment patterns. **(A)** Visual representation of ratio of Tat over Control and **(B)** Meth over Control.

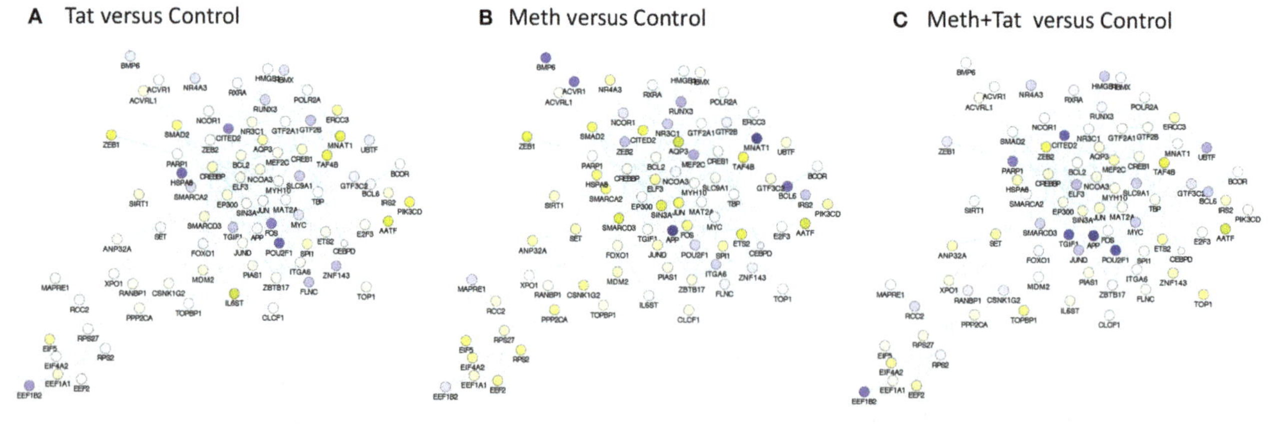

FIGURE 6 | TBP-centered genomic neighborhood derived from pathway-based network association of genes with RNA Pol recruitment patterns affected by HIV-1 Tat or Meth. A sub-network was generated from the pathway-based association study through targeting and selecting the TBP gene and its first neighbors, through physical interaction edges. Colors designate significantly decreased (blue), and increased (yellow) RNA Pol II recruitment patterns, based on the ratio between **(A)** Tat over Control, **(B)** Meth over Control, and **(C)** Meth+Tat over Control.

The confirmation of the disruption in TBP expression included the examination of potentially remaining splice variants (**Table 3**), where we observed only residual expression of TBP_4, but complete clearance of TBP_7 splice variant.

In order to estimate the impact of TBP depletion on the response to HIV-1 Tat, alone and in the context of Meth exposure, a TBP-regulated gene network was identified in the RNA Pol II gene list, with Biogrid Homo sapiens 3.4 gene

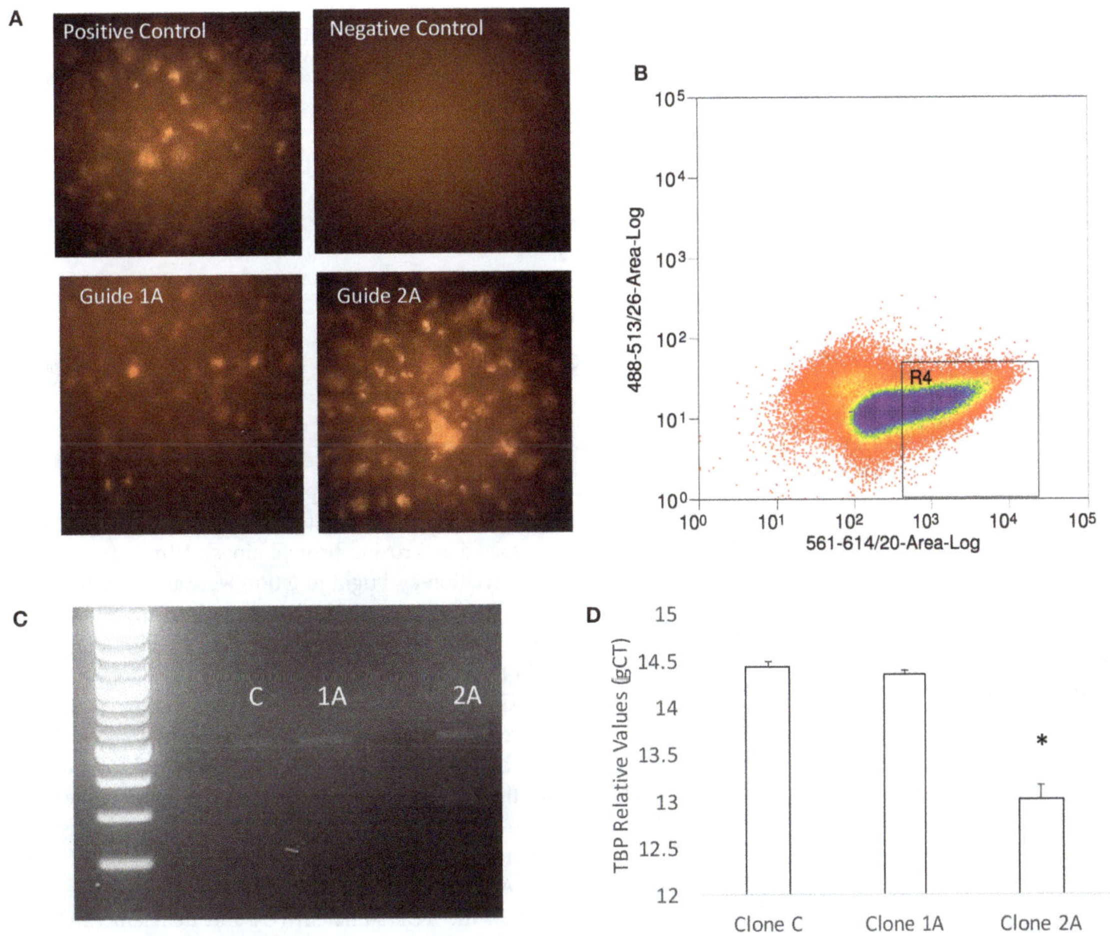

FIGURE 7 | Generation of a TBP-deficient THP1 clone. **(A)** Seventy-two hours after exposure to gesicles containing the TBP guide sequence and Cas9, positively transfected cells were visualized under a fluorescence-microscope for detection of intracellular red fluorescence signal originated from the Cherry Picker reporter on the gesicles' surface. Positive control provided by the manufacturer was compared with a negative control performed with empty gesicles, and two clones that received the guide sequence. Clone 1A showed low efficiency, and clone 2A was highly positive. **(B)** The Cherry Picker-positive cells were gated based on fluorescence intensity, and sorted using a BD FACSJazz (BD Biosciences, San Diego, CA). **(C)** The TBP mutation was confirmed in clone 2A using DNA hybridization with Guide-It Resolvase on a gel-purified genomic TBP sequence, and with **(D)** qRT-PCR. Results are the average ± standard error of 2 experiments performed in triplicate.

network. We then used iRegulon (56) in Cytoscape environment, to reverse-engineer the TBP transcriptional regulatory network through the detection of enriched TATA box motifs and their optimal sets of targets in the RNA Pol II data, pooled from all experimental conditions performed in TBP-sufficient clones (**Figure 8** and **Supplementary Table 1**). The resulting TBP targetome contained 1,811 genes identified in THP1 cells. The expression levels of these genes was estimated by RNA seq performed in the control THP1 clones (C), and in the clone that was depleted of TBP gene expression using Crispr/Cas9, upon the stimulation with HIV-1 Tat, or with Tat plus Meth. **Figure 8A** shows that control C clones stimulated with Tat had a global upregulation of the genes in that network (gene nodes with yellow color), suggesting a significant effect orchestrated through TBP. In **Figure 8B**, the TBP targetome gene network in the TBP-deficient clone 2A that has either similar (white nodes) or lower baseline expression (blue nodes) when compared to control clone C. Interestingly, the genes in the TBP targetome were significantly suppressed in Tat-stimulated TBP-deficient clone 2A compared to clone C, as revealed by the higher number and intensity of blue colored nodes in the network, and confirming that these genes, under Tat stimulation, were predominantly transcribed via Tata box promoter element, and in a TBP-dependent manner (**Figure 8C**). However, when Tat was incubated together with Meth, the genes in the TBP targetome were upregulated even in clone 2A, bypassing the TBP deficiency, as shown by the higher number of yellow colored nodes, and suggesting that in the context of Meth exposure, a diversification of transcriptional factors plays a role in activating the same promoters (**Figure 8D**), as a potential mechanism of exacerbated consequences in HIV and drug abuse.

In order to further estimate the impact of TBP in Tat stimulation and the effect of Meth, global changes in the TBP targetome genes were calculated by the sum of fold changes in all 1811 genes, in clones C and 2A, upon Tat, plus and minus Meth stimulation (**Figure 9**). The strategy showns that Tat globally

TABLE 3 | TBP splice variant reads in Control and 2A clones.

Feature ID	Transcript ID	Experiment - Range	C clone (unique transcript reads)	2A clone (unique transcript reads)	Kahl's *Z*-test *p* value
TBP_1	ENST00000421512	1	33	0	0.000703333
TBP_2	ENST00000446829	0	0	0	1
TBP_3	ENST00000616883	12	12	1	0.001138457
TBP_4	ENST00000230354	76	361	24	0.01604091
TBP_5	ENST00000423353	0	0	0	1
TBP_6	ENST00000540980	0	0	0	1
TBP_7	ENST00000392092	143	489	0	0.000164347

The potential of residual TBP expression through alternative splice was estimated in the Control and 2A clones using RNA seq. The number of reads in both clones and p values are reported.

TABLE 4 | KEGG pathway analysis of genes that failed to upregulate in response to Tat in TBP-deficient 2A clones.

Genes Pathway	*p* value	Benjamini
Proteoglycans in cancer	0.00043	0.067
Hedgehog signaling pathway	0.00076	0.059
Axon guidance	0.001	0.052
Signaling pathways regulating pluripotency of stem cells	0.0018	0.07
Central carbon metabolism in cancer	0.0038	0.11
FoxO signaling pathway	0.0052	0.13
Transcriptional misregulation in cancer	0.0067	0.14
HTLV-I infection	0.01	0.18
Basal cell carcinoma	0.012	0.2
Tight junction	0.026	0.34
Wnt signaling pathway	0.026	0.34
Pathways in cancer	0.027	0.32
Hippo signaling pathway	0.039	0.41
Mineral absorption	0.043	0.42
AMPK signaling pathway	0.046	0.42
Notch signaling pathway	0.048	0.41
Progesterone-mediated oocyte maturation	0.05	0.4

increased TATA-box bearing genes by an average of 8.6%, in the control clone (CT/CPhi), but failed to do it so in the clone 2A (2AT/2APhi). However, Tat in combination with Meth increased the same genes in the TBP-defficient clone 2A by an average of 29% (2AMT/2APhi).

These findings may have profound implications to the character of the inflammatory pathogenesis in HIV-infected Meth abusers. A prediction of the involvement of TBP-regulated genes in molecular pathways was examined using BinGO (57, 58) (**Figure 10** and **Supplementary Table 2**). TBP-regulated genes are predominantly involved in immune and inflammatory pathways, but also in epigenetic, regulatory and metabolic pathways. In **Figure 10**, large circles report overrepresentation, and orange color report higher perturbation, to allow the visualization of stronger effects on innate immune and epigenetic function, as well as regulation (adjusted $p = 0.00136$, $p = 0.000601$, respectively). Within the whole TBP targetome, genes that failed to be upregulated in clone 2A upon Tat stimulation were functionally associated to the nucleus, DNA-binding, transcription, nucleotide binding, developmental protein and cytoskeleton (Benjamini $p < 0.01$), but genes involved in tyrosine-protein kinase, Wnt-signaling, ATP binding, methylation and tight junction were also represented (Benjamini $p < 0.05$). Main identified TBP-controlled pathways using this strategy were assessed in KEGG, and are shown in **Table 4**.

Genes that play a role in inflammatory pathology, and that have been described to have an involvement in HIV pathogenesis, in the brain and elsewhere, were selected for a closer validation of the role of TBP in Tat stimulation, and of the ability of Meth as a co-morbidity to enhance those same genes through other transcription factors. A detailed examination of genes that have a TATA box promoter element and their changes in response to Tat in the TBP-sufficient (C) and deficient (2A) clones reveals two classes of genes, which seem to segregate based on their expression levels in unstimulated controls (**Figure 11**). The genes in **Figure 11A**, which are not detectable in the unstimulated clone C or clone 2A, are highly induced by Tat in clone C, but not in clone 2A, suggesting that the transcription of these genes upon HIV-1 Tat stimulation is primarily triggered via the TATA box promoter domain, under TBP control. On the other hand, the stimulation with Tat in the presence of Meth, or Meth alone, was able to increase these transcripts in both clones, and bypassing the TBP deficiency in clone 2A, confirming a diversification of transcription factor usage by the drug, alone or in the context of HIV Tat. Examples include genes involved in blood brain barrier permeability, inflammation and immune regulation, neuroprotection and metabolic outcomes, such as CD163, Claudins 5 and 9 (CLDN5 and CLDN9), FoxP3, Brain-derived neurotrophic factor (BDNF), Insulin growth factor 1 Receptor (IGF1R), Retinoic acid receptor alpha (RARA), and the important kinase CDK9. The genes in **Figure 10B** also present TATA box promoter element, and were detected in the TBP targetome, but differed from the genes represented in **Figure 11A** by being constitutively expressed in unstimulated cells, regardless of the TBP expression. Interestingly, these genes were not responsive to Tat, or to Meth. This was the case for instance of CXCL2, Tumor necrosis factor receptor superfamily member 25 (TNFRsF25), and the T-box 2 transcription factor (TBX2).

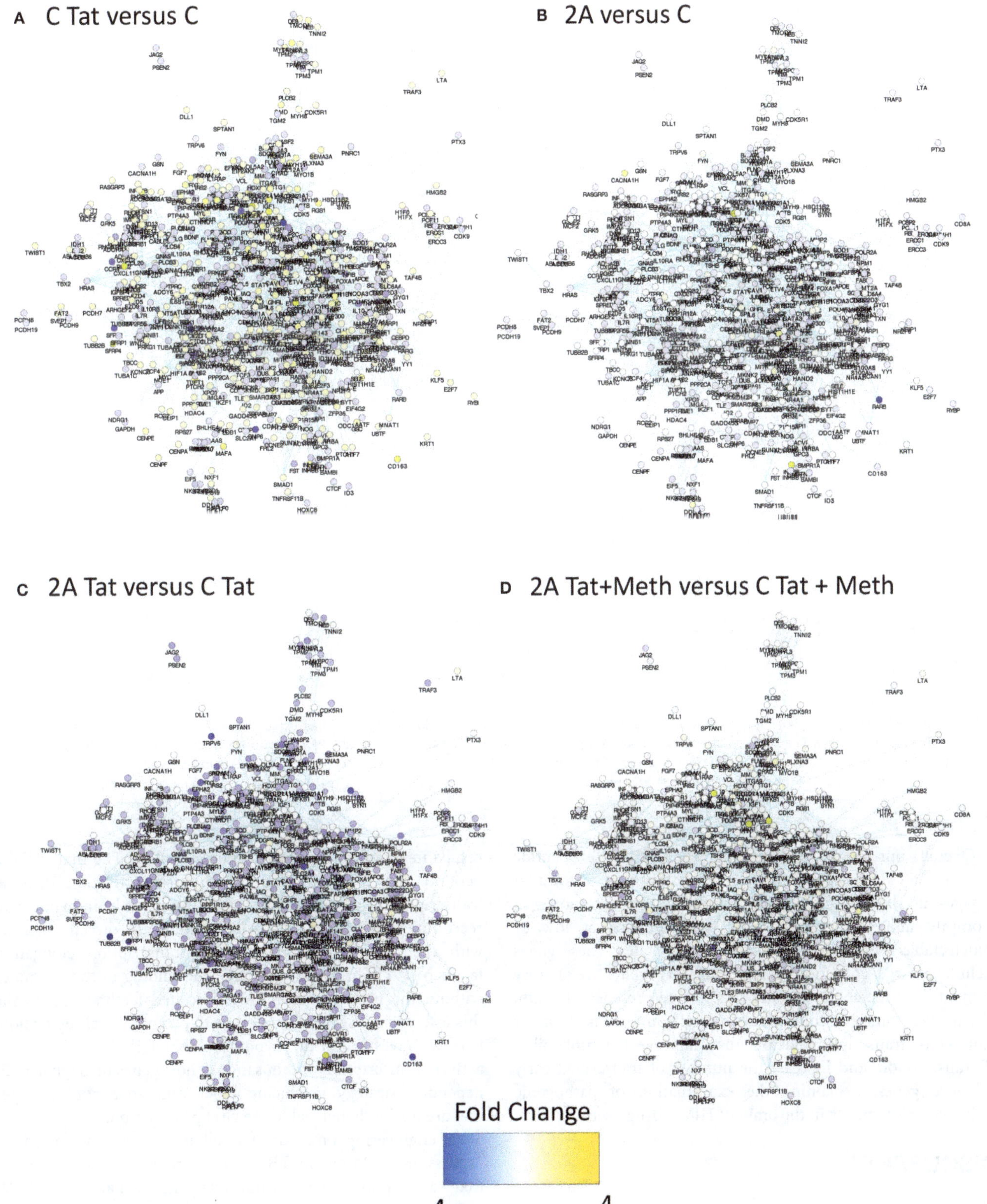

FIGURE 8 | Impact of TBP deficiency on the expression of genes in the TBP targetome following stimulation with Tat, in the presence and in the absence of Meth. The genes that contain Tata box promoter elements and their relationship was estimated in Homo sapiens 3.4 Biogrid default network using iRegulon, with TBP as a factor, and filtered to contain genes that were significantly represented in THP1 cells based on RNA Pol II recruitment capacity at any given experimental condition.

(Continued)

FIGURE 8 | The produced mega-network containing 1811 genes was denominated TBP targetome, and used to determine the effect of TBP depletion on Tat stimulation, alone or in the context of Meth. For that, RNA seq was performed in the control clone C and in the TBP-deficient clone 2A, stimulated with 10 μg/ml of HIV Tat, alone or together with 60 μM of Meth. The expression changes were estimated 24 h after stimulation. Yellow tones represent upregulation, and blue tones represent downregulation. **(A)** Clone C treated with Tat was compared to clone C treated with vehicle, showing that the majority of the genes in this network are yellow, indicating that Tat upregulates genes with a TBP binding domain. **(B)** Vehicle-treated clones 2A and C were compared, showing little or no change in color, indicating that they do not differ at baseline. **(C)** Clone 2A stimulated with Tat was compared to clone C stimulated with Tat, showing that most genes are in blue nodes indicating that clone 2A had a lower expression than clone C, upon Tat stimulation. **(D)** Clone 2A treated with Tat+Meth was compared with clone C also treateated with Tat+Meth, where nodes with no color change or yellow indicate that in the presence of Meth, the TBP deficient clone 2A either does not differ from clone C or further increases the expression of genes with a TBP binding promoter domain.

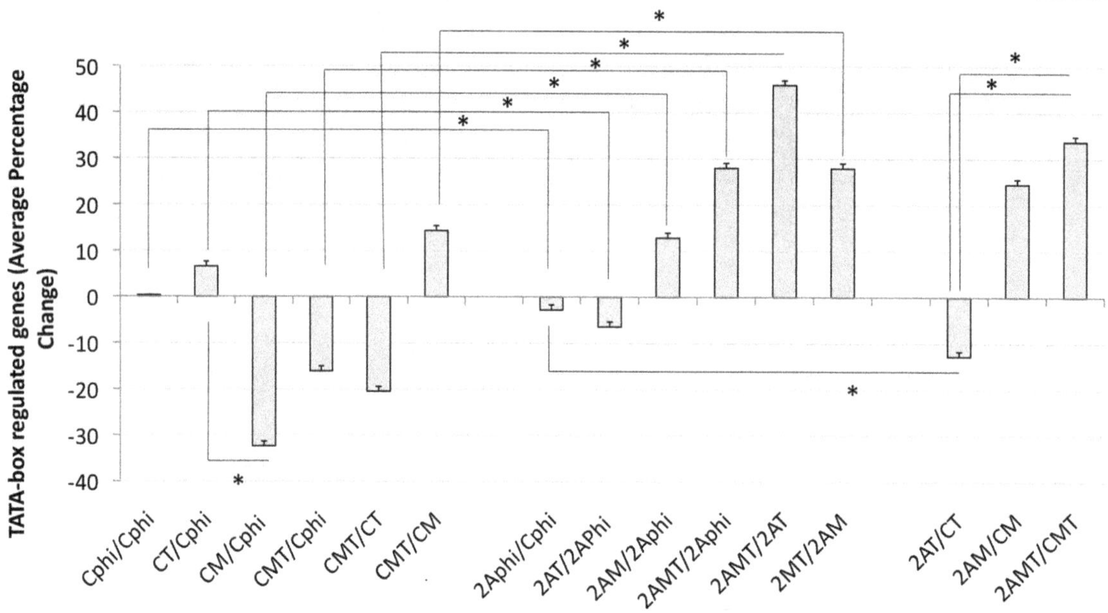

FIGURE 9 | Global changes in the TBP targetome in TBP-sufficient and –deficient monocyte clones after Tat stimulation with or without Meth. The sum of all fold changes in genes that have a Tata box promoter element upon designated stimulations. C is Control clone and 2A is the TBP-defficient clone. T refers to Tat stimulation, M to Meth stimulation, and MT is their combination. Phi refers to control function. Results represent the average ± standard deviation of expression of 1,811 genes included in the TBP megatargetome identified in iRegulon. *$p < 0.05$ in assigned comparisons, using ANOVA and Bonferroni's *post hoc* test.

Overall, our results indicate that the HIV-1 Tat peptide acts through the usage of TBP as a transcription factor that engages in the Tata-box binding motif in the promoter of promptly inducible genes, which are expressed at low or undetectable levels in unstimulated resting states. These genes include a large collection of inflammatory genes, regulatory elements and metabolic components. In the presence of Meth, which is a common comorbidity of HIV infection, a larger number of transcription factors may increase the probability of transcription, and increase the number of transcribed early response genes, explaining the exacerbation of pathogenic hallmarks, particularly in the brain of HIV+ drug users.

DISCUSSION

The role of the Tata-box promoter domain in HIV transcription has been suggested (23). In addition, single nucleotide polymorphisms in its sequence located in the long-terminal repeat (LTR) in the viral transcription complex, which confers a low affinity to TBP, the Tata-box binding transcription factor, results in significantly slower replication (59). The main HIV-1 peptide that is responsible for the transactivation of viral transcription, Tat, performs its task by directly inducing and recruiting TBP to the LTR, via its ability to directly interact with the cellular cofactor positive transcription elongation factor b (P-TEFb), which bridges TBP binding to the promoter without the need of other TBP-associated factors (23). While this is a mechanism that is relevant to promote viral replication, here we investigated the hypothesis that HIV-1 Tat is able to activate transcription of thousands of host genes through a TBP-dependent strategy, producing hyper-inflammatory phenotypes that are further beneficial to the viral propagation.

By engineering a macrophage cell line that is deficient on the expression of dominant TBP splice variants, we demonstrated that transcriptional changes induced by the incubation with HIV-1 Tat favor inducible genes that have the Tata-box promoter sequence in their promoters. We also showed that such effect is achieved through the dominant usage of TBP as a transcription factor. Other transcription factors that may be triggered, cJun, interferon regulatory factor 2 (IRF2), cFos and POU6F1, also

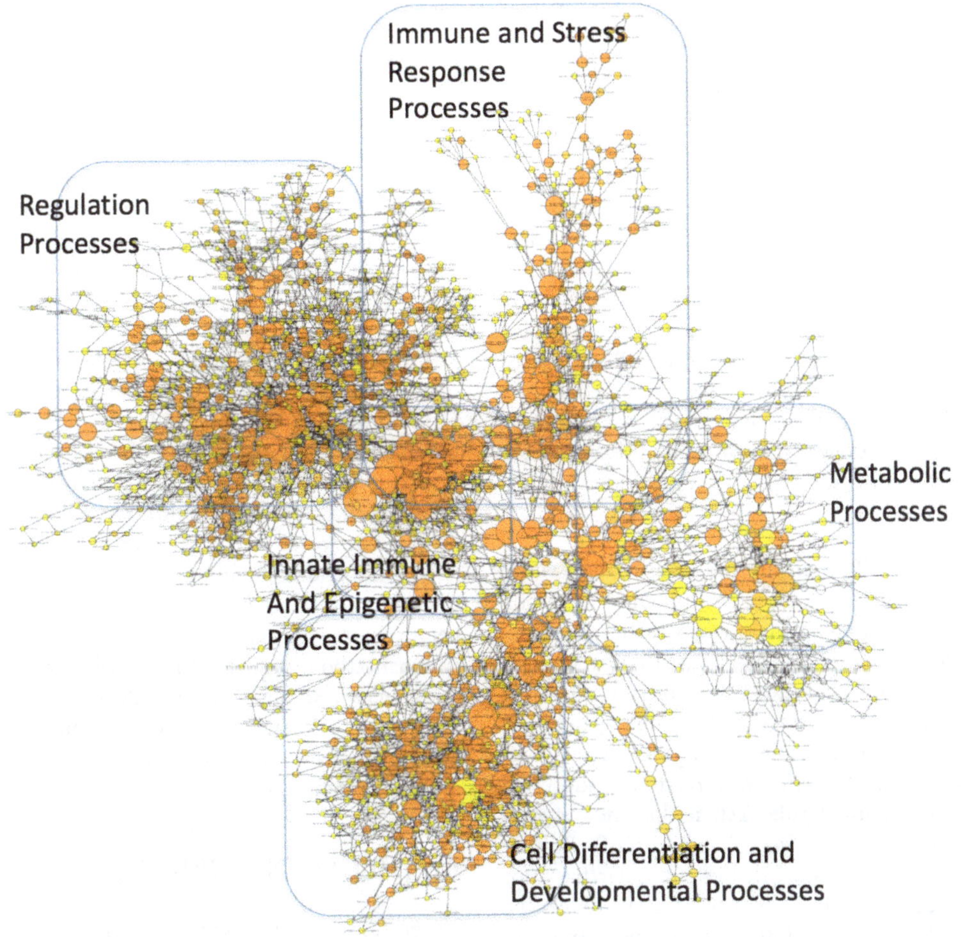

FIGURE 10 | Mapping of functional categories identified in genes of the TBP targetome. Gene Ontology (GO) analysis was performed using BinGO. The circles' size show overrepresentation, and colors report perturbation, orange being high, and yellow, low.

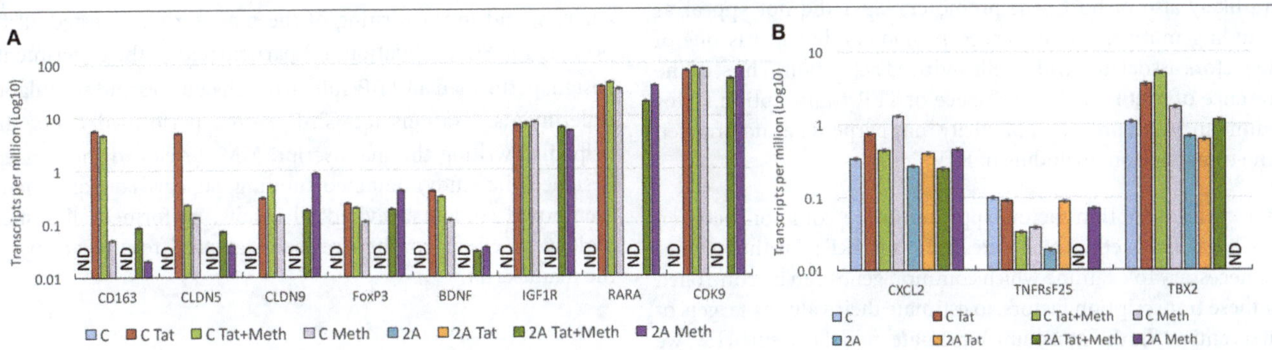

FIGURE 11 | Effect of TBP transcription factor in the upregulation of gene transcripts in response to Tat and Meth. Gene transcript counts are represented in log10 of transcripts per million (TPM). The axis in log allows the appreciation of genes that are increased with different intensities for comparison of their behaviors in response to stimulation. **(A)** Representative TBP targets illustrating the changes in genes that are undetectable in unstimulated cells and responsive to Tat and/or Meth. **(B)** Representative hits illustrating the behavior of genes that are constitutively transcribed in unstimulated cells, and not responsive to Tat and/or Meth. ND, Not detectable.

appear to be triggered, as their binding motifs are identified in the promoters of genes with increased RNA Pol recruitment, and can be controlling different sets of genes. These findings may have important implications for understanding mechanisms of pathogenesis in HIV infection, and potentially for therapy. We also showed that the exposure of macrophages to a stimulant drug, Meth, together with HIV-1 Tat, is able to activate the same gene promoters, which is revealed by the efficient recruitment of RNA Pol. However, this happens through a distinctive and more diversified usage of transcriptional factors. The absence of TAF9 in Meth-stimulated cells, and the results of the analysis of consensus promoter sequences in TBP-sufficient cells stimulated with Tat plus Meth, support that an alternative to TBP is triggered by Meth, it can potentially co-exist with TBP in the context of HIV-1 Tat, but ultimately support promoter activation through different motifs. This may suggest that co-morbidities represent a factor of complexity in therapies that target transcriptional machineries.

We have shown that TBP and Tat are translocated within 5 min into the cell nucleus, when in the presence of Meth, which may have important implications to the viral transcription. However, we did not test the effects of TBP disruption on viral transcription or replication, but exclusively on the effects of Tat as a factor that enhances transcription of host genes. The identification of TBP as a the most frequently aligned promoter motif in genes with RNA Pol efficiently recruited, suggested that TBP played an important role. Yet, it does not explain the basis for the interaction between Tat and TBP. Further experiments are necessary to establish the molecular basis for that interaction in the context of absence of TAR, or on the effects over the LTR. Although TBP was the most frequent transcription factor motif, other transcription motifs were also significant, such as cJun/cFos, IRF2, and POU6F1. In other systems, Sp-1 has been suggested as a Tat molecular partner, bridged by Cyclin T1/CDK9 complexes, which can promote transcription of the virus in a TAR-independent fashion (60–62), and likely also of host gene promoters. Sp-1 did not appear as a binding motif in Tat-enhanced promoters, but it was one of the factors associated with Meth-induced activation. Thus, in the presence of Meth, or in the absence of TBP, transcription factor redundancy and promoter plasticity may perpetuate and broaden gene transcription, including of HIV.

Two transcription factors appeared to be common between HIV-1 Tat and Meth, which were Egr-1, and IRF4. Further studies are necessary to examine which common genes can be controlled by these transcription factors, to estimate their value as targets of intervention. In the non-human primate model of neuroHIV, we have previously demonstrated that a decrease in Egr-1 expression in neurons is associated with neurological deficits in the context of inflammation (63). Its role in cell transcriptional regulation has been described (64). IRF4, on the other hand, is a positive regulator of inflammation (65, 66), converge as a common epigenetic switch.

Our results suggest that the occurrence of additional cellular stimulus in HIV-1 may deviate transcription factor usage, by promoting diversity. However, a role for TBP inhibitors should not be ruled out as a strategy to ameliorate stimulant drug users. For instance, it has been suggested that although the Tata-box promoter domain sequences are selectively used by TBP *in vivo*, the binding can be modulated by TBP inhibitors such as TBA-associated factor 1 (TAF1) (67–69). In addition, Tat in combination with Meth enhanced the acute translocation of Tat into the cellular nucleus, which may have implications to the viral transcription, not examined here.

Overall, we have found a key role for TBP in the induction of genes containing the TATA-box core promoter element by the HIV Tat peptide, characterized by early response, inflammatory and metabolic genes. We have also determined the effect of the interactions between Tat and Meth, a common co-morbidity of HIV infection, on diversifying the collection of transcription factors able to redundantly act on the activation of promoters, RNA Pol recruitment and ultimately transcription of genes with important implications in inflammatory pathology. Our findings help explain aggravated phenotypes associated to inflammation and to metabolic disorders that are commonly observed in HIV+ individuals with substance use disorders, but also suggest that in these individuals, targeting elements of the transcriptional machinery posits the risk of failure, while dealing with additional molecular complexities.

AUTHOR CONTRIBUTIONS

RT performed the Crispr/Cas9 disruption of TBP expression, tested and selected the positive clones, and performed all the *in vitro* stimulations. JAN performed the fixation of cells for RNA Pol ChIP assay. AL performed THP1-deficient cells PCRs. LAC provided guidance for the design and execution of Crispr/Cas9-based TBP disruption, reviewed all the results, helped in the analysis, and in the writing of the manuscript. JJ tested all the primers for PCR validation. LB participated in the experimental design, performed all TBP-sufficient cell cultures and stimulation experiments, fixations for ChIP assays, performed PCRs, and helped in writing the manuscript. MM developed the concept, designed the study, obtained funding, supervised experiments, menthored students, revised all results, performed all systems biology-based approaches, revised statistical results, and wrote the manuscript.

ACKNOWLEDGMENTS

We want to thank Drs. Paul Labhart and Madeleine Lisa Craske (Active Motif Inc., Carlsbad, CA), for technical support and help with troubleshooting. We thank Daniel Ryan (SDBRI) and Nikki

Bortell for critically reviewing the manuscript, Christine Auciello and Fazila Kiyam for administrative support.

SUPPLEMENTARY MATERIAL

Supplementary Table 1 | TBP megatargetome-RNA Pol ChIP average peak values in genes that have a TATA-box binding motif in the core promoter element. Cross linking for RNA Pol II ChIP was performed 15 min after stimulation with HIV Tat (10 ng/ml), Meth (60 μM), or Tat+Meth, for determination of gene intervals, and average peak ratios.

Supplementary Table 2 | The effect of TBP disruption in the response to Tat and/or Meth. RNA-seq was performed in TBP-defficient clone 2A and compared to TBP-sufficient clone C. T = Tat stimulation, M = Meth stimulation, MT = Meth+Tat. Gene IDs, Transcript ID, chromosomes and gene intervals are provided. This experiment was performed in triplicate.

Supplementary Figure S1 | TBP nuclear translocation. The PMA-differentiated THP1 cells were stimulated with Meth (60 μM), and/or HIV Tat (10 ng/ml) for examination of TBP nuclear translocation 5, 15, 30, and 60 min following stimulation, by immunocytochemistry. TBP was stained in red, and nuclei were visualized with DAPI (blue). Confocal images were used for the determination of a translocation index, as the percentage of total TBP staining that was co-localized with DAPI. Representative images of **(A)** Controls and Tat stimulation, **(B)** Tat+Meth stimulation. This experiment was performed three times in triplicate.

REFERENCES

1. Basova L, Najera JA, Bortell N, Wang D, Moya R, Lindsey A, et al. Dopamine and its receptors play a role in the modulation of CCR5 expression in innate immune cells following exposure to Methamphetamine: implications to HIV infection. *PLoS ONE* (2018) 13:e0199861. doi: 10.1371/journal.pone.0199861
2. Bosshart H, Heinzelmann M. THP-1 cells as a model for human monocytes. *Ann Transl Med.* (2016) 4:438. doi: 10.21037/atm.2016.08.53
3. Fauci AS. Host factors and the pathogenesis of HIV induced disease. *Nature* (1996) 384:529–34. doi: 10.1038/384529a0
4. Lindl KA, Marks DR, Kolson DL, Jordan-Sciutto KL. HIV-associated neurocognitive disorder: pathogenesis and therapeutic opportunities. *J Neuroimmune Pharmacol.* (2010) 5:294–309. doi: 10.1007/s11481-010-9205-z
5. Marcondes MC, Flynn C, Watry DD, Zandonatti M, Fox HS. Methamphetamine increases brain viral load and activates natural killer cells in simian immunodeficiency virus-infected monkeys. *Am J Pathol.* (2010) 177:355–61. doi: 10.2353/ajpath.2010.090953
6. Nath A, Maragos WF, Avison MJ, Schmitt FA, Berger JR. Acceleration of HIV dementia with methamphetamine and cocaine. *J Neurovirol.* (2001) 7:66–71. doi: 10.1080/135502801300069737
7. Najera JA, Bustamante EA, Bortell N, Morsey B, Fox HS, Ravasi T, et al. Methamphetamine abuse affects gene expression in brain-derived microglia of SIV-infected macaques to enhance inflammation and promote virus targets. *BMC Immunol.* (2016) 17:7. doi: 10.1186/s12865-016-0145-0
8. Bortell N, Morsey B, Basova L, Fox HS, Marcondes MC. Phenotypic changes in the brain of SIV-infected macaques exposed to methamphetamine parallel macrophage activation patterns induced by the common gamma-chain cytokine system. *Front Microbiol.* (2015) 6:900. doi: 10.3389/fmicb.2015.00900
9. Debaisieux S, Rayne F, Yezid H, Beaumelle B. The ins and outs of HIV-1 Tat. *Traffic* (2012) 13:355–63. doi: 10.1111/j.1600-0854.2011.01286.x
10. Rayne F, Debaisieux S, Bonhoure A, Beaumelle B. HIV-1 Tat is unconventionally secreted through the plasma membrane. *Cell Biol Int.* (2010) 34:409–13. doi: 10.1042/CBI20090376
11. Rayne F, Debaisieux S, Tu A, Chopard C, Tryoen-Toth P, Beaumelle B. Detecting HIV-1 Tat in cell culture supernatants by ELISA or Western Blot. *Methods Mol Biol.* (2016) 1354:329–42. doi: 10.1007/978-1-4939-3046-3_22
12. Vendeville, Rayne F, Bonhoure A, Bettache N, Montcourrier P, Beaumelle B. HIV-1 Tat enters T cells using coated pits before translocating from acidified endosomes and eliciting biological responses. *Mol Biol Cell* (2004) 15:2347–60. doi: 10.1091/mbc.e03-12-0921
13. Carey AN, Liu X, Mintzopoulos D, Paris JJ, Muschamp JW, McLaughlin JP, et al. Conditional Tat protein expression in the GT-tg bigenic mouse brain induces gray matter density reductions. *Prog Neuro Psychopharmacol Biol Psychiatry* (2013) 43:49–54. doi: 10.1016/j.pnpbp.2012.12.018
14. Carey AN, Sypek EI, Singh HD, Kaufman MJ, McLaughlin JP. Expression of HIV-Tat protein is associated with learning and memory deficits in the mouse. *Behav Brain Res.* (2012) 229:48–56. doi: 10.1016/j.bbr.2011.12.019
15. Kesby JP, Najera JA, Romoli B, Fang Y, Basova L, Birmingham A, et al. HIV-1 TAT protein enhances sensitization to methamphetamine by affecting dopaminergic function. *Brain Behav Immun.* (2017) 65:210–21. doi: 10.1016/j.bbi.2017.05.004
16. Bannwarth S, Gatignol A. HIV-1 TAR RNA: the target of molecular interactions between the virus and its host. *Curr HIV Res.* (2005) 3:61–71. doi: 10.2174/1570162052772924
17. Brady J, Kashanchi F. Tat gets the "green" light on transcription initiation. *Retrovirology* (2005) 2:69. doi: 10.1186/1742-4690-2-69
18. Davidson A, Leeper TC, Athanassiou Z, Patora-Komisarska K, Karn J, Robinson JA, et al. Simultaneous recognition of HIV-1 TAR RNA bulge and loop sequences by cyclic peptide mimics of Tat protein. *Proc Natl Acad Sci USA.* (2009) 106:11931–6. doi: 10.1073/pnas.0900629106
19. Naryshkin NA, Gait MJ, Ivanovskaya MG. RNA recognition and regulation of HIV-1 gene expression by viral factor Tat. *Biochemistry* (1998) 63: 489–503.
20. Richter, Ping YH, Rana TM. TAR RNA loop: a scaffold for the assembly of a regulatory switch in HIV replication. *Proc Natl Acad Sci USA.* (2002) 99:7928–33. doi: 10.1073/pnas.122119999
21. Wei P, Garber ME, Fang SM, Fischer WH, Jones KA. A novel CDK9-associated C-type cyclin interacts directly with HIV-1 Tat and mediates its high-affinity, loop-specific binding to TAR RNA. *Cell* (1998) 92:451–62. doi: 10.1016/S0092-8674(00)80939-3
22. Bieniasz PD, Grdina TA, Bogerd HP, Cullen BR. Recruitment of cyclin T1/P-TEFb to an HIV type 1 long terminal repeat promoter proximal RNA target is both necessary and sufficient for full activation of transcription. *Proc Natl Acad Sci USA.* (1999) 96:7791–6. doi: 10.1073/pnas.96.14.7791
23. Raha T, Cheng SW, Green MR. HIV-1 Tat stimulates transcription complex assembly through recruitment of TBP in the absence of TAFs. *PLoS Biol.* (2005) 3:e44. doi: 10.1371/journal.pbio.0030044
24. Verrijzer CP, Yokomori K, Chen JL, Tjian R. Drosophila TAFII150: similarity to yeast gene TSM-1 and specific binding to core promoter DNA. *Science* (1994) 264:933–41. doi: 10.1126/science.8178153
25. Kim YS, Panganiban AT. Examination of TAR-independent Trans activation by human immunodeficiency virus type 1 Tat in human glial cells. *J Neurosci Res.* (1996) 43:652–66. doi: 10.1002/(SICI)1097-4547(19960315)43:6<652::AID-JNR2>3.0.CO;2-D
26. Pu H, Tian J, Flora G, Lee YW, Nath A, Hennig B, et al. HIV-1 Tat protein upregulates inflammatory mediators and induces monocyte invasion into the brain. *Mol Cell Neurosci.* (2003) 24:224–37. doi: 10.1016/S1044-7431(03)00171-4
27. Toborek M, Lee YW, Pu H, Malecki A, Flora G, Garrido R, et al. HIV-Tat protein induces oxidative and inflammatory pathways in brain endothelium. *J Neurochem.* (2003) 84:169–79. doi: 10.1046/j.1471-4159.2003.01543.x
28. Roebuck KA, Rabbi MF, Kagnoff MF. HIV-1 Tat protein can transactivate a heterologous TATAA element independent of viral promoter sequences and the trans-activation response element. *AIDS* (1997) 11:139–46. doi: 10.1097/00002030-199702000-00002

29. Veschambre P, Simard P, Jalinot P. Evidence for functional interaction between the HIV-1 Tat transactivator and the TATA box binding protein in vivo. *J Mol Biol.* (1995) 250:169–80. doi: 10.1006/jmbi.1995.0368
30. Andras IE, Pu H, Deli MA, Nath A, Hennig B, Toborek M. HIV-1 Tat protein alters tight junction protein expression and distribution in cultured brain endothelial cells. *J Neurosci Res.* (2003) 74:255–65. doi: 10.1002/jnr.10762
31. Ben Haij N, Planes R, Leghmari K, Serrero M, Delobel P, Izopet J, et al. HIV-1 Tat protein induces production of proinflammatory cytokines by human dendritic cells and monocytes/macrophages through engagement of TLR4-MD2-CD14 complex and activation of NF-kappaB pathway. *PLoS ONE* (2015) 10:e0129425. doi: 10.1371/journal.pone.0129425
32. Ben Haij N, Leghmari K, Planes R, Thieblemont N, Bahraoui E. HIV-1 Tat protein binds to TLR4-MD2 and signals to induce TNF-alpha and IL-10. *Retrovirology* (2013) 10:123. doi: 10.1186/1742-4690-10-123
33. Leghmari K, Bennasser Y, Bahraoui E. HIV-1 Tat protein induces IL-10 production in monocytes by classical and alternative NF-kappaB pathways. *Eur J Cell Biol.* (2008) 87:947–62. doi: 10.1016/j.ejcb.2008.06.005
34. Contreras X, Bennasser Y, Bahraoui E. IL-10 production induced by HIV-1 Tat stimulation of human monocytes is dependent on the activation of PKC beta(II) and delta isozymes. *Microbes Infect.* (2004) 6:1182–90. doi: 10.1016/j.micinf.2004.06.008
35. Bennasser Y, Badou A, Tkaczuk J, Bahraoui E. Signaling pathways triggered by HIV-1 Tat in human monocytes to induce TNF-alpha. *Virology* (2002) 303:174–80. doi: 10.1006/viro.2002.1676
36. Bennasser Y, Contreras X, Moreau M, Le Clerc C, Badou A, Bahraoui E. HIV-1 Tat protein induces IL-10 production by human monocytes: implications of the PKC and calcium pathway. *J Soc Biol.* (2001) 195:319–26. doi: 10.1051/jbio/2001195030319
37. Vives E, Charneau P, van Rietschoten J, Rochat H, Bahraoui E. Effects of the Tat basic domain on human immunodeficiency virus type 1 transactivation, using chemically synthesized Tat protein and Tat peptides. *J Virol.* (1994) 68:3343–53.
38. Hahn S, Buratowski S, Sharp PA, Guarente L, Isolation of the gene encoding the yeast TATA binding protein TFIID: a gene identical to the SPT15 suppressor of Ty element insertions. *Cell* (1989) 58:1173–81. doi: 10.1016/0092-8674(89)90515-1
39. Hahn S, Buratowski S, Sharp PA, Guarente L. Yeast TATA-binding protein TFIID binds to TATA elements with both consensus and nonconsensus DNA sequences. *Proc Natl Acad Sci US A.* (1989) 86:5718–22. doi: 10.1073/pnas.86.15.5718
40. Yang C, Bolotin E, Jiang T, Sladek FM, Martinez E. Prevalence of the initiator over the TATA box in human and yeast genes and identification of DNA motifs enriched in human TATA-less core promoters. *Gene* (2007) 389:52–65. doi: 10.1016/j.gene.2006.09.029
41. Suzuki Y, Tsunoda T, Sese J, Taira H, Mizushima-Sugano J, Hata H, et al. Identification and characterization of the potential promoter regions of 1031 kinds of human genes. *Genome Res.* (2001) 11:677–84. doi: 10.1101/gr.GR-1640R
42. Tullai JW, Schaffer ME, Mullenbrock S, Sholder G, Kasif S, Cooper GM. Immediate-early and delayed primary response genes are distinct in function and genomic architecture. *J Biol Chem.* (2007) 282:23981–95. doi: 10.1074/jbc.M702044200
43. Marban C, Su T, Ferrari R, Li B, Vatakis D, Pellegrini M, et al. Genome-wide binding map of the HIV-1 Tat protein to the human genome. *PLoS ONE* (2011) 6:e26894. doi: 10.1371/journal.pone.0026894
44. Reeder JE, Kwak YT, McNamara RP, Forst CV, D'Orso I. HIV Tat controls RNA Polymerase II and the epigenetic landscape to transcriptionally reprogram target immune cells. *Elife* (2015) 4:e08955. doi: 10.7554/eLife.08955
45. Kashanchi F, Piras G, Radonovich MF, Duvall JF, Fattaey A, Chiang CM, et al. Direct interaction of human TFIID with the HIV-1 transactivator tat. *Nature* (1994) 367:295–9. doi: 10.1038/367295a0
46. Majello B, Napolitano G, Lania L. Recruitment of the TATA-binding protein to the HIV-1 promoter is a limiting step for Tat transactivation. *AIDS* (1998) 12:1957–64. doi: 10.1097/00002030-199815000-00006
47. Wilson JM, Kalasinsky KS, Levey AI, Bergeron C, Reiber G, Anthony RM, et al. Striatal dopamine nerve terminal markers in human, chronic methamphetamine users. *Nat Med.* (1996) 2:699–703. doi: 10.1038/nm0696-699
48. Xu S, Grullon S, Ge K, Peng W. Spatial clustering for identification of ChIP-enriched regions (SICER) to map regions of histone methylation patterns in embryonic stem cells. *Methods Mol Biol.* (2014) 1150:97–111. doi: 10.1007/978-1-4939-0512-6_5
49. Chekmenev DS, Haid C, Kel AE. P-Match: transcription factor binding site search by combining patterns and weight matrices. *Nucleic Acids Res.* (2005) 33:W432–7. doi: 10.1093/nar/gki441
50. Kel AE, Gossling E, Reuter I, Cheremushkin E, Kel-Margoulis OV, Wingender E. MATCH: A tool for searching transcription factor binding sites in DNA sequences. *Nucleic Acids Res.* (2003) 31:3576–9. doi: 10.1093/nar/gkg585
51. Zuris JA, Thompson DB, Shu Y, Guilinger JP, Bessen JL, Hu JH, et al. Cationic lipid-mediated delivery of proteins enables efficient protein-based genome editing *in vitro* and *in vivo*. *Nat Biotechnol.* (2015) 33:73–80. doi: 10.1038/nbt.3081
52. Fu Y, Foden JA, Khayter C, Maeder ML, Reyon D, Joung JK, et al. High-frequency off-target mutagenesis induced by CRISPR-Cas nucleases in human cells. *Nat Biotechnol.* (2013) 31:822–6. doi: 10.1038/nbt.2623
53. Lin S, Staahl BT, Alla RK, Doudna JA. Enhanced homology-directed human genome engineering by controlled timing of CRISPR/Cas9 delivery. *Elife* (2014) 3:e04766. doi: 10.7554/eLife.04766
54. Mali P, Aach J, Stranges PB, Esvelt KM, Moosburner M, Kosuri S, et al. CAS9 transcriptional activators for target specificity screening and paired nickases for cooperative genome engineering. *Nat Biotechnol.* (2013) 31:833–8. doi: 10.1038/nbt.2675
55. Hsu PD, Scott DA, Weinstein JA, Ran FA, Konermann S, Agarwala V, et al. DNA targeting specificity of RNA-guided Cas9 nucleases. *Nat Biotechnol.* (2013) 31:827–32. doi: 10.1038/nbt.2647
56. Janky R, Verfaillie A, Imrichova H, Van de Sande B, Standaert L, Christiaens V, et al. iRegulon: from a gene list to a gene regulatory network using large motif and track collections. *PLoS Comput Biol.* (2014) 10:e1003731. doi: 10.1371/journal.pcbi.1003731
57. Blake JA, Harris MA. The Gene Ontology (GO) project: structured vocabularies for molecular biology and their application to genome and expression analysis. *Curr Protoc Bioinformatics* (2002) Chapter 7:Unit 7.2. doi: 10.1002/0471250953.bi0702s23
58. Harris MA, Clark J, Ireland A, Lomax J, Ashburner M, Foulger R, et al. The Gene Ontology (GO) database and informatics resource. *Nucleic Acids Res.* (2004) 32:D258–61. doi: 10.1093/nar/gkh036
59. Suslov VV, Ponomarenko PM, Efimov VM, Savinkova LK, Ponomarenko MP, Kolchanov NA. SNPs in the HIV-1 TATA box and the AIDS pandemic. *J Bioinform Comput Biol.* (2010) 8:607–25. doi: 10.1142/S0219720010004677
60. Berkhout B, Gatignol A, Rabson AB, Jeang KT. TAR-independent activation of the HIV-1 LTR: evidence that tat requires specific regions of the promoter. *Cell* (1990) 62:757–67. doi: 10.1016/0092-8674(90)90120-4
61. Loregian A, Bortolozzo K, Boso S, Sapino B, Betti M, Biasolo MA, et al. The Sp1 transcription factor does not directly interact with the HIV-1 Tat protein. *J Cell Physiol.* (2003) 196:251–7. doi: 10.1002/jcp.10271
62. Loregian A, Bortolozzo K, Boso S, Caputo A, Palu G. Interaction of Sp1 transcription factor with HIV-1 Tat protein: looking for cellular partners. *FEBS Lett.* (2003) 543:l61–5. doi: 10.1016/S0014-5793(03)00399-5
63. Gersten M, Alirezaei M, Marcondes MC, Flynn C, Ravasi T, Ideker T, et al. An integrated systems analysis implicates EGR1 downregulation in simian immunodeficiency virus encephalitis-induced neural dysfunction. *J Neurosci.* (2009) 29:12467–76. doi: 10.1523/JNEUROSCI.3180-09.2009
64. Sarkar R, Verma SC. Egr-1 regulates RTA transcription through a cooperative involvement of transcriptional regulators. *Oncotarget* (2017) 8:91425–44. doi: 10.18632/oncotarget.20648
65. Achuthan A, Cook AD, Lee MC, Saleh R, Khiew HW, Chang MW, et al. Granulocyte macrophage colony-stimulating factor induces CCL17 production via IRF4 to mediate inflammation. *J Clin Invest.* (2016) 126:3453–66. doi: 10.1172/JCI87828
66. Lech M, Weidenbusch M, Kulkarni OP, Ryu M, Darisipudi MN, Susanti HE, et al. IRF4 deficiency abrogates lupus nephritis despite enhancing

systemic cytokine production. *J Am Soc Nephrol.* (2011) 22:1443–52. doi: 10.1681/ASN.2010121260

67. Basehoar AD, Zanton SJ, Pugh BF. Identification and distinct regulation of yeast TATA box-containing genes. *Cell* (2004) 116:699–709. doi: 10.1016/S0092-8674(04)00205-3
68. Chitikila, Huisinga KL, Irvin JD, Basehoar AD, Pugh BF. Interplay of TBP inhibitors in global transcriptional control. Mol *Cell* (2002) 10:871–82. doi: 10.1016/S1097-2765(02)00683-4
69. Jackson-Fisher AJ, Chitikila C, Mitra M, Pugh BF. A role for TBP dimerization in preventing unregulated gene expression. *Mol Cell* (1999) 3:717–27. doi: 10.1016/S1097-2765(01)80004-6

7

Long-Term Delivery of an Anti-SIV Monoclonal Antibody With AAV

José M. Martinez-Navio[1†], Sebastian P. Fuchs[1†], Desiree E. Mendes[1], Eva G. Rakasz[2], Guangping Gao[3], Jeffrey D. Lifson[4] and Ronald C. Desrosiers[1]*

[1] Department of Pathology, Miller School of Medicine, University of Miami, Miami, FL, United States, [2] Wisconsin National Primate Research Center, University of Wisconsin, Madison, WI, United States, [3] Gene Therapy Center, University of Massachusetts Medical School, Worcester, MA, United States, [4] AIDS and Cancer Virus Program, Frederick National Laboratory for Cancer Research, Frederick, MD, United States

***Correspondence:**
Ronald C. Desrosiers
r.desrosiers@med.miami.edu

† These authors have contributed equally to this work and share first authorship

Long-term delivery of anti-HIV monoclonal antibodies using adeno-associated virus (AAV) holds promise for the prevention and treatment of HIV infection. We previously reported that after receiving a single administration of AAV vector coding for anti-SIV antibody 5L7, monkey 84-05 achieved high levels of AAV-delivered 5L7 IgG1 *in vivo* which conferred sterile protection against six successive, escalating dose, intravenous challenges with highly infectious, highly pathogenic SIVmac239, including a final challenge with 10 animal infectious doses (1). Here we report that monkey 84-05 has successfully maintained 240–350 μg/ml of anti-SIV antibody 5L7 for over 6 years. Approximately 2% of the circulating IgG in this monkey is this one monoclonal antibody. This monkey generated little or no anti-drug antibodies (ADA) to the AAV-delivered antibody for the duration of the study. Due to the nature of the high-dose challenge used and in order to rule out a potential low-level infection not detected by regular viral loads, we have used ultrasensitive techniques to detect cell-associated viral DNA and RNA in PBMCs from this animal. In addition, we have tested serum from 84-05 by ELISA against overlapping peptides spanning the whole envelope sequence for SIVmac239 (PepScan) and against recombinant p27 and gp41 proteins. No reactivity has been detected in the ELISAs indicating the absence of naturally arising anti-SIV antibodies; moreover, the ultrasensitive cell-associated viral tests yielded no positive reaction. We conclude that macaque 84-05 was effectively protected and remained uninfected. Our data show that durable, continuous antibody expression can be achieved after one single administration of AAV and support the potential for lifelong protection against HIV from a single vector administration.

Keywords: gene therapy, AAV vector, long-term expression, broadly neutralizing antibodies, HIV/SIV cure, immunotherapy, prophylaxis, rhesus monkeys

INTRODUCTION

Gene therapy has come of age. Almost 50 years after its inception, gene therapy is now considered a promising treatment option for several human diseases including cancer, genetic disorders and infectious disease (2). Gene therapies can work by several mechanisms: replacing defective genes with healthy ones, adding new genes to help the body fight or treat disease, or deactivating problematic genes (3). Importantly, for any of these gene therapy approaches, achieving long-term delivery of the transgene remains a key, infrequently realized goal. Recombinant adeno-associated virus (AAV) vectors have been widely used for such gene delivery applications because of their safety and cost-efficiency: a single injection can result in long-term expression of the transgene product (4). Also, recombinant AAV is ideal as a delivery vehicle in some additional respects: the only protein expressed from it comes from the inserted transgene; it can effectively transduce terminally differentiated non-dividing cells; and it shows little or no integration into host genome sequences (5–10).

One potentially important application of the AAV system is the delivery of broadly neutralizing antibodies as a gene therapy approach against HIV (1, 11–14). For that purpose, recombinant AAVs encoding neutralizing antibodies are inoculated into the host and the antibody or antibodies of interest will then be directly expressed from the transduced cells. Thus, the immune system is bypassed in the sense that no immune response to an immunogen or vaccine is needed; the desired final products (broadly neutralizing antibodies) are delivered directly to the host. This approach against HIV has been made realistically possible in recent years thanks to the isolation and characterization of a remarkable collection of potent, broadly-neutralizing, monoclonal antibodies from select individuals (15–17). These antibodies have been extensively characterized in the laboratory and some have moved to clinical trials, where they have shown activity (18–22). They have the potential to prevent infection and also serve as a therapeutic approach complementing or even substituting antiretroviral drugs (11, 14, 18, 20–25). Importantly, the use of AAV voids the need for repeated administrations of purified antibody to maintain therapeutic levels in circulation. Due to its simplicity and ease of deployment, the approach is ideal for global use (26).

One main problem has been encountered in the applicability of this approach. Host antibodies generated against the delivered antibody (generally known as anti-drug antibodies or ADAs) can reduce its functionality and concentration thus drastically reducing its effectiveness (1, 11, 24, 27–32). The large repertoire of endogenously generated antibodies present in any individual has gone through a complex checks and balances system to be allowed into circulation (33). The antibodies being made in one individual are different from the antibodies being made in another individual (34). In addition, the potent broadly-neutralizing anti-HIV antibodies that one would want to use for these applications are typically highly evolved over a prolonged period of time. Due to years of affinity maturation, they exhibit unusually high levels of somatic hypermutation in the variable domains and many have accumulated unusual structural features (35, 36) which are generally required for potent neutralization and breadth (37). This high level of mutation likely enhances the immunogenicity of these antibodies when delivered to a host other than the one in which those particular sequences originated. Interestingly, when characterizing the humoral responses to the AAV-delivered antibodies we and others have found that the variable regions were predominantly or exclusively targeted (1, 11, 28, 30). We have also reported a highly significant correlation of the magnitude of the host anti-antibody response with the distance from germline of the AAV-delivered antibody: the more mutated, the more immunogenic (28). ADAs are in fact a common problem with many gene therapy approaches (38, 39). However, if the hurdle of the ADAs can be overcome, the promise of the AAV-delivery of antibodies against HIV could be realized (12). Here, we report that monkey 84-05 has maintained 240–350 μg/ml of anti-SIV antibody 5L7 for over 6 years in the absence of detectable ADAs. Our data show that durable, continuous antibody expression can be achieved after a single administration of AAV and support the potential for lifelong protection against HIV from a single vector administration.

MATERIALS AND METHODS

Macaque 84-05

The animal used in this study is a *Mamu B*08*-neg *B*17*-neg female Indian-origin rhesus macaque (*Macaca mulatta*), originally housed at the New England Primate Research Center in a biosafety level 3 animal containment facility in accordance with the standards of the Association for Assessment and Accreditation of Laboratory Animal Care and the Harvard Medical School Animal Care and Use Committee. Research was conducted according to the principles described in the *Guide for the Care and Use of Laboratory Animals* and was approved by the Harvard Medical School Animal Care and Use Committee (40). Macaque 84-05 tested negative for the presence of antibodies to HIV and AAV1 capsid prior to AAV administration. At the time this manuscript was written, the monkey was 14 years old and weighted 6.4 kg. She was administered AAV encoding for 5L7 antibody when she was 7 years old and weighted 5.5 kg (1). At week 108 (about 2 years) post-AAV administration, the monkey was transferred to and subsequently housed at the Wisconsin National Primate Research Center and cared for in accordance with the guidelines of the Weatherall Report under a protocol approved by the University of Wisconsin Graduate School Animal Care and Use Committee.

Recombinant AAV

Coding sequences were designed *in silico*, codon-optimized and gene-synthesized (GenScript). 5L7 immunoadhesin sequences (11) served as a template and full-length antibodies were constructed by adding CH1 domain and CL domain of rhesus IgG to the already known immunoadhesin sequences. 5L7 sequences originate from recombinant anti-SIV Fab sequences (347-23h) derived from the bone marrow of SIV-infected rhesus monkeys (41). The rhesus IgG1 sequence used is based on accession no. AAF14058 and AAQ57555. Rhesus kappa light chain was designed using the constant light domain sequence from AAD02577. Synthesized fragments were then cloned into the NotI site of our AAV vector plasmids (1, 42). Production of recombinant AAVs was conducted as described previously (43). In short, HEK-293 cells were transfected with a select AAV vector plasmid and two helper plasmids to allow generation of infectious AAV particles. After harvesting transfected cells and cell culture supernatant, AAV was purified by three sequential CsCl centrifugation steps. Vector genome number was assessed by Real-Time PCR, and the purity of the preparation was verified by electron microscopy and silver-stained SDS-PAGE. The AAV genomes were encapsidated with the AAV1 serotype.

Monkey 84-05 received recombinant AAV1 encoding the anti-SIV antibody 5L7, using a total dose of 1.6×10^{13} particles (2.9×10^{12} AAV vector genomes per kilogram of body weight). AAV administration was conducted by a one-time inoculation of four deep intramuscular injections (two separate 0.5 ml injections into both quadriceps).

Recombinant 5L7 Antibody

5L7 recognizes gp120 and gp140 forms of the SIVmac239 envelope glycoprotein (28) and binds conformational epitopes involving the V3-V4 region (41). HEK-293T cells were expanded and then transfected with recombinant AAV vector plasmid coding for 5L7 antibody. Cells were washed after 4 h with pre-warmed PBS and then transferred to serum-free medium (Invitrogen). Afterwards, the antibody-containing medium was harvested, precleared by centrifugation, and filtered through a 0.22 μm-pore-size membrane. Then, IgG was affinity-purified using protein A Sepharose 4 Fast Flow (GE Healthcare), concentrated and desalted, followed by protein quantification with a Nanodrop UV spectrometer (Thermo Fisher Scientific). Antibody purity was confirmed by sodium dodecyl sulfate-polyacrylamide gel electrophoresis (SDS-PAGE) and subsequent Coomassie blue staining (Thermo Fisher Scientific).

In vivo 5L7 Antibody Quantification and Anti-Drug Antibody (ADA) Responses

AAV-delivered 5L7 antibody was quantitated by standard ELISA using plate bound SIVmac239 gp140 (Immune Tech) to capture the antibody from pre-diluted serum samples and then HRP-conjugated secondary anti-rhesus IgG (Southern Biotech) as the detection method. Absorbance at 450 nm was compared to a serial dilution of purified 5L7 produced in HEK 293T cells, and the amount of antibody in serum was interpolated based on the standard curve. To measure host humoral responses to the AAV-delivered 5L7 antibody, purified recombinant 5L7 was used to coat plates. Then, serum samples from monkey 84-05 were tested at a 1:20 dilution and ADA responses were detected by means of an anti-lambda HRP-conjugated secondary antibody (Southern Biotech) in a regular ELISA (28). This secondary did not cross-react with 5L7 coated on the plates since 5L7 bears a kappa light chain. This allowed us to readily detect those anti-antibodies with a lambda light chain, which have been reported to reflect humoral responses in our previous studies (1, 28). Levels of AAV-delivered 5L7, and the corresponding ADAs, were measured for a total of 340 weeks.

PepScan

PepScan or ELISA against a panel of 218 peptides overlapping the entire SIVmac239 envelope protein was used to detect antibody responses to the viral spike. Fifteen-mer-length peptides, each successive peptide overlapped by 11 amino acids, were obtained from the NIH AIDS Research and Reference Reagent Program. Peptides were properly resuspended and used to coat ELISA plates at 40 μg/ml in phosphate-buffered saline (PBS). Plates were then washed, blocked and incubated for 1 h at 37°C with a 1:20 dilution of the corresponding monkey sera or 5L7 antibody diluted to 2 μg/ml. Binding antibodies were detected with an HRP-conjugated goat anti-human IgG antibody (SouthernBiotech) diluted 1:1,000 in 5% non-fat powdered milk in PBS and developed with soluble tetramethylbenzidine (TMB) reagent (Calbiochem, Gibbstown, NJ). The reaction was stopped by the addition of 50 μl of acidic stop solution (SouthernBiotech, Birmingham, AL), and the optical density at 450 nm was measured using a Wallac Victor plate reader (Perkin-Elmer, Waltham, MA).

Antibody Responses to p27 and gp41

Antibody responses against p27 and gp41 were quantitated by regular ELISA using SIVmac239 p27 purified recombinant protein (Catalog# 13446; obtained through the NIH AIDS Reagent Program, Division of AIDS, NIAID, NIH) and recombinant SIV gp41 (Catalog# 5019; ImmunoDX) to coat plates at 10 μg/ml in PBS. Plates were then washed, blocked and incubated for 1 h at 37°C with a 1:20 dilution of the corresponding monkey sera or 5L7 antibody diluted to 2 μg/ml. Antibodies binding the p27 antigen or the gp41 were detected with a goat anti-monkey secondary antibody (Catalog# 2015-05, Santa Cruz) and developed with TMB High Sensitivity Substrate Solution (Catalog# 421501, Biolegend). The reaction was stopped by the addition of 50 μl of acidic stop solution (SouthernBiotech, Birmingham, AL), and the optical density at 450 nm was measured using a Wallac Victor plate reader (Perkin-Elmer, Waltham, MA).

Viral Load Monitoring

Plasma SIV RNA was measured using a gag-targeted quantitative real-time/digital PCR method with 6 replicate reactions analyzed per extracted sample for an assay threshold of 30 SIV RNA copies/ml (44). Cell-associated SIV RNA and DNA were measured by quantitative hybrid real-time/digital RT-PCR and PCR assays (45, 46).

RESULTS

Over 6 Years of Continuous Antibody Expression *in vivo*

Monkey 84-05 received a single administration of AAV on September 6th, 2012. As we reported at that time (1), starting at week 44 post-AAV inoculation and then every 3 weeks, this animal was repeatedly challenged with highly pathogenic, highly infectious SIVmac239 for a total of six intravenous administrations (see schematics in **Figure 1A**). The first four challenges were performed with 1 animal infectious dose (AID), followed by challenge with 2 AID and then a final 10 AID challenge. Viral load measurements in plasma from 84-05 were negative (<30 copies/ml), indicating the animal successfully resisted all six challenges (1). The antibody levels achieved remarkable values of ~270 μg/ml (1). We now report long-term follow-up on levels of 5L7 antibody and the corresponding ADAs in circulation. As shown in **Figure 1B**, macaque 84-05 has successfully maintained 240–350 μg/ml of anti-SIV antibody 5L7 for over 340 weeks (>6 years). Moreover, this animal has

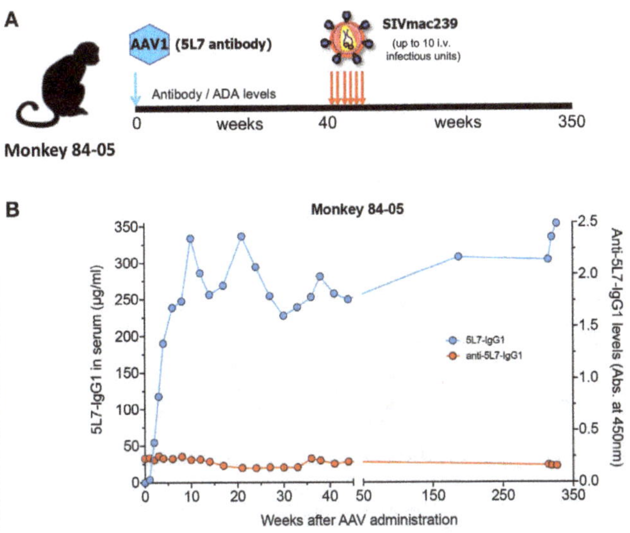

FIGURE 1 | 5L7 antibody levels and the corresponding anti-antibodies (ADAs) in serum following AAV administration. **(A)** Schematic of the experiment in which rhesus monkey 84-05 received intramuscular administration of AAV1 coding for antibody 5L7 and was subsequently challenged with SIVmac239 (six times: 4 times with a 1 animal infectious doses followed by a 2x dose challenge and a final 10x dose challenge). **(B)** 5L7 antibody levels (blue; plotted on left axis) and anti-5L7 antibody levels (red; plotted on right axis) in serum from monkey 84-05, quantified by ELISA.

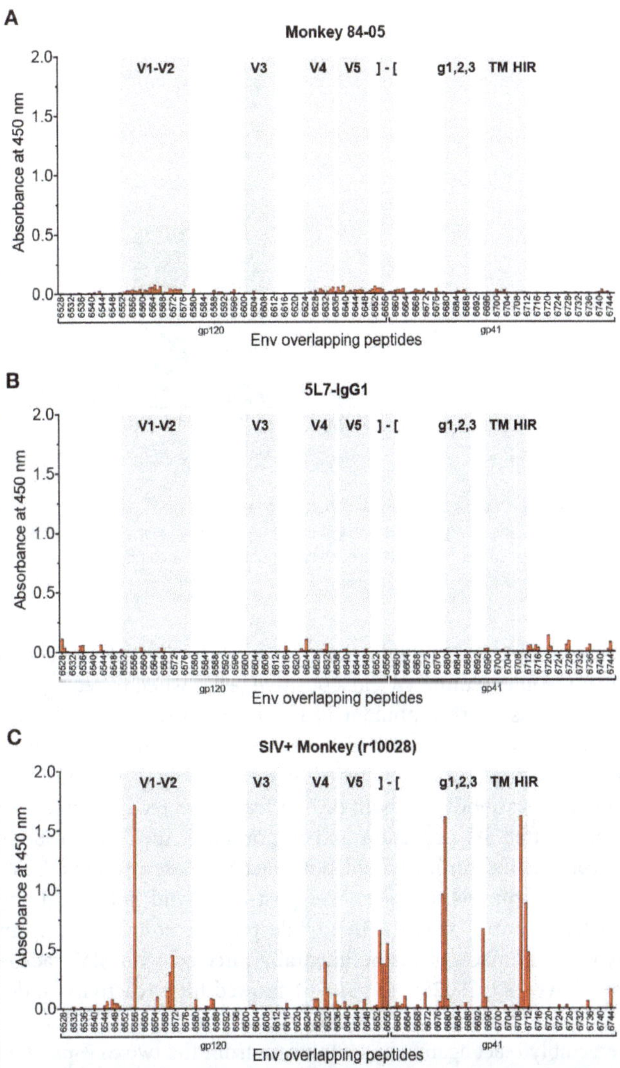

FIGURE 2 | Analysis of antibody responses by PepScan. PepScan (ELISA against overlapping peptides) spanning the whole envelope sequence for SIVmac239, performed with **(A)** serum from 84-05 (week 328 post-AAV) at a 1:20 dilution; **(B)** recombinant purified 5L7 antibody at a concentration of 2 µg/ml; and **(C)** serum from a rhesus monkey experimentally infected with SIVmac239 (week 12 post-SIV infection) at a 1:20 dilution. Note: regions of interest are shadowed in gray and indicated as follows: variable regions 1–2, 3, 4, and 5 are labeled V1–V2, V3, V4, and V5, respectively; the cleavage site and beginning of gp41 are represented by brackets; g123 indicates the location of the N-linked carbohydrate sites found in gp41; TM is the transmembrane domain of gp41; and HIR stands for highly immunogenic region. Data from SIV+ monkey in panel **(C)** is representative of many such SIV+ monkeys tested previously (47, 48).

shown little or no ADA responses to the AAV-delivered 5L7 antibody (**Figure 1B**).

Negative Envelope PepScan

Due to the nature of the high-dose challenge employed, and the high levels of anti-envelope reactivity found in serum of this animal, one could speculate about a potential low-level infection not detected by regular viral load measurements, which could lead to development of endogenous anti-Env responses, resulting in an overestimation of the concentration of 5L7 antibody in the anti-SIVmac239 gp140 ELISA employed (see Materials and Methods). In order to rule out this potential scenario, we tested serum from 84-05 by PepScan (ELISA against overlapping peptides spanning the whole envelope sequence for SIVmac239) (47, 48). One of the most sensitive measures of infection is seroconversion. Established immunodominant regions of the envelope, i.e., the variable loops V1–V2 and V3, the C terminus of gp120, some peptides in the ectodomain of gp41, and the highly immunogenic region (HIR) at the beginning of the cytoplasmic tail of gp41(47–49) are the regions frequently targeted by antibodies. As shown in **Figure 2A**, the serum from this animal did not detectably react to any of the peptides in the SIVmac239 envelope PepScan. Importantly, and as expected, recombinant purified antibody 5L7 (which is known to bind a conformational epitope involving the V3-V4 region of the envelope (11, 41) and should therefore not bind the linear epitopes present in the PepScan), did not detectably bind any of the tested peptides (**Figure 2B**). Conversely, when positive control serum from a SIV-infected macaque (r10028) was tested on a PepScan in the same conditions, strong reactivity was shown to the immunodominant regions cited above (**Figure 2C**).

No Detectable Antibody Responses to p27 or gp41 by ELISA

With the high levels of 5L7 antibody consistently found in serum of 84-05, meaning high reactivity to gp120, assessing

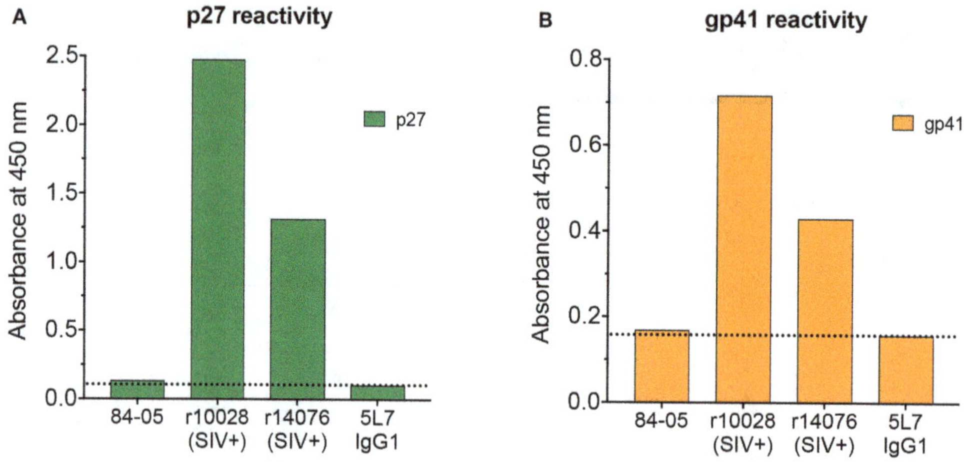

FIGURE 3 | Analysis of antibody responses to p27 and gp41. Serum from 84-05 (week 328 post-AAV) at a 1:20 dilution was tested by ELISA against recombinant purified proteins p27 **(A)** gp41 and **(B)** sera from two rhesus monkeys experimentally infected with SIVmac239 (week 12 post-SIV infection) at a 1:20 dilution were used as positive controls, and recombinant purified 5L7 as a negative.

a potential low-level infection can be complicated since that serum would definitely yield a positive result when tested against whole virus or recombinant gp120 by ELISA, the benchmark assays. An alternate method to test potential seroconversion is by measuring ELISA reactivity to p27 and gp41 recombinant proteins. Antibodies to both p27 and gp41 are readily detectable shortly after SIV infection and importantly, the 5L7 antibody present in the serum would not react to these proteins. Tests of serum from 84-05 (week 328 post-AAV) did not reveal any reactivity to p27 (**Figure 3A**), while positive control sera from two rhesus macaques experimentally infected with SIVmac239 for 12 weeks (r10028 and r14076) showed high reactivity under the same conditions. Similarly, serum from 84-05 did not detectably react against gp41, but sera from the two SIV-positive monkeys did (**Figure 3B**). Purified 5L7 antibody tested in parallel did not significantly bind to either p27 or gp41 (**Figure 3**).

Absence of Cell-Associated Viral DNA or RNA

To further rule out a potential low-level infection that could not be detected by the aforementioned ELISA-based tests, we used ultrasensitive techniques to detect cell-associated viral DNA and RNA in PBMCs from 84-05. We did not detect SIV gag RNA or DNA in the analysis of a combined total of 1.17×10^8 cell equivalents obtained over a 2-week period (week 340 and week 342; **Table 1**) with a nominal sensitivity of 1 copy per reaction.

TABLE 1 | Ultrasensitive detection of cell-associated viral DNA and RNA in PBMCs.

	Week 340[a]	Week 342[b]
Cell associated viral DNA	<1 DNA copies/10^6 cells	<1 DNA copies/10^6 cells
Cell associated viral RNA	<1 RNA copies/10^6 cells	<1 RNA copies/10^6 cells

[a] A total of 7.4×10^7 cells were analyzed for this time point and [b] a total of 4.3×10^7 cells were analyzed for this time point. Both with a nominal sensitivity of 1 copy per reaction.

DISCUSSION

Here we describe continuous, prolonged, high level delivery of an antibody to a rhesus monkey using AAV vector over 6 years of longitudinal measurements. Approximately 2% of the IgG in monkey 84-05 is derived from the vector that we inoculated more than 6 years previous. This result is consistent with the belief that muscle cells essentially do not turn over (50) and thus represent a potentially long term stable source of AAV-delivered antibody. It seems likely that monkey 84-05 will continue to produce similar levels of this antibody for the rest of its life. Importantly, this animal withstood six successive challenges with SIVmac239, including a final challenge with 10 animal infectious doses (1). By different means we show here that monkey 84-05 was effectively protected and remained uninfected: these include testing seroconversion in three different ways and the use of ultrasensitive techniques to detect cell-associated viral DNA and RNA. Due to the difficulties associated with proving curative and/or protective interventions (51), additional tests were considered such as *in vivo* CD8+ T-cell depletion and attempts at adoptive transfer of infection to naïve rhesus macaques. However, we did not want to put this precious monkey at any risk with the CD8 depletion; and, surprisingly, adoptive transfer may not be as sensitive as one would think (14).

The absence of an ADA response is almost certainly a key factor in the continuous production of the transgene product in monkey 84-05. Other examples of AAV delivery of protein to monkeys over a prolonged period have been documented in the reports of Rivera et al. (52) and Guilbaud et al. (53). Both of these reports used periodic induction of expression of an erythropoietin identical in sequence to the monkey's own erythropoietin over 5 or more years of study. Additional examples include the persistent expression of dopamine-synthesizing enzymes in the putamen reported in one monkey for 15 years in a primate model of Parkinson's disease (54); the sustained expression of human α-L-iduronidase, an important enzyme required for the lysosomal degradation of glycosaminoglycans, reported for almost 4 years after intrathecal cervical AAV9 gene delivery in four one-month-old rhesus monkeys (55); the sustained expression of alpha-1 antitrypsin for over 5 years after one AAV vector administration in alpha-1 antitrypsin deficient patients (56); and the successful expression for 3.5 years obtained in two dogs of a dystrophin gene in a canine model for human Duchenne muscular dystrophy using AAV6 and a brief course of immunosuppressants (57), or in a similar study for over 2 years in two dogs using AAV8 in the absence of immunosuppression (58). Remarkably our animal 84-05 never received any immunosuppressant. The hemophilia gene therapy arena also has good examples of long-term delivery with AAV for up to a decade of Factor IX in hemophilic humans (59) and of Factor VIII in hemophilic dogs (60). For more examples on long-term delivery with AAV of hemophilia factors, please see the following references (61–68). The long-term delivery described in our report here is significant as the first such report for very long-term delivery of an antibody, particularly given the serious difficulties that have been encountered when AAV has been used to deliver antibodies that are significantly diverged from germ line or contain unusual features (1, 14, 28, 30, 31). The findings give hope that long-term delivery of therapeutic antibodies via AAV can be consistently achieved if the ADA problem can be overcome.

What may be responsible for the absence of ADAs in 84-05 and the continued high level of production of the transgene product over this prolonged period? Factors that have been shown to influence whether, or not, ADAs are observed following AAV-mediated expression of a transgene product include the following: the particular sequence of the transgene product (69); whether the recipient is already making a similar or identical protein (39); the serotype of AAV used (38); and targeted delivery or targeted expression at particular sites or in particular tissues or cells (54, 70–76). AAV-delivered 5L7 antibody certainly has the potential to be immunogenic in rhesus monkeys since 50% of monkeys receiving it have had robust ADA responses (1). Might there be particular genetic determinants that restrict an ADA response to the 5L7 antibody in some monkeys but not others? Might the antibody repertoire present in an individual at any one time influence to what extent the 5L7 antibody may be recognized as foreign? Might 5L7 just be on the cusp of self/non-self recognition? These questions remain unanswered at least for the time being.

Like the Miami monkey (14, 77, 78), monkey 84-05 stands out as a shining example of what is possible in the realm of AAV delivery of monoclonal antibodies in the fight against HIV. The Miami monkey has maintained high levels of two anti-HIV monoclonal antibodies and complete virologic suppression of SHIV infection for more than 4 years of follow-up without any repeated administrations and without any other antiviral therapies. It is likely that the ADA problem with AAV-delivered antibodies will need to be overcome for this approach to become a consistent reality in the context of human HIV infection. A recently-published human trial of AAV to deliver the human anti-HIV monoclonal antibody PG9 revealed readily detectable ADAs in 10 of 13 recipients in the four highest dose groups and zero measurable delivery of the PG9 antibody (31, 79). We feel that monkey modeling will need to play a key role in the development of successful strategies. Our group is currently focused on simple, easy-to-apply strategies for creating tolerance in monkeys to AAV-delivered monoclonal antibodies. If satisfactory delivery methods are found, it becomes possible to envision long-term control of viral replication in the absence of antiretroviral treatment by delivering a combination of antibodies in people, and long-lasting protection when this approach is used in a prophylactic setting. The long-term expression reported here highlights the potential of AAV-mediated antibody expression for impacting HIV-1 infections worldwide.

ETHICS STATEMENT

The animal study was reviewed and approved by The Harvard Medical School Animal Care and Use Committee and The University of Wisconsin Graduate School Animal Care and Use Committee.

AUTHOR CONTRIBUTIONS

The study was conceived and designed and the manuscript was composed by JM-N, SF, and RD. The experiments were performed by JM-N, SF, DM, ER, GG, and JL. Reagents that were used in the study were generated by JM-N, SF, DM, ER, GG, and JL. Data analysis was performed by JM-N, SF, DM, ER, GG, JL, and RD.

ACKNOWLEDGMENTS

The authors thank Kimberly L. Weisgrau and Jessica Furlott for technical assistance; the Gene Therapy Core at the University of Massachusetts Medical School for excellent AAV vector preparation; the Wisconsin National Primate Research Center veterinary staff for professional animal care; Nancy Schultz-Darken, Wendy Newton, and Eric Alexander for animal experiment planning and conduct; and William J. Bosche, Randy Fast, Michael Hull, Kelli Oswald, and Rebecca Shoemaker of the Quantitative Molecular Virology Core in the AIDS and Cancer Virus Program of the Frederick National Laboratory for Cancer Research for expert technical assistance with viral quantitation.

REFERENCES

1. Fuchs SP, Martinez-Navio JM, Piatak MJr, Lifson JD, Gao G, Desrosiers RC. AAV-delivered antibody mediates significant protective effects against SIVmac239 challenge in the absence of neutralizing activity. *PLoS Pathog.* (2015) 11:e1005090. doi: 10.1371/journal.ppat.1005090
2. Dunbar CE, High KA, Joung JK, Kohn DB, Ozawa K, Sadelain M. Gene therapy comes of age. *Science.* (2018) 359:eaan4672. doi: 10.1126/science.aan4672
3. FDA. *U.S. Food and Drug Administration - What is Gene Therapy?* (2018). Available online at: https://www.fda.gov/vaccines-blood-biologics/cellular-gene-therapy-products/what-gene-therapy
4. Hastie E, Samulski RJ. Adeno-associated virus at 50: a golden anniversary of discovery, research, and gene therapy success-a personal perspective. *Hum Gene Ther.* (2015) 26:257–65. doi: 10.1089/hum.2015.025
5. Goncalves MA. Adeno-associated virus: from defective virus to effective vector. *Virol J.* (2005) 2:43. doi: 10.1186/1743-422X-2-43
6. Daya S, Berns KI. Gene therapy using adeno-associated virus vectors. *Clin Microbiol Rev.* (2008) 21:583–93. doi: 10.1128/CMR.00008-08
7. McCarty DM. Self-complementary AAV vectors; advances and applications. *Mol Ther.* (2008) 16:1648–56. doi: 10.1038/mt.2008.171
8. Schultz BR, Chamberlain JS. Recombinant adeno-associated virus transduction and integration. *Mol Ther.* (2008) 16:1189–99. doi: 10.1038/mt.2008.103
9. Mingozzi F, High KA. Therapeutic *in vivo* gene transfer for genetic disease using AAV: progress and challenges. *Nat Rev Genet.* (2011) 12:341–55. doi: 10.1038/nrg2988
10. Wang D, Tai PWL, Gao G. Adeno-associated virus vector as a platform for gene therapy delivery. *Nat Rev Drug Discov.* (2019) 18:358–78. doi: 10.1038/s41573-019-0012-9
11. Johnson PR, Schnepp BC, Zhang J, Connell MJ, Greene SM, Yuste E, et al. Vector-mediated gene transfer engenders long-lived neutralizing activity and protection against SIV infection in monkeys. *Nat Med.* (2009) 15:901–6. doi: 10.1038/nm.1967
12. Fuchs SP, Desrosiers RC. Promise and problems associated with the use of recombinant AAV for the delivery of anti-HIV antibodies. *Mol Ther Methods Clin Dev.* (2016) 3:16068. doi: 10.1038/mtm.2016.68
13. Brady JM, Baltimore D, Balazs AB. Antibody gene transfer with adeno-associated viral vectors as a method for HIV prevention. *Immunol Rev.* (2017) 275:324–33. doi: 10.1111/imr.12478
14. Martinez-Navio JM, Fuchs SP, Pantry SN, Lauer WA, Duggan NN, Keele BF. Deno-associated virus delivery of anti-HIV monoclonal antibodies can drive long-term virologic suppression. *Immunity.* (2019) 50:567–75 e5. doi: 10.1016/j.immuni.2019.02.005
15. Sok D, Burton DR. Recent progress in broadly neutralizing antibodies to HIV. *Nat Immunol.* (2018) 19:1179–88. doi: 10.1038/s41590-018-0235-7
16. Dashti A, DeVico AL, Lewis GK, Sajadi MM. Broadly neutralizing antibodies against HIV: back to blood. *Trends Mol Med.* (2019) 25:228–40. doi: 10.1016/j.molmed.2019.01.007
17. Haynes BF, Burton DR, Mascola JR. Multiple roles for HIV broadly neutralizing antibodies. *Sci Transl Med.* (2019) 11:eaaz2686. doi: 10.1126/scitranslmed.aaz2686
18. Caskey M, Klein F, Lorenzi JC, Seaman MS, West AP Jr, Buckley N, et al. Viraemia suppressed in HIV-1-infected humans by broadly neutralizing antibody 3BNC117. *Nature.* (2015) 522:487–91. doi: 10.1038/nature14411
19. Bar KJ, Sneller MC, Harrison LJ, Justement JS, Overton ET, Petrone ME, et al. Effect of HIV antibody VRC01 on viral rebound after treatment interruption. *N Engl J Med.* (2016) 375:2037–50. doi: 10.1056/NEJMoa1608243
20. Scheid JF, Horwitz JA, Bar-On Y, Kreider EF, Lu CL, Lorenzi JC, et al. HIV-1 antibody 3BNC117 suppresses viral rebound in humans during treatment interruption. *Nature.* (2016) 535:556–60. doi: 10.1038/nature18929
21. Caskey M, Schoofs T, Gruell H, Settler A, Karagounis T, Kreider EF, et al. Antibody 10-1074 suppresses viremia in HIV-1-infected individuals. *Nat Med.* (2017) 23:185–91. doi: 10.1038/nm.4268
22. Mendoza P, Gruell H, Nogueira L, Pai JA, Butler AL, Millard K, et al. Combination therapy with anti-HIV-1 antibodies maintains viral suppression. *Nature.* (2018) 561:479–84. doi: 10.1038/s41586-018-0531-2
23. Balazs AB, Chen J, Hong CM, Rao DS, Yang L, Baltimore D. Antibody-based protection against HIV infection by vectored immunoprophylaxis. *Nature.* (2011) 481:81–4. doi: 10.1038/nature10660
24. Gardner MR, Kattenhorn LM, Kondur HR, von Schaewen M, Dorfman T, Chiang JJ, et al. AAV-expressed eCD4-Ig provides durable protection from multiple SHIV challenges. *Nature.* (2015) 519:87–91. doi: 10.1038/nature14264
25. Gardner MR, Fellinger CH, Kattenhorn LM, Davis-Gardner ME, Weber JA, Alfant B. AAV-delivered eCD4-Ig protects rhesus macaques from high-dose SIVmac239 challenges. *Sci. Transl. Med.* (2019) 11:eaau5409. doi: 10.1126/scitranslmed.aau5409
26. Hollevoet K, Declerck PJ. State of play and clinical prospects of antibody gene transfer. *J Transl Med.* (2017) 15:131. doi: 10.1186/s12967-017-1234-4
27. Saunders KO, Wang L, Joyce MG, Yang ZY, Balazs AB, Cheng C, et al. Broadly neutralizing human immunodeficiency virus type 1 antibody gene transfer protects nonhuman primates from mucosal simian-human immunodeficiency virus infection. *J Virol.* (2015) 89:8334–45. doi: 10.1128/JVI.00908-15
28. Martinez-Navio JM, Fuchs SP, Pedreno-Lopez S, Rakasz EG, Gao G, Desrosiers RC. Host anti-antibody responses following adeno-associated virus-mediated delivery of antibodies against HIV and SIV in rhesus monkeys. *Mol Ther.* (2016) 24:76–86. doi: 10.1038/mt.2015.191
29. Welles HC, Jennewein MF, Mason RD, Narpala S, Wang L, Cheng C, et al. Vectored delivery of anti-SIV envelope targeting mAb via AAV8 protects rhesus macaques from repeated limiting dose intrarectal swarm SIVsmE660 challenge. *PLoS Pathog.* (2018) 14:e1007395. doi: 10.1371/journal.ppat.1007395
30. Gardner MR, Fetzer I, Kattenhorn LM, Davis-Gardner ME, Zhou AS, Alfant B, et al. Anti-drug antibody responses impair prophylaxis mediated by AAV-delivered HIV-1 broadly neutralizing antibodies. *Mol Ther.* (2019) 27:650–60. doi: 10.1016/j.ymthe.2019.01.004
31. Priddy FH, Lewis DJM, Gelderblom HC, Hassanin H, Streatfield C, LaBranche C, et al. Adeno-associated virus vectored immunoprophylaxis to prevent HIV in healthy adults: a phase 1 randomised controlled trial. *Lancet HIV.* (2019) 6:e230–9. doi: 10.1016/S2352-3018(19)30003-7
32. van den Berg FT, Makoah NA, Ali SA, Scott TA, Mapengo RE, Mutsvunguma LZ. AAV-mediated expression of broadly neutralizing and vaccine-like antibodies targeting the HIV-1 envelope V2 region. *Mol Ther Methods Clin Dev.* (2019) 14:100–12. doi: 10.1016/j.omtm.2019.06.002
33. Wardemann H, Yurasov S, Schaefer A, Young JW, Meffre E, Nussenzweig MC. Predominant autoantibody production by early human B cell precursors. *Science.* (2003) 301:1374–7. doi: 10.1126/science.1086907
34. Wang C, Liu Y, Cavanagh MM, Le Saux S, Qi Q, Roskin KM, et al. B-cell repertoire responses to varicella-zoster vaccination in human identical twins. *Proc Natl Acad Sci USA.* (2015) 112:500–5. doi: 10.1073/pnas.1415875112
35. Scheid JF, Mouquet H, Ueberheide B, Diskin R, Klein F, Oliveira TY, et al. Sequence and structural convergence of broad and potent HIV antibodies that mimic CD4 binding. *Science.* (2011) 333:1633–7. doi: 10.1126/science.1207227
36. Klein F, Mouquet H, Dosenovic P, Scheid JF, Scharf L, Nussenzweig MC. Antibodies in HIV-1 vaccine development and therapy. *Science.* (2013) 341:1199–204. doi: 10.1126/science.1241144
37. Klein F, Diskin R, Scheid JF, Gaebler C, Mouquet H, Georgiev IS, et al. Somatic mutations of the immunoglobulin framework are generally required for broad and potent HIV-1 neutralization. *Cell.* (2013) 153:126–38. doi: 10.1016/j.cell.2013.03.018
38. Mingozzi F, High KA. Immune responses to AAV vectors: overcoming barriers to successful gene therapy. *Blood.* (2013) 122:23–36. doi: 10.1182/blood-2013-01-306647
39. Herzog RW. Complexity of immune responses to AAV transgene products - example of factor IX. *Cell Immunol.* (2019) 342:103658. doi: 10.1016/j.cellimm.2017.05.006
40. National Research Council IoLAR. Commission on Life Sciences (1996). *Guide for the Care and Use of Laboratory Animals.* Washington, DC: The National Academies Press. doi: 10.17226/5140
41. Johnson WE, Sanford H, Schwall L, Burton DR, Parren PW, Robinson JE, et al. Assorted mutations in the envelope gene of simian

immunodeficiency virus lead to loss of neutralization resistance against antibodies representing a broad spectrum of specificities. *J Virol.* (2003) 77:9993–10003. doi: 10.1128/JVI.77.18.9993-10003.2003

42. Fuchs SP, Martinez-Navio JM, Gao G, Desrosiers RC. Recombinant AAV vectors for enhanced expression of authentic IgG. *PLoS ONE.* (2016) 11:e0158009. doi: 10.1371/journal.pone.0158009
43. Mueller C, Ratner D, Zhong L, Esteves-Sena M, Gao G. Production and discovery of novel recombinant adeno-associated viral vectors. *Curr Protoc Microbiol.* (2012) Chapter 14:Unit14D.1. doi: 10.1002/9780471729259.mc14d01s26
44. Li H, Wang S, Kong R, Ding W, Lee FH, Parker Z, et al. Envelope residue 375 substitutions in simian-human immunodeficiency viruses enhance CD4 binding and replication in rhesus macaques. *Proc Natl Acad Sci USA.* (2016) 113:E3413–22. doi: 10.1073/pnas.1606636113
45. Hansen SG, Piatak M Jr, Ventura AB, Hughes CM, Gilbride RM, Ford JC, et al. Immune clearance of highly pathogenic SIV infection. *Nature.* (2013) 502:100–4. doi: 10.1038/nature12519
46. Hansen SG, Piatak M, Ventura AB, Hughes CM, Gilbride RM, Ford JC, et al. Addendum: immune clearance of highly pathogenic SIV infection. *Nature.* (2017) 547:123–4. doi: 10.1038/nature22984
47. Yuste E, Bixby J, Lifson J, Sato S, Johnson W, Desrosiers R. Glycosylation of gp41 of simian immunodeficiency virus shields epitopes that can be targets for neutralizing antibodies. *J Virol.* (2008) 82:12472–86. doi: 10.1128/JVI.01382-08
48. Martinez-Navio JM, Desrosiers RC. Neutralizing capacity of monoclonal antibodies that recognize peptide sequences underlying the carbohydrates on gp41 of simian immunodeficiency virus. *J Virol.* (2012) 86:12484–93. doi: 10.1128/JVI.01959-12
49. Postler TS, Martinez-Navio JM, Yuste E, Desrosiers RC. Evidence against extracellular exposure of a highly immunogenic region in the C-terminal domain of the simian immunodeficiency virus gp41 transmembrane protein. *J Virol.* (2012) 86:1145–57. doi: 10.1128/JVI.06463-11
50. Spalding KL, Bhardwaj RD, Buchholz BA, Druid H, Frisen J. Retrospective birth dating of cells in humans. *Cell.* (2005) 122:133–43. doi: 10.1016/j.cell.2005.04.028
51. Yukl SA, Boritz E, Busch M, Bentsen C, Chun TW, Douek D, et al. Challenges in detecting HIV persistence during potentially curative interventions: a study of the berlin patient. *PLoS Pathog.* (2013) 9:e1003347. doi: 10.1371/journal.ppat.1003347
52. Rivera VM, Gao GP, Grant RL, Schnell MA, Zoltick PW, Rozamus LW, et al. Long-term pharmacologically regulated expression of erythropoietin in primates following AAV-mediated gene transfer. *Blood.* (2005) 105:1424–30. doi: 10.1182/blood-2004-06-2501
53. Guilbaud M, Devaux M, Couzinie C, Le Duff J, Toromanoff A, Vandamme C, et al. Five years of successful inducible transgene expression following locoregional adeno-associated virus delivery in nonhuman primates with no detectable immunity. *Hum Gene Ther.* (2019) 30:802–13. doi: 10.1089/hum.2018.234
54. Sehara Y, Fujimoto KI, Ikeguchi K, Katakai Y, Ono F, Takino N, et al. Persistent expression of dopamine-synthesizing enzymes 15 years after gene transfer in a primate model of parkinson's disease. *Hum Gene Ther Clin Dev.* (2017) 28:74–9. doi: 10.1089/humc.2017.010
55. Hordeaux J, Hinderer C, Buza EL, Louboutin JP, Jahan T, Bell P, et al. Safe and sustained expression of human iduronidase after intrathecal administration of adeno-associated virus serotype 9 in infant rhesus monkeys. *Hum Gene Ther.* (2019) 30:957–66. doi: 10.1089/hum.2019.012
56. Mueller C, Gernoux G, Gruntman AM, Borel F, Reeves EP, Calcedo R, et al. 5 Year expression and neutrophil defect repair after gene therapy in alpha-1 antitrypsin deficiency. *Mol Ther.* (2017) 25:1387–94. doi: 10.1016/j.ymthe.2017.03.029
57. Wang Z, Storb R, Halbert CL, Banks GB, Butts TM, Finn EE, et al. Successful regional delivery and long-term expression of a dystrophin gene in canine muscular dystrophy: a preclinical model for human therapies. *Mol Ther.* (2012) 20:1501–7. doi: 10.1038/mt.2012.111
58. Le Guiner C, Servais L, Montus M, Larcher T, Fraysse B, Moullec S, et al. Long-term microdystrophin gene therapy is effective in a canine model of Duchenne muscular dystrophy. *Nat Commun.* (2017) 8:16105. doi: 10.1038/ncomms16105
59. Buchlis G, Podsakoff GM, Radu A, Hawk SM, Flake AW, Mingozzi F, et al. Factor IX expression in skeletal muscle of a severe hemophilia B patient 10 years after AAV-mediated gene transfer. *Blood.* (2012) 119:3038–41. doi: 10.1182/blood-2011-09-382317
60. Nguyen GN, Everett JK, Raymond H, Kafle S, Merricks EP, Kazazian HH. Long-Term AAV-Mediated Factor VIII Expression in Nine Hemophilia A Dogs: A 10 Year Follow-up Analysis on Durability, Safety and Vector Integration *In 61st American Society of Hematology Annual Meeting and Exposition.* Orlando, FL (2019) 134:611. doi: 10.1182/blood-2019-126007
61. Niemeyer GP, Herzog RW, Mount J, Arruda VR, Tillson DM, Hathcock J, et al. Long-term correction of inhibitor-prone hemophilia B dogs treated with liver-directed AAV2-mediated factor IX gene therapy. *Blood.* (2009) 113:797–806. doi: 10.1182/blood-2008-10-181479
62. Finn JD, Ozelo MC, Sabatino DE, Franck HW, Merricks EP, Crudele JM, et al. Eradication of neutralizing antibodies to factor VIII in canine hemophilia A after liver gene therapy. *Blood.* (2010) 116:5842–8. doi: 10.1182/blood-2010-06-288001
63. Sabatino DE, Lange AM, Altynova ES, Sarkar R, Zhou S, Merricks EP, et al. Efficacy and safety of long-term prophylaxis in severe hemophilia A dogs following liver gene therapy using AAV vectors. *Mol Ther.* (2011) 19:442–9. doi: 10.1038/mt.2010.240
64. Crudele JM, Finn JD, Siner JI, Martin NB, Niemeyer GP, Zhou S, et al. AAV liver expression of FIX-padua prevents and eradicates FIX inhibitor without increasing thrombogenicity in hemophilia B dogs and mice. *Blood.* (2015) 125:1553–61. doi: 10.1182/blood-2014-07-588194
65. Callan MB, Haskins ME, Wang P, Zhou S, High KA, Arruda VR. Successful phenotype improvement following gene therapy for severe hemophilia A in privately owned dogs. *PLoS ONE.* (2016) 11:e0151800. doi: 10.1371/journal.pone.0151800
66. George LA, Sullivan SK, Giermasz A, Rasko JEJ, Samelson Jones BJ, Ducore J, et al. Hemophilia B gene therapy with a high-specific-activity factor IX variant. *N Engl J Med.* (2017) 377:2215–27. doi: 10.1056/NEJMoa1708538
67. Rangarajan S, Walsh L, Lester W, Perry D, Madan B, Laffan M, et al. AAV5-factor VIII gene transfer in severe hemophilia A. *N Engl J Med.* (2017) 377:2519–30. doi: 10.1056/NEJMoa1708483
68. Batty P, Lillicrap D. Advances and challenges for hemophilia gene therapy. *Hum Mol Genet.* (2019) 28:R95–101. doi: 10.1093/hmg/ddz157
69. Cao O, Hoffman BE, Moghimi B, Nayak S, Cooper M, Zhou S, et al. Impact of the underlying mutation and the route of vector administration on immune responses to factor IX in gene therapy for hemophilia B. *Mol Ther.* (2009) 17:1733–42. doi: 10.1038/mt.2009.159
70. Mitchell AM, Nicolson SC, Warischalk JK, Samulski RJ. AAV's anatomy: roadmap for optimizing vectors for translational success. *Curr Gene Ther.* (2010) 10:319–40. doi: 10.2174/156652310793180706
71. Mays LE, Wilson JM. The complex and evolving story of T cell activation to AAV vector-encoded transgene products. *Mol Ther.* (2011) 19:16–27. doi: 10.1038/mt.2010.250
72. Wang D, Zhong L, Nahid MA, Gao G. The potential of adeno-associated viral vectors for gene delivery to muscle tissue. *Expert Opin Drug Deliv.* (2014) 11:345–64. doi: 10.1517/17425247.2014.871258
73. Boisgerault F, Mingozzi F. The skeletal muscle environment and its role in immunity and tolerance to AAV vector-mediated gene transfer. *Curr Gene Ther.* (2015) 15:381–94. doi: 10.2174/1566523215666150630121750
74. Kattenhorn LM, Tipper CH, Stoica L, Geraghty DS, Wright TL, Clark KR, et al. Adeno-associated virus gene therapy for liver disease. *Hum Gene Ther.* (2016) 27:947–61. doi: 10.1089/hum.2016.160
75. Bartolo L, Li Chung Tong S, Chappert P, Urbain D, Collaud F, Colella P. Dual muscle-liver transduction imposes immune tolerance for muscle transgene engraftment despite preexisting immunity. *JCI Insight.* (2019) 4:127008. doi: 10.1172/jci.insight.127008
76. Fuchs SP, Martinez-Navio JM, Rakasz EG, Gao G, Desrosiers RC. Liver-directed but not muscle-directed AAV-antibody gene transfer limits humoral immune responses in rhesus monkeys. *Mol Ther Methods Clin Dev.* (2019) 16:94–102. doi: 10.1016/j.omtm.2019.11.010
77. Haigwood NL, Hessell AJ. Antibodies tip the balance towards an HIV cure. *Trends Immunol.* (2019) 40:375–7. doi: 10.1016/j.it.2019.03.008
78. Liberatore RA, Ho DD. The miami monkey: a sunny alternative to the berlin patient. *Immunity.* (2019) 50:537–9. doi: 10.1016/j.immuni.2019.02.010
79. Caskey M. Delivery of anti-HIV bNAbs by viral vectors. *Lancet HIV.* (2019) 6:e207–8. doi: 10.1016/S2352-3018(19)30041-4

8

Neuroanatomical Changes Underlying Vertical HIV Infection in Adolescents

Xiao Yu[1†], Lei Gao[1†], Haha Wang[1], Zhuang Yin[1], Jian Fang[1], Jing Chen[2], Qiang Li[3], Haibo Xu[1] and Xien Gui[3*]*

[1] Department of Radiology, Zhongnan Hospital of Wuhan University, Wuhan University, Wuhan, China, [2] Publicity Department, Zhongnan Hospital of Wuhan University, Wuhan University, Wuhan, China, [3] Training Centre of AIDS Prevention and Cure of Hubei Province, Zhongnan Hospital of Wuhan University, Wuhan University, Wuhan, China

***Correspondence:**
Haibo Xu
xuhaibo1120@hotmail.com
Xien Gui
znact@126.com

† These authors have contributed equally to this work

Purpose: The aim of this study was to investigate how human immunodeficiency virus (HIV) affects brain development in adolescents, what are susceptible brain regions, and how these brain structural changes correlate with cognitive abilities.

Methods: We used structural magnetic resonance imaging to examine gray matter volume and cortical thickness in 16 HIV-infected children (mean age = 13.63 years) and 25 HIV-exposed uninfected children (mean age = 13.32 years), 12 of them were subjected to a 1-year repetitive magnetic resonance scan of the brain. Five neurocognitive tests were performed on each subject to assess cognitive performance in different areas.

Results: Cross-sectional studies showed that the gray matter volume of HIV-infected children was widely reduced (mainly in the bilateral frontal, temporal, and insular regions, and cerebellum). The changes in cortical thickness were mainly due to thinning of the right temporal lobe and thickening of the left occipital lobe. Longitudinal studies showed that the gray matter volume reduction of HIV-infected children after 1 year mainly occurs in the advanced functional area of the right prefrontal, parietal lobe and the motor area, cortical thinning of brain regions were sensorimotor cortex and the limbic system. The gray matter volume of the bilateral cerebellum was positively correlated with the performance of the Wisconsin Card Sorting Test, while the cortical thickness of the right dorsolateral prefrontal cortex was negatively correlated with this test.

Conclusion: This study found that HIV-infected pubertal children showed a delayed cortical maturation with atrophy. This abnormal pattern of cortical development may be the structural basis for cognitive impairment in HIV-infected children.

Keywords: AIDS, brain development, structural MRI, HIV exposure, children, mother-to-child transmission

INTRODUCTION

Acquired immune deficiency syndrome (AIDS)-related encephalopathy is one of the most serious complications of AIDS and is more common in children than in adults (1). At present, there are nearly 2 million children living with human immunodeficiency virus (HIV) in the world, almost all newly infected children are infected through mother-to-child transmission (2). Effective antiretroviral therapy (ART) can significantly reduce mortality and the incidence of HIV encephalopathy (3). Although the children's HIV/AIDS has been transformed into chronic, controllable disease patterns, due to the HIV virus, antiretroviral drugs and a variety of environmental factors, a series of neuropsychological defects can still appear on HIV-infected (HIV+) children, sometimes even after the treatment has fully been accepted (4).

Currently, some studies have reported and summarized the neurocognitive impairment and behavioral abnormality in children infected with HIV. For example, language barriers, delayed motor development, poor school performance, etc., and some may even have psychological problems such as anxiety and depression (5, 6). Although highly active antiretroviral therapy can improve the cognitive function of HIV+ children in the long run (7), there are also studies showing that cognitive impairment will exist for a long time (8). It will affect their future learning, work performance and social practice, we need to focus on long-term outcomes of nervous system development to inform treatment options and guide early intervention treatment strategy to prevent deterioration of cognitive function.

The rapid development of neuroimaging has provided us with a powerful tool for studying brain development in children. Current structural magnetic resonance imaging (MRI) studies have observed some changes in brain structure in HIV+ children and adolescents, including subcortical volume, shape deformation (9), gyrification, and overall or regional gray matter volume (GMV) reduction (10, 11), but there are very few longitudinal research on cortical development. A longitudinal study observed persistent damage to human white matter development in HIV+ children, regardless of whether they received antiretroviral therapy or viral suppression at an early stage (12). Furthermore, many studies have used the emerging MRI technology to reveal the characteristics of brain structure, function and the influence of cognitive factors in children with HIV/AIDS, but the future impact of these developmental abnormalities are still unclear, brain regions vulnerable to HIV or antiretroviral drugs have also not been identified (13–15).

Some studies have shown that the developmental maturity of brain structure is consistent with the development of individual cognitive ability (16, 17). We hypothesized that HIV would have less influence on the development of brain regions related to primary functions such as sensory and motor domains, but have a greater impact on the development of brain regions related to advanced cognition such as decision-making and reasoning. We attempted to conduct cross-sectional and longitudinal studies through high-resolution structural MRI to observe which brain regions HIV may preferentially affect and to combine multiple domains of neuropsychological cognitive testing to observe the correlation between brain structural changes and cognitive ability.

Abbreviations: AIDS, acquired immune deficiency syndrome; HIV, human immunodeficiency virus; HIV+, HIV-infected; MRI, magnetic resonance imaging; GMV, gray matter volume; HEU, HIV-exposed uninfected; VBM, voxel-based morphometric; CT, cortical thickness; MNI, Montreal neurological institute; FWE, Family Wise Error; TFCE, threshold-free cluster enhancement; OFC, orbital frontal cortex.

MATERIALS AND METHODS

Subjects

We recruited 16 HIV+ adolescents (mean age ± SD, 13.63 ± 1.83 years; range, 11–17 years; mean CD4 count ± SD, 558.87 ± 199.89 cells/mm^3; range, 276–940), the viral load of them did not reach the lower limit of detection (<20 copies/ml). The presence of HIV+ children was confirmed by Western blot. We also recruited 25 age- and gender-matched HIV-Exposed Uninfected (HEU) subjects (mean age ± SD, 13.32 ± 1.62 years; range,11–17 years). All HIV+ adolescents were infected by mother-to-child transmission during pregnancy, childbirth or through breastfeeding. HEU subjects' fathers, mothers, or parents also suffered from HIV infections. The socioeconomic status, cultural background and ethnic background of the two communities were similar. Detailed population information and clinical measures are listed in **Table 1**. All subjects were enrolled from Training Centre of AIDS Prevention and Cure of Hubei Province. The inclusion criteria for HIV+ subjects included HIV acquisition during the fetal or neonatal period, currently treated with ART, and right-handed. For the control subjects, the inclusion criteria included confirmation of HIV negative status by ELISA and right-handedness.

Exclusion criteria for all subjects included those younger than 11 years of age or over 17 years of age, with acute medical illnesses, current or past medical or neurological diseases, psychiatric illnesses, mental retardation, current alcohol or drug abuse, HIV encephalopathy and opportunistic infections, MRI contraindications, claustrophobia, metabolic disorders or other brain diseases (not AIDS-related). We used the exclusion criteria, which included HIV-related encephalopathy to rule out space-occupying masses, other lesions or obvious cortical atrophy in the brain of HIV+ adolescents, so that we got the difference in anatomical gray matter covariance between the two groups. Only one individual in the HIV+ group was excluded because of age 7. For the control subjects, the exclusion criteria also included serious educational difficulties and a chronic medication other than asthma medication.

The study was approved by the Medical Ethics Committee of Zhongnan Hospital of Wuhan University, and a written and informed consent was made from all participants or their guardians in accordance with the Helsinki Declaration of 1975 (and as revised in 1983), following a complete description of the measurements. These methods were carried out in accordance with the approved guidelines and regulations.

Neuropsychological Tests

In order to more comprehensively assess the cognitive abilities of the subjects, we selected five tests based on the Frascati criteria (21). (1) Word Semantics Test: to examine written language comprehension, especially at the level of sentences. (2) Verbal Working Memory Test (present audio): comes from the digital memory span subtest of Wechsler Intelligence Scale. (3) Wisconsin Card Sorting Test: to examine executive control capabilities. (4) Picture Memory Test. (5) Indicate the Midpoint Test of the Line Segment: focus on sensory

TABLE 1 | Demographics and results of neuropsychological tests.

	HIV+ group	HEU group	*p*-value	Cohen' *d*(ES)	Power
Number of subjects (*n*)	16	25	–	–	–
Sex (male/female)	8/8	12/13	0.915	–	–
Age (years)	13.63 ± 1.83	13.32 ± 1.62	0.589	0.176	0.135
BMI (kg/m^2)	18.27 ± 2.66	18.29 ± 3.06	0.873	0.008	0.053
Education (years)	7.31 ± 2.20	7.16 ± 1.51	0.799	0.081	0.081
Ethnicity (Han/Tujia)	15/1	24/1	0.904	–	–
Longitudinal data (*n*)	5 (31.25%)	7 (28.0%)	–	–	–
Mother-to-child transmission	16 (100%)	25 (100%)	–	–	–
CD4 count (cells/mm^3)	558.87 ± 199.89	–	–	–	–
COGNITIVE DOMAIN					
Vocabulary/language (*n*)	4 (26.67%)	0 (0%)	0.17	–	–
Working memory/attention (*n*)	3 (23.08%)	0 (0%)	0.269	–	–
Executive/abstraction (*n*)	7 (46.67%)	0 (0%)	**0.015**	–	–
Memory/learning and recall (n)	1 (6.67%)	0 (0%)	0.733	–	–
Sensory perceptual/motor skills (*n*)	0 (0%)	0 (0%)	–	–	–

HIV+, HIV-infected; HEU, HIV-exposed uninfected; ES, effect size; BMI, Body Mass Index, Values are n (% of total) or mean ± standard-deviation. Cognitive results of individuals in HIV+ group failed to follow the normal distribution test, thus we used the rank sum test. Significance at $P < 0.05$.

perceptual and motor skills. We conducted all tests online using the professional "Multi-Dimensional Psychology" platform (http://www.dweipsy.com/lattice/). All these tests and MRI scans were carried out within a month of study enrollment for each participant.

MRI Acquisition

High-resolution T1-weighted structural MRI scans were acquired on the 3.0 T scanner (Siemens, Prisma, Germany), which was stationed at the Department of Radiology, the Zhongnan Hospital of Wuhan University, using a multi-echo magnetization prepared rapid gradient echo (MPRAGE) pulse sequence (repetition time = 5,000 ms, echo time = 2.88 ms, inversion time = 700 ms, flip angle = 4°, slice thickness = 1.00 mm, and matrix size = 256 × 256) that yielded 176 axial slices with an in-plane resolution of 1.0 × 1.0 mm. We visually inspected the cerebral microbleeds foci measured by susceptibility-weighted imaging (SWI), and white matter hyperintensity by T2- fluid-attenuated inversion recovery (FLAIR) images through all the subjects. We also excluded any subject that exhibited obvious gray and white matter lesion imaged by SWI and FLAIR.

Brain Morphometry Analysis

In this study, we analyzed two morphological brain measures, the gray matter volume [via voxel-based morphometric (VBM) analysis] and cortical thickness (CT) analysis. All data processing uses Statistical Parametric Mapping software (SPM12; Wellcome Department of Cognitive Neurology, London, UK; http://www.fl.ion.ucl.ac.uk/spm) and Computational Anatomy Toolbox (CAT12, http://dbm.neuro.uni-jena.de/vbm/) based on MATLAB (MathWorks, Natick, MA, USA). The data preprocessing mainly included: (1) experienced radiologists screen data with obvious abnormalities, excluding data with large artifacts and obvious lesions; (2) the original T1 images were manually reoriented to match the AC-PC plane, (3) segmented into gray matter, white matter, and cerebrospinal fluid using the standard unified segmented model (18, 19) in the CAT12, (4) nonlinearly normalized into standard Montreal Neurological Institute (MNI) space using a pediatric template for 12- to 18-year-old children from the Imaging Research Center at Cincinnati Children's Hospital Medical Center (CCHMC), (5) the normalized segmentations were then modulated to ensure that the relative volumes of gray matter were retained, (6) the modulated images were re-sampled to 1.5 × 1.5 × 1.5 mm^3 and smoothed with an 8 mm full-width at half-maximum (FWHM) Gaussian kernel, (7) to control for deviations, we included an additional quality check based on heterogeneity measurements of the sample as implemented in CAT; using the covariance of voxel-based data to identify the outliers who were two or more standard deviations outside of the GMV sample distributions, and one patient and one control were excluded based on this criterion, (8) finally, exclude voxels with a gray matter value <0.15 to eliminate the potential edge effects between the gray matter and white matter.

The CT was also computed by using the CAT12, all the parameters were set by default in the CAT12, except for the brain template using a pediatric template for 12- to 18-year-old children from the Imaging Research Center at Cincinnati Children's Hospital Medical Center (CCHMC) (https://irc.cchmc.org/software/pedbrain.php). Briefly, this automated method (20) allows for central surface reconstructions and CT measurement in one step, then the topological defects of cortical surface mesh were repaired by using a spherical harmonic method. Prior to the statistical analyses, the individual CT maps were smoothed by using a Gaussian filter with full-width at half-maximum of 15 mm.

For the longitudinal analysis of GMV and CT, we also used the CAT12 default parameters with the pediatric template and performed the analysis under the longitudinal analysis module to obtain subtle changes at the individual level between the two-time points (1 year before and after).

Statistical Analysis

For clinical and behavioral data, statistical analysis was conducted using IBM SPSS version 20 (IBM SPSS Inc., Chicago, IL, USA) and G*Power 3.1.9.3. The significance threshold was set to $p < 0.05$. For the brain morphological parameters (gray matter volume and cortical thickness), cross-sectional between-group comparisons were tested in SPM12 using independent two-sample t-tests, with age and gender as covariates, longitudinal comparisons were carried by flexible design 2×2 analysis of variance (ANOVA). The significance threshold was set to $p < 0.05$ with a cluster level Family Wise Error (FWE) correction and threshold-free cluster enhancement (TFCE) multiple comparison-corrected.

TABLE 2 | Between-group comparison on gray matter volume.

Contrast	Brain regions	Extent	t-value	MNI Coordinates		
				x	y	z
HIV + < HEU	Frontal_Inf_Tri_R	359	−4.7245	37.5	16.5	28.5
	Frontal_Inf_Oper_L	181	−3.8543	−48	12	13.5
	Temporal_Mid_R	158	−3.8214	45	−58.5	4.5
	Cerebelum_Crus1_L	334	−3.6533	−36	−69	−34.5
	Parietal_Inf_L	146	−3.5301	−27	−61.5	39
	Cerebelum_Crus1_R	378	−3.3279	39	−61.5	−37.5
	Cuneus_R	86	−3.2899	7.5	−81	18
	Insula_L	276	−3.251	−28.5	27	6
	Temporal_Pole_Sup_L	132	−3.1098	−51	6	−3
	Frontal_Mid_2_L	139	−3.0554	−31.5	19.5	60
	Frontal_Inf_Oper_L	124	−2.9471	−39	4.5	25.5
	Frontal_Sup_2_L	88	−2.9143	−18	33	39
	Insula_R	72	−2.9079	34.5	30	0
	Temporal_Sup_L	66	−2.7822	−52.5	−9	−3
	Angular_R	50	−2.7661	30	−60	40.5

HIV+, HIV-infected; HEU, HIV-exposed uninfected; MNI, Montreal Neurological Institute; L, left; R, right. All regions were corrected by FWE cluster level p < 0.05.

RESULTS

Demographics and Neuropsychological Tests

For demographic and clinical data, the HIV+ and HEU controls were comparable on age, gender, and education ($p > 0.05$, **Table 1**). For cognitive testing, the HIV+ group performed significantly worse in the Wisconsin card classification test (execution and abstraction functions) than their HEU controls ($p = 0.015$, **Table 1**). In addition, we also noted that 5 of the adolescents in the HIV+ group scored at least 2 items below the mean of the control group minus a standard deviation of one time, which can be diagnosed asymptomatic neurocognitive impairment according to Frascati criteria (21).

Between-Group Comparison on Gray Matter Volume

We first investigated the between-group differences on GMV by using VBM. This analysis revealed a significant reduction in the GMV across broad regions, including bilateral superior cerebellar, frontal, temporal, insular, angular regions, and right cuneus, in the HIV+ individuals, these results were corrected by FWE cluster level $p < 0.05$ (**Table 2**; **Figure 1**).

Between-Group Comparison on Cortical Thickness

We next reported the between-group differences on surface-based metrics of CT. Individuals with HIV showed significantly thicker cortices in left occipital (the middle and inferior gyri) and right olfactory sulcus, also, significantly thinner cortices in the temporal (the middle and the pole parts) and orbitofrontal regions. The results were corrected by FWE cluster level $p < 0.05$ (**Table 3**; **Figure 2**).

Longitudinal Changes in Gray Matter Volume

Based on the cross-sectional results, an important aim of this study is to investigate the longitudinal brain develop trajectory.

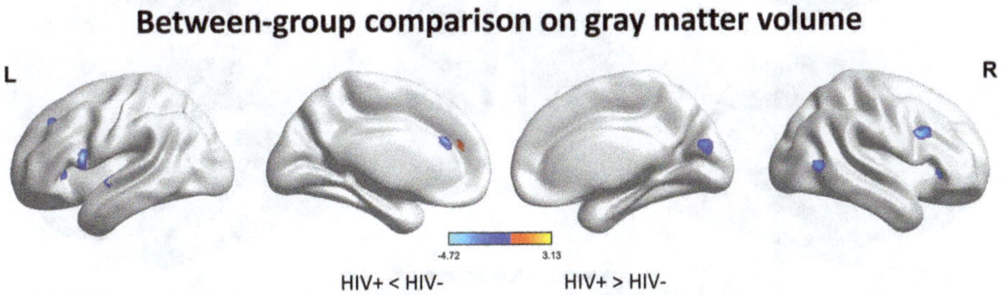

FIGURE 1 | Between-group comparison on gray matter volume (GMV). Clusters showing significantly (corrected $P < 0.05$) lower (blue) and higher (red) GMV in HIV+ children compared to controls. But the red region isn't successfully positioned in the template. This figure was rendered using BrainNet Viewer (http://www.nitrc.org/projects/bnv/).

Using a 2 × 2 ANOVA, we then contrasted the development patterns between the two groups.

For the GMV, generally, the HIV+ group showed changes in GMV over a wider range of brain regions and was dominated by a significant decrease in GMV after 1 year. These regions mainly included decreased GMV in the bilateral frontal, supplementary, parietal, and occipital regions; and increased GMV in the right inferior temporal, inferior occipital and orbital frontal cortex (OFC) regions (**Table 4**; **Figure 3A**).

TABLE 3 | Between-group comparison on cortical thickness.

Contrast	Cortical regions	Side	Size	*P*-value
HIV + > HEU	42% G_occipital_middle 24% S_oc_middle_and_Lunatus 21% G_and_S_occipital_inf 9% Pole_occipital 2% G_pariet_inf-Angular 2%S_oc_sup_and_transversal	L	611	0.00960
	100% G_cingul-Post-ventral	L	1	0.04800
	42% S_orbital_med-olfact 38% G_rectus 15%G_subcallosal	R	79	0.04260
HIV+<HEU	74% G_orbital 26%S_orbital_lateral	L	19	0.04740
	100% G_orbital	L	15	0.04640
	44% G_temporal_middle 32% Pole_temporal 12% S_temporal_inf 11% G_temp_sup-Lateral 1%S_temporal_sup	R	214	0.02880
	66% G_orbital 22% S_orbital_med-olfact 11% G_rectus 1%G_and_S_frontomargin	R	73	0.03380

HIV+, HIV-infected; HEU, HIV-exposed uninfected; L, left; R, right. All regions were corrected by FWE cluster level p <0.05.

TABLE 4 | Volume change of gray matter in HIV+ group after 1 year.

Contrast	Brain regions	Extent	*t*-value	MNI coordinates		
				x	y	z
Positive	Temporal_Inf_R	144	5.440	44	−56	−14
	Occipital_Inf_R	144	4.362	51	−75	−14
	OFCmed_R	134	5.293	21	27	−20
Negative	Frontal_Mid_2_L	306	−8.717	−30	54	6
	Occipital_Sup_R	292	−7.799	27	−69	42
	Supp_Motor_Area_R	2409	−7.215	5	15	50
	Frontal_Sup_Medial_R	2409	−6.253	6	38	51
	Parietal_Sup_R	172	−6.944	38	−50	56
	Precuneus_L	755	−6.851	−8	−47	63
	Paracentral_Lobule_R	755	−4.995	12	−35	48
	Parietal_Inf_L	315	−6.177	−44	−42	51
	Postcentral_L	315	−4.796	−53	−15	36
	Frontal_Sup_2_L	292	−5.973	−18	54	26
	Parietal_Inf_L	281	−5.877	−27	−69	42
	Frontal_Inf_Oper_L	296	−5.857	−50	8	15
	Postcentral_R	113	−5.798	56	−6	29
	Frontal_Sup_2_R	442	−5.697	24	54	27
	Frontal_Mid_2_R	442	−4.432	39	50	14
	Postcentral_R	286	−5.620	47	−35	54
	Cingulate_Post_L	96	−5.516	−6	−50	32
	Precuneus_R	95	−5.365	8	−50	51
	Frontal_Mid_2_L	154	−5.351	−30	47	21
	SupraMarginal_R	69	−5.146	65	−17	27
	Cerebelum_Crus1_L	50	−5.038	−45	−48	−41
	Supp_Motor_Area_R	335	−4.992	3	−11	62
	Frontal_Sup_2_R	81	−4.660	15	47	41
	Temporal_Sup_R	51	−4.435	56	−14	8
	Cerebelum_4_5_L	57	−4.291	−6	−47	−5
	Parietal_Inf_L	54	−4.237	−53	−44	36
	Frontal_Sup_2_L	50	−4.075	−18	42	44
	Precentral_L	71	−4.003	−38	0	60

HIV+, HIV-infected; MNI, Montreal Neurological Institute; L, left; R, right. All regions were corrected by FWE cluster level p < 0.05.

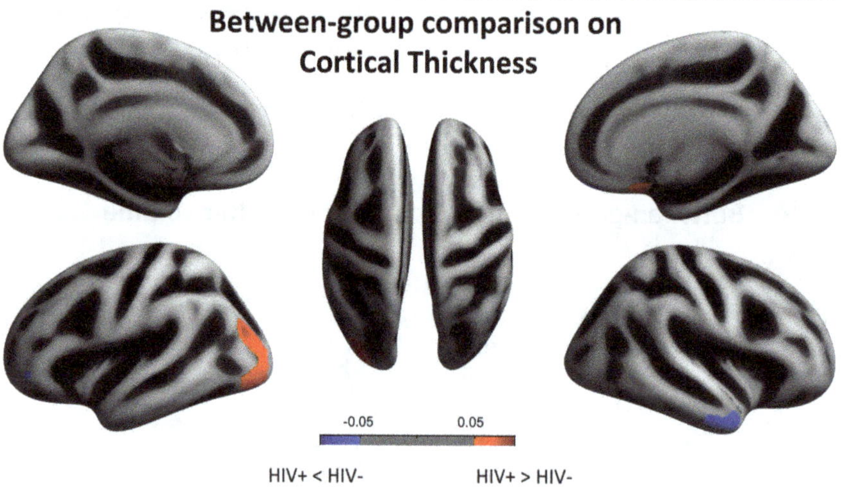

FIGURE 2 | Between-group comparison on cortical thickness (CT). Clusters showing significantly (corrected $P < 0.05$) lower (blue) and higher (red) CT in HIV+ children compared to controls. These figures were rendered using BrainNet Viewer (http://www.nitrc.org/projects/bnv/).

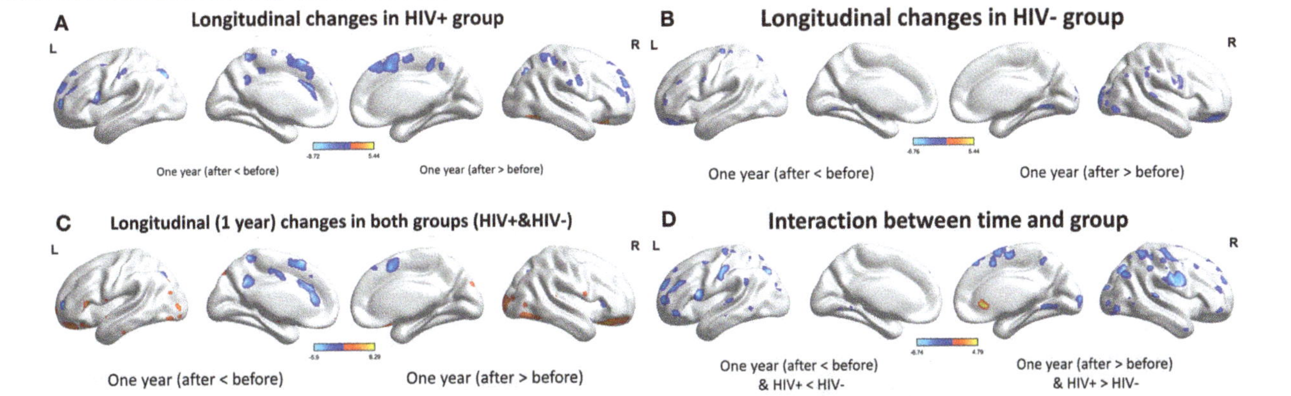

FIGURE 3 | Longitudinal changes on gray matter volume (GMV) after 1 year. Clusters showing significantly (corrected $P < 0.05$) lower (blue) and higher (red) GMV changes after 1 year. **(A)** Clusters showing many lower and few higher GMV regions in HIV+ group children. **(B)** Clusters only showing significantly lower GMV regions in HEU group children. **(C)** Put together the two groups for statistical analysis and showing significantly changes of GMV after 1 year. **(D)** In assessing the time and interactions between the two groups, clusters showing widely areas of GMV significantly reduced. These figures were rendered using BrainNet Viewer (http://www.nitrc.org/projects/bnv/).

The HEU group showed only areas with significantly reduced GMV after 1 year, mainly in the bilateral temporal lobe, left inferior frontal gyrus, right anterior OFC, and right parietal lobe (postcentral, angular, and superior parietal gyrus) and right occipital lobe, part of the basal ganglia nuclei (putamen, thalamus), bilateral cerebellum (**Table 5**; **Figure 3B**).

The two groups were put together for statistical analysis and showed that after 1 year, the GMV of multiple brain regions increased significantly, mainly including bilateral frontal lobes (the right OFC, the left inferior frontal cortex, the right precentral cortex, etc), and the right temporal lobe, bilateral upper cerebellar and parietal-occipital lobes, right amygdala, and thalamus; areas of markedly reduced GMV mainly include right medial OFC, left supplemental motor area, left cingulate gyrus, and temporal-occipital cortex (**Table 6**; **Figure 3C**). In assessing the time and interactions between the two groups, it was shown that the volume of gray matter in a wide area was significantly reduced, mainly including the bilateral parietal lobes (above gyrus, supramarginal gyrus, and precuneus), and bilateral multiple other lobes; significant gray matter volume increase only in the right cingulate anterior (**Table 7**; **Figure 3D**).

Longitudinal Changes on Cortical Thickness

For the cortical measures, the longitudinal results showed extensive cortical thinning in both the HIV+ and HEU groups after 1 year. In the HIV+ group, the bilateral cingulate gyrus, the postcentral gyrus, the parietal lobe and the left superior frontal gyrus, the calcarine, the angular gyrus, the precentral gyrus, the inferior frontal gyrus, the right paracentral lobes, the frontal pole, the central sulcus, and the inferior parietal lobule were displayed (**Table 8**; **Figure 4A**).

The HEU group showed significant cortical thinning mainly around the bilateral central sulcus and mainly in the frontal lobe, left occipital lobe and the right temporal lobe, significantly thickened cortex mainly in the left olfactory sulcus, orbital gyrus

TABLE 5 | Volume change of gray matter in HEU group after 1 year.

Contrast	Brain regions	Extent	*t*-value	MNI coordinates		
				x	y	z
Negative	Temporal_Pole_Sup_L	5516	−6.760	−60	8	−5
	Frontal_Inf_Oper_L	5516	−5.867	−54	20	32
	Postcentral_R	4111	−5.767	65	0	30
	Temporal_Pole_Mid_R	4111	−5.650	50	24	−27
	Temporal_Pole_Sup_R	4111	−5.417	62	11	−6
	OFCant_R	2130	−5.588	47	53	−14
	Precuneus_R	98	−5.308	2	−66	62
	Supp_Motor_Area_R	170	−5.105	9	2	75
	Angular_R	1266	−5.008	56	−68	35
	Parietal_Sup_R	1266	−4.506	35	−74	53
	Parietal_Sup_R	1266	−4.469	51	−39	59
	Frontal_Mid_2_R	357	−4.989	45	12	56
	Precentral_R	357	−3.925	42	−8	66
	Thalamus_R	413	−4.890	15	−20	5
	Lingual_L	1601	−4.130	−15	−66	−9
	Cerebelum_4_5_L	1601	−3.965	−11	−50	−23
	Occipital_Sup_R	1146	−4.669	23	−102	9
	Occipital_Mid_R	1146	−4.498	33	−90	26
	Occipital_Mid_R	1146	−4.086	39	−93	2
	Calcarine_L	123	−4.591	5	−98	0
	Temporal_Pole_Mid_L	269	−4.044	−20	15	−39
	Temporal_Sup_R	79	−4.429	66	−53	20
	Occipital_Inf_R	70	−4.388	44	−78	−9
	Thalamus_L	386	−4.288	−17	−27	2
	Putamen_R	940	−4.349	27	12	−8
	Putamen_R	940	−4.255	30	−5	11
	Precentral_L	306	−4.309	−30	−21	69
	Lingual_R	186	−4.254	15	−65	−6
	Temporal_Inf_L	72	−4.231	−69	−33	−20
	Cerebelum_4_5_R	553	−4.139	18	−45	−26
	Parietal_Inf_L	70	−4.125	−38	−63	51
	Occipital_Sup_L	77	−3.911	−18	−98	15

HEU, HIV-exposed uninfected; MNI, Montreal Neurological Institute; L, left; R, right. All regions were corrected by FWE cluster level $p < 0.05$.

TABLE 6 | Volume change of gray matter in HIV+ and HEU groups after 1 year.

Contrast	Brain regions	Extent	*t*-value	MNI coordinates		
				x	y	z
Positive	OFCpost_R	3035	5.829	23	23	−27
	Temporal_Inf_R	1626	4.445	56	−45	−29
	Cerebelum_6_R	1626	3.393	18	−62	−30
	Temporal_Pole_Sup_R	1996	5.278	57	18	−14
	Precentral_R	1996	4.207	66	5	18
	Temporal_Sup_R	1996	4.155	66	0	−5
	Occipital_Inf_R	630	5.100	50	−75	−12
	Temporal_Inf_R	630	4.142	45	−56	−14
	Occipital_Mid_L	2366	4.276	−33	−87	2
	Parietal_Sup_L	2366	4.011	−29	−72	57
	Frontal_Inf_Oper_L	1136	4.559	−54	20	33
	Frontal_Inf_Tri_L	1136	4.434	−59	26	6
	Frontal_Mid_2_L	1136	4.238	−48	50	6
	Amygdala_R	931	3.584	32	−5	−14
	Cerebelum_4_5_L	1443	4.258	−29	−27	−33
	Frontal_Sup_Medial_L	556	3.275	0	68	12
	Temporal_Sup_R	212	3.985	66	−51	23
	OFCant_L	197	3.831	−21	30	−18
	Occipital_Sup_R	463	3.819	26	−101	9
	Occipital_Inf_R	463	3.105	30	−87	−8
	Cerebelum_9_R	129	3.530	18	−41	−53
	Putamen_R	249	3.528	26	12	−8
	Parietal_Sup_L	58	3.528	−24	−57	74
	Postcentral_L	69	3.522	−36	−32	72
	Occipital_Mid_R	141	3.506	36	−89	24
	Frontal_Sup_Medial_L	114	3.476	−17	66	−2
	Parietal_Inf_R	54	3.438	42	−63	57
	Thalamus_L	74	3.286	−20	−27	0
Negative	Frontal_Mid_2_L	247	−5.901	−29	54	6
	Precuneus_L	100	−5.162	−8	−47	63
	Supp_Motor_Area_L	1270	−4.985	−6	20	56
	Cingulate_Mid_L	1270	−4.004	0	−2	39
	Cingulate_Mid_L	1270	−3.695	−11	−20	47
	Temporal_Sup_L	115	−4.479	−50	−42	18
	Cingulate_Post_L	248	−4.388	−6	−48	32
	Occipital_Mid_L	291	−4.161	−26	−62	38
	Cerebelum_8_R	57	−4.073	12	−69	−45
	Insula_R	63	−3.784	38	26	3
	Occipital_Sup_R	174	−3.739	26	−69	42
	Temporal_Sup_L	141	−3.438	−42	−15	−6
	Cerebelum_9_R	54	−3.395	2	−53	−56
	Temporal_Sup_R	51	−3.256	44	−8	−8
	OFCmed_R	3035	3.958	18	26	−24

HIV+, HIV-infected; HEU, HIV-exposed uninfected; MNI, Montreal Neurological Institute. All regions were corrected by FWE cluster level $p < 0.05$.

and the right inferior orbital sulcus and the right gyrus rectus (**Table 9**; **Figure 4B**).

The two groups were put together for statistical analysis, the areas of the cortical thickening were more obvious, mainly in the

TABLE 7 | Interactions between groups and time points of gray matter volume.

Contrast	Brain regions	Extent	*t*-value	MNI coordinates		
				x	y	z
Positive	Cingulate_Ant_R	100	4.936	5	27	−3
Negative	Occipital_Sup_R	676	−6.745	27	−69	44
	Frontal_Sup_2_L	2897	−6.375	−27	56	8
	Frontal_Mid_2_L	2897	−5.558	−44	41	29
	Frontal_Inf_Tri_L	2897	−4.869	−56	35	12
	SupraMarginal_R	4756	−6.233	65	−17	27
	Parietal_Sup_R	4756	−5.901	38	−50	56
	Postcentral_R	4756	−5.317	54	−26	56
	Vermis_10	221	−5.884	−2	−45	−38
	Parietal_Inf_L	84	−5.858	−44	−42	51
	Temporal_Pole_Sup_L	774	−5.560	−57	9	−6
	Frontal_Inf_Oper_L	774	−4.651	−51	9	15
	Occipital_Inf_R	213	−5.559	33	−83	−11
	Supp_Motor_Area_R	549	−5.552	9	2	75
	Parietal_Inf_L	428	−5.363	−51	−26	47
	Frontal_Sup_Medial_R	494	−5.327	9	38	56
	Cerebelum_4_5_L	902	−5.290	−6	−47	−5
	Lingual_L	902	−4.408	−15	−63	−12
	Cerebelum_Crus1_L	168	−5.261	−29	−80	−26
	OFCant_R	239	−5.039	45	51	−15
	Precuneus_R	420	−4.979	8	−50	51
	Precentral_L	436	−4.966	−41	0	62
	Frontal_Sup_Medial_L	131	−4.938	−6	54	44
	Supp_Motor_Area_R	124	−4.898	6	15	50
	Frontal_Sup_2_R	287	−4.855	27	59	24
	Angular_R	280	−4.850	53	−66	35
	Cerebelum_4_5_R	481	−4.829	9	−60	−5
	Frontal_Mid_2_R	241	−4.765	39	54	18
	Parietal_Inf_L	380	−4.732	−38	−62	53
	Precuneus_R	63	−4.695	3	−66	60
	Cerebelum_Crus2_R	443	−4.590	42	−78	−44
	Temporal_Mid_R	113	−4.542	65	−2	−21
	Temporal_Sup_L	171	−4.511	−65	−27	6
	SupraMarginal_L	355	−4.497	−59	−50	26
	Temporal_Sup_R	85	−4.447	65	−8	8
	Occipital_Sup_R	126	−4.441	24	−93	20
	Frontal_Sup_2_R	77	−4.410	23	12	68
	Temporal_Mid_R	402	−4.355	65	−42	9
	Temporal_Mid_R	335	−4.330	53	−66	8
	Parietal_Sup_L	66	−4.289	−21	−66	59
	Occipital_Mid_L	69	−4.262	−29	−87	21
	Precentral_L	182	−4.256	−27	−23	71
	Frontal_Sup_2_L	100	−4.254	−20	44	45
	Occipital_Mid_R	87	−4.246	38	−95	0
	Temporal_Pole_Mid_R	193	−4.211	51	9	−35
	Frontal_Sup_Medial_R	83	−4.103	11	69	2
	Temporal_Mid_L	80	−4.092	−60	−54	−5
	Thalamus_R	137	−3.943	17	−18	8
	Thalamus_L	214	−3.885	−6	−6	8
	Frontal_Inf_Tri_R	122	−3.882	53	38	17

Two groups = HIV-infected group and HIV-exposed uninfected group, MNI, Montreal Neurological Institute; L, left; R, right. All regions were corrected by FWE cluster level $p < 0.05$.

TABLE 8 | Cortical thickness change in HIV+ group after 1 year.

Contrast	Cortical regions	Side	Size	P-value
Positive	92% G_oc-temp_med-Parahip 8%S_collat_transv_ant	L	490	0.00287
	28% S_occipital_ant 22% S_temporal_inf 17% G_and_S_occipital_inf 13% S_temporal_sup 12% G_temporal_middle 4% G_occipital_middle 4%G_temporal_inf	R	1205	0.00032
	75% S_front_inf 25%G_front_middle	R	306	0.00029
Negative	56% G_front_sup 15% G_front_middle 8% G_and_S_frontomargin 6% G_and_S_cingul-Ant 5% G_and_S_transv_frontopol 4% S_orbital_lateral 3% S_front_sup 2% S_front_inf 1%S_front_middle	L	3546	0.00006
	66% S_calcarine 11% G_cingul-Post-ventral 8% S_parieto_occipital 8% G_oc-temp_med-Lingual 6%G_precuneus	L	2371	0.00000
	82% G_postcentral 8% S_postcentral 8% S_central 2%G_and_S_paracentral	L	851	0.00139
	48% G_pariet_inf-Angular 27% S_intrapariet_and_P_trans 19% G_pariet_inf-Supramar 7%S_postcentra	L	847	0.00000
	55% G_precentral 45%S_precentral-sup-part	L	671	0.00043
	77% S_front_inf 17% G_front_middle 5% G_front_inf-Opercular 2%G_front_inf-Triangul	L	482	0.00036
	51%G_cingul-Post-dorsal 36% S_cingul-Marginalis 12% G_and_S_cingul-Mid-Post 2% G_precuneus	L	335	0.00103
	56% S_intrapariet_and_P_trans 26% G_parietal_sup 18%S_postcentral	L	325	0.00095
	28% G_and_S_paracentral 26% G_front_sup 18% G_postcentral 17% S_central 10%G_precentral	R	2247	0.00085
	27% G_and_S_transv_frontopol 23% G_front_middle 21% G_front_sup 13% G_and_S_frontomargin 13% S_front_middle 2%G_and_S_cingul-Ant	R	1644	0.00000
	54% S_central 26% G_precentral 18%G_postcentral	R	1271	0.00173
	69% G_and_S_cingul-Mid-Post 31%G_front_sup	R	750	0.00070
	55% S_postcentral 40% S_interm_prim-Jensen 4%S_intrapariet_and_P_trans	R	688	0.00011
	83% S_subparietal 13% G_precuneus 4%G_cingul-Post-dorsal	R	581	0.00130
	100%S_intrapariet_and_P_trans	R	408	0.00006

HIV+, HIV-infected; L, left; R, right. All regions were corrected by FWE cluster level p <0.05.

bilateral middle occipital gyrus, the parietal lobe (angle gyrus), the frontal lobe (near the right inferior frontal gyrus) and the right middle temporal gyrus. Cortical thinning was mainly in the right frontal lobe (**Table 10**; **Figure 4C**). In the evaluation of the time and the interaction between the two groups, the cortical thinning in a wide area was shown, mainly around the bilateral central sulcus, the insular, the frontal lobe (mainly in the middle gyrus), the cingulate sulcus. Significant cortical thickening only showed in bilateral orbital gyrus and the right parahippocampal gyrus (**Table 11**; **Figure 4D**).

The Relationship Between Brain Morphological Metrics and Behavior

Finally, we analyzed the association between behavioral performance and brain morphological measures in HIV+ adolescents. Because there was a significant difference in Wisconsin Card Classification Test between the two groups, we performed a nonparametric correlation analysis on the Wisconsin Card Classification scores of the HIV+ group and the morphological measures with significant between-group differences on the cross-sectional analysis. For the GMV, the gray matter volume of the bilateral cerebellum in the HIV+ group was significantly positively correlated with the Wisconsin Card Classification Test score ($r = 0.681$, $p = 0.005$). For the CT, the cortical thickness of HIV+'s right rostral middle frontal ($r = -0.646$, $p = 0.009$) and right superior frontal gyri was significantly negatively correlated with the Wisconsin Card Classification Test score.

DISCUSSION

Cross-sectionally, we found a wide reduction in cortical volume and changes in cortical thickness with thinning of the right temporal lobe and thickening of the left occipital lobe in HIV+ individuals during adolescence. Longitudinally, the reduction in gray matter volume and thinning of the cortex in HIV+ individuals occurred mainly in different functional areas of the frontal and parietal lobe, which was significantly different from the pattern of their HEU controls.

Cross-sectionally, the alterations in the advanced cortices including the OFC and primary sensorimotor cortices as found

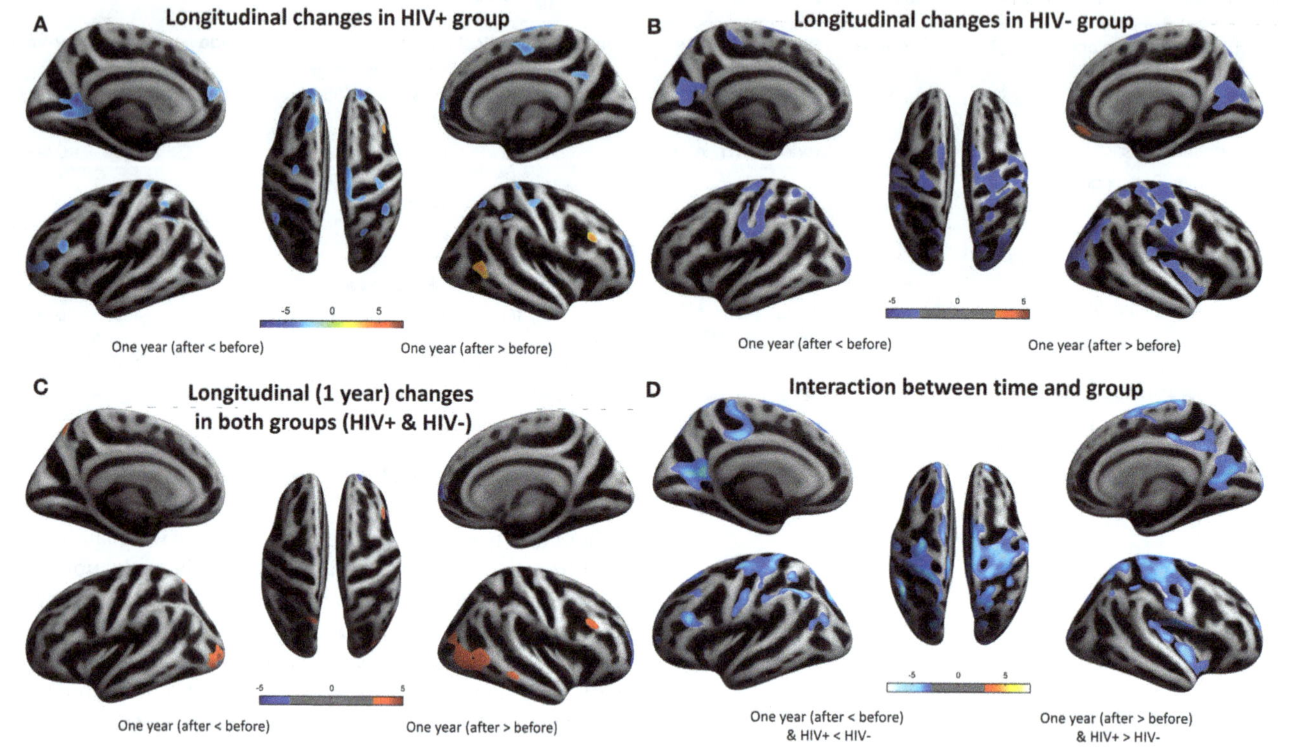

FIGURE 4 | Longitudinal changes on cortical thickness (CT) after 1 year. Clusters showing significantly (corrected $P < 0.05$) lower (blue) and higher (red) CT changes after 1 year. **(A)** Clusters showing lower and higher CT regions in HIV+ group children. **(B)** Clusters showing significantly lower and higher CT regions in HEU group children. **(C)** Put together the two groups for statistical analysis and showing significantly lower regions more obviously than higher regions of CT after 1 year. **(D)** In assessing the time and interactions between the two groups, clusters showing widely areas of CT significantly reduced.

here are generally consistent with our hypothesis and earlier reports (22, 23). The HIV virus can rapidly enter the central nervous system (CNS) and cause encephalitis within a few days after the exposure (24). In the early stages of the disease, HIV induces the CNS inflammatory T-cell response with vasculitis and leptomeningitis, directly damage oligodendrocytes, neurons, and white matter (25). The same process can be observed in the cerebral cortex of AIDS patients, thereby inducing neuronal apoptosis. Immunoreactive gliosis and neuronal loss can even cause diffuse poliodystrophy (26, 27). These pathological changes should explain why our GMV cross-sectional results only show a decrease in gray matter volume in multiple brain regions, mainly in the bilateral frontal, temporal, insular, and cerebellar cortical regions.

A major novelty of this study is the using of longitudinal structural brain data to examine brain development during early puberty after HIV exposure. Longitudinally, we found that the brain maturation in HIV-infected and non-HIV-infected children follows a general pattern, but unique changes have taken place in terms of developmental speed, spatial range, etc. The human brain decreases its gray matter in late childhood or adolescence in typical healthy development (28, 29). Our longitudinal VBM results also showed this trend, however, the GMV loss pattern of HIV+ children are significantly different from that of the controls over 1 year, the topographies of this loss including the right frontal, superior parietal, and sensorimotor regions. Changes in the OFC have been suggested with pronounced negative emotions (30). The difference in volume changes in the right OFC after 1 year suggests that this brain area may be one of the key brain areas affected by HIV. The OFC is an important limbic brain region responsible for emotion, decision making and reward evaluation, which collectively with basal ganglia, amygdala and the medial prefrontal cortex form an limbic-emotion circuit (31). It is generally believed that the functional imbalance of this circuit is related to the pathogenesis of obsessive-compulsive disorder (32, 33).

The neuroanatomical features are significantly controlled over genetic and environmental factors. GMV is a function of surface area and cortical thickness, the cortical surface area has been reported to more likely to be regulated by a genetic factor than the cortical thickness (34). A human study has shown that a decrease in synaptic density in healthy children between the ages of 2 and 16 years is accompanied by a slight decrease in neuronal density (35). We can consider that thinning of the cortex during adolescence represents the concurrent process of synapses, axons, dendritic pruning, and myelination. It plays an important role in improving the connectivity between brain networks and improving signal transmission efficiency. The thinning of association cortices is seen as a reliable marker of maturity in healthy children (36, 37). The difference in

TABLE 9 | Cortical thickness change in HEU group after 1 year.

Contrast	Cortical regions	Side	Size	*P*-value
Positive	51% S_orbital_med-olfact 34% G_orbital 11% S_orbital-H_Shaped 5%G_rectus	L	619	0.00013
	54% S_suborbital 32% G_rectus 13% G_and_S_cingul-Ant 2%G_front_sup	R	449	0.00073
Negative	41% G_postcentral 32% S_central 16% S_postcentral 7% G_pariet_inf-Supramar 3%G_and_S_subcentral	L	5583	0.00055
	68% G_parietal_sup 10% G_occipital_sup 8% G_precuneus 6% S_intrapariet_and_P_trans 5% S_oc_sup_and_transversal 3%G_and_S_paracentral	L	2688	0.00004
	53% S_parieto_occipital 24% S_calcarine 15% G_precuneus 6% G_cuneus 1%G_cingul-Post-dorsal	L	2637	0.00085
	43% G_occipital_middle 29% Pole_occipital 20% S_oc_middle_and_Lunatus 7% S_oc_sup_and_transversal 1%G_and_S_occipital_inf	L	2249	0.00049
	50% G_precentral 43% S_central 6%S_precentral-sup-part	L	1875	0.00086
	55% G_pariet_inf-Angular 31% G_pariet_inf-Supramar 10% S_postcentral 2% G_occipital_middle 2%S_oc_sup_and_transversal	L	1728	0.00169
	58%S_cingul-Marginalis 18%G_and_S_paracentral 15%G_and_S_cingul-Mid-Post 4% G_cingul-Post-dorsal 2% G_front_sup 2%G_precuneus	L	1657	0.00109
	100%G_front_sup	L	1163	0.00064
	53%G_oc-temp_lat-fusifor 32%S_oc-temp_med_and_Lingual 9% G_oc-temp_med-Lingual 6%S_collat_transv_post	L	853	0.00052
	100% G_parietal_sup	L	577	0.00044
	10%G_postcentral 9% S_central 9% G_precentral 6% G_parietal_sup 6% S_postcentral 5% G_pariet_inf-Supramar 5% G_occipital_middle 5% S_circular_insula_inf 5% Lat_Fis-post 5% Pole_occipital 5% G_and_S_subcentral 5% G_front_sup 4% G_occipital_sup 4% G_pariet_inf-Angular 3% S_oc_sup_and_transversal 2% G_Ins_lg_and_S_cent_ins 2% G_temp_sup-Plan_tempo 2% S_oc_middle_and_Lunatus 2% G_precuneus 1% G_insular_short 1%G_temp_sup-G_T_transv	R	29750	0.00024
	48% S_parieto_occipital 27% S_calcarine 21% G_cuneus 3%G_precuneus	R	2817	0.00030
	61% G_temp_sup-Lateral 24% G_temp_sup-G_T_transv 10% S_temporal_transverse 4%G_temp_sup-Plan_polar	R	522	0.00204
	100% G_and_S_paracentral	R	305	0.00246
	62% G_front_middle 38%S_front_inf	R	302	0.00156

HEU, HIV-exposed uninfected; L, left; R, right. All regions were corrected by FWE cluster level p <0.05.

cortical thickness between children with HIV and uninfected HEU children was predominantly in the association cortex with a few areas of excessive thinning, which may be the result of excessive synaptic pruning or abnormal plasticity. However, cross-sectional results are unavoidably affected by individual differences and groups. Our longitudinal study will overcome these limitations.

Neuroimaging has provided evidence of temporal hierarchy on typical brain development, with the primary cortices develop first and the association cortices continue to develop until the early three-decade of life. Sowell et al. mapped gray matter density in 176 typical development individuals aged 7 to 87 years and found that there was a significant non-linear decrease in gray matter density with age, especially on the lateral/dorsal frontal and parietal cortices. The primary sensorimotor regions, such as the visual, auditory, and the somatomotor cortices, begin to myelination at an early stage and exhibits a more linear developmental pattern, while the myelinization of the advanced functional cortex of the frontoparietal regions can continue into adulthood. In particular, the language cortex at the temporal cortex has the longest maturation process (16), and finally mature brain regions (frontal lobes) that involve advanced functions such as executive function and attention, but in this process not some brain regions are fully mature and other brain regions begin to develop (17). These studies indicate that the order of cortical maturation is consistent with the development of related cognitive abilities. Cortical thinning should occur first in the sensorimotor area, followed by the associated area, and finally in the more advanced cortical area. In our study, HIV+ children showed cortical maturation in multiple brain regions from primary to advanced functional regions after 1 year, but the brain regions involved were mostly sensory motor

TABLE 10 | Cortical thickness change in HIV+ and HEU groups after 1 year.

Contrast	Cortical regions	Side	Size	*P*-value
Positive	39% S_oc_middle_and_Lunatus 31% G_occipital_middle 15% Pole_occipital 14%G_and_S_occipital_inf	L	1687	0.00011
	66% G_parietal_sup 34%G_precuneus	L	820	0.00070
	32% G_occipital_middle 17% S_occipital_ant 12% S_oc_middle_and_Lunatus 12% G_and_S_occipital_inf 10% S_temporal_inf 9% G_temporal_middle 3% G_temporal_inf 3% S_temporal_sup 2%S_oc_sup_and_transversal	R	2912	0.00021
	99% G_pariet_inf-Angular	R	632	0.00253
	70% S_front_inf 30%G_front_middle	R	418	0.00023
	49% G_front_inf-Opercular 25% Lat_Fis-ant-Vertical 24% S_circular_insula_sup 1%G_front_inf-Triangul	R	361	0.00114
	100% G_temporal_middle	R	359	0.00096
Negative	44% G_and_S_transv_frontopol 26% G_and_S_frontomargin 23% G_front_middle 7%S_front_middle	R	764	0.00037
	59% G_front_sup 30% G_and_S_cingul-Ant 11%G_and_S_transv_frontopol	R	435	0.00011

HIV+, HIV-infected, HEU, HIV-exposed uninfected; L, left; R, right. All regions were corrected by FWE cluster level p <0.05.

cortex and limbic systems. The range and extent of the HIV+ group's cortical maturation are significantly lower than that in HEU children. This pattern of high-function-associated cortical lagging development (especially in the left parietal lobe and bilateral occipital lobes) may be the basis for the manifestation of neurocognitive abnormalities and atypical brain development.

Cortical morphometry of neuroimaging has revealed atypical development in several brain diseases including schizophrenia and hyperactivity disorder, etc. (38). In a longitudinal study of children with schizophrenia, the developmental pattern of temporally and spatially thinning of the cerebral cortex was shown and was first detected in the parietal cortex associated with visual space and associative thinking. And this pattern of gray matter loss is related to the severity of mental symptoms (39). However, Shaw et al. showed that 223 children with attention-deficit/hyperactivity disorder (ADHD) showed that the age at which the peak cortical thickness was reached significantly later than that of normal children, especially in the prefrontal cortex. It indicates that there is a significant development delay in cortical maturation in children with ADHD (40). The different results of these studies suggest that changes in the basic maturation model of the cerebral cortex may be the basis of neurodevelopmental

TABLE 11 | Interactions between groups and time points of cortical thickness.

Contrast	Cortical regions	Side	Size	*P*-value
Positive	57% G_orbital 23% S_orbital_med-olfact 20%S_orbital-H_Shaped	L	261	0.00025
	52% G_orbital 34% S_orbital-H_Shaped 15%S_orbital_med-olfact	R	810	0.00156
	92% G_oc-temp_med-Parahip 8%S_oc-temp_med_and_Lingual	R	207	0.00184
Negative	13% G_postcentral 12% S_central 11% G_parietal_sup 9% S_calcarine 8% G_pariet_inf-Angular 8% S_parieto_occipital 8% G_pariet_inf-Supramar 7% G_precentral 4% S_postcentral 4% S_temporal_sup 3% G_precuneus 3% S_intrapariet_and_P_trans 2% S_precentral-sup-part 2% G_occipital_sup 2% G_and_S_paracentral 1%G_cuneus	L	18597	0.00000
	90% G_front_sup 6% G_front_middle 3%S_front_sup	L	3533	0.00038
	40% S_cingul-Marginalis 18% G_and_S_paracentral 12% G_and_S_cingul-Mid-Post 11% G_precuneus 9% S_subparietal 7% G_cingul-Post-dorsal 4%G_front_sup	L	3215	0.00014
	54% S_central 18% G_precentral 9% G_postcentral 6% S_precentral-inf-part 6% G_and_S_subcentral 4% S_precentral-sup-part 2%G_front_middle	L	2387	0.00066
	31% S_circular_insula_inf 25% S_circular_insula_sup 20% S_circular_insula_ant 15% G_insular_short 10%G_Ins_lg_and_S_cent_ins	L	1696	0.00139
	48% S_front_inf 25% G_front_inf-Opercular 19% G_front_middle 7%G_front_inf-Triangul	L	1067	0.00008
	42% G_front_middle 33% G_and_S_frontomargin 15% S_orbital_lateral 5% S_front_inf 3% S_front_middle 3%G_orbital	L	721	0.00088
	54% S_intrapariet_and_P_trans 33% G_parietal_sup 13%S_postcentral	L	669	0.00045

(Continued)

TABLE 11 | Continued

Contrast	Cortical regions	Side	Size	*P*-value
	44% S_oc-temp_med_and_Lingual 37% G_oc-temp_lat-fusifor 19%G_oc-temp_med-Lingual	L	585	0.00234
	99% G_front_middle 1%S_front_sup	L	467	0.00177
	23% S_central 18% G_postcentral 16% G_precentral 13% G_front_sup 12% S_postcentral 8% G_and_S_paracentral 4% G_pariet_inf-Supramar 3% S_precentral-sup-part 1%G_and_S_cingul-Mid-Post	R	17427	0.00005
	26% S_circular_insula_inf 22% Lat_Fis-post 17% G_and_S_subcentral 8% G_Ins_lg_and_S_cent_ins 7% G_temp_sup-G_T_transv 6% G_insular_short 4% G_front_inf-Opercular 2% S_temporal_transverse 2% G_temp_sup-Lateral 2% S_circular_insula_ant 1%G_temp_sup-Plan_tempo	R	7725	0.00017
	27% S_subparietal 21% S_parieto_occipital 21% S_calcarine 9% G_precuneus 9% G_cuneus 5% G_cingul-Post-dorsal 4% S_cingul-Marginalis 2% G_oc-temp_med-Lingual 2%G_and_S_cingul-Mid-Post	R	5913	0.00019
	66% G_parietal_sup 20% S_intrapariet_and_P_trans 14% G_precuneus 1%S_postcentral	R	3429	0.00013
	49% Pole_occipital 17% G_occipital_middle 14% S_oc_sup_and_transversal 8% G_pariet_inf-Angular 6% G_occipital_sup 4% S_oc_middle_and_Lunatus 2%S_temporal_sup	R	2109	0.00176
	79% G_occipital_sup 8% S_oc_sup_and_transversal 5% G_cuneus 4% S_intrapariet_and_P_trans 3% G_parietal_sup 1%S_parieto_occipital	R	949	0.00037
	64% G_front_middle 28% S_front_middle 7% G_and_S_transv_frontopol 1%G_front_sup	R	408	0.00012
	61% G_oc-temp_lat-fusifor 39%S_oc-temp_med_and_Lingual	R	368	0.00124
	100%G_pariet_inf-Angular	R	362	0.00075
	80% G_front_middle 20%S_front_inf	R	226	0.00209

Two groups = HIV-infected group and HIV-exposed uninfected group; L, left; R, right. All regions were corrected by FWE cluster level p <0.05.

disorders. This process, together with social psychology and environmental factors, affects the development of individual cognitive abilities. The independent and interactive effects of these various factors may play an important role in brain structural changes and HIV-associated neurocognitive disorders in HIV+ patients. In the future, more in-depth clinical and basic research is needed to determine the pathophysiological mechanisms and potential therapeutic targets (41, 42).

Finally, we need to emphasize the role of white matter damage in the morphometric changes of HIV+. These cortical morphological changes found in this study may be partly due to the contribution of white matter damage. The axonal and myelin development of white matter has an important influence on the coordinated development of the gray matter. Recently, several studies have also pointed out that damage of the white matter structural connectivity that link the frontal, temporal, and occipital regions, as we reported, constitutes the basis of damage in HIV transmitted infection children, which suggests that the white matter damage may also be the basis for abnormal development of gray matter morphology in these population, but the relationship between them is still an open question, both for the typical development and HIV infected children. This relationship can be further analyzed and explored in future research (12, 43–45).

LIMITATIONS

There are several limitations in this study. Firstly, because the data of this type of population is extremely rare, the sample size is very small, even if this study is obtained by using an unique opportunity. Secondly, the results reported in this paper only involved 1-year follow-up, and further follow-up is needed to obtain a detailed description of their developmental trajectories, and relevant research is continuing. In addition, because the subjects in this study were from different regions of the country, it is not very easy to completely and accurately obtain their previous complications.

CONCLUSION

This cross-sectional and longitudinal study found that HIV-infected pubertal children showed a delayed cortical maturation (mainly in the left parietal lobe and bilateral occipital lobe) with atrophy (mainly occurs in the right frontal lobe, parietal lobe of the higher functional areas and multiple motor areas). This abnormal pattern of cortical development may be the structural basis for cognitive impairment in HIV+ children. Longer-term longitudinal studies are needed in the future to verify and improve this conclusion.

ETHICS STATEMENT

The study was approved by the Medical Ethics Committee of Zhongnan Hospital of Wuhan University, and a written and informed consent was made from all participants or their guardians in accordance with the Helsinki Declaration of 1975 (and as revised in 1983), following a complete description of the measurements. These methods were carried out in accordance with the approved guidelines and regulations.

AUTHOR CONTRIBUTIONS

XY designed this study and wrote the paper, LG analyzed data, and contributed to writing of the paper. XY, HW, ZY, JF, JC, and QL performed experiments together. HX and XG guided the entire experimental process.

ACKNOWLEDGMENTS

We thank all the children and their parents for being willing to take part in this study.

REFERENCES

1. Tardieu M, Le Chenadec J, Persoz A, Meyer L, Blanche S, Mayaux MJ. HIV-1-related encephalopathy in infants compared with children and adults. *Neurology.* (2000) 54:1089–95. doi: 10.1212/WNL.54.5.1089
2. World Health Organization. *Global update on the Health Sector Response to HIV*, 2014, World Health Organization. (2014).
3. Patel K, Ming X, Williams PL, Robertson KR, Oleske JM, Seage GR, et al. Impact of HAART and CNS-penetrating antiretroviral regimens on HIV encephalopathy among perinatally infected children and adolescents. *AIDS.* (2009) 23:1893–901. doi: 10.1097/QAD.0b013e32832dc041
4. Cohen S, Ter Stege JA, Geurtsen GJ, Scherpbier HJ, Kuijpers TW, Reiss P, et al. Poorer cognitive performance in perinatally HIV-infected children versus healthy socioeconomically matched controls. *Clin Infect Dis.* (2015) 60:1111–9. doi: 10.1093/cid/ciu1144
5. Baillieu N, Potterton J. The extent of delay of language, motor, and cognitive development in HIV-positive infants. *J Neurol Phys Ther.* (2008) 32:118–21. doi: 10.1097/NPT.0b013e3181846232
6. Abubakar A. Infections of the Central Nervous System and Child Development in Sub-Saharan Africa. In: Abubakar A, van de Vijver FJR, editors. *Handbook of Applied Developmental Science in Sub-Saharan Africa.* Springer Science+Business Media LLC (2017). doi: 10.1007/978-1-4939-7328-6_7
7. Lindsey JC, Malee KM, Brouwers P, Hughes MD. Neurodevelopmental functioning in HIV-infected infants and young children before and after the introduction of protease inhibitor-based highly active antiretroviral therapy. *Pediatrics.* (2007) 119:681–93. doi: 10.1542/peds.2006-1145
8. Nozyce ML, Lee SS, Wiznia A, Nachman S, Mofenson LM, Smith ME, et al. A behavioral and cognitive profile of clinically stable HIV-infected children. *Pediatrics.* (2006) 117:763–70. doi: 10.1542/peds.2005-0451
9. Lewis-de Los Angeles CP, Alpert KI, Williams PL, Malee K, Huo Y, Csernansky JG, et al. Deformed subcortical structures are related to past HIV disease severity in youth with perinatally acquired HIV infection. *Pediatr Infect Dis Soc.* (2016) 5(Suppl. 1):S6–14. doi: 10.1093/jpids/piw051
10. Lewis-de Los Angeles CP, Williams PL, Huo Y, Wang SD, Uban KA, Herting MM, et al. Lower total and regional gray matter brain volumes in youth with perinatally-acquired HIV infection: associations with HIV disease severity, substance use, and cognition. *Brain Behav Immun.* (2017) 62:100–9. doi: 10.1016/j.bbi.2017.01.004
11. Nwosu EC, Robertson FC, Holmes MJ, Cotton MF, Dobbels E, Little F, et al. Altered brain morphometry in 7-year old HIV-infected children on early ART. *Metab Brain Dis.* (2018) 33:523–35. doi: 10.1007/s11011-017-0162-6
12. Jankiewicz M, Holmes MJ, Taylor PA, Cotton MF, Laughton B, van der Kouwe A, et al. White matter abnormalities in children with HIV infection and exposure. *Front Neuroanat.* (2017) 11:88. doi: 10.3389/fnana.2017.00088
13. Hoare J, Ransford GL, Phillips N, Amos T, Donald K, Stein DJ. Systematic review of neuroimaging studies in vertically transmitted HIV positive children and adolescents. *Metab Brain Dis.* (2014) 29:221–9. doi: 10.1007/s11011-013-9456-5
14. Thompson PM, Jahanshad N. Novel neuroimaging methods to understand how HIV affects the brain. *Curr HIV/AIDS Rep.* (2015) 12:289–98. doi: 10.1007/s11904-015-0268-6
15. Blokhuis C, Kootstra NA, Caan MW, Pajkrt D. Neurodevelopmental delay in pediatric HIV/AIDS: current perspectives. *Neurobehav HIV Med.* (2016) 7:1–13. doi: 10.2147/NBHIV.S68954
16. Sowell ER, Peterson BS, Thompson PM, Welcome SE, Henkenius AL, Toga AW. Mapping cortical change across the human life span. *Nat Neurosci.* (2003) 6:309–15. doi: 10.1038/nn1008
17. Gogtay N, Giedd JN, Lusk L, Hayashi KM, Greenstein D, Vaituzis AC, et al. Dynamic mapping of human cortical development during childhood through early adulthood. *Proc Natl Acad Sci USA.* (2004) 101:8174–9. doi: 10.1073/pnas.0402680101
18. Ashburner J, Friston K J. Unified segmentation. *Neuroimage.* (2005) 26:839–51. doi: 10.1016/j.neuroimage.2005.02.018
19. Tohka J, Zijdenbos A, Evans A. Fast and robust parameter estimation for statistical partial volume models in brain MRI. *Neuroimage.* (2004) 23:84–97. doi: 10.1016/j.neuroimage.2004.05.007
20. Dahnke R, Yotter RA, Gaser C. Cortical thickness and central surface estimation. *Neuroimage.* (2013) 65:336–48. doi: 10.1016/j.neuroimage.2012.09.050
21. Antinori A, Arendt G, Becker JT, Brew BJ, Byrd DA, Cherner M, et al. Updated research nosology for HIV-associated neurocognitive disorders. *Neurology.* (2007) 69:1789–99. doi: 10.1212/01.WNL.0000287431.88658.8b
22. Thompson PM, Dutton RA, Hayashi KM, Toga AW, Lopez OL, Aizenstein HJ, et al. Thinning of the cerebral cortex visualized in HIV/AIDS reflects CD4+ T lymphocyte decline. *Proc Natl Acad Sci USA.* (2005) 102:15647–52. doi: 10.1073/pnas.0502548102
23. Pfefferbaum A, Rogosa DA, Rosenbloom MJ, Chu W, Sassoon SA, Kemper CA, et al. Accelerated aging of selective brain structures in HIV infection: a controlled, longitudinal MRI study. *Neurobiol Aging.* (2014) 35:1755–68. doi: 10.1016/j.neurobiolaging.2014.01.008
24. Valcour V, Chalermchai T, Sailasuta N, Marovich M, Lerdlum S, Suttichom D, et al. Central nervous system viral invasion and inflammation during acute HIV infection. *J Infect Dis.* (2012) 206:275–82. doi: 10.1093/infdis/jis326
25. Gray F, Scaravilli F, Everall I, Chretien F, An S, Boche D, et al. Neuropathology of early HIV-1 infection. *Brain Pathol.* (1996) 6:1–15. doi: 10.1111/j.1750-3639.1996.tb00775.x
26. Soontornniyomkij V. *Neuropathology of HIV-1 Disease[M].* New York, NY: Springer (2017). p. 143–208.
27. Ozdener H. Molecular mechanisms of HIV-1 associated neurodegeneration. *J Biosci.* (2005) 30:391–405. doi: 10.1007/BF02703676
28. Giedd JN, Blumenthal J, Jeffries NO, Castellanos FX, Liu H, Zijdenbos A, et al. Brain development during childhood and adolescence: a longitudinal MRI study. *Nat Neurosci.* (1999) 2:861–3. doi: 10.1038/13158
29. Lenroot RK, Gogtay N, Greenstein DK, Wells EM, Wallace GL, Clasen LS, et al. Sexual dimorphism of brain developmental trajectories during childhood and adolescence. *Neuroimage.* (2007) 36:1065–73. doi: 10.1016/j.neuroimage.2007.03.053
30. Miller EK, Cohen JD. An integrative theory of prefrontal cortex function. *Ann Rev Neurosci.* (2001) 24:167–202. doi: 10.1146/annurev.neuro.24.1.167
31. Krawczyk DC. Contributions of the prefrontal cortex to the neural basis of human decision making. *Neurosci Biobehav Rev.* (2002) 26:631–64 doi: 10.1016/S0149-7634(02)00021-0
32. Macmaster FP, O'Neill J, Rosenberg DR. Brain imaging in pediatric obsessive compulsive disorder. *J Am Acad Child Adolesc Psychiatry.* (2008) 47:1262–72. doi: 10.1097/CHI.0b013e318185d2be
33. Saxena S, Rauch SL. Functional neuroimaging and the neuroanatomy of obsessive-compulsive disorder. *Psychiatr Clinics North Am.* (2000) 23:563–86. doi: 10.1016/S0193-953X(05)70181-7

34. Winkler AM, Kochunov P, Blangero J, Almasy L, Zilles K, Fox PT, et al. Cortical thickness or gray matter volume? The importance of selecting the phenotype for imaging genetics studies. *Neuroimage.* (2010) 53:1135–46. doi: 10.1016/j.neuroimage.2009.12.028
35. Huttenlocher PR. Synaptic density in human frontal cortex - developmental changes and effects of aging. *Brain Res.* (1979) 163:195–205. doi: 10.1016/0006-8993(79)90349-4
36. Tau GZ, Peterson BS. Normal development of brain circuits. *Neuropsychopharmacology.* (2010) 35:147–68. doi: 10.1038/npp.2009.115
37. Giedd JN, Keshavan M, Paus T. Why do many psychiatric disorders emerge during adolescence? *Nat Rev Neurosci.* (2008) 9:947–57. doi: 10.1038/nrn2513
38. Kessler RC, Berglund P, Demler O, Jin R, Merikangas KR, Walters EE. Lifetime prevalence and age-of-onset distributions of DSM-IV disorders in the National Comorbidity Survey Replication. *Arch Gen Psychiatry.* (2005) 62:593–602. doi: 10.1001/archpsyc.62.6.593
39. Thompson PM, Vidal C, Giedd JN, Gochman P, Blumenthal J, Nicolson R, et al. Mapping adolescent brain change reveals dynamic wave of accelerated gray matter loss in very early-onset schizophrenia. *Proc Natl Acad Sci USA.* (2001) 98:11650–5. doi: 10.1073/pnas.201243998
40. Shaw P, Eckstrand K, Sharp W, Blumenthal J, Lerch JP, Greenstein D, et al. Attention-deficit/hyperactivity disorder is characterized by a delay in cortical maturation. *Proc Natl Acad Sci USA.* (2007) 104:19649–54. doi: 10.1073/pnas.0707741104
41. Thames AD, Kuhn TP, Mahmood Z, Bilder RM, Williamson TJ, Singer EJ, et al. Effects of social adversity and HIV on subcortical shape and neurocognitive function. *Brain Imag Behav.* (2018) 12:96–108. doi: 10.1007/s11682-017-9676-0
42. Womersley JS, Seedat S, Hemmings SMJ. Childhood maltreatment and HIV-associated neurocognitive disorders share similar pathophysiology: a potential sensitisation mechanism? *Metab Brain Dis.* (2017) 32:1717–33. doi: 10.1007/s11011-017-0062-9
43. Ackermann C, Andronikou S, Saleh MG, Laughton B, Alhamud AA, van der Kouwe A, et al. Early antiretroviral therapy in HIV-infected children is associated with diffuse white matter structural abnormality and corpus callosum sparing. *Am J Neuroradiol.* (2016) 37:2363–9. doi: 10.3174/ajnr.A4921
44. Fennema-Notestine C, Ellis RJ, Archibald SL, Jernigan TL, Letendre SL, Notestine RJ, et al. Increases in brain white matter abnormalities and subcortical gray matter are linked to CD4 recovery in HIV infection. *J Neurovirol.* (2013) 19:393–401. doi: 10.1007/s13365-013-0185-7
45. Zhu T, Zhong J, Hu R, Tivarus M, Ekholm S, Harezlak J, et al. Patterns of white matter injury in HIV infection after partial immune reconstitution: a DTI tract-based spatial statistics study. *J Neurovirol.* (2013) 19:10–23. doi: 10.1007/s13365-012-0135-9

9

HIVconsv Vaccines and Romidepsin in Early-Treated HIV-1-Infected Individuals: Safety, Immunogenicity and Effect on the Viral Reservoir (Study BCN02)

Beatriz Mothe[1,2,3†], Miriam Rosás-Umbert[1,4†], Pep Coll[1], Christian Manzardo[5], Maria C. Puertas[1], Sara Morón-López[1], Anuska Llano[1], Cristina Miranda[2], Samandhy Cedeño[1], Miriam López[2], Yovaninna Alarcón-Soto[6], Guadalupe Gómez Melis[6], Klaus Langohr[6], Ana M. Barriocanal[4,7], Jessica Toro[2], Irene Ruiz[5], Cristina Rovira[5], Antonio Carrillo[7], Michael Meulbroek[8], Alison Crook[9], Edmund G. Wee[9], Jose M. Miró[5], Bonaventura Clotet[1,2,3,4], Marta Valle[4,10], Javier Martinez-Picado[1,3,11], Tomáš Hanke[9,12], Christian Brander[1,3,11†], José Moltó[2,7†] and the BCN02 Study Investigators*

[1] IrsiCaixa AIDS Research Institute-HIVACAT, Badalona, Spain, [2] Fundació Lluita contra la Sida, Infectious Diseases Department, Hospital Universitari Germans Trias i Pujol, Badalona, Spain, [3] Faculty of Medicine, Universitat de Vic-Central de Catalunya (UVic-UCC), Vic, Spain, [4] Department of Cellular Biology, Physiology and Immunology, Universitat Autonoma de Barcelona (UAB), Barcelona, Spain, [5] Hospital Clinic- IDIBAPS, University of Barcelona, Barcelona, Spain, [6] Departament d'Estadística i Investigació Operativa, Universitat Politècnica de Catalunya/BARCELONATECH, Barcelona, Spain, [7] Department of Infectious Diseases, Germans Trias i Pujol Research Institute, Badalona, Spain, [8] Projecte dels NOMS-Hispanosida, BCN Checkpoint, Barcelona, Spain, [9] The Jenner Institute, University of Oxford, Oxford, United Kingdom, [10] Pharmacokinetic/Pharmacodynamic Modeling and Simultation, Institut de Recerca de l'Hospital de la Santa Creu i Sant Pau-IIB Sant Pau, Barcelona, Spain, [11] ICREA, Barcelona, Spain, [12] Joint Research Center for Human Retrovirus Infection, Kumamoto University, Kumamoto, Japan

***Correspondence:**
Beatriz Mothe
bmothe@irsicaixa.es

† These authors have contributed equally to this work

Kick&kill strategies combining drugs aiming to reactivate the viral reservoir with therapeutic vaccines to induce effective cytotoxic immune responses hold potential to achieve a functional cure for HIV-1 infection. Here, we report on an open-label, single-arm, phase I clinical trial, enrolling 15 early-treated HIV-1-infected individuals, testing the combination of the histone deacetylase inhibitor romidepsin as a latency-reversing agent and the MVA.HIVconsv vaccine. Romidepsin treatment resulted in increased histone acetylation, cell-associated HIV-1 RNA, and T-cell activation, which were associated with a marginally significant reduction of the viral reservoir. Vaccinations boosted robust and broad HIVconsv-specific T cells, which were strongly refocused toward conserved regions of the HIV-1 proteome. During a monitored ART interruption phase using plasma viral load over 2,000 copies/ml as a criterium for ART resumption, 23% of individuals showed sustained suppression of viremia up to 32 weeks without evidence for reseeding the viral reservoir. Results from this pilot study show that the combined kick&kill intervention was safe and suggest a role for this strategy in achieving an immune-driven durable viremic control.

Keywords: romidepsin, HDAC inhibitor, kick&kill strategy, HIVconsv, early-treatment

INTRODUCTION

Current antiretroviral therapy (ART) effectively suppresses HIV-1 replication, thus preventing disease progression. However, the infection remains chronic given that a latent HIV-1 reservoir, established early after infection, persists despite suppressive ART (1). Upon ART discontinuation, integrated replication-competent proviruses in the reservoir drive a rapid viral rebound (2). Therapeutic vaccination has been proposed as a possible approach to induce an effective immune control able to contain rebounding virus (3).

Most therapeutic vaccines tested in the past expressed one or several HIV-1 proteins, which expanded HIV-1-specific $CD8^+$ cytotoxic T lymphocyte (CTL) responses to varying levels. However, the responses were ineffective in controlling viremia after ART interruption, likely because of their suboptimal magnitude, breadth, width, specificity, and/or polyfunctionality (4–8), raising the need for novel immunogens and delivery methods to tackle HIV-1 diversity and the virus' ability to escape. New vaccines strategies are being developed to maximize the vaccine coverage of circulating viruses using multivalent mosaic immunogens designed *in silico* (9, 10). Alternatively, vaccines designs are tested that aim to focus the CTL responses toward more conserved and protective regions of the virus, which are less likely to mutate and escape the T-cell response (11–15). Among the latter, the HIVconsv immunogen is one of the most advanced vaccine candidates in clinical development. HIVconsv immunogen consists of a chimeric protein assembled from 14 highly conserved domains derived from HIV-1 genes Gag, Pol, Vif, and Env alternating, for each domain, the consensus sequence of the four major HIV-1 clades A, B, C, and D (12). Upon delivery to both HIV-1-negative and positive individuals by heterologous prime/boost regimens as DNA or in simian adenovirus of chimpanzee (ChAdV) and poxvirus MVA vectors, HIVconsv vaccines were safe and induced $CD8^+$ T cells with broad inhibitory capacity of HIV-1 *in vitro*, but showed no effect on the viral reservoir (16–23).

To overcome the limitations of therapeutic vaccines -administered alone- in targeting the viral reservoir, vaccines are combined with latency reversing agents (LRA) in the so called kick&kill strategies (24). This approach intends to activate transcription of HIV-1 using small molecules able to disrupt the viral latency and facilitate effective sensing and clearance of infected cells by vaccine-elicited HIV-1-specific CTL (25, 26). Histone deacetylase inhibitors (HDACi) have been proposed as potential HIV-1 LRA (27–31). Romidepsin (RMD; Istodax®, Celgene Ltd.) is a potent HDACi approved for the treatment of cutaneous and peripheral T-cell lymphomas, which has been shown to induce HIV-1 transcription both *in vitro* and *in vivo* (32, 33). The REDUC trial combined RMD with Vacc-4x and rhuGM-CSF in chronically suppressed HIV-1-positive individuals, resulting in a mean reduction of 39.7% in total HIV-1 DNA (34). However, this intervention failed to delay viral rebound after ART interruption, suggesting that the reservoir-purge effect was not sufficient and/or the vaccine-induced response was unable to eliminate cells actively replicating HIV-1. In fact, the increase in cell-associated HIV-1 RNA inversely correlated with time to rebound, supporting that, in the absence of an enhanced HIV-1-specific CTL response, viral reactivation might facilitate viral rebound once ART is interrupted (35).

Here, in this single-arm, open-label, phase I, proof-of-concept study, referred to as BCN02 trial (NCT02616874), we assessed the safety, tolerability, immunogenicity and effect on the viral reservoir of a kick&kill strategy consisting of the combination of HIVconsv vaccines with RMD in suppressed early-treated HIV-1-infected individuals. Participants were rolled-over from the therapeutic vaccine trial BCN01 (NCT01712425), in which individuals who started ART during acute/recent HIV-1 infection had received a prime/boost regimen of the ChAdV63.HIVconsv and MVA.HIVconsv vaccines (CM) (20). Three years after, BCN01 participants who had shown sustained viral suppression and who accepted to participate in BCN02 study were immunized with two doses of MVA.HIVconsv, before and after three weekly-doses of RMD, followed by a monitored antiretroviral pause (MAP) for a period of 32 weeks to assess the ability of the intervention to control viral rebound.

MATERIALS AND METHODS

Study Design and Interventions

The BCN02 clinical trial was an investigator initiated phase I, open-label, single-arm, multicenter, single-country study to assess the safety, tolerability and efficacy of a combined kick&kill strategy in suppressed HIV-1-infected patients that had initiated ART during acute/recent HIV-infection. Individuals were rolled over from vaccine trial BCN01 (20) and invited to participate after 3 years on suppressive ART. A complete list of inclusion/exclusion criteria is available in the Study Protocol (**Appendix**). The study took place between February 2016 and October 2017 at two HIV-1 units from universitary hospitals (Hospital Universitari Germans Trias i Pujol -HUGTIP, Badalona and Hospital Clínic, Barcelona) and a community center (BCN-Checkpoint, Barcelona). Before inclusion in the study, all participants signed an informed consent previously discussed, reviewed and approved by the Community Advisory Board of the Barcelona-based vaccine program (HIVACAT). The study was approved by the institutional ethical review board of the participating institutions (Reference Nr AC-15-108-R) and by the Spanish Regulatory Authorities; and was conducted in accordance to the principles of the Helsinki Declaration and local personal data protection law (LOPD 15/1999). The MVA.HIVconsv vaccine was GMP manufactured at IDT Biologika GmbH, Germany, and supplied for the study under an investigator initiated clinical trial contract agreement. Risk of Genetically Modified Organism release to the environment was evaluated by the Spanish Ministry of Environment (B/ES/12/09). RMD was supplied for the study by Celgene Ltd. (Couvet, Switzerland) under an investigator initiated clinical trial contract agreement.

The BCN02 trial design is summarized in **Figure 1A**. After their inclusion in the study (week 0), all participants received a first dose of 2×10^8 plaque-forming units (pfu) of MVA.HIVconsv (MVA_1) administered intramuscularly, followed

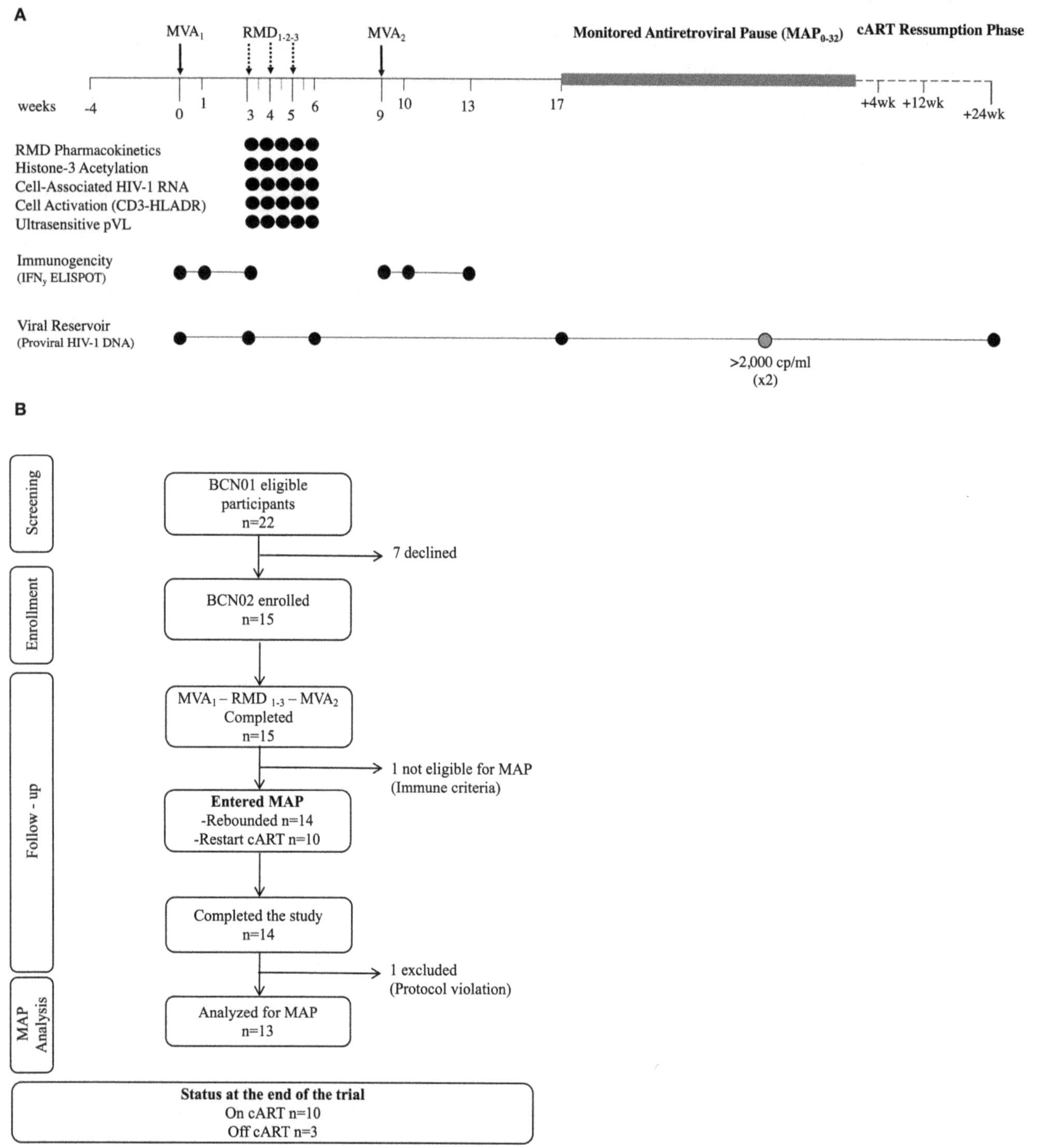

FIGURE 1 | Trial design. **(A)** Schematic study design. **(B)** Consolidated Standards of Reporting Trials (CONSORT) flow diagram for the trial. *Viral rebound during MAP was defined as pVL >20 copies/ml and #criteria for ART resumption included pVL over 2,000 copies/ml in two consecutive determinations, $CD4^+$ cell counts decrease over 50% and/or below 500 cells/mm^3 and/or development of clinical symptoms suggestive of an acute retroviral syndrome. MVA, MVA.HIVconsv vaccine; RMD, romidepsin; MAP, monitored antiretroviral pause; ART, antiretroviral therapy; pVL, plasma HIV-1 viral load.

by three weekly doses of RMD of 5 mg/m^2 BSA infused intravenously over 4 hours (RMD$_{1-2-3}$), and by a second dose of 2×10^8 pfu of MVA.HIVconsv (MVA$_2$) 4 weeks after RMD$_3$ to compensate for any potential impairment in the previous vaccine-induced response caused by RMD. Following RMD prescription information, participants received prophylactic antiemetic treatment with ondasetron before and during 3 days after each RMD dose.

Eight weeks after MVA_2 (week 17), eligible participants initiated a MAP for a maximum of 32 weeks (MAP_{0-32}) or until any ART resumption criteria were met. To be eligible for the MAP, participants had to maintain undetectable HIV-1 pVL and meet the immune futility criteria, defined as showing a net increase in HIVconsv-specific immune response with MVA_2 boost measured in an *ex vivo* IFN-γ ELISPOT assay. During MAP, participants were allowed to choose either the hospital units or BCN-Checkpoint community center for the follow up visits. Symptoms suggestive of acute retroviral syndrome and sexually transmitted diseases were solicited and viral load was tested using the finger-tip Xpert HIV-1 Qual kit (Cepheid, Sunnyvale, CA, US) in all visits. When a positive result was obtained in the Xpert HIV-1 Qual, participants were called in for a confirmatory quantitative pVL within the next 24 h. If pVL was confirmed to be over 20 copies/ml, a visit was scheduled 3 days after to closely monitor viral rebound and be able to offer prompt ART resumption if required. Details on viral load management during MAP are described in the Study Protocol (**Appendix**). After ART ressumption, participants were followed at 4, 12, and 24 weeks to assure that they re-attained viral suppression.

Study Population

BCN02 participants were adult (≥18 years) HIV-1-infected individuals, who had initiated ART >6 months after estimated date of HIV-1 acquisition and who had received a prime/boost heterologous vaccination regimen using ChAdV63.HIVconsv-MVA.HIVconsv in the parental BCN01 study (20). To be eligible for BCN02, participants had to maintain optimal HIV-1 suppression during at least 3 years and $CD4^+$ cell counts ≥500 cells/mm^3 at BCN02 baseline visit. Main exclusion criteria included active hepatitis B or C, history of AIDS-defining disease, treatment for cancer or lymphoproliferative disease within 1 year before study entry or use of immunosuppressants within the 3 months prior to the screening visit. Concomitant treatment with strong CYP3A4 inhibitors was not permitted, but switching ART to a non-boosted integrase-inhibitor raltegravir- or dolutegravir-based regimen at least 4 weeks before baseline visit was allowed for those patients receiving ART containing ritonavir or cobicistat at screening.

Study Endpoints

The primary endpoint of this study was to assess the safety, tolerability and the effect on the viral reservoir size of the combined treatment with HIVconsv vaccines and RMD given as a latency reversing agent. Secondary endpoints included the extent and specificity of the CTL response and the effect of the intervention in controlling viral rebound after ART interruption. Other secondary endpoints included RMD pharmacokinetics and the effects of RMD on histone acetylation in lymphocytes, induction of viral transcription, changes in T-cell activation surface markers, and quantification of plasma viremia.

Safety and tolerability were evaluated by the development of grade ≥3 and serious adverse events (AE). Local and systemic AE were solicited prospectively for a minimum of 7 days following each immunization and RMD administration. Both local and systemic AE were graded according to the Division of AIDS (DAIDS) Table for Grading the Severity of Adult and Pediatric Adverse Events, version 2.0, November 2014, accessible online at https://rsc.niaid.nih.gov/sites/default/files/daids-ae-grading-table-v2-nov2014.pdf. AE were specified as unrelated, unlikely, probably or definitely related to the investigational products by the investigator.

Determination of RMD Pharmacokinetics

The concentration of RMD in plasma was determined, for RMD_1, at the end of the infusion (4 h) and 4.5, 5, 6, 8, 12, and 24 h after and, for RMD_2 and RMD_3, at the end of the infusion and 12 h after. RMD concentrations were measured by liquid chromatography-mass spectrometry/mass spectrometry (LC-MS/MS), according to a validated method. A population pharmacokinetic model for RMD was developed using non-linear mixed-effects modeling with the computer program NONMEM version 7.3 (Icon Development Solution, Ellicot City, MD) (36). Bayesian estimates of the individual parameters of RMD were used to simulate individual drug concentrations, and RMD area under the concentration-time curve (AUC0-inf) was calculated for each individual on each occasion using a non-compartmental approach (Winnonlin software; Phoenix, version 7.0).

Flow Cytometry Determination of acH3 and Activation of T Cells

The levels of histone H3 acetylation in lymphocytes (based on FSC/SCC scatter) were determined by flow cytometry from samples taken before (0 h) and at the end of each RMD infusion (RMD_{1-2-3}) (4 h), at 8 and 24 h (+1 day) RMD_1, and at 72 h (+3 days) and 7 days after (RMD_{1-2-3}). Cryopreserverd PBMC were thawed 4 h before use, and 500,000 cells were blocked with 600 ul of PBS/10% FBS for 20 min and stained with polyclonal rabbit anti-acetyl histoneH3 (10 μg/ml, MerckMillipore #06-599) or normal rabbit serum (control stain, LifeTechnologies #10510) for 30 min. Cells were washed and subsequently incubated with donkey anti-rabbit IgG(H+L) (6 μg/mL, LifeTechnologies #A21206) for 30 min at room temperature in the dark. Cells were washed, re-suspended in 150 μl PBS and analyzed. ~50,000 events were acquired per sample. The median fluorescence intensity (MFI) for each sample was calculated by substracting the background MFI (isotype control stain) from the anti-acetyl histoneH3 stain.

Activation of T cells was determined based upon HLA-DR expression on $CD3^+$ T cells. Cryopreserved PBMC were thawed, and 1,000,000 cells were stained with CD3 APC-Cy7, CD4 FITC, CD8 BV510 and HLA-DR PECy7 (BioLegend #344818, 300538, 301048, and 307616, respectively). Cells were collected on an LSRII instrument (BD), and data analyzed according to the gating criteria shown in **Supplementary Figure 1** using FlowJo 10 software.

Quantification of Cell-Associated (CA) HIV-1 RNA in CD4+ T Cells

Cell-associated HIV-1 RNA was quantified in peripheral $CD4^+$ T cells by ddPCR (One-Step RT-ddPCR Advanced Kit for Probes, BioRad) from samples taken before (0 h) and at the end of each RMD infusion (4 h), at 8 and 24 h (+1 day) after RMD_1, and 72 h (+3 days) and 7 days after RMD_{1-2-3}. CA HIV-1 RNA was quantified using two different primers/probe sets annealing to the 5′LTR and GAG conserved regions of HIV-1, to circumvent potential primer mismatch in individuals' viral sequence as previously described (37). HIV-1 transcription levels were normalized to the housekeeping gene TATA-binding protein (TBP) and shown as relative to levels before RMD_1.

Ultra-Sensitive Determination of Residual Viremia

To evaluate HIV-1 RNA below 20 copies/ml, 4–8 ml of plasma samples taken before (0 h) and at the end of each RMD infusion (4 h), at 8 and 24 h (+1 day) after RMD_1, and 72 h (+3 days) and 7 days after RMD_{1-2-3} were ultracentrifugated at 170,000 g at 4°C for 30 min and viral RNA was extracted automatically using the m2000sp Abbot device. HIV-1 RNA copies were quantified using the Abbott Real-Time HIV-1 assay (Abbott Molecular Inc.) and in-house calibration curve sets as described (38). The limit of detection (2 HIV-1 RNA copies/mL) was calculated relative to the plasma volume.

Vaccine Immunogenicity

Total HIV-1 and HIVconsv-specific T cells were assessed *ex vivo* using cryopreserved PBMC obtained the day of vaccination and 1 week afterwards, 3 weeks after MVA_1, and 4 weeks after MVA_2 using an IFN-γ-detecting enzyme-linked immunoabsorbent spot assay (ELISPOT IFN-γ Mabtech kit). 15-mer peptides overlapping by 11 amino acid were combined into 6 pools of 32–33 peptides per pool corresponding to the HIVconsv vaccine insert (P1-P6, total $n = 166$ peptides, IN pools) (**Figure 3A**) and 12 pools of 39–67 peptides per pool spanning the rest of the HIV-1 viral protein sequences (OUT pools for "outside the immunogen," obtained through the NIH AIDS Reagent Program). All peptides pools were tested in duplicates. The final concentration of individual peptides in the ELISPOT assay was 1.57 μg/ml. Medium only was used as no-peptide negative control in quadruplicate wells, and PHA (50 μg/ml) and a CEF peptide pool (2 μg/ml) consisting of 23 previously defined human $CD8^+$ T-cell epitopes from cytomegalovirus, Epstein-Barr virus and influenza virus (C.T.L. OH, USA) were added as positive controls.

To address the breadth of the vaccine-induced response at the peak immunogenicity time point, an IFN-γ ELISPOT assay with *in vitro* expanded T cells was performed on stored samples from week 10 and 13 to test individual overlapping peptides covering the HIVconsv immunogen sequence ($n = 166$ OLP). Briefly, cryopreserved PBMC were thawed and incubated for 3 h at 37°C in R10 before stimulation with an anti-CD3 monoclonal antibody during 2–4 weeks in RPMI 1640 supplemented with FBS and penicillin/streptomycin with 50 U/ml of recombinant IL-2 (39). Before their use in ELISPOT assays, the expanded cells were washed twice with R10 and incubated overnight at 37 °C in the absence of IL-2 and individual OLP were added at 5 μg/ml. 100,000 cells were used per well as in the direct *ex vivo* assay.

Spots were counted using an automated Cellular Technology Limited (C.T.L., OH, USA) ELISPOT Reader Unit. The threshold for positive responses was set at $\geq$50 SFC/10^6 PBMC (5 spots per well), > the mean number of SFC in negative control wells plus 3 SD of the negative control wells, or > 3× the mean of negative control wells, whichever was higher. To avoid overestimating the breadth of responses, positive responses to two consecutive 15-mer overlapping peptide were counted as one response. The highest magnitude of the sequential responses was taken as the magnitude for each identified response.

Quantification of HIV-1 Reservoir

To quantify the size of the peripheral blood proviral reservoir, lysed extracts from $CD4^+$ T cells were used to measure total CA HIV-1 DNA by ddPCR. Primers and probes for the RPP30 cellular gene were used for input normalization.

Statistical Analysis

Qualitative variables were represented as mean absolute and relative frequencies, whereas quantitative variables were represented as mean or median and range. Safety endpoints are summarized by the number and percentage of participants reporting local and systemic AE and their grading. The Wilcoxon signed rank test was used to test whether the viral reservoir and the immune parameter changed as an effect of the intervention, without correction for multiple comparisons. The maximum breadth of the T-cell response per individual was estimated as the number of P1-P6 pools eliciting a positive response throughout the study and the number of individual OLP eliciting a response at peak immunogenicity time point from the mapping assay. Reservoir size and immunogenicity were analyzed using GraphPad Prism (v5.01) for Mac OS X (San Diego, CA).

To evaluate the effect of the intervention on viral rebound, a positive pre-defined efficacy signal was established if at least over 20% of patients remained with pVL below 2,000 copies/ml at week 12 of MAP, considering previous data suggesting that early treatment initiation could favor delayed viral rebound/spontaneous viral control in up to 15% of individuals (40). However, BCN02 was an exploratory pilot trial and, due to the absence of a control arm and its final small sample size, the nature of this study only allowed to detect trends in virological effects, which collectively, could be useful to design future studies. To detect possible factors associated to the viremic control observed during the MAP phase, univariate log-binomial regression models were used (41). This model uses the logarithm as a link function, and is a generalized lineal model for a binary outcome where the error terms follows a binomial distribution. The effect size measure of the model is the relative risk. Because of the low number of MAP-C ($n = 3$), multivariate log-binomial regression models were not fitted. The significance threshold for all univariate analyses was set at a two-sided $\alpha = 0.05$. The analyses were performed with R Core Team (42) (v3.0.2).

RESULTS

Participants Enrolled in the Study

Between February 29th and September 15th 2016, 15 out of the 22 eligible BCN01 participants were enrolled in BCN02. Seven declined to participate due to their inability to attend all the scheduled visits. Baseline characteristics of trial participants are summarized in **Table 1**. All 15 participants received two doses MVA.HIVconsv (MVA_{1-2}) and three doses of romidepsin (RMD_{1-2-3}) as shown in the study chronogram (**Figure 1A**), and were included in the safety, immunogenicity and reservoir analyses. One participant was not eligible for MAP due to immune futility pre-defined criteria and 14 participants underwent a MAP for a maximum of 32 weeks. Retrospective analyses of stored plasma samples obtained during MAP revealed the presence of antiretroviral drugs in some samples from one participant, whose MAP data were censored for the viral rebound kinetics analyses (**Figure 1B**).

Safety of MVA.HIVconsv and RMD Administrations

All participants reported adverse events (AE) related to both study investigational medicinal products. A total of 333 AE were recorded during the study intervention phase, 129 after MVA_{1-2} and 204 after RMD_{1-2-3}, which were mostly mild or moderate (grade 1-2) ($n = 318$, 95%). The most frequent AE related to MVA.HIVconsv, summarized in **Table 2**, were local pain at the injection site and a flu-like syndrome consisting of fatigue, headache, myalgia, and/or low-grade temperature (<38°C). Regarding AE related to RMD (**Table 3**), the most common grade 1–2 events were headache, fatigue, and gastro-intestinal symptoms. Despite prophylactic ondansetron treatment, 4 (27%) individuals vomited the days of RMD administration. One participant experienced a grade 4 AE consisting in a sepsis by *Shigella sonnei* that required hospital admission for 24 h, thus fulfilling the criteria of serious adverse event (SAE). The symptoms started within 4 h after RMD_3 and therefore, the SAE was considered as possibly related to RMD.

No laboratory abnormalities related to MVA_{1-2} were reported. All laboratory abnormalities related to RMD were grade 1-2 ($n = 22$), the most frequent being hypophosphatemia (8 events) and thrombocytopenia (5 events), except from one case of grade 4 creatinine kinase elevation with normal eGFR which resolved within 7 days without sequelae. Noteworthy, $CD4^+$ T-cell counts showed a transient decrease by a median of 248 cells/mm^3 3 days after each RMD administration which was not fully recovered by day 7 after RMD_3 (**Supplementary Figure 2**). Overall, both MVA.HIVconsv and RMD at the regimen and dose administered in this study were well-tolerated and safety profiles were consistent with data previously reported (20, 34).

During the MAP, 12 (86%) participants reported a total of 58 AE, which were all grade 1-2 and not suggestive of acute retroviral syndrome (not shown). Grade 1 anxiety was observed in one participant who repeatedly declined psychological support (same participant with protocol violation during the MAP).

RMD Pharmacokinetics and Pharmacodynamics

Pharmacokinetics of RMD was comparable to previously described data (43). A population pharmacokinetic model adequately describing RMD concentrations in plasma was developed (36). According to the individual profiles simulated using the model, each infusion was followed by a rapid and polyexponential decline in RMD concentrations in plasma, reaching nearly undetectable levels by 24 h after dosing (**Figure 2A**).

Regarding the direct effect of RMD on chromatin and induction of viral transcription, histone H3 acetylation (acH3)

TABLE 1 | Demographic, clinical, and treatment characteristics of study patients at study entry ($n = 15$).

Age (years)	43 (33–51)
Gender (M/F), *n*	14/1
MSM/HTS, *n*	14/1
Time since HIV-1 acquisition to ART (days)	92 (28–164)
Pre ART log_{10} HIV-1 RNA (copies/ml)	4.9 (3.2–5.8)
Time on ART (years)	3.23 (3.03–3.77)
ART regimen, *n (%)*	
TDF/FTC/RAL	11 (73)
ABC/3TC/RAL	2 (13)
ABC/3TC/DTG	2 (13)
$CD4^+$ T-cell counts (cells/mm^3)	728 (416–1,408)
Ratio CD4/CD8	1.37 (0.97–1.93)

Median (range) is shown unless otherwise described. M, male; F, female; MSM, men who have sex with men; HTS, heterosexual; ART, antiretroviral therapy; TDF, Tenofovir Disoproxil Fumarate; FTC, Emtricitabine; RAL, Raltegravir; ABC, Abacavir; 3TC, Lamivudine; DTG, Dolutegravir.

TABLE 2 | Summary of adverse events related to MVA.HIVconsv vaccinations ($n = 15$).

	Grade 1 *n*	Grade 2 *n*	Grade 3 *n*	Grade 4 *n*	Total *n (%)*
Injection site reaction					
Local pain	7	4	2	0	13 (87)
Redness	1	0	0	0	1 (7)
Induration	0	0	0	0	0 (0)
Systemic adverse events					
Fatigue	7	4	2	0	13 (87)
Headache	5	3	1	0	9 (60)
Myalgia	4	3	2	0	9 (60)
Fever	5	0	0	0	5 (33)
Anorexia	3	0	1	0	4 (27)
Sweating	2	2	0	0	4 (27)
Nausea	2	0	1	0	3 (20)
Abdominal pain	0	1	1	0	2 (13)
Flatulence	1	0	0	0	1 (7)
Somnolence	1	0	0	0	1 (7)

TABLE 3 | Summary of adverse events related to RMD_{1-2-3} treatment ($n = 15$).

	Grade 1 *n*	Grade 2 *n*	Grade 3 *n*	Grade 4 *n*	Total *n* (%)
Headache	9	5	0	0	14 (93)
Fatigue	9	5	0	0	14 (93)
Nausea	4	7	0	0	11 (73)
Anorexia	8	1	0	0	9 (60)
Abdominal pain	5	2	0	0	7 (47)
Metallic taste	5	1	0	0	6 (40)
Constipation	4	2	0	0	6 (40)
Abdominal distension	4	1	0	0	5 (33)
Vomits	4	0	0	0	4 (27)
Sweating	2	2	0	0	4 (27)
Palpitations	3	0	0	0	3 (20)
Myalgia	1	1	0	0	2 (13)
Rash	0	2	0	0	2 (13)
Dry mouth	1	0	0	0	1 (7)
ECG: ST-elevation	1	0	0	0	1 (7)
Anxiety	0	1	0	0	1 (7)
Libido decrease	0	1	0	0	1 (7)
Somnolence	1	0	0	0	1 (7)
Sepsis by *Shigella sonnei* (SAE)	0	0	0	1	1 (7)
Hypotension	0	1	0	0	1 (7)

increased rapidly during each RMD infusion, remained high during 4 h, and returned to baseline values 3 days after each dose (**Figure 2B**), which is consistent with previous reports (33, 34). HIV-1 transcription transiently increased in parallel, with changes more pronouned after RMD_2 and RMD_3 (**Figure 2C**). These changes were more evident without normalization for house-keeping genes (**Supplementary Figure 3**) possibly reflecting the general increase in histone acetylation levels (44) induced by RMD. Increases in T-cell activation, measured by the proportion of $CD3^+$/HLA-DR^+ cells, were observed 3 days after each RMD dose. Over the course of the three RMD doses, T-cell activation increased in a progressive manner and was maintained up to 1 week after RMD_3 (**Figure 2D**), suggesting a cumulative effect of RMD.

To evaluate changes in levels of quantifiable plasma HIV-1 RNA, an ultrasensitive single copy assay was used. Kinetics of plasma HIV-1 RNA levels did not follow a clear pattern (**Figure 2E**), despite the increasing percentage of participants with detectable low-level viremia at the end of each RMD dose (**Supplementary Figure 4**). Collectively, we reproduced effects on acH3, HIV-1 transcription and T cell activation previously reported in chronically infected individuals (34), suggesting that a lower viral reservoir level achieved by early-treatment initiation does not preclude the reactivation potential of RMD.

MVA.HIVconsv Immunogenicity

Total HIV-1 and HIVconsv-specific T cells were assessed *ex vivo* by an IFN-γ-detecting enzyme-linked immunoabsorbent spot (ELISPOT) assay using 6 peptide pools covering the HIVconsv immunogen sequence (P1-P6) on week 0 (day of MVA_1), 1, 3 (day of RMD_1), 9 (day of MVA_2), 10, and 13. A total of 90 samples were obtained, of which 3 (3%) were censored due to low positive controls and/or high background. All 15 participants showed an absolute increase in HIVconsv-specific IFN-γ-producing T cells during the study, either after MVA_1 (Wilcoxon signed-rank, $p = 0.0007$) or after MVA_2 (Wilcoxon signed-rank, $p = 0.0017$) (**Figure 3B**). Median (range) total frequencies of HIVconsv-specific T cells reached 1,965 (530-6,901) spot-forming cells (SFC)/10^6 PBMC at the peak immunogenicity time point, which represented an absolute median increase of 1,600 (300–6,621) SFC/10^6 PBMC from baseline (Wilcoxon signed-rank, $p < 0.0001$).

Over the intervention phase, participants responded to median (range) of 5 (2–6) peptide pools (**Supplementary Figure 5**). To map the maximum vaccine-induced breadth at peak immunogenicity time point (weeks 10–13), *in vitro* expanded T cells responding toward individual OLPs covering the HIVconsv immunogen were assessed. Median (range) of 8 (3–16) IFN-γ-producing responses to individual OLPs were found, with a dominance in Pol-specific T cells, consistent with the immunogen composition (**Figure 3C**).

The dominance of HIVconsv-specific responses was calculated at each time point as the percentage of HIVconsv-specific T-cell frequencies divided by the total HIV-1 proteome-specific T-cell frequencies. At the moment of HIV diagnoses, HIVconsv responses were subdominant (<10% being HIVconsv-specfic) and peaked after the CM vaccination reaching a median (range) of 58% (7%−100%) of the total anti-HIV-1 T-cell responses (BCN01 parental study) (20). In BCN02, 2 years from the last HIVconsv vaccination, the increase in the frequency of HIVconsv-specific T-cell responses after MVA_1 or MVA_2 further shifted the patterns of T-cell immuno-dominance toward HIVconsv with median (range) of 85% (54%–100%) of the total anti-HIV-1 T-cell responses at peak immunogenicity time point being HIVconsv specific (**Figure 3D**).

Effects on the HIV-1 Reservoir

All participants had detectable viral reservoirs, as measured by total $CD4^+$ T cell-associated HIV-1 DNA, throughout the study. Results from 2 samples out of a total of 60 were considered invalid and were censored. At BCN02 study entry, median (range) reservoir size was of 140 (17–752) HIV-1 DNA copies/10^6 $CD4^+$ T-cells (**Figure 4**). Proviral DNA showed a tendency to further decrease from baseline to week 17 (Wilcoxon signed-rank, $p = 0.0599$, **Figure 4**) to median (range) levels of 120 (11-680) copies/10^6 $CD4^+$ Tcells.

Monitored Antiretroviral Pause (MAP)

Participants undergoing MAP were monitored weekly for the first 12 weeks and every 2 weeks thereafter for a maximum of 32 weeks (MAP_{0-32}). Criteria for ART resumption included pVL over 2,000 copies/ml in two consecutive determinations, $CD4^+$ cell counts decrease over 50% and/or below 500 cells/mm^3 and/or development of clinical symptoms suggestive of an acute retroviral syndrome.

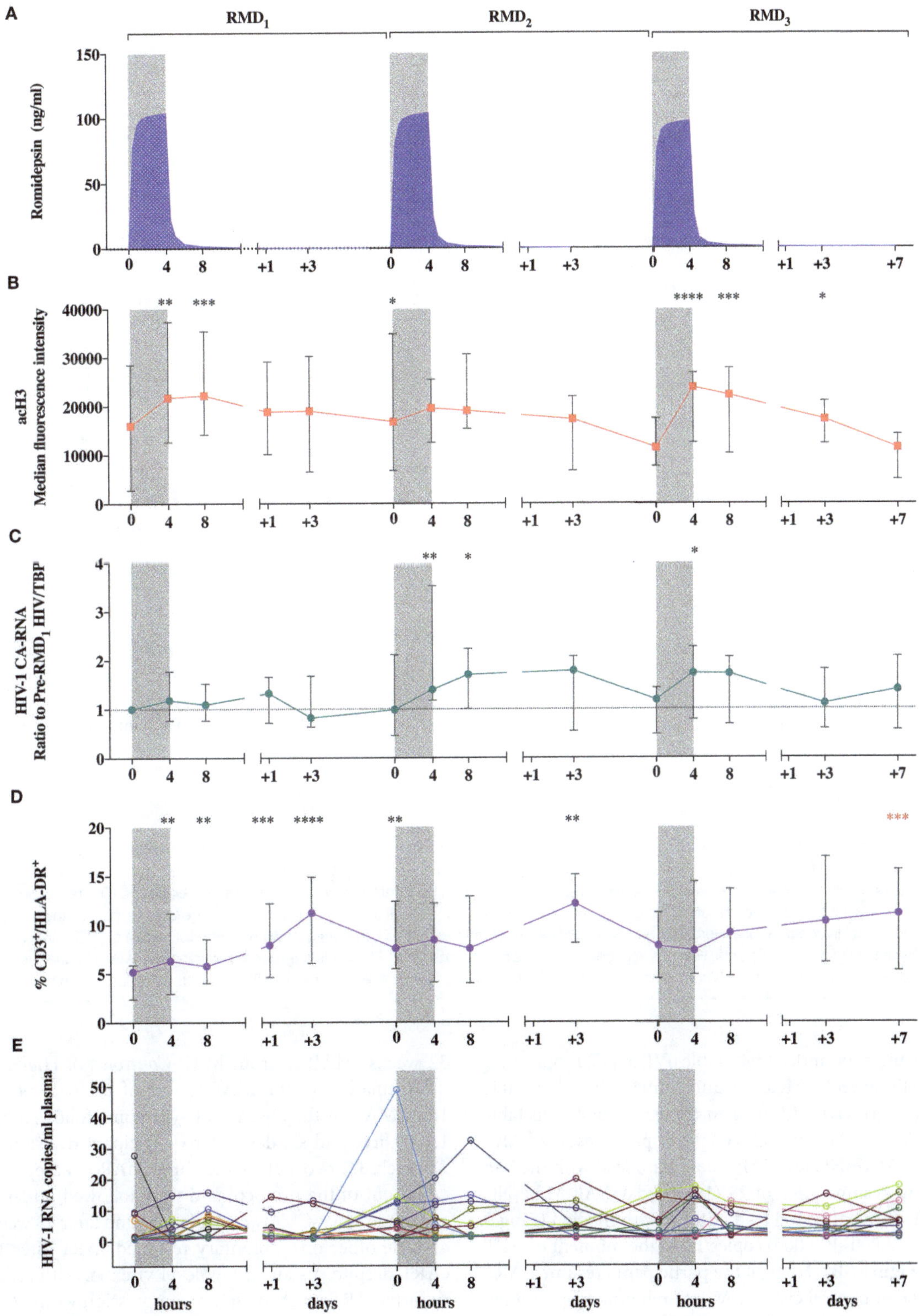

FIGURE 2 | Pharmacokinetic and pharmacodynamic effects of RMD. **(A)** Mean individual predictions of RMD plasma concentrations. **(B)** Levels of histone H3 acetylation in peripheral lymphocytes. **(C)** Viral transcription levels expressed as changes from pre-RMD_1 levels of cell-associated HIV-1 RNA in peripheral $CD4^+$ T-cells. **(D)** Levels of T-cell activation ($CD3^+/HLA\text{-}DR^+$ cells). **(E)** individual determinations of pVL. Median of frequencies and IQR (error bars) are represented. Wilcoxon signed-rank *p*-values compare each represented time point with the corresponding values preceding each RMD administration. $^*p < 0.05$. $^{**}p < 0.01$. $^{***}p < 0.001$ and $^{****}p < 0.0001$. The *p* value resulting from the comparison between the value at day 0 of RMD_1 and 7 days after RMD_3 is shown in red.

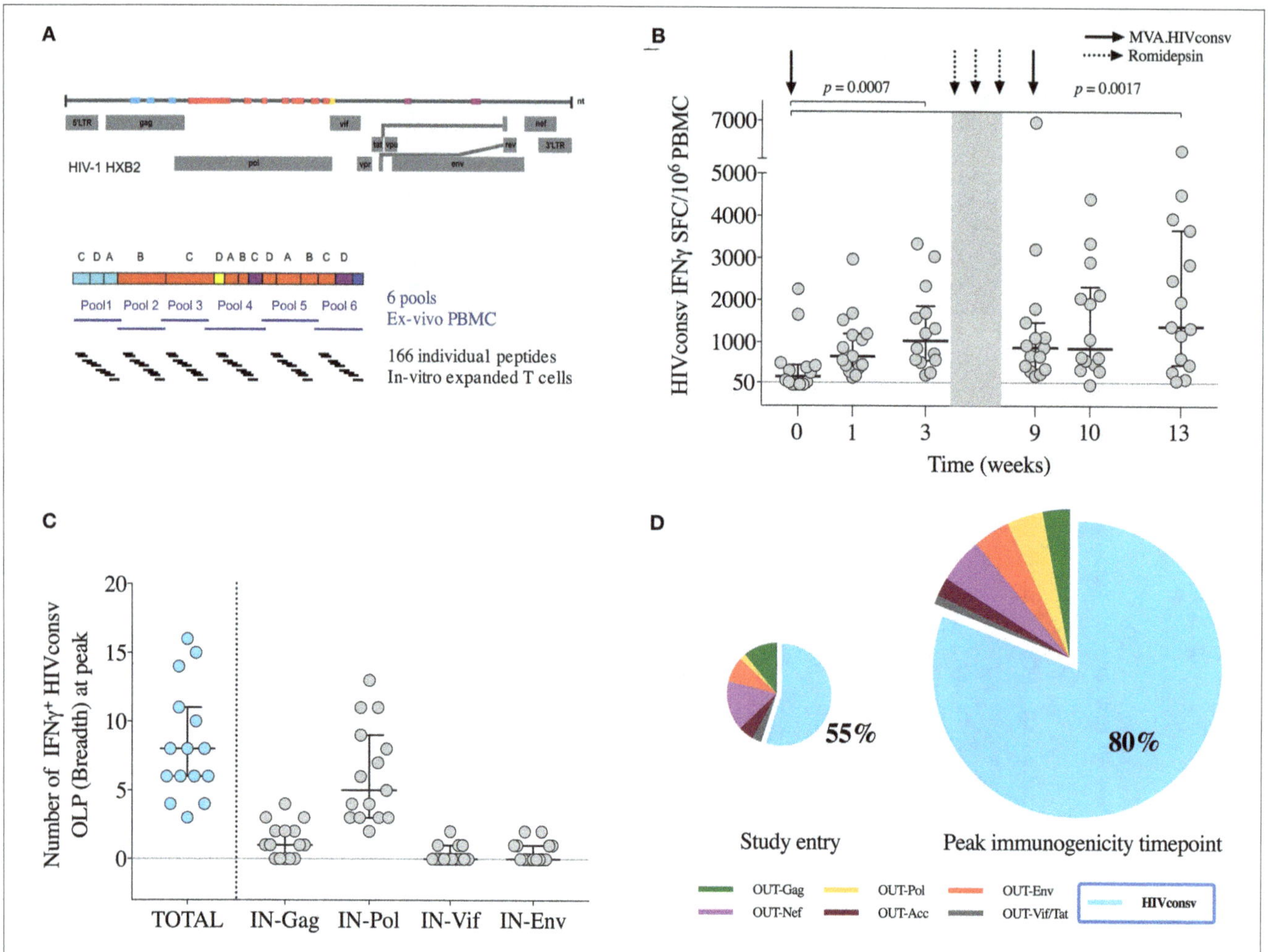

FIGURE 3 | Vaccine immunogenicity. **(A)** Schematic representation of the selected regions in the HIV-1 proteome from different clades included in the HIVconsv immunogen and distribution of 6 peptide pools (P1-P6) and individual overlapping 15-mer peptides (OLP) used in the IFN-γ ELISPOT assays. **(B)** Magnitude (sum of SFU/10^6 PBMC to pools P1-P6) of vaccine-induced responses over the BCN02 study. Horizontal and error bars represent median and IQR, respectively, and p-values correspond to comparisons between the indicated time points using the Wilcoxon signed-rank test. **(C)** Breadth of vaccine-elicited responses toward individual OLP included in the indicated HIVconsv regions. Horizontal and error bars represent median and IQR, respectively. **(D)** Average distribution of total HIV-1 T-cells according to their specificity at the indicated time points. HIVconsv-specific responses are shown in blue. Pie charts are scaled according to the total frequencies of responses. IN are peptide pools corresponding to the HIVconsv vaccine insert and OUT peptide pools spanning the rest of HIV-1 proteome "outside the immunogen".

All participants rebounded (detectable pVL over 20 copies/ml) during MAP (**Figure 5A**). Median (range) time to first detectable pVL was 13 (7–35) days with median (range) of first detectable pVL of 122 (28–3,410) copies/ml. Ten participants resumed ART before MAP_{12} (MAP-NC for MAP-*Non-controllers*) with median (range) time to resume ART of 28 (16–59) days. All MAP-NC resumed ART due to the viral load criteria, with median (range) pVL of 19,250 (2,900–179,000) copies/ml at the moment of ART resumption (**Figure 5B**). None of the participants resumed ART due to immune or clinical criteria. A "late-rebounder" presented the first detectable pVL 5 weeks after ART interruption (MAP_5, pVL of 59 copies/ml) and was able to maintain viral load below 2,000 for 3 more weeks, resuming ART at MAP_8. In addition to the "late-rebounder," 3 (23%) other participants remained off ART with sustained pVL <2,000 copies/ml for a total of 32 weeks (MAP-C, from MAP-*Controllers*). Highest peak pVL determination in the MAP-C was of 3,110 copies/ml at week 12 of MAP in the absence of symptoms followed by 2,460 and 1,100 three and six days later (participant decision to stay off). At week 32, two out of the three MAP-C accepted to stay off cART out of the protocol and were followed under standard of care. One MAP-C showed a late rebound after 48 weeks off cART and the other one, voluntary resumed cART after 1.5 years off cART despite sustained low-level viremia. All participants who restarted ART reached viral re-suppression within 6 months. No evidence of emergence of drug resistance was detected.

To assess re-seeding of the viral reservoir during the MAP, total HIV-1 DNA was measured at MAP_0 ($n = 13$), on the day of ART resumption ($n = 10$), and 6 months after for the 10 MAP-NC ($n = 8$ available), and at MAP_{32} for the three MAP-C. We did

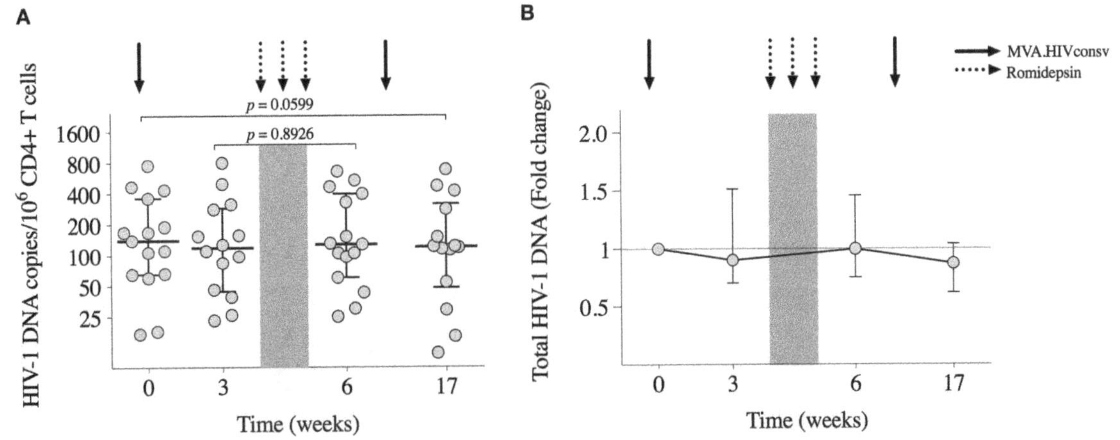

FIGURE 4 | Viral reservoir. **(A)** Total HIV-1 DNA copies/10^6 $CD4^+$ T cells for each participant are shown at study entry (week 0), week 3 (day of RMD_1), and week 6 (1 week after RMD_3) and at week 17 (8 weeks after MVA_2). Horizontal and error bars represent median and IQR, respectively, and *p*-values correspond to comparisons between the indicated time points using the Wilcoxon signed-rank test. **(B)** Changes in proviral DNA throughout the study with respect to baseline (week 0), which is considered to be 1.

not observe any significant change in total HIV-1 DNA during MAP in participants with early ART resumption (Wilcoxon signed-rank, $p = 0.5759$ for MAP-NC) and, noteworthy, nor in the three participants with sustained low level viremia for 32 weeks. Moreover, one of the three MAP-C showed a 2-fold reduction in the HIV-1 DNA (from 34 at MAP_0 to 16 copies/10^6 $CD4^+$ cells at MAP_{32}, **Figure 5C**). This was the only participant undergoing MAP carrying HLA alleles associated with natural HIV control (HLA-B*27:01/HLA-B*51:01) (45, 46).

Factors Influencing Viral Rebound Kinetics

Supplementary Table 1 shows the summary of variables explored to explain the binary outcome defined as MAP-NC vs. MAP-C. The estimated relative risks obtained from the log-binomial models for different covariates analyzed are shown in **Figure 5D**.

Univariate log-binomial regression models used to detect factors associated with virologic control during MAP revealed that pVL before ART initiation (pre-ART pVL) was the only factor statistically significantly associated with control of viral rebound after ART interruption. For each log increase on the pre-ART pVL, the probability of becoming a MAP-C decreased by 66% (RR 0.34; 95% CI 0.14, 0.79). Interestingly, albeit not statistically significant in the univariate models, the 3 MAP-C had among the lowest reservoir levels at treatment interruption time point (16, 54 and 122 copies/10^6 $CD4^+$ T cells) –consistent with lower pre-ART pVL– and showed the highest shift in CTL immunodominance pattern after vaccination (>700 HIVconsv-specific SFC/10^6 PBMCs and >75% of HIVconsv dominance at peak immunogenicity time point, **Supplementary Figure 6**).

DISCUSSION

In this single-arm, open-label, phase I, proof-of-concept trial performed in HIV-1-infected ART-suppressed individuals treated during acute/recent HIV-1 infection, we show that combination of the HIVconsv vaccines with RMD as a latency reversing agent was safe, highly immunogenic, and induced bursts of viral transcription. The combined intervention resulted in a tendency toward a reduction in proviral DNA levels and was followed by a prolonged viremic control in 23% of participants after ART interruption without evidence of reservoir re-seeding.

Early-treated individuals typically show less immune exhaustion (47) and reduced frequency of immune-escaped viral variants compared to individuals initiating ART at later stages of HIV-1 infection (48), offering a potentially favorable setting to induce a protective immune response upon therapeutic vaccinations. In the parental BCN01 trial, a prime/boost vaccine regimen with ChAdV63.HIVconsv and MVA.HIVconsv induced high frequencies of T cells with high *in vitro* suppressive capacity that markedly shifted the focus of the $CD8^+$ CTL response toward HIVconsv sequences that are subdominant during natural infection (20). In the BCN02 trial, after 3 years of viral suppression and 2 years since the last vaccination in BCN01, booster MVA.HIVconsv vaccinations were still immunogenic and further increased breadth, magnitude and immunodominance of CTL responses toward HIVconsv sequences.

Along with a strong vaccine-elicited CTL activity ("kill"), the ability to simultaneously induce reactivation of the viral reservoir ("kick") is a critical feature for the success of the kick&kill strategy (24). A 3-dose regimen of weekly RMD at 5 mg/m^2 BSA was selected based on results from previous trials (33, 34). Consistently, we observed a direct *in vivo* effect of RMD in histone 3 acetylation upon each RMD dose, which was followed by changes in cell-associated HIV-1 RNA levels. Conversely, a placebo-controlled dose-escalating trial (ACTG 5315) testing 3 RMD doses (5 mg/m^2 BSA) administered every two weeks in chronically suppressed individuals, did not show changes in viral transcription (49). The weekly administration regimen and the

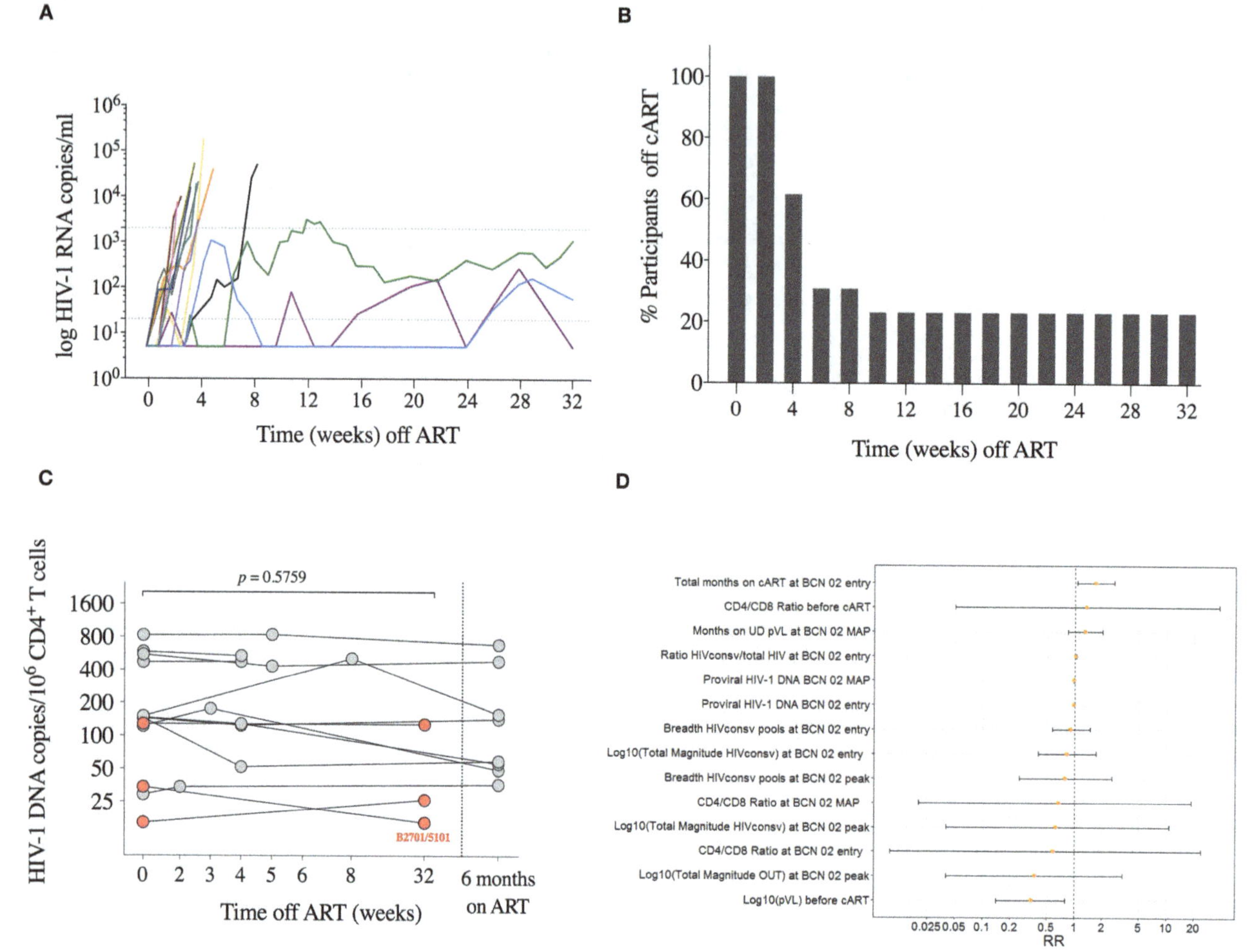

FIGURE 5 | Monitored antiretroviral pause. **(A)** Individual pVL during MAP is shown for each participant in different colors ($n = 13$). Lines are interrupted on day of ART resumption. Dotted lines represent detection limit and threshold for ART resumption (20 and 2,000 copies/ml, respectively). **(B)** Proportion of individuals remaining off ART during MAP. **(C)** Total HIV-1 DNA copies/10^6 $CD4^+$ T cells are shown for each participant at MAP initiation, at day of ART ressumption, and 24 weeks after ART. *P*-value corresponds to comparison between MAP initiation and the day of ART resumption for each individual using the Wilcoxon signed-rank test. Individuals with sustained low-level viremia over 32 weeks are shown in red. **(D)** Estimated relative risks and 95% confidence intervals for the durable control of pVL during MAP obtained from univariate log-binomial regression models.

intensive sampling after each RMD dose in our study allowed us to detect increases in CA HIV-1 RNA above 2-fold in 80% of individuals at any time point after RMD administrations. These changes were followed by consistent increases in T cell activation markers, which remarkably, were maintained one week after RMD3, likely reflecting a direct and cumulative effect of weekly RMD dosing and an effective induction of viral transcription. Noteworthy, changes above 2.1-fold in CA-RNA have been estimated to occur in <5% of repeated measurements in an individual (50).

Despite the induction of viral transcription, the kinetics of plasma HIV-1 RNA followed an unclear pattern, similar to previous studies showing variable changes in plasma viremia following LRA administration (34, 51, 52). This variability might reflect suboptimal potency of the agents tested so far and/or the reactivation of predominantly defective proviruses. In the context of the current study, elimination of reactivated cells by vaccine-elicited T cells may have additionally blunted quantification of plasma viremia.

A critical objective of the use of LRA in a kick&kill strategy is to mobilize and ultimately reduce the viral reservoir. Our findings showed that, despite robust immunogenicity of HIVconsv vaccines and at least partial reactivation of the viral reservoir induced by RMD, the net effect on the proviral DNA levels was modest. All participants had detectable levels of HIV-1 DNA at the time of treatment interruption although a tendency toward a decrease by 19.3% from baseline to week 17 (Wilcoxon signed-rank, $p = 0.0599$) was detected. Conversely, a mean 39.7% decrease in reservoir size was observed in the REDUC trial (34). This discrepancy between REDUC and BCN02 results may be explained by the inclusion of early-treated individuals in our study, in which already baseline levels of proviral DNA were substantially lower, challenging the quantification of the effects of the intervention on HIV-1 DNA levels. We acknowledge that the translation of HIV-1 protein expression into antigen presentation—even in case of defective proviruses (1)—upon LRA reactivation is poorly understood. Likewise, the ability of LRA-induced HIV-1 protein expression to effectively induce recognition and killing by $CD8^+$ T cells remains to be fully elucidated (53) and therefore, the potential effects of further RMD administrations on the viral reservoir are to be determined. A potential significant toxicity—suggested in *in vitro* assays (54)—on vaccine-induced T cells might also have limited our capability to observe a further reduction in the reservoir size in our study. This hypothesis is consistent with the fact that HIVconsv vaccines induced higher levels of activated T cells compared to Vacc-4x vaccination in the REDUC trial. Nevertheless, the potential toxicity of RMD *in vivo*, its relationship with RMD exposure and, ultimately, whether vaccine-induced T cells were able to sensor and remove infected cells in response to HIV-1 reactivation remains to be determined.

To attain a functional cure, a persistent immune-mediated control of residual HIV-1 might be as relevant as achieving an absolute reduction on the proviral DNA levels. In this regard, the three BCN02 MAP-C, were among the subjects with both lower viral reservoir levels at MAP and higher vaccine-induced responses. In our study, having lower pre-ART pVL was the only outstanding marker associated with viral control during MAP, which correlates with the size of the viral reservoir after ART suppression. These relationships are consistent with previous studies suggesting a role of a low viral reservoir on analytical treatment interruptions (ATI) outcomes (55, 56). Furthermore, after ART discontinuation, MAP-C did not show an initial burst in pVL followed by a fast post-peak control as described in several post treatment controllers (PTC) (8, 57). Collectively, the findings from this and other studies suggest that a small reservoir size, resulting from early ART or another intervention, may be essential to achieve sustained post-intervention control (55) but also, that a potent vaccine-induced immune pressure might contribute to prevent a peak burst of viremia and maintain suppressed viremia for a substantial period of time. This control, mediated by immune pressure, is supported by the absence of re-seeding of the viral reservoir in the BCN02 MAP-C, in contrast to reports from previous ATI trials (58, 59).

The interpretation of the outcome of kick&kill studies may be confounded by individuals controlling HIV rebound after treatment interruption without the need for a prior therapeutic intervention. The prevalence and mechanisms driving such PTC in natural HIV infection are not well-understood. A recent metanalysis (CHAMP study) including 14 interruption trials estimated a 13% rate of PTC among early-treated individuals (57). Importantly, and in contrast to the three BCN02 MAP-C who did not show a transient high burst of viremia, 32% of the 61 PTCs analyzed in the CHAMP metanalysis had peaks of viremia ranging from 1,000 to over 10,000 copies/ml within the first 24 weeks after treatment interruption. Thus, in addition to the different behavior of the 3 MAP-C (23%) with respect to the PTC, according to this metanalysis, the BCN02 trial may have missed additional MAP-C due to the conservative ART resumption criteria used (two consecutive pVL over 2,000 copies/ml).

The safety and tolerability profiles of MVA.HIVconsv and RMD were similar to those reported in previous studies (19, 20, 34). However, there was a SAE in one participant. This case highlights the need for planning intensive monitoring in this kind of pilot trials, even if not powered to detect low-frequency AE, and points toward the need for a trade-off between the number of participants potentially put at risk in well-powered controlled trials and for caution with the use of uncompletely characterized agents in large numbers of individuals. Given that natural PTC rates are considered to be up to 13% in early-treated individuals, powering trials to show viral control efficacy after an ATI becomes challenging (60). Despite frequent clinical monitoring for pVL and access to psychological support, protocol violation during MAP occurred in one individual, probably due to anxiety secondary to the antiretroviral interruption. This case warrants close psychological management in longer term ATIs.

We fully acknowledge the limitations of the small sample size and lack of a control arm in the present study. Therefore, we interpret these results with caution and regard this study only as hypothesis-generating trial for future interventions. BCN02 eligibility was restricted to vaccinated participants in the parental open-label BCN01 trial. This intrinsic restriction limited the sample size to a small number of previously vaccinated individuals and precluded the inclusion of a control arm. At the time of trial design, interventional trials including an ATI were typically small and included very conservative ART resumption criteria (58, 61). Furthermore, ATI acceptability by participants, risks of HIV-1 transmission to others in the absence of available PrEP, and potential viral re-seeding upon treatment interruption were of special concern in early-treated individuals, who had limited viral reservoirs both in size and diversity (48).

Altogether, the results from this pilot study suggest a potential role for kick&kill strategies in inducing durable immune-mediated HIV-1 control in a proportion of early-treated individuals. In view of these results, future controlled studies to identify the mechanisms underlying sustained HIV-1 suppression are warranted.

ETHICS STATEMENT

The studies involving human participants were reviewed and approved by Hospital Germans Trias i Pujol and Hospital Clínic (AC-15-108-R). The patients/participants provided their written informed consent to participate in this study.

AUTHOR CONTRIBUTIONS

BM, JM, BC, and CB conceived and designed the study. CMa, TH, JMM, JM-P, AB, PC, MM, and MV contributed to the study design. CMi, CMa, IR, JT, ACa, MR-U, and MP contributed contributed to data management. BM, MR-U, MP, ML, SM-L, AL,

JM, PC, ACa, CMi, SC, AB, and CMa performed the experiments. JM, BM, MP, MV, YA-S, GM, and KL undertook the statistical analysis. ACr and TH contributed with reagents, materials, analysis tools. BM, JM, and CB drafted the manuscript. TH, MR-U, CMa, MP, SM-L, JM-P, JMM, MV, and BC participated in study analyses and revised the manuscript critically for important intellectual content. All authors reviewed and approved the final version of the manuscript.

INVESTIGATORS MEMBERS OF THE BCN02

IrsiCaixa AIDS Research Institute-HIVACAT, Hospital Universitari Germans Trias i Pujol, Badalona, Spain: Susana Benet, Christian Brander, Samandhy Cedeño, Bonaventura Clotet, Pep Coll, Anuska Llano, Javier Martinez-Picado, Marta Marszalek, Sara Morón-López, Beatriz Mothe, Roger Paredes, Maria C. Puertas, Miriam Rosás-Umbert, Marta Ruiz-Riol. Fundació Lluita contra la Sida, Infectious Diseases Department, Hospital Universitari Germans Trias i Pujol, Badalona, Spain: Roser Escrig, Silvia Gel, Miriam López, Cristina Miranda, José Moltó, Jose Muñoz, Nuria Perez-Alvarez, Jordi Puig, Boris Revollo, Jessica Toro. Germans Trias i Pujol Research Institute, Badalona, Spain: Ana María Barriocanal, Cristina Perez-Reche. Clinical Pharmacology Unit, Hospital Universitari Germans Trias i Pujol, Badalona, Spain: Magí Farré. Pharmacokinetic/pharmacodynamic modeling and simultation, Institut de Recerca de l'Hospital de la Santa Creu i Sant Pau-IIB Sant Pau, Barcelona, Spain: Marta Valle. Hospital Clinic-HIVACAT, IDIBAPS, University of Barcelona, Barcelona, Spain: Christian Manzardo, Juan Ambrosioni, Irene Ruiz, Cristina Rovira, Carmen Ligero, Emma Fernández, and Jose M. Miró. Projecte dels NOMS-Hispanosida, BCN Checkpoint, Barcelona, Spain: Antonio Carrillo, Michael Meulbroek, Ferran Pujol and Jorge Saz. The Jenner Institute, The Nuffield Department of Medicine, University of Oxford, UK: Nicola Borthwick, Alison Crook, Edmund G. Wee and Tomáš Hanke.

FUNDING

BCN02 study was an investigator-initiated study funded by the ISCIII PI15/01188 grant, the HIVACAT Catalan research program for an HIV vaccine and the Fundació Gloria Soler. Some sub-analyses were partly funded by the European Union's Horizon 2020 research and innovation program under grant agreement 681137-EAVI2020 and by NIH grant P01-AI131568. The GMP manufacture of the MVA.HIVconsv vaccines was jointly funded by the Medical Research Council (MRC) UK and the UK Department for International Development (DFID) under the MRC/DFID Concordat agreements (G0701669) and kindly provided through an IIS agreement. Romidepsin was kindly provided by Celgene Ltd through an IIS agreement. BM held a post-doctoral fellowship grant from ISCIII (JR 13/00024) from 2014–16. CMa held a post-doctoral research grant (PERIS-2016/2020) from the Departament de Salut de la Generalitat de Catalunya, Barcelona, Spain during the conduct of the study. SM-L held a Ph.D. grant from DGR (2013FI_B 00275) from 2013–16. JM received a 80:20 research grant from IDIBAPS, Barcelona, Spain, during 2017–21. GM, KL, and YS have been partially supported by Grant MTM2015-64465-C2-1-R from Ministerio de Economía y Competitividad.

ACKNOWLEDGMENTS

We would like to thank i2e3 for providing medical writing support. We especially thank Agueda Fernandez, Rafaela Ayen, Lucía Gómez and Carmen Ligero for their technical assistance. Special thanks to all the volunteers participating in this study for their perseverance and dedication.

REFERENCES

1. Bruner KM, Murray AJ, Pollack RA, Soliman MG, Laskey SB, Capoferri AA, et al. Defective proviruses rapidly accumulate during acute HIV-1 infection. *Nat Med.* (2016) 22:1043–9. doi: 10.1038/nm.4156
2. Davey RT Jr, Bhat N, Yoder C, Chun TW, Metcalf JA, Dewar RN, et al. HIV-1 and T cell dynamics after interruption of highly active antiretroviral therapy (HAART) in patients with a history of sustained viral suppression. *Proc Natl Acad Sci USA.* (1999) 96:15109–14. doi: 10.1073/pnas.96.26.15109
3. Mothe B, Brander C. HIV T-cell vaccines. In: editors. *Advances in Experimental Medicine and Biology, Vol. 1075.* Springer: New York LLC (2018). p. 31–51. doi: 10.1007/978-981-13-0484-2_2
4. Autran B, Murphy RL, Costagliola D, Tubiana R, Clotet B, Gatell J, et al. Greater viral rebound and reduced time to resume antiretroviral therapy after therapeutic immunization with the ALVAC-HIV vaccine (vCP1452). *AIDS.* (2008) 22:1313–22. doi: 10.1097/QAD.0b013e3282fdce94
5. Schooley RT, Spritzler J, Wang H, Lederman MM, Havlir D, Kuritzkes DR, et al. AIDS clinical trials group 5197: a placebo-controlled trial of immunization of HIV-1–infected persons with a replication-deficient adenovirus type 5 vaccine expressing the HIV-1 core protein. *J Infect Dis.* (2010) 202:705–16. doi: 10.1086/655468
6. Harrer T, Plettenberg A, Arastéh K, Van Lunzen J, Fätkenheuer G, Jaeger H, et al. Safety and immunogenicity of an adjuvanted protein therapeutic HIV-1 vaccine in subjects with HIV-1 infection: a randomised placebo-controlled study. *Vaccine.* (2014) 32:2657–65. doi: 10.1016/j.vaccine.2013.10.030
7. Evans TG, Keefer MC, Weinhold KJ, Wolff M, Montefiori D, Gorse GJ, et al. A canarypox vaccine expressing multiple human immunodeficiency virus type 1 genes given alone or with Rgp120 elicits broad and durable $CD8^+$ cytotoxic T lymphocyte responses in seronegative volunteers. *J Infect Dis.* (1999) 180:290–8. doi: 10.1086/314895
8. Sneller MC, Justement JS, Gittens KR, Petrone ME, Clarridge KE, Proschan MA, et al. A randomized controlled safety/efficacy trial of therapeutic vaccination in HIV-infected individuals who initiated antiretroviral therapy early in infection. *Sci Transl Med.* (2017) 9:eaan8848. doi: 10.1126/scitranslmed.aan8848
9. Fischer W, Perkins S, Theiler J, Bhattacharya T, Yusim K, Funkhouser R, et al. Polyvalent vaccines for optimal coverage of potential T-cell epitopes in global HIV-1 variants. *Nat Med.* (2007) 13:100–6. doi: 10.1038/nm1461

10. Theiler J, Yoon H, Yusim K, Picker LJ, Fruh K, Korber B. Epigraph: a vaccine design tool applied to an HIV therapeutic vaccine and a pan-filovirus vaccine. *Sci Rep.* (2016) 6:33987. doi: 10.1038/srep33987
11. Mothe B, Hu X, Llano A, Rosati M, Olvera A, Kulkarni V, et al. A human immune data-informed vaccine concept elicits strong and broad T-cell specificities associated with HIV-1 control in mice and macaques. *J Transl Med.* (2015) 13:60. doi: 10.1186/s12967-015-0392-5
12. Létourneau S, Im EJ, Mashishi T, Brereton C, Bridgeman A, Yang H, et al. Design and pre-clinical evaluation of a universal HIV-1 vaccine. *PLoS ONE.* (2007) 2:e984. doi: 10.1371/journal.pone.0000984
13. Rolland M, Nickle DC, Mullins JI. HIV-1 group M conserved elements vaccine. *PLoS Pathog.* (2007) 3:e157. doi: 10.1371/journal.ppat.0030157
14. Ondondo B, Murakoshi H, Clutton G, Abdul-Jawad S, Wee EG, Gatanaga H, et al. Novel conserved-region T-cell mosaic vaccine with high global HIV-1 coverage is recognized by protective responses in untreated infection. *Mol Ther.* (2016) 24:832–42. doi: 10.1038/mt.2016.3
15. Gaiha GD, Rossin EJ, Urbach J, Landeros C, Collins DR, Nwonu C, et al. Structural topology defines protective CD8 $^+$ T cell epitopes in the HIV proteome. *Science.* (2019) 364:480–4. doi: 10.1126/science.aav5095
16. Borthwick N, Ahmed T, Ondondo B, Hayes P, Rose A, Ebrahimsa U, et al. Vaccine-elicited human T cells recognizing conserved protein regions inhibit HIV-1. *Mol Ther.* (2014) 22:464–75. doi: 10.1038/mt.2013.248
17. Hayton EJ, Rose A, Ibrahimsa U, Del Sorbo M, Capone S, Crook A, et al. Safety and tolerability of conserved region vaccines vectored by plasmid DNA, simian adenovirus and modified vaccinia virus ankara administered to human immunodeficiency virus type 1-uninfected adults in a randomized, single-blind phase I trial. *PLoS ONE.* (2014) 9:e101591. doi: 10.1371/journal.pone.0101591
18. Mutua G, Farah B, Langat R, Indangasi J, Ogola S, Onsembe B, et al. Broad HIV-1 inhibition in vitro by vaccine-elicited CD8$^+$ T cells in African adults. *Mol Ther Methods Clin Dev.* (2016) 3:16061. doi: 10.1038/mtm.2016.61
19. Hancock G, Morón-López S, Kopycinski J, Puertas MC, Giannoulatou E, Rose A, et al. Evaluation of the immunogenicity and impact on the latent HIV-1 reservoir of a conserved region vaccine, MVA.HIVconsv, in antiretroviral therapy-treated subjects. *J Int AIDS Soc.* (2017) 20:1–11. doi: 10.7448/IAS.20.1.21171
20. Mothe B, Manzardo C, Sanchez-Bernabeu A, Coll P, Morón-López S, Puertas MC, et al. Therapeutic vaccination refocuses T-cell responses towards conserved regions of HIV-1 in early treated individuals (BCN 01 study). *Clin Med.* (2019) 11:65–80. doi: 10.1016/j.eclinm.2019.05.009
21. Hartnell F, Brown A, Capone S, Kopycinski J, Bliss C, Makvandi-Nejad S, et al. A novel vaccine strategy employing serologically different chimpanzee adenoviral vectors for the prevention of HIV-1 and HCV coinfection. *Front Immunol.* (2018) 9:3175. doi: 10.3389/fimmu.2018.03175
22. Borthwick NJ, Lane T, Moyo N, Crook A, Shim JM, Baines I, et al. Randomized phase I trial HIV-CORE 003: depletion of serum amyloid P component and immunogenicity of DNA vaccination against HIV-1. Borrow R, ed. *PLoS ONE.* (2018) 13:e0197299. doi: 10.1371/journal.pone.0197299
23. Fidler S, Stöhr W, Pace M, Dorrell L, Lever A, Pett S, et al. Antiretroviral therapy alone versus antiretroviral therapy with a kick and kill approach, on measures of the HIV reservoir in participants with recent HIV infection (the RIVER trial): a phase 2, randomised trial. *The Lancet.* (2020) 395:888–98. doi: 10.1016/S0140-6736(19)32990-3
24. Shan L, Deng K, Shroff NS, Durand CM, Rabi SA, Yang HC, et al. Stimulation of HIV-1-specific cytolytic T lymphocytes facilitates elimination of latent viral reservoir after virus reactivation. *Immunity.* (2012) 36:491–501. doi: 10.1016/j.immuni.2012.01.014
25. Sengupta S, Siliciano RF. Targeting the latent reservoir for HIV-1. *Immunity.* (2018) 48:872–95. doi: 10.1016/j.immuni.2018.04.030
26. Pankrac J, Klein K, Mann JFS. Eradication of HIV-1 latent reservoirs through therapeutic vaccination. *AIDS Res Ther.* (2017) 14:45. doi: 10.1186/s12981-017-0177-4
27. Rasmussen TA, Schmeltz Søgaard O, Brinkmann C, Wightman F, Lewin SR, Melchjorsen J, et al. Comparison of HDAC inhibitors in clinical development: effect on HIV production in latently infected cells and T-cell activation. *Hum Vaccin Immunother.* (2013) 9:993–1001. doi: 10.4161/hv.23800
28. Bullen CK, Laird GM, Durand CM, Siliciano JD, Siliciano RF. New ex vivo approaches distinguish effective and ineffective single agents for reversing HIV-1 latency in vivo. *Nat Med.* (2014) 20:425–9. doi: 10.1038/nm.3489
29. Shan L, Xing S, Yang H-C, Zhang H, Margolick JB, Siliciano RF. Unique characteristics of histone deacetylase inhibitors in reactivation of latent HIV-1 in Bcl-2-transduced primary resting CD4$^+$ T cells. *J Antimicrob Chemother.* (2014) 69:28–33. doi: 10.1093/jac/dkt338
30. Archin NM, Liberty AL, Kashuba AD, Choudhary SK, Kuruc JD, Crooks AM, et al. Administration of vorinostat disrupts HIV-1 latency in patients on antiretroviral therapy. *Nature.* (2012) 487:482–5. doi: 10.1038/nature11286
31. Lehrman G, Hogue IB, Palmer S, Jennings C, Spina CA, Wiegand A, et al. Depletion of latent HIV-1 infection *in vivo*: a proof-of-concept study. *Lancet.* (2005) 366:549–55. doi: 10.1016/S0140-6736(05)67098-5
32. Wei DG, Chiang V, Fyne E, Balakrishnan M, Barnes T, Graupe M, et al. Histone deacetylase inhibitor romidepsin induces HIV expression in CD4 T cells from patients on suppressive antiretroviral therapy at concentrations achieved by clinical dosing. *PLoS Pathog.* (2014) 10:e1004071. doi: 10.1371/journal.ppat.1004071
33. Søgaard OS, Graversen ME, Leth S, Olesen R, Brinkmann CR, Nissen SK, et al. The depsipeptide romidepsin reverses HIV-1 latency *in vivo*. Siliciano RF, ed. *PLoS Pathog.* (2015) 11:e1005142. doi: 10.1371/journal.ppat.1005142
34. Leth S, Schleimann MH, Nissen SK, Højen JF, Olesen R, Graversen ME, et al. Combined effect of Vacc-4x, recombinant human granulocyte macrophage colony-stimulating factor vaccination, and romidepsin on the HIV-1 reservoir (REDUC): a single-arm, phase 1B/2A trial. *Lancet HIV.* (2016) 3:e463–72. doi: 10.1016/S2352-3018(16)30055-8
35. Moron-Lopez S, Kim P, Søgaard OS, Tolstrup M, Wong JK, Yukl SA. Characterization of the HIV-1 transcription profile after romidepsin administration in ART-suppressed individuals. *AIDS.* (2019) 33:425–31. doi: 10.1097/QAD.0000000000002083
36. Moltó J, Perez C, Valle M, Mothe B, Miranda C, Farré M, et al. Population pharmacokinetics of romidepsin as a latency reactivating agent in HIV-infected adults. In: *18th International Workshop on Clinical Pharmacologyof Antiviral Therapy.* Chicago: IL (2017).
37. Morón-López S, Puertas MC, Gálvez C, Navarro J, Carrasco A, Esteve M, et al. Sensitive quantification of the HIV-1 reservoir in gut-associated lymphoid tissue. Roques P, ed. *PLoS ONE.* (2017) 12:e0175899. doi: 10.1371/journal.pone.0175899
38. Gupta RK, Abdul-Jawad S, McCoy LE, Mok HP, Peppa D, Salgado M, et al. HIV-1 remission following CCR5Δ32/Δ32 haematopoietic stem-cell transplantation. *Nature.* (2019) 568:244–8. doi: 10.1038/s41586-019-1027-4
39. Kawana-Tachikawa A, Llibre JM, Bravo I, Escrig R, Mothe B, Puig J, P et al. Effect of maraviroc intensification on HIV-1-specific T cell immunity in recently HIV-1-infected individuals. *PLoS ONE.* (2014) 9:e87334. doi: 10.1371/journal.pone.0087334
40. Sáez-Cirión A, Bacchus C, Hocqueloux L, Avettand-Fenoel V, Girault I, Lecuroux C, et al. Post-treatment HIV-1 controllers with a long-term virological remission after the interruption of early initiated antiretroviral therapy ANRS VISCONTI study. *PLoS Pathog.* (2013) 9:e1003211. doi: 10.1371/journal.ppat.1003211
41. Wacholder S. Binomial regression in GLIM: estimating risk ratios and risk differences. *Am J Epidemiol.* (1986) 123:174–84. doi: 10.1093/oxfordjournals.aje.a114212
42. R Core Team. *R: A Language and Environment for Statistical Computing.* (2017). Available online at: https://www.r-project.org/ (accessed February 1, 2017).
43. Woo S, Gardner ER, Chen X, Ockers SB, Baum CE, Sissung TM, et al. Population pharmacokinetics of romidepsin in patients with cutaneous T-cell lymphoma and relapsed peripheral T-cell lymphoma. *Clin Cancer Res.* (2009) 15:1496–503. doi: 10.1158/1078-0432.CCR-08-1215
44. Mogal A, Abdulkadir SA. Effects of histone deacetylase inhibitor (HDACi) trichostatin-A (TSA) on the expression of housekeeping genes. *Mol Cell Probes.* (2006) 20:81–6. doi: 10.1016/j.mcp.2005.09.008
45. Gao X, Bashirova A, Iversen AK, Phair J, Goedert JJ, Buchbinder S, et al. AIDS restriction HLA allotypes target distinct intervals of HIV-1 pathogenesis. *Nat Med.* (2005) 11:1290–92. doi: 10.1038/nm1333
46. Carrington M, O'Brien SJ. The influence of HLA genotype on AIDS. *Annu Rev Med.* (2003) 54:535–51. doi: 10.1146/annurev.med.54.101601.152346

47. Robb ML, Ananworanich J. Lessons from acute HIV infection. *Curr Opin HIV AIDS.* (2016) 11:555–60. doi: 10.1097/COH.0000000000000316
48. Deng K, Pertea M, Rongvaux A, Wang L, Durand CM, Ghiaur G, et al. Broad CTL response is required to clear latent HIV-1 due to dominance of escape mutations. *Nature.* (2015) 517:381–5. doi: 10.1038/nature14053
49. McMahon D, Zheng L, Cyktor JC, Aga E, Macatangay BJ, Godfrey C, et al. Multidose IV romidepsin: no increased HIV-1 expression in persons on ART, ACTG A5315. *Conference Retrovirus and Opportunistic Infections, March 4–7 2019, Seattle (#26).* Seattle: Washington (2019).
50. Leth S, Nymann R, Jørgensen S, Olesen R, Rasmussen TA, Østergaard L, et al. HIV-1 transcriptional activity during frequent longitudinal sampling in aviremic patients on antiretroviral therapy. *AIDS.* (2016) 30:713–21. doi: 10.1097/QAD.0000000000000974
51. Elliott JH, McMahon JH, Chang CC, Lee SA, Hartogensis W, Bumpus N, et al. Short-term administration of disulfiram for reversal of latent HIV infection: a phase 2 dose-escalation study. *Lancet HIV.* (2015) 2:e520–29. doi: 10.1016/S2352-3018(15)00226-X
52. Rasmussen TA, Tolstrup M, Brinkmann CR, Olesen R, Erikstrup C, Solomon A, et al. Panobinostat, a histone deacetylase inhibitor, for latentvirus reactivation in HIV-infected patients on suppressive antiretroviral therapy: a phase 1/2, single group, clinical trial. *Lancet HIV.* (2014) 1:e13–21. doi: 10.1016/S2352-3018(14)70014-1
53. Ruiz A, Blanch-Lombarte O, Jimenez-Moyano E, Ouchi D, Mothe B, Peña R, et al. Antigen production after latency reversal and expression of inhibitory receptors in $CD8^+$ T cells limit the killing of HIV-1 reactivated cells. *Front Immunol.* (2019) 9:3162. doi: 10.3389/fimmu.2018.03162
54. Jones RB, O'Connor R, Mueller S, Foley M, Szeto GL, Karel D, et al. Histone deacetylase inhibitors impair the elimination of HIV-infected cells by cytotoxic T-lymphocytes. *PLoS Pathog.* (2014) 10:e1004287. doi: 10.1371/journal.ppat.1004287
55. Li JZ, Etemad B, Ahmed H, Aga E, Bosch RJ, Mellors JW, et al. The size of the expressed HIV reservoir predicts timing of viral rebound after treatment interruption. *AIDS.* (2016) 30:343–53. doi: 10.1097/01.aids.0000499516.66930.89
56. Williams JP, Hurst J, Stöhr W, Robinson N, Brown H, Fisher M, et al. HIV-1 DNA predicts disease progression and post-treatment virological control. *Elife.* (2014) 3:e03821. doi: 10.7554/eLife.03821
57. Namazi G, Fajnzylber JM, Aga E, Bosch RJ, Acosta EP, Sharaf R, et al. The control of HIV after antiretroviral medication pause (CHAMP) study: posttreatment controllers identified from 14 clinical studies. *J Infect Dis.* (2018) 218:1954–63. doi: 10.1093/infdis/jiy479
58. Colby DJ, Trautmann L, Pinyakorn S, Leyre L, Pagliuzza A, Kroon E, et al. Rapid HIV RNA rebound after antiretroviral treatment interruption in persons durably suppressed in fiebig I acute HIV infection. *Nat Med.* (2018) 24:923–6. doi: 10.1038/s41591-018-0026-6
59. Huiting ED, Gittens K, Justement JS, Shi V, Blazkova J, Benko E, et al. Impact of treatment interruption on HIV reservoirs and lymphocyte subsets in individuals who initiated antiretroviral therapy during the early phase of infection. *J Infect Dis.* (2019) 220:270–74. doi: 10.1093/infdis/jiz100
60. Julg B, Dee L, Ananworanich J, Barouch DH, Bar K, Caskey M, et al. Recommendations for analytical antiretroviral treatment interruptions in HIV research trials—report of a consensus meeting. *Lancet HIV.* (2019) 6:e259–68. doi: 10.1016/S2352-3018(19)30052-9
61. Anderson JL, Fromentin R, Corbelli GM, Østergaard L, Ross AL. Progress towards an HIV cure: update from the (2014). International AIDS society symposium. *AIDS Res Hum Retroviruses.* (2015) 31:36–44. doi: 10.1089/aid.2014.0236

10

In vivo Effects of Romidepsin on T-Cell Activation, Apoptosis and Function in the BCN02 HIV-1 Kick&Kill Clinical Trial

Miriam Rosás-Umbert[1,2], Marta Ruiz-Riol[1], Marco A. Fernández[3], Marta Marszalek[1], Pep Coll[1], Christian Manzardo[4], Samandhy Cedeño[1], José M. Miró[4], Bonaventura Clotet[1,5,6,7], Tomáš Hanke[8,9], José Moltó[5,6], Beatriz Mothe[1,6,7], Christian Brander[1,7,10] and the BCN02 study group*

[1] IrsiCaixa AIDS Research Institute-HIVACAT, Badalona, Spain, [2] Department of Cellular Biology, Physiology and Immunology, Universitat Autònoma de Barcelona (UAB), Barcelona, Spain, [3] Flow Cytometry Facility, Health Sciences Research Institute Germans Trias i Pujol, Badalona, Spain, [4] Hospital Clinic- IDIBAPS, University of Barcelona, Barcelona, Spain, [5] Fundació Lluita contra la Sida, Hospital Universitari Germans Trias i Pujol, Badalona, Spain, [6] Department of Infectious Diseases, Hospital Germans Trias i Pujol, Badalona, Spain, [7] Centre for Health and Social Care Research (CESS), Faculty of Medicine, University of Vic – Central University of Catalonia (UVic – UCC), Vic, Spain, [8] The Jenner Institute, University of Oxford, Oxford, United Kingdom, [9] Joint Research Center for Human Retrovirus Infection, Kumamoto University, Kumamoto, Japan, [10] ICREA, Pg. Lluis Companys, Barcelona, Spain

***Correspondence:**
Beatriz Mothe
bmothe@irsicaixa.es

Romidepsin (RMD) is a well-characterized histone deacetylase inhibitor approved for the treatment of cutaneous T-cell lymphoma. *in vitro* and *in vivo* studies have demonstrated that it is able to induce HIV-1 gene expression in latently infected $CD4^+$ T cells from HIV-1^+ individuals on suppressive antiretroviral therapy. However, *in vitro* experiments suggested that RMD could also impair T-cell functionality, particularly of activated T cells. Thus, the usefulness of RMD in HIV-1 kick&kill strategies, that aim to enhance the immune system elimination of infected cells after inducing HIV-1 viral reactivation, may be limited. In order to address whether the *in vitro* observations are replicated *in vivo*, we determined the effects of RMD on the total and HIV-1-specific T-cell populations in longitudinal samples from the BCN02 kick&kill clinical trial (NCT02616874). BCN02 was a proof-of-concept study in 15 early treated HIV-1^+ individuals that combined MVA.HIVconsv vaccination with three weekly infusions of RMD given as a latency reversing agent. Our results show that RMD induced a transient increase in the frequency of apoptotic T cells and an enhanced activation of vaccine-induced T cells. Although RMD reduced the number of vaccine-elicited T cells secreting multiple cytokines, viral suppressive capacity of $CD8^+$ T cells was preserved over the RMD treatment. These observations have important implications for the design of effective kick&kill strategies for the HIV-1 cure.

Keywords: romidepsin, HDAC inhibitor, kick&kill strategy, therapeutic vaccine, latency reversing agent (LRA)

INTRODUCTION

Current antiretroviral therapy (ART) effectively suppresses HIV-1 replication in plasma, but it is not able to completely eliminate the virus from infected individuals. Cessation of antiretroviral treatment results in a rebound of plasma viremia within 3–4 weeks in most individuals (1). This rapid viral rebound after treatment interruption is due to the existence of a latent viral reservoir and the inability of the immune system to effectively contain viral replication. To date, numerous strategies have been pursued to achieve a functional cure or virus eradication, including early ART initiation, ART intensification (2–6), passive administration of antibodies (7), therapeutic vaccination (8–13) and gene therapy (14, 15), among others.

HIV-1 kick&kill strategies are based on the use of latency reversing agents (LRA) to induce production of HIV-1 proteins in latently infected cells and render these cells susceptible to vaccine-induced virus-specific cytolytic T lymphocytes (CTL). The interest in LRA able to reactivate the latent provirus has increased over the past decade, with histone deacetylation inhibitors (HDACi) being some of the best characterized agents both *in vitro* and *in vivo*. The inhibitory effect of HDACi on histone deacetylation results in a higher degree of acetylated histones, causing opening of chromosomes and increased gene transcription. In *ex vivo* isolated cells from ART-suppressed HIV-1-infected individuals, exposure to HDACi resulted in reactivation of the integrated HIV-1 and led to viral protein expression by latently infected cells (16–18). Some HDACi, such as vorinostat (SAHA), panobinostat, and romidepsin (RMD) have also been tested for their *in vivo* potential to reverse HIV-1 latency (19–22). RMD, a cyclic depsipeptide naturally produced by *Chromobacterium violaceum*, is a pan-HDACi that inhibits class I HDACs. RMD was clinically developed as an anti-cancer drug and is approved for the treatment of cutaneous T-cell lymphoma (23). Furthermore, RMD has been shown to induce HIV-1 gene expression in latently infected cells *in vitro* (18, 24) and *in vivo*, when administrated alone (22) and in combination with therapeutic vaccine Vacc-4x (25) in chronically-infected ART-suppressed individuals. Although it was first thought that reactivation of the virus itself would lead to robust immune activation and control of the rebounding virus, it is generally accepted that prior stimulation of the immune effector response by a therapeutic vaccine and/or an immune checkpoint inhibitor, may be needed in order to efficiently eliminate infected cells after LRA exposure (26). Therefore, different immunotherapies are being investigated together with LRAs to test their combined effect, especially combination treatments that include T-cell vaccines.

The proof-of-concept BCN02 trial evaluated a kick&kill strategy that combined the HIVconsv T-cell vaccines with the HDACi RMD in a cohort of early-treated, HIV-1-infected individuals. Fifteen participants of BCN01 (12), who previously received simian adenovirus-vectored vaccine ChAdV63.HIVconsv and MVA.HIVconsv, were invited 2–3 years later to receive two more dosing of the MVA.HIVconsv vaccine before (MVA_1) and after (MVA_2) three weekly-doses of RMD (RMD_{1-2-3}) followed by a monitored antiretroviral pause (MAP) for a period of 32 weeks (NCT02616874). The combined strategy was proven to be safe and vaccination was highly immunogenic. RMD treatment resulted in marked increases in histone acetylation and cell-associated HIV-1 RNA levels compatible with induction of viral transcription. However, the ultimate reduction of the viral reservoir in the BCN02 trial was overall minimal (27). Aside from effects on virus reactivation, for a successful purge of the viral reservoir, it is critical that the LRA used in such strategies does not have any detrimental effects on the vaccine-induced immune cells (28, 29). Here, we assessed the *in vivo* impact of three weekly RMD doses on total and vaccine-induced T cells in longitudinal samples from the BCN02 trial (**Figure 1**).

MATERIALS AND METHODS

Study and Samples

The BCN02 clinical trial (NCT02616874) was a phase I, open-label, single-arm, multicenter study in Spain (27). The study was approved by the institutional ethical review board of the participating institutions (Reference Nr AC-15-108-R) and by the Spanish Regulatory Authorities (EudraCT 2015-002300-84) and was conducted in accordance with the principles of the Helsinki Declaration and local personal data protection law (LOPD 15/1999). Fifteen participants were immunized with MVA.HIVconsv (MVA_1, 2×10^8 pfu intramuscularly), followed by three weekly-doses of romidepsin (RMD_{1-2-3}, 5 mg/m^2 body-surface area; BSA) and a second MVA.HIVconsv boost vaccination (MVA_2, 2×10^8 pfu i.m.) before undergoing a monitored antiretroviral pause (MAP) 8 weeks later and for a maximum of 32 weeks. Cryopreserved peripheral blood

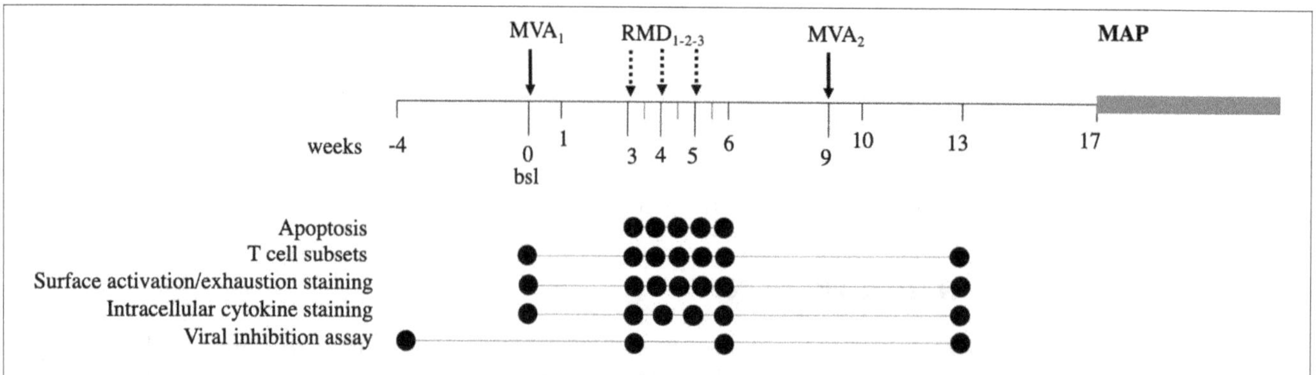

FIGURE 1 | Study design. The BCN02 study was a single arm, open label, proof-of-concept study to address safety and effect on the viral reservoir of a kick&kill strategy combining MVA.HIVconsv vaccines with the HDACi RMD. Timepoints used for the analysis presented here are indicated for each assay by filled circles.

mononuclear cells (PBMC) were stored before, at the end and after 8, 24 h (only for RMD_1), and 3 and 7 days after all RMD doses for immunological and virological studies.

Flow Cytometry

Apoptosis Measurement

PBMC viability was measured using a Pacific Blue™ Annexin V Apoptosis Detection Kit with 7-AAD (BioLegend). Lineage surface markers (CD3, CD4, and CD8) and activation markers (HLA-DR, CD25, and CD69) were included in the staining.

Briefly, 1×10^6 of isolated PBMC were washed in PBS with 1% FBS and resuspend in 100 μl of surface staining solution (CD3, CD4, CD8, CD25, CD69, HLA-DR) and incubated for 20 min. After 2 washes with 300 μl of PBS with 1% FBS, cells were resuspended in 100 μl of Annexin V Binding Buffer with the corresponding Annexin V and 7-AAD. After 15 min of incubation, 250 μl of Binding Buffer was added to each tube and acquired on a LSRII BD cytometer. The percentages of apoptotic and live cells were analyzed using FlowJo software. The gating strategy is summarized in **Supplementary Figure 1**.

T Cells and HIVconsv-Specific T-Cell Lineage, Activation and Cytokine Detection

PBMCs were thawed and stimulated with anti-CD49d and anti-CD28 antibodies (BD) in presence/absence of three peptides pools (containing 58, 54, and 54 peptides) covering the HIVconsv immunogen protein in the presence of GolgiStop for 5 h. Cultures were then stored overnight at 4°C until staining. Cells were stained first with a viability stain (Aqua Live/Dead Fixable Dead Cell Stain kit, Invitrogen), followed by T cell lineage and maduration/activation markers (using anti-CD3-APC Cy7, anti-CD4 PECy5; anti-CD8 PerCP, anti-CCR7 B711, anti-CD45RA BV785, anti-HLA-DR BV650, anti-PD-1 BV605, anti-CD69 APC, and anti-CD25 PEDazzle594 chromogen-conjugated monoclonal antiobodies; BioLegend) and dump channel (using anti-CD19-V450 for B-cells and anti-CD14-V450 mAbs for monocytes; BioLegend) surface staining. Following the fixation and permeabilization step (Fix and Perm kit, Invitrogen), intracellular staining with conjugated antibodies specific for cytokines (IFN-γ A700; Invitrogen, IL-2 PECy7, TNF-α FITC; BiolLegend and MIP1-β PE; RD Systems) was performed. Approximately 10^5 cells were acquired on an LSRFortessa BD instrument, and analysis was performed using FlowJo 10 software. The gating strategy is summarized in **Supplementary Figure 2**.

Intracellular cytokine staining analyses were done applying boolean gates in FlowJo 10, subtracting unstimulated signals using Pestle v1.7 program and represented using SPICE v5.35 software (provided by the National Institute of Health, Mario Roeder, ImmunoTechnology Section, Vaccine Research Center, NIAID, NIH, Bethesda) (30).

Viral Inhibition Assay

$CD8^+$ T-cell mediated viral inhibition capacity was measured at 1:1 and 1:10 CD8 effector to CD4 target ratios. Cryopreserved PBMCs were obtained from timepoints before the BCN02 intervention and $CD8^+$ cells were depleted by magnetic bead separation (MACS Milteny Biotec). $CD8^+$-depleted cells ($CD4^+$-enriched fraction) were stimulated with PHA (5 μg/ml) in RPMI plus 10% fetal bovine serum (R10) and antibiotics (penicillin 100 U/mL and streptavidin 100 μg/ml). After 3 days of stimulation, the CD4-enriched fraction was infected by spinoculation with HIV-1_{BaL} and HIV-1_{IIIB} laboratory-adapted strains at a multiplicity of infection (MOI) of 0.01 as reported previously (12, 31). HIV-infected cells were cultured in duplicates or triplicates in R10 medium with 20 U/ml of IL-2 in 96-well round-bottomed plates, alone or together with unstimulated $CD8^+$ T cells obtained by positive magnetic bead separation the same day from an additional vial of frozen PBMC from screening (week −4), 3 weeks after MVA_1 (week 3, postMVA_1), 1 week after RMD_3 (week 6, postRMD_3), 4 weeks after MVA_2 (week 13, postMVA_2) timepoints. Cultures at different CD8:CD4 ratios (E:T = 1:1 and 1:10) were harvested after 6 days. Cells were stained first with Aqua Live/Dead stained for surface markers (CD3 APC-H7, BD Biosciences, CD4 PerCP, BD Biosciences, and CD8 APC, BD Biosciences), then permeabilized (FIX & PERM® Cell Permeabilization Kit, ThermoFisher). Cells were then fixed (FIX & PERM® Cell Permeabilization Kit, ThermoFisher) at room temperature and finally stained with anti-Gag p24 antibody (KC-57-FITC; Beckman Coulter). $CD8^+$ T-cell antiviral activity is expressed as % inhibition = [(fraction of $p24^+$ cells in $CD4^+$ T cells cultured alone)−(fraction of $p24^+$ cells in $CD4^+$ T cells cultured with $CD8^+$ T cells)]/(fraction of $p24^+$ in $CD4^+$ T cells cultured alone) × 100. At least 100,000 cells were collected on a LSRII BD cytometer and analysis was performed using FlowJo 10 software.

Statistical Analysis

GraphPad Prism version 7 for Windows (San Diego, CA) was used for statistical analysis. Mann-Whitney test and Wilcoxon matched paired test were used for unpaired and paired comparisons, respectively. Significant values were considered for $p < 0.05$.

RESULTS

Increased Apoptosis After RMD Exposure

Since RMD was previously described to have a toxic effect *in vitro* (28, 29), especially on activated T cells, we first measured the effect of RMD on cell viability both in total $CD8^+$ and $CD4^+$ T cells and in activated, HLA-DR^+ expressing cells in PBMC from the BCN02 participants. Viability in total T cells was assessed by flow cytometry by Annexin V/7AAD staining before and after the three RMD doses. Increases in the number of apoptotic $CD8^+$ T cells (Annexin V^+) were detected at 24 h after RMD_1 (Wilcoxon signed-rank, $p = 0.0151$) and 3 days after each RMD dose (Wilcoxon signed-rank, RMD_1 $p = 0.0413$, RMD_2 $p = 0.0181$, and RMD_3 $p = 0.0833$, respectively, **Figure 2A**). A similar pattern was observed in $CD4^+$ T cells, with apoptotic cells being significantly increased 3 days after RMD_2 and RMD_3 (Wilcoxon signed-rank, RMD_2 $p = 0.0067$ and RMD_3 $p = 0.0413$, respectively, **Figure 2B**). One week after RMD_3 the levels of apoptotic cells in both $CD8^+$ T cells and $CD4^+$ were not restored

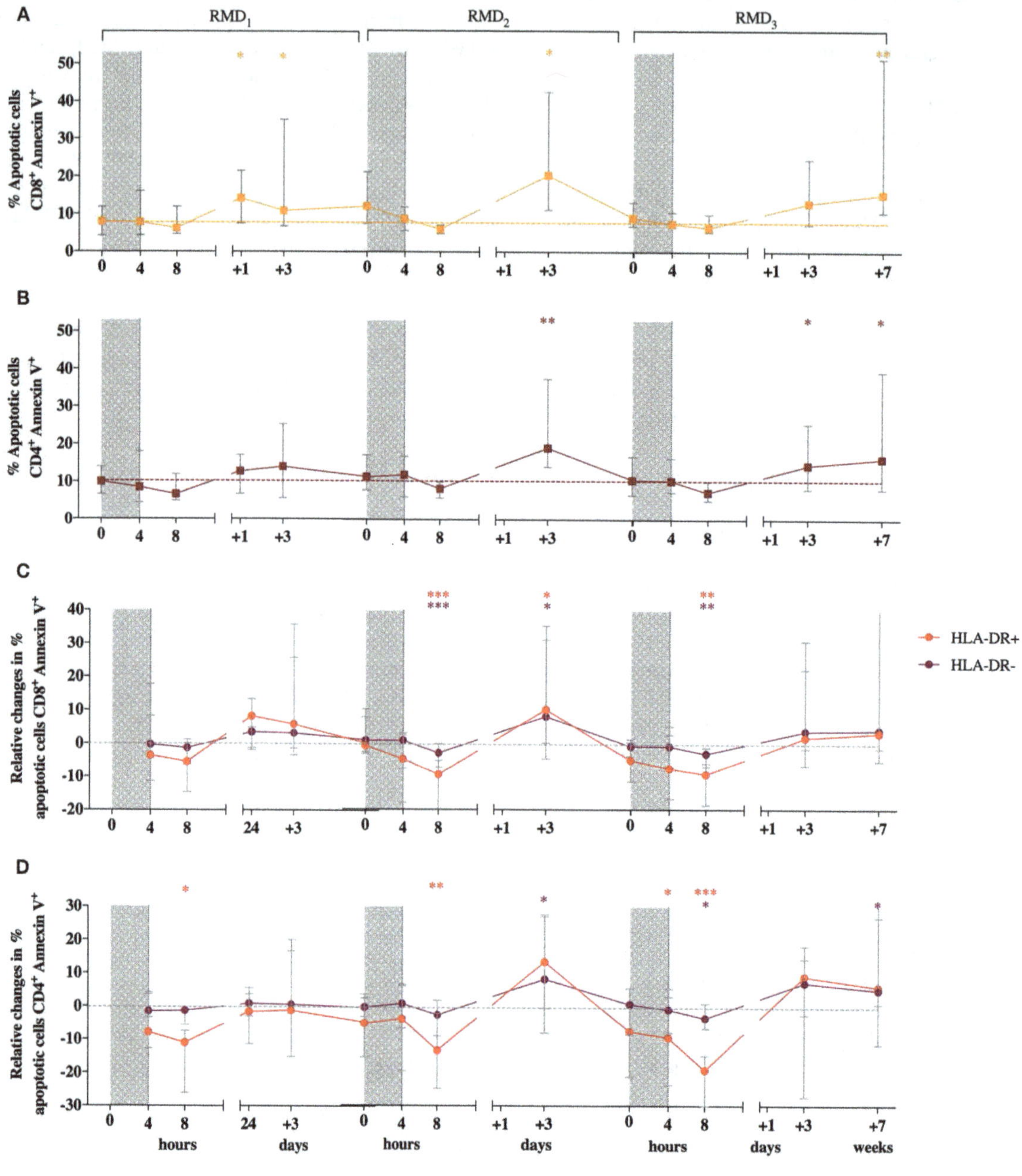

FIGURE 2 | Effect of RMD on the viability on T cells. Apoptotic cells (Annexin V^+/$7AAD^+$ and Annexin V^+/$7AAD^-$) percentages are shown for $CD8^+$ **(A)** and $CD4^+$ T cells **(B)**. Changes relative to baseline in the percentage of apoptosis in HLA-DR^+ (in red) and HLA-DR^- cells (in purple) are shown for $CD8^+$ **(C)** and $CD4^+$ **(D)** T cells. RMD administration cycles are indicated by gray bars. Sampling time points at 4 h, 8 h, 3 days, and 7 days after each RMD administration are indicated. Median with interquartile range is shown. *P*-values ($^*p < 0.05$, $^{**}p < 0.01$, $^{***}p < 0.001$) are indicative for the corresponding timepoint compared to pre-RMD_1.

to pre-RMD levels ($p = 0.0054$ for $CD8^+$ and $p = 0.0181$ for $CD4^+$), suggestive of an accumulative toxic effect of RMD.

As activated T cell have been found to be particularly sensitive to RMD exposure (28), levels of apoptosis in $CD4^+$ and $CD8^+$ T cell with high or low expression of the activation marker HLA-DR were assessed. Changes in the percentage of apoptotic cells relative to baseline during RMD exposure was comparable between HLA-DR^+ and HLA-DR^- CD8 T cells (**Figures 2C,D**). The same results were observed in CD4+ T cells. Therefore, non- activated HLA-DR^- cells had the same susceptibility to induction of apoptosis due to RMD exposure as the activated HLA-DR^+ cells.

$CD8^+$ and $CD4^+$ Naïve Populations Increase After MVA_1 and Up to 24 h After 1st Romidepsin Exposure Followed by a Shift to Memory Phenotypes

As activation status did not impact susceptibility of T cells to RMD-induced apoptosis, we next assessed whether RMD could

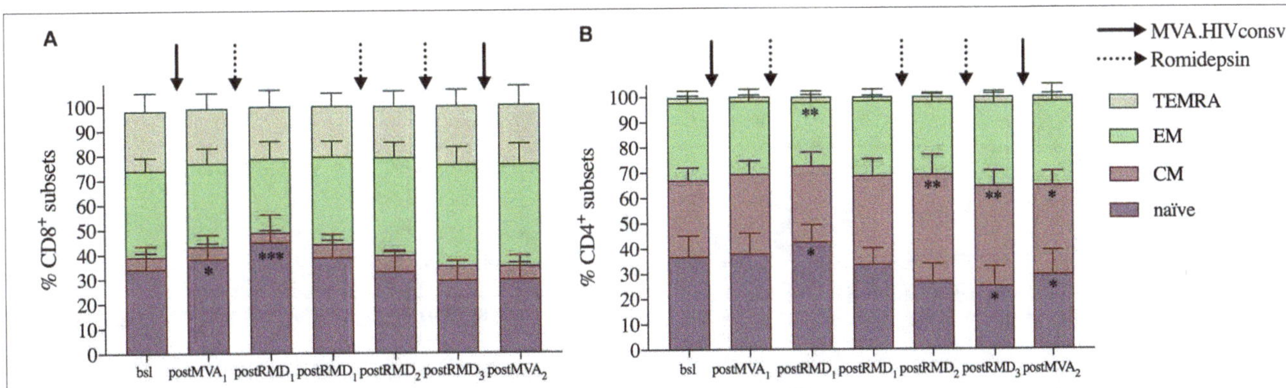

FIGURE 3 | Evolution of T-cell subsets over the course of the intervention. Averages of relative frequency of $CD8^+$ **(A)** and $CD4^+$ **(B)** T-cell subsets based on CCR7 and CD45RA expression are shown. TEMRA: highly differentiated effector cells expressing CD45RA ($CCR7^-/CD45RA^+$), EM: effector memory cells ($CCR7^-/CD45RA^-$), CM: central memory ($CCR7^+/CD45RA^-$), and naïve ($CCR7^+/CD45RA^+$). *P*-values (*$p < 0.05$, **$p < 0.01$, ***$p < 0.001$) are indicative for the corresponding timepoint compared with values from baseline samples prior to MVA_1.

affect the distribution of different T-cell differentiation subsets in the peripheral blood. Flow cytometry was used to measure the frequency of $CD4^+$ and $CD8^+$ differentiation subsets defined by CCR7 and CD45RA expression at each timepoint. Three weeks after MVA_1, the frequency of naïve $CD8^+$ T cells increased from median frequency of 30.5–35.2% and up to 49.6% 24 h after RMD_1 (Wilcoxon signed-rank $p = 0.0122$ and $p = 0.0005$, respectively, **Figure 3A**). Similar results were observed for naïve $CD4^+$ T cells, which increased from 33% at baseline to 35.2% 3 weeks after MVA_1 and up to 41.7% at 24 h after RMD_1 (Wilcoxon signed-rank $p = 0.0227$ and $p = 0.0110$, respectively, **Figure 3B**). The frequency of $CD8^+$ and $CD4^+$ naïve cells were not further increased after RMD_2 or RMD_3, as their frequency actually decreased after RMD_2 and RMD_3. At the same time, the median frequency of $CD8^+$ effector memory and $CD4^+$ central memory T cells progressively increased over RMD_{1-2-3}. T-cell differentiation subsets were not further changed 4 weeks after MVA_2 compared to subset population observed after RMD doses.

RMD Treatment Increases T-Cell Activation Especially of the HIVconsv-Specific T Cells

In order to assess the effect of RMD on T-cell activation and exhaustion markers, we evaluated the frequency of $CD4^+$ and $CD8^+$ T cells expressing HLA-DR, CD69, CD25, and PD-1. A peak in the frequency of $CD8^+HLA\text{-}DR^+$ T cells was observed 3 days after RMD_1 (Wilcoxon signed-rank, $p < 0.0001$) and increased levels were maintained over the course of the 3 RMD doses, as their median frequency more than doubled (4.1% at baseline to 9.6% 1 week after RMD_3, Wilcoxon signed-rank, $p = 0.0002$, **Figure 4A**). The same results were observed in $CD4^+$ T cells, with levels of HLA-DR expression increasing 3 days after RMD_1 (Wilcoxon signed-rank, $p < 0.0001$) and with twice as many HLA-DR expressing cells at day 7 after RMD_3 (median 3.1% at baseline to 6.3%, Wilcoxon signed-rank, $p = 0.0017$, **Figure 4A**) compared to baseline. The largest increase in percentage of cells expressing HLA-DR in both $CD4^+$ and $CD8^+$ T cells was observed in effector memory (EM) and highly differentiated effector cells expressing CD45RA (TEMRA) (**Supplementary Figure 3**).

Importantly, upon *in vitro* stimulation with peptides derived from the vaccine immunogen, changes in the $HLA\text{-}DR^+$ in expression were already detected after MVA_1. Both, HIVconsv-specific $CD8^+$ and $CD4^+$ T cells, defined upon *in vitro* antigen-specific stimulation and detection based on their ability to produce cytokines (IL-2, MIP1-β, TNF-α, IFN-γ) in response to antigen specific stimulation, showed detectable increases of $HLA\text{-}DR^+$ expression earlier and up to higher levels compared to the changes seen in total $CD8^+$ and $CD4^+$ T cells (**Figure 4A**). The percentage of $HLA\text{-}DR^+$ among HIVconsv-specific $CD8^+$ cells increased from median of 5.1% at baseline to 10.11% 3 weeks after MVA_1, and up to 21% 3 days after RMD_1 (Wilcoxon signed-rank $p = 0.0245$ and $p = 0.0002$, **Figure 4B**) and percentage of $HLA\text{-}DR^+$, HIVconsv-specific $CD4^+$ cells increased from median of 4.2% at baseline to 8.3% 3 weeks after MVA_1, and up to 21.8% 3 days after RMD_1 (Wilcoxon signed-rank $p = 0.5614$ and $p = 0.0023$, **Figure 4C**). High levels of activation were maintained during all RMD doses (**Figures 4C,D**) and reached the peak 3 days after RMD_3 suggestive of an additive effect of RMD on the activation of vaccine-stimulated $CD4^+$ and $CD8^+$ T cells.

As changes in *in vivo* histone acetylation and induction of viral transcription occur rapidly after RMD exposure (22, 27), we assessed the expression of early activation markers CD69 and CD25 in $CD4^+$ and $CD8^+$ T cells. Increases in the expression of CD69 in $CD4^+$ T cells were observed upon each RMD dosing, with significant increases seen after RMD_2 and RMD_3 in the CM subset (from baseline levels of 2.5 to 7.1% (RMD_2 $p = 0.0107$) and 6.7% (RMD_3 $p = 0.0479$) and in the TEMRA subset (baseline levels of 2.7 to 9% (RMD_2 $p = 0.0203$) and 6.6% (RMD_3 $p = 0.0315$), respectively (**Supplementary Figure 4B**). As with HLA-DR surface staining, expression of CD69 returned to baseline levels 4 weeks after last vaccination. No significant changes were observed in CD69 expression on $CD8^+$ T cells (**Supplementary Figure 4A**) nor in the expression of CD25 on $CD8^+$ or $CD4^+$ T cells over the course of the intervention.

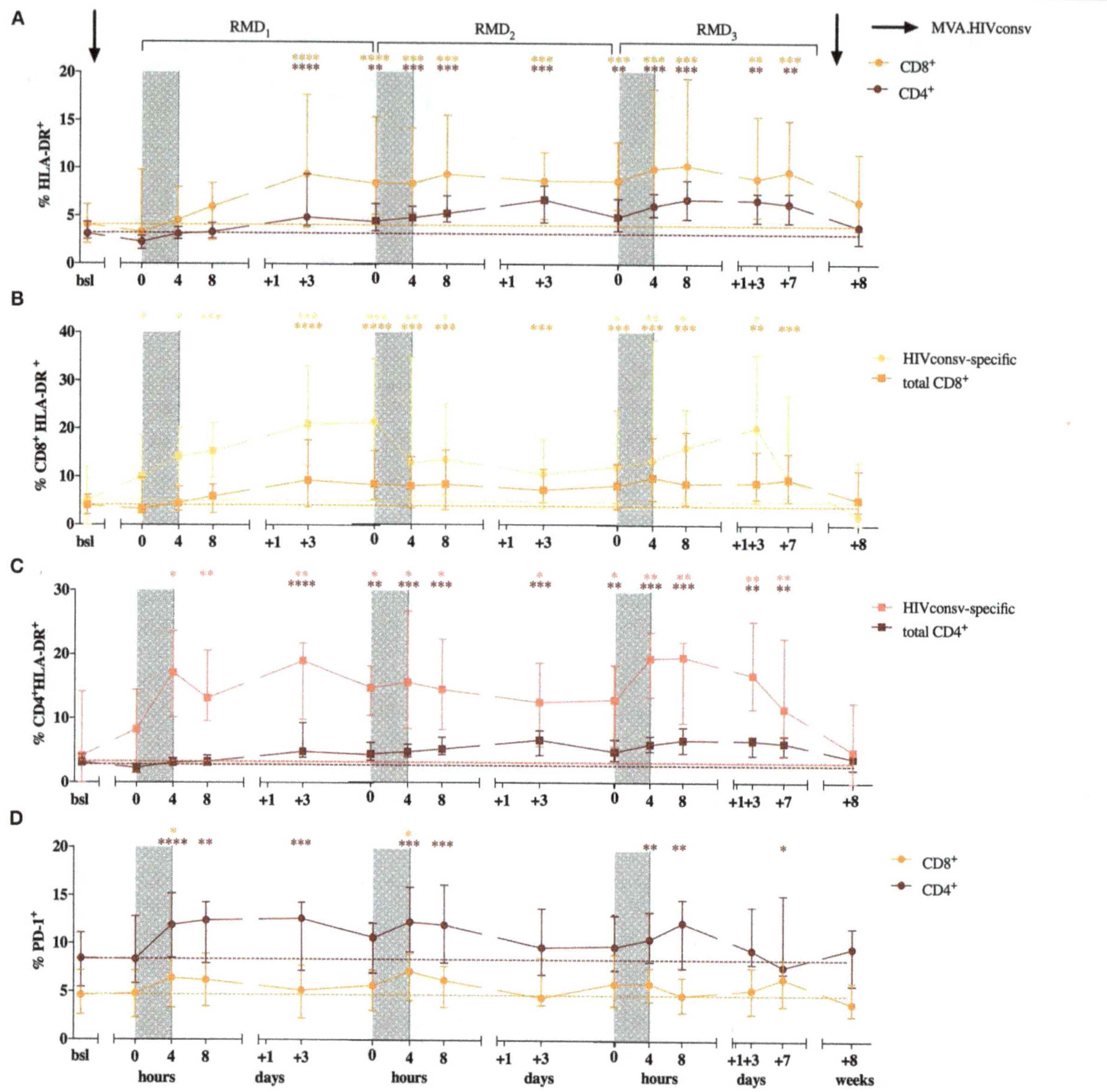

FIGURE 4 | $CD4^+$ and $CD8^+$ T cell activation status over the course of the intervention. Percentage of HLA-DR expression is shown for $CD8^+$ in orange and $CD4^+$ T cells in purple **(A)**. Levels of HLA-DR are shown for $CD8^+$ **(B)** and $CD4^+$ T cells **(C)** in HIVconsv specific and total T cells. HIVconsv-specific T cells were defined upon *in vitro* antigen-specific stimulation and detection based on their ability to produce cytokines (IL-2, MIP1-β, TNF-α, IFN-γ) in response to stimulation. Percentage of PD-1 is shown for $CD8^+$ in orange and $CD4^+$ T cells in purple **(D)**. Median with interquartile range is shown. *P*-values ($^*p < 0.05$, $^{**}p < 0.01$, $^{***}p < 0.001$, $^{****}p < 0.0001$) are indicative for the corresponding timepoint compared with baseline.

The expression of PD-1^+ increased rapidly in $CD8^+$ T cells from median baseline levels of 4.6–6.4, 7.2, and 6.1% at 4 h after the end of RMD_{1-2-3} treatment (Wilcoxon singed-rank, $p = 0.0215$, $p = 0.0238$, and $p = 0.0574$, respectively, **Figure 4D**). The same kinetics was observed in $CD4^+$ T cells where the frequency of PD-1 expressing cells raised from median baseline levels of 8.5–11.9, 12.35, and 10.7% at 4 h after RMD_{1-2-3} (Wilcoxon singed-rank, $p = 0.0004$, $p = 0.0002$, and $p = 0.0046$, respectively, **Figure 4D**). However, in contrast to the additive effect of RMD_{1-2-3} on T-cell activation markers, changes in PD-1 expression in both $CD8^+$ and $CD4^+$ T cells were transient, and the levels of PD-1 expression were consistently restored to baseline levels within 3 days after each RMD dose.

Polyfunctionality of HIVconsv-Specific Responses Increases After MVA_1 and Decreases Over RMD Treatment

Considering the effect of RMD on the expression of markers of cell death, exhaustion and activation, we assessed the

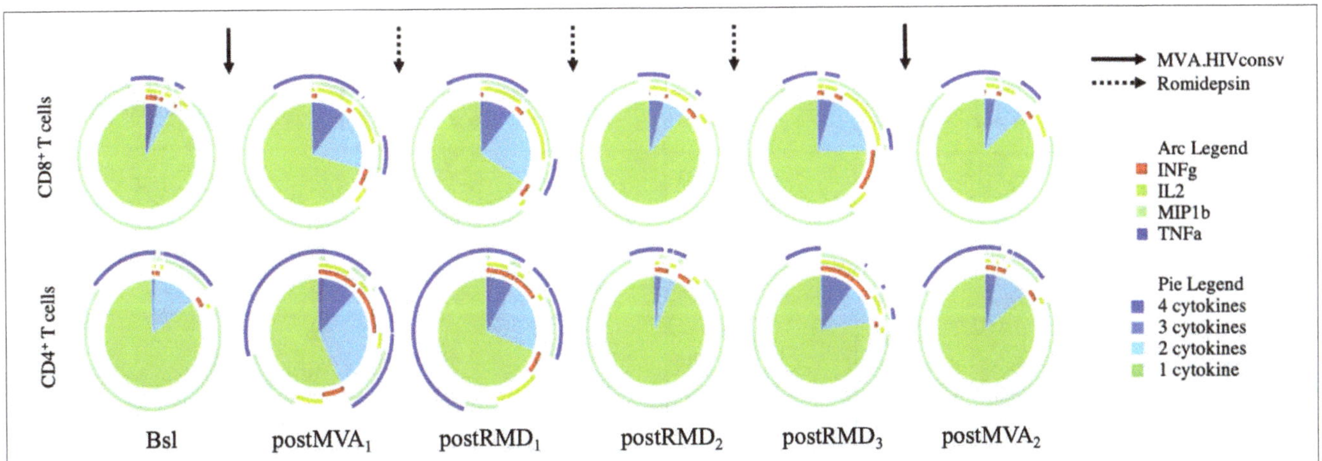

FIGURE 5 | Longitudinal assessment of the T-cell cytokine production over the course of the intervention. Polyfunctionality of CD8+ and CD4+ T cells was analyzed by Boolean gating. Pie charts illustrate relative proportion of each of the different subsets (cells producing 1, 2, 3, or 4 cytokines, respectively).

effect of RMD on the functionality of vaccine-elicited T cells. Polyfunctionality of HIVconsv-specific T cells was measured by stimulation of PBMC with the HIVconsv peptides and enumeration of the cells producing IFN-γ, IL-2, MIP1-β, and/or TNF-α by flow cytometry. As shown in **Figure 5**, MVA_1 vaccination increased relative polyfunctionality in both $CD4^+$ and $CD8^+$ HIVconsv-specific T cells. Three weeks after MVA_1 ($postMVA_1$), the highest increase in polyfunctionality was observed in vaccine immunogen-specific $CD4^+$ T cells that produced 2, 3, and 4 cytokines (post MVA_1, **Figure 5**), with a particular increase in INF-γ secreting cells. On the other hand, vaccine-specific $CD8^+$ T cells produced INF-γ, IL-2, and TNF-α and were mostly polyfunctional, producing 2 or 3 cytokines. However, during the treatment with RMD, the polyfunctionality was reduced to baseline levels in both HIVconsv-specific $CD4^+$ and $CD8^+$ T cells and the final MVA_2 vaccination was not able to re-boost functionality profiles (post MVA_2, **Figure 5** and **Supplementary Figure 5**). These results suggest that RMD treatment might have impaired functionality of vaccine-induced responses and prevented their subsequent booster vaccination effect.

$CD8^+$ Cells Maintain Antiviral Activity of After the RMD Treatment

To further study the functionality of vaccine-induced T cells during the intervention, we measured the *in vitro* antiviral capacity of $CD8^+$ T cells. The *in vitro* replication inhibition capacity of PBMC-derived $CD8^+$ T cells was measured by standard viral inhibition assay (VIA) (12, 31) using autologous $CD4^+$ T cells infected with two laboratory-adapted HIV-1 strains BaL (R5 tropic virus) and IIIB (X4 tropic virus). Virus replication was measured by flow cytometry as the percentage of HIV-1 Gag p24-positive $CD4^+$ cells. $CD8^+$ T-cell inhibitory capacity was determined at screening, 3 weeks after MVA_1 ($postMVA_1$), 1 week after RMD_3 ($postRMD_3$), and 4 weeks after MVA_2 ($postMVA_2$). In contrast to the changes in cytokine production/polyfunctionality detected by flow cytometry, neither MVA_1 nor RMD_{1-2-3} altered the inhibition activity, which was median of 64, 52, and 53,5% at the screening, $postMVA_1$ and $postRMD_3$ time points at the E:T ratio 1:1, respectively, against HIV-1_{BaL} and median 46, 44, and 43% at the screening, $postMVA_1$ and $postRMD_3$ time points, respectively, against HIV-1_{IIIB}. In fact, there was a weak, but statistically significant increase in the inhibitory capacity against HIV-1_{BaL} after the second MVA vaccination given 4 weeks after RMD_3 from median of 64% at baseline to 69% at $postMVA_2$ at the E:T ratio 1:1 and from median of 11% at baseline to 21% at $postMVA_2$, for the E:T ratio1:10 (Wilcoxon signed-rank, $p = 0.0200$) (**Figure 6A**) and against HIV-1_{IIIB} from median of 12% at baseline to 16% at $postMVA_2$, for at the 1:10 E:T ratio (Wilcoxon signed-rank, $p = 0.0156$) (**Figure 6B**). These data indicate that antiviral activity, measured by VIA with laboratory-adapted viral strains, was not negatively impacted during RMD treatment.

DISCUSSION

The BCN02 study was an HIV-1 kick&kill proof-of-concept trial combining MVA.HIVconsv vaccines with the HDACi RMD given as an LRA to the previous ChAdV63.HIVconsv-MVA.HIVconsv regimen recipients from the parental BCN01 trial (12). The immune analyses in BCN02 showed a highly significant shift of HIV-1-specific T-cell responses toward conserved regions of HIV-1 covered by the immunogen and marked increases in histone acetylation and induction of viral transcription *in vivo* by RMD. However, the reduction of the viral reservoir after these interventions was overall minimal (27). Already low baseline levels of viral reservoir in the early-treated participants enrolled in the BCN02 study likely limited latency reversal activity of RMD and/or a potential toxicity of RMD (28, 32) on vaccine-induced T cells might have precluded the capability to observe a more pronounced reduction in the size of the viral reservoir. To address the latter possibility, we here evaluated the effect that the HDACi RMD had on the T-cell viability, activation and

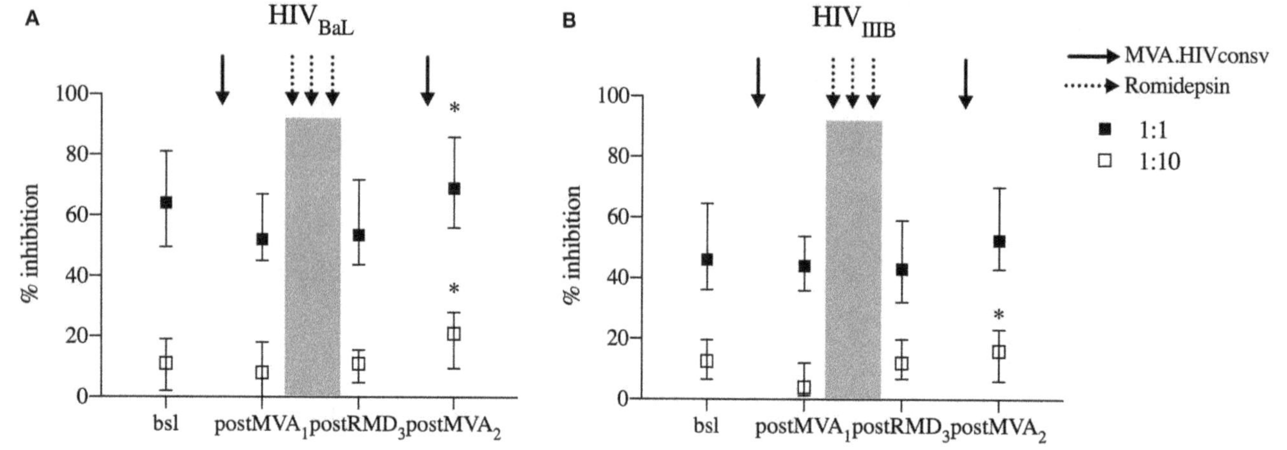

FIGURE 6 | *In vitro* viral replication inhibition capacity. Levels of $CD8^+$ viral inhibitory capacity are shown for HIV-1_{BaL} **(A)** and HIV-1_{IIIB} **(B)** at two E/T ratios (effector/target ratio) 1:1 and E/T 1:10 in individuals that underwent the intervention ($n = 14$ for HIV-1_{BaL} and $n = 15$ for HIV-1_{IIIB}). *P*-values (*$p < 0.05$) are indicative for the corresponding timepoint compared with respective bsl.

functionality throughout the intervention that included RMD given in a three weekly 5 mg/m^2 BSA regimen.

Our data document a *in vivo* toxic effect of RMD on T cells 3 days after each RMD exposure. Although these effects were transient and viability of T cells was partially recovered 7 days after RMD_1 and RMD_2, there was an additive increase in apoptosis over the full RMD regimen, which was not fully restored by 7 days after RMD_3. Jones et al. and Zhao et al. have described increases in cell death upon long term (18- and 72- h period) *in vitro* exposure to RMD, but no cytotoxic effect were observed when T cells were exposed to RMD for 4 h only, which is more similar to the *in vivo* regimen where the terminal half-life ($t_{1/2}$) of RMD is estimated to be ~3 h (28, 32). Indeed, Clutton et al. exposed *ex vivo* PBMC to RMD for 3 h, washed them and cultivated them further in the absence of RMD for 3 days in order to mimic *in vivo* exposure, and reported that the cell viability was not changed after 3 or 24 h, but was significantly reduced at 48 and 72 h (33). These results concur with our observations showing a peak of apoptotic T cells 3 days after each RMD infusion and could explain the transient decreases in peripheral $CD4^+$ T-cell counts observed in BCN02 (27). Also, the cumulative effect on viability observed after 3 RMD doses is in line with the delayed effects of RMD suggested by Clutton.

As RMD may induce T-cell activation resulting from reservoir reactivation and viral antigen presentation, which could also drive increase in exhaustion levels prior to the induction of apoptosis, we evaluated the frequency of activated $CD4^+$ and $CD8^+$ T cells. Indeed, the additive increase in HLA-DR^+ activation markers in both $CD8^+$ and $CD4^+$ T cells over RMD treatment, especially in HIVconsv-specific T cells, was already observed after the first MVA.HIVconsv vaccination. Moreover, as the increased expression of HLA-DR was mostly observed in T effector memory cells and the fact that HIVconsv-specific T cells showed higher levels of HLA-DR expression, the data suggest that there could be a different memory distribution among HIVconsv-specific T cells compared to the total T cell population. These changes are in line with the increase in the magnitude of the immunogen-specific responses upon vaccination (27). However, the magnitudes of vaccine-specific responses were not increased further during RMD administration, suggesting that viral reactivation did not contribute in a major way to the increased levels of cell activation during RMD. In contrast, RMD treatment changed levels of CD69 and PD-1 more rapidly albeit transiently, peaking at 4 h after the end of each RMD dose. In line with our observation on CD69 longitudinal expression, an increase in $CD69^+$ expression was previously described upon RMD, panobinostat and vorinostat treatments *in vitro* (18, 24) and also *in vivo* given alone (22) or in combination with a vaccine (34). This enhanced expression of PD-1 and CD69 could be the result of a generalized increased expression of the host genes induced by the action of RMD. So far, little is known about the effect of RMD and other LRA on the host genome gene expression profiles. There is an urgent need to better understand these effects and, especially, to clarify how they can affect the antiviral immunity against HIV-1 (35) or, in fact, fueling it.

Although it was previously described that RMD can impair T-cell and NK function *in vitro* (28, 29, 36, 37), Søgaard et al. presented *in vivo* data from the REDUC trial, indicating that RMD did not alter the proportion of HIV-1-specific T cells nor inhibited T-cell cytokine production (22), at least in the peripheral blood. Nonetheless, there appears to be a trend toward decreased HIV-specific T cell responses after RMD treatment, which may have not reached statistical significance due to the limited group size. On another note, vaccine-induced responses in the REDUC trial were weaker compared to the responses induced in the BCN02 trial (12, 27), possibly due to weaker vaccine vectors/immunogens employed in the REDUC trial. In addition, REDUC did not include early-treated individuals with relatively intact immunity, and the detection of reduced polyfunctionality of vaccine-induced T-cells could have been limited. In BCN02, the first MVA.HIVconsv vaccination enhanced polyfunctionality, especially in $CD4^+$ T cells, in line with previous reports showing that MVA-vectored vaccination can improve the polyfunctionality and T effector memory phenotype in $CD4^+$ T cells more so than in $CD8^+$ T cells (38). This increased effector function profile induced by MVA_1 was reduced upon RMD treatment but did not lead to a net reduction of the latent reservoir compared to baseline.

Our data also indicate that despite fluctuations in activation, maturation phenotypes and polyfunctionality, RMD treatment did not impair the *in vitro* antiviral capacity of $CD8^+$ T cells. While some *in vitro* studies have shown a diminished inhibitory capacity when $CD8^+$ T cells were exposed to RMD, but not to other HDACi (39, 40), such an effect was not observed *in vivo* in clinical trials using RMD. In the REDUC trial, the viral inhibition assay showed a trend toward increased inhibitory activity post-immunization that was lost after RMD exposure, but overall, antiviral capacity did not significantly change over time. Similarly, we did not see a reduction in the antiviral capacity of T cells over the course of RMD_{1-2-3}, suggesting that the preservation of the antiviral capacity may depend on the balance between the deleterious effects of RMD and the potency of the employed vaccination strategy.

Of note, our results highlight that there is no direct comparability between assays used to characterize CTL functionality, including multiparametric flow cytometry and *in vitro* inhibition assays. In particular, in our study, the polyfunctionality of $CD8^+$ T cells decreased slightly during RMD treatment, while *in vitro* VIA activity was maintained. In addition, the MVA_2 boost vaccination did not augment the proportion of cell secreting multiple cytokines, while a moderately increased *in vitro* suppressive capacity was observed. These data are consistent with other studies, which showed a disconnection between cytokine secretion and antiviral capacity (41, 42), indicating that polyfunctionality of HIV-1-specific $CD8^+$ T cells (at least as measured in standard assays) is not directly associated with viral suppression capacity (31, 43, 44). This lack of consistency between the two techniques could be due to the cytokines measured in standard protocols for intracellular cytokine assays: whilst IFN-γ, IL-2, MIP1-β, and TNF-α are used to measure functionality of HIV-1-specific T cells, evaluating secretion of granzyme B and perforin could be more accurate when assessing T-cell killing activity and may provide better concordance with VIA activity (45). However, whether antiviral capacity measured by standard *in vitro* VIA assay using laboratory-adapted viral strains will translate into effective *in vivo* killing or reactivated, HIV-1 infected cells remain to be determined as well. In addition, further work using autologous virus might be more representative of the physiological conditions in kick&kill strategies. Finally, viral suppression capacity was measured in total bulk $CD8^+$ T cells while cytokine secretion was measured in vaccine specific cells, which could have been more susceptible to *in vivo* effects by RMD.

This present study has a number of limitations, which include a small sample size and the lack of control arms, both placebo and single intervention arms to discern the effects exerted by RMD or the vaccine alone. Thus, the presented results need to be interpreted with caution. Still, the present study shows that RMD has a transient effect on T-cell viability, exhaustion and increased cell activation in an additive way over three weekly doses. Although this can result in a decrease of polyfunctionality of vaccine-induced HIVconsv-specific responses, the *in vitro* replication inhibition capacity of $CD8^+$ T cells was not impaired and should not preclude effective killing upon RMD-induced viral reactivation. As RMD increased higher levels of HIV-1 transcription on the RMD_2 and RMD_3 dose, it is tempting to speculate that increasing the number the RMD doses could result in further increased in levels of reservoir reactivation without overly inhibiting the antiviral capacity of $CD8^+$ T cells. Regardless whether this would occur *in vivo* with longer term RMD administration, the present data indicate that timing and order of LRA and T-cell immunotherapy regimens are critical in order to achieve the clearance of reactivated latently HIV-1-infected cells. Larger controlled clinical trials are needed to further investigate combinations of LRA and immune intervention in order to find the best strategy to achieve a functional cure of HIV-1.

ETHICS STATEMENT

This study was carried out in accordance with the recommendations of and approval by the Ethics Committee of the Hospital Universitari Germans Trias i Pujol (Badalona, Spain). All subjects provided their written informed consent to participate. The study was conducted according to the principles expressed in the Declaration of Helsinki.

AUTHOR CONTRIBUTIONS

MR-U, MR-R, BM, and CB conceived and designed the study and drafted the manuscript. MF, MM, PC, CM, SC, JMM, BC, TH, and JM contributed to the study design. MR-U, MR-R, and MF performed the experiments. All authors revised the manuscript critically for important intellectual content and approved the final version of the manuscript.

ACKNOWLEDGMENTS

Special thanks to all volunteers participating in this study for their perseverance and dedication, without whom the phase I clinical trial would not have been possible.

Members of the BCN 02 Study Group

IrsiCaixa AIDS Research Institute-HIVACAT, Hospital Universitari Germans Trias i Pujol, Badalona, Spain: Susana Benet, Christian Brander, Samandhy Cedeño, Bonaventura Clotet, Pep Coll, Anuksa Llano, Javier Martinez-Picado, Marta Marszalek, Sara Morón-López, Beatriz Mothe, Roger Paredes, Maria C. Puertas, Miriam Rosás-Umbert, Marta Ruiz-Riol.

Fundació Lluita contra la Sida, Hospital Universitari Germans Trias i Pujol, Badalona, Spain: Roser Escrig, Silvia Gel, Miriam López, Cristina Miranda, José Moltó, Jose Muñoz, Nuria Perez-Alvarez, Jordi Puig, Boris Revollo, Jessica Toro.

Germans Trias i Pujol Research Institute, Badalona, Spain: Ana Maria Barriocanal, Magi Farré, Cristina Perez-Reche.

Pharmacokinetic/pharmacodynamic modeling and simultation, Institut de Recerca de l'Hospital de la Santa Creu i Sant Pau-IIB Sant Pau, Barcelona, Spain: Marta Valle. Hospital Clinic-HIVACAT, IDIBAPS, University of Barcelona, Spain: Christian Manzardo (currently working at Hospital Universitari Arnau de Vilanova, Lleida, Spain), Juan Ambrosioni, Irene Ruiz, Cristina Rovira, Carmen Ligero and Jose M. Miro.

Projecte dels noms, BCN Checkpoint, Barcelona, Spain: Antonio Carrillo, Michael Meulbroek, Ferran Pujol and Jorge Saz.

The Jenner Institute, The Nuffield Department of Medicine, University of Oxford, UK: Nicola Borthwick, Alison Crook, Edmund G. Wee and Tomáš Hanke.

REFERENCES

1. El-Sadr WM, Abrams D, Losso M, General De Agudos H-T, Ramos Mejia JM, Rappoport C. CD4+ count-guided interruption of antiretroviral treatment. *N Engl J Med.* (2006) 355:2283–96. doi: 10.1056/NEJMoa062360
2. Buzón JM, Massanella M, Llibre JM, Esteve A, Dahl V, Puertas MC, et al. HIV-1 replication and immune dynamics are affected by raltegravir intensification of HAART-suppressed subjects. *Nat Med.* (2010) 16:460–5. doi: 10.1038/nm.2111
3. Llibre JM, Buzón MJ, Massanella M, Esteve A, Dahl V, Puertas MC, et al. Treatment intensification with raltegravir in subjects with sustained HIV-1 viraemia suppression: a randomized 48-week study. *Antivir Ther.* (2011) 17:355–64. doi: 10.3851/IMP1917
4. Gutiérrez C, Díaz L, Vallejo A, Hernández-Novoa B, Abad M, Madrid N, et al. Intensification of antiretroviral therapy with a CCR5 antagonist in patients with chronic HIV-1 infection: effect on t cells latently infected. *PLoS ONE.* (2011) 6:e27864. doi: 10.1371/journal.pone.0027864
5. Vallejo A, Gutierrez C, Hernandez-Novoa B, Diaz L, Madrid N, Abad-Fernandez M, et al. The effect of intensification with raltegravir on the HIV-1 reservoir of latently infected memory CD4 T cells in suppressed patients. *AIDS.* (2012) 26:1885–94. doi: 10.1097/QAD.0b013e3283584521
6. Gandhi RT, Coombs RW, Chan ES, Bosch RJ, Zheng L, Margolis DM, et al. No effect of raltegravir intensification on viral replication markers in the blood of HIV-1-infected patients receiving antiretroviral therapy. *J Acquir Immune Defic Syndr.* (2012) 59:229–35. doi: 10.1097/QAI.0b013e31823fd1f2
7. Lynch RM, Boritz E, Coates EE, DeZure A, Madden P, Costner P, et al. Virologic effects of broadly neutralizing antibody VRC01 administration during chronic HIV-1 infection. *Sci Transl Med.* (2015) 7:319ra206. doi: 10.1126/scitranslmed.aad5752
8. Sneller MC, Justement JS, Gittens KR, Petrone ME, Clarridge KE, Proschan MA, et al. A randomized controlled safety/efficacy trial of therapeutic vaccination in HIV-infected individuals who initiated antiretroviral therapy early in infection. *Sci Transl Med.* (2017) 9:eaan8848. doi: 10.1126/scitranslmed.aan8848
9. García F, Climent N, Guardo AC, Gil C, León A, Autran B, et al. A dendritic cell-based vaccine elicits T cell responses associated with control of HIV-1 replication. *Sci Transl Med.* (2013) 5:166ra2. doi: 10.1126/scitranslmed.3004682
10. Autran B, Murphy RL, Costagliola D, Tubiana R, Clotet B, Gatell J, et al. Greater viral rebound and reduced time to resume antiretroviral therapy after therapeutic immunization with the ALVAC-HIV vaccine (vCP1452). *AIDS.* (2008) 22:1313–22. doi: 10.1097/QAD.0b013e3282fdce94
11. Schooley RT, Spritzler J, Wang H, Lederman MM, Havlir D, Kuritzkes DR, et al. AIDS clinical trials group 5197: a placebo-controlled trial of immunization of HIV-1-infected persons with a replication-deficient adenovirus type 5 vaccine expressing the HIV-1 core protein. *J Infect Dis.* (2010) 202:705–16. doi: 10.1086/655468
12. Mothe B, Manzardo C, Sanchez-Bernabeu A, Coll P, Morón-López S, Puertas MC, et al. Therapeutic vaccination refocuses T-cell responses towards conserved regions of HIV-1 in early treated individuals (BCN 01 study). *EClinicalMedicine.* (2019) 11:65–80. doi: 10.1016/j.eclinm.2019.05.009
13. Hancock G, Morón-López S, Kopycinski J, Puertas MC, Giannoulatou E, Rose A, et al. Evaluation of the immunogenicity and impact on the latent HIV-1 reservoir of a conserved region vaccine, MVA.HIVconsv, in antiretroviral therapy-treated subjects. *J Int AIDS Soc.* (2017) 20:21171. doi: 10.7448/IAS.20.1.21171
14. Tebas P, Stein D, Tang WW, Frank I, Wang SQ, Lee G, et al. Gene editing of CCR5 in autologous CD4 T cells of persons infected with HIV. *N Engl J Med.* (2014) 370:901–10. doi: 10.1056/NEJMoa1300662
15. Wang CX, Cannon PM. The clinical applications of genome editing in HIV. *Blood.* (2016) 127:2546–52. doi: 10.1182/blood-2016-01-678144
16. Ververis K, Karagiannis TC. Potential non-oncological applications of histone deacetylase inhibitors. *Am J Transl Res.* (2011) 3:454–67.
17. Archin NM, Liberty AL, Kashuba AD, Choudhary SK, Kuruc JD, Crooks AM, et al. Administration of vorinostat disrupts HIV-1 latency in patients on antiretroviral therapy. *Nature.* (2012) 487:482–5. doi: 10.1038/nature11286
18. Wei DG, Chiang V, Fyne E, Balakrishnan M, Barnes T, Graupe M, et al. Histone deacetylase inhibitor romidepsin induces HIV expression in CD4 T cells from patients on suppressive antiretroviral therapy at concentrations achieved by clinical dosing. *PLoS Pathog.* (2014) 10:e1004071. doi: 10.1371/journal.ppat.1004071
19. Rasmussen TA, Tolstrup M, Brinkmann CR, Olesen R, Erikstrup C, Solomon A, et al. Panobinostat, a histone deacetylase inhibitor, for latent-virus reactivation in HIV-infected patients on suppressive antiretroviral therapy: a phase 1/2, single group, clinical trial. *Lancet HIV.* (2014) 1:e13–21. doi: 10.1016/S2352-3018(14)70014-1
20. Elliott JH, Wightman F, Solomon A, Ghneim K, Ahlers J, Cameron MJ, et al. Activation of HIV transcription with short-course vorinostat in HIV-infected patients on suppressive antiretroviral therapy. *PLoS Pathog.* (2014) 10:e1004473. doi: 10.1371/journal.ppat.1004473
21. Archin NM, Bateson R, Tripathy MK, Crooks AM, Yang K-H, Dahl NP, et al. HIV-1 expression within resting CD4+ T cells after multiple doses of vorinostat. *J Infect Dis.* (2014) 210:728–35. doi: 10.1093/infdis/jiu155
22. Søgaard OS, Graversen ME, Leth S, Olesen R, Brinkmann CR, Nissen SK, et al. The depsipeptide romidepsin reverses HIV-1 latency *in vivo*. *PLoS Pathog.* (2015) 11:1–22. doi: 10.1371/journal.ppat.1005142
23. Kim YH, Demierre M-F, Kim EJ, Lerner A, Rook AH, Duvic M, et al. Clinically meaningful reduction in pruritus in patients with cutaneous T-cell lymphoma treated with romidepsin. *Leuk Lymphoma.* (2013) 54:284–289. doi: 10.3109/10428194.2012.711829
24. Rasmussen TA, Søgaard OS, Brinkmann C, Wightman F, Lewin SR, Melchjorsen J, et al. Comparison of HDAC inhibitors in clinical development: Effect on HIV production in latently infected cells and T-cell activation. *Hum Vaccines Immunother.* (2013) 9:993–1001. doi: 10.4161/hv.23800
25. Leth S, Schleimann MH, Nissen SK, Højen JF, Olesen R, Graversen ME, et al. Combined effect of Vacc-4x, recombinant human granulocyte macrophage colony-stimulating factor vaccination, and romidepsin on the HIV-1 reservoir (REDUC): a single-arm, phase 1B/2A trial. *Lancet HIV.* (2016) 3:e463–72. doi: 10.1016/S2352-3018(16)30055-8
26. Shan L, Deng K, Shroff NS, Durand CM, Rabi SA, Yang HC, et al. Stimulation of HIV-1-Specific cytolytic T lymphocytes facilitates elimination

of latent viral reservoir after virus reactivation. *Immunity*. (2012) 36:491–501. doi: 10.1016/j.immuni.2012.01.014
27. Mothe B. Therapeutic vaccines after early ART: impact on reservoir. In: *Oral session on Therapeutic Vaccines and Cure Strategies at the Joint Keystone Symposia on HIV Vaccines and Functional Cures and the Eradication of HIV, 2019 Mar 24–28*. Whistler, BC (2019).
28. Jones RB, Connor RO, Mueller S, Foley M, Szeto GL, Karel D, et al. Histone deacetylase inhibitors impair the elimination of HIV-infected cells by cytotoxic T-Lymphocytes. (2014) 10:e1004287. doi: 10.1371/journal.ppat.1004287
29. Jones RB, Mueller S, Connor RO, Rimpel K, Sloan D, Karel D, et al. A subset of latency-reversing agents expose HIV-infected resting CD4 + T-cells to recognition by cytotoxic T-lymphocytes. (2016) 12:1–25. doi: 10.1371/journal.ppat.1005545
30. Roederer M, Nozzi JL, Nason MC. SPICE: exploration and analysis of post-cytometric complex multivariate datasets. *Cytometry A*. (2011) 79:167–74. doi: 10.1002/cyto.a.21015
31. Yang H, Wu H, Hancock G, Clutton G, Sande N, Xu X, et al. Antiviral inhibitory capacity of CD8+ T cells predicts the rate of CD4+ T-cell decline in HIV-1 infection. *J Infect Dis*. (2012) 206:552–61. doi: 10.1093/infdis/jis379
32. Zhao M, De Crignis E, Rokx C, Verbon A, van Gelder T, Mahmoudi T, et al. T cell toxicity of HIV latency reversing agents. *Pharmacol Res*. (2019) 139:524–34. doi: 10.1016/j.phrs.2018.10.023
33. Clutton G, Xu Y, Baldoni PL, Mollan KR, Kirchherr J, Newhard W, et al. The differential short- and long-term effects of HIV-1 latency-reversing agents on T cell function. *Sci Rep*. (2016) 6:30749. doi: 10.1038/srep30749
34. Tapia G, Højen JF, Ökvist M, Olesen R, Leth S, Nissen SK, et al. Sequential Vacc-4x and romidepsin during combination antiretroviral therapy (cART): Immune responses to Vacc-4x regions on p24 and changes in HIV reservoirs. *J Infect*. (2017) 75:555–71. doi: 10.1016/j.jinf.2017.09.004
35. Ruiz-Riol M, Brander C. Can we just kick-and-kill HIV: possible challenges posed by the epigenetically controlled interplay between HIV and host immunity. *Immunotherapy*. (2019) 11:931–5. doi: 10.2217/imt-2019-0092
36. Pace M, Williams J, Kurioka A, Gerry AB, Jakobsen B, Klenerman P, et al. Histone deacetylase inhibitors enhance CD4 T Cell susceptibility to NK cell killing but reduce NK Cell function. *PLoS Pathog*. (2016) 12:e1005782. doi: 10.1371/journal.ppat.1005782
37. Garrido C, Spivak AM, Soriano-Sarabia N, Checkley MA, Barker E, Karn J, et al. HIV latency-reversing agents have diverse effects on natural killer cell function. *Front Immunol*. (2016) 7:356. doi: 10.3389/fimmu.2016.00356
38. Gómez CE, Perdiguero B, García-Arriaza J, Cepeda V, Sánchez-Sorzano CÓ, Mothe B, et al. A phase I randomized therapeutic MVA-B vaccination improves the magnitude and quality of the T cell immune responses in HIV-1-infected subjects on HAART. *PLoS ONE*. (2015) 10:e0141456. doi: 10.1371/journal.pone.0141456
39. Sung JA, Lam S, Garrido C, Archin N, Rooney CM, Bollard CM, et al. Expanded cytotoxic T-cell lymphocytes target the latent HIV reservoir. *J Infect Dis*. (2015) 212:258–63. doi: 10.1093/infdis/jiv022
40. Walker-Sperling VE, Pohlmeyer CW, Veenhuis RT, May M, Luna KA, Kirkpatrick AR, et al. Factors associated with the control of viral replication and virologic breakthrough in a recently infected HIV-1 controller. *EBioMedicine*. (2017) 16:141–9. doi: 10.1016/j.ebiom.2017.01.034
41. Payne RP, Kløverpris H, Sacha JB, Brumme Z, Brumme C, Buus S, et al. Efficacious early antiviral activity of HIV Gag- and Pol-specific HLA-B*2705-restricted CD8 + T Cells. *J Virol*. (2010) 84:10543–57. doi: 10.1128/JVI.00793-10
42. Salido J, Ruiz MJ, Trifone C, Figueroa MI, Caruso MP, Gherardi MM, et al. Phenotype, polyfunctionality, and antiviral activity of *in vitro* stimulated CD8+ T-cells from HIV+ subjects who initiated cART at different time-points after acute infection. *Front Immunol*. (2018) 9:2443. doi: 10.3389/fimmu.2018.02443
43. Ruiz-Riol M, Llano A, Ibarrondo J, Zamarreño J, Yusim K, Bach V, et al. Alternative effector-function profiling identifies broad HIV-specific T-cell responses in highly HIV-exposed individuals who remain uninfected. *J Infect Dis*. (2015) 211:936–46. doi: 10.1093/infdis/jiu534
44. Rosas-Umbert M, Llano A, Olvera A, Ruiz-riol M, Rocafort M, Cobarsi P, et al. Mechanisms of abrupt loss of virus control in a cohort of previous HIV controllers. *J Virol*. (2019) 93:e01436-18. doi: 10.1128/JVI.01436-18
45. Migueles SA, Osborne CM, Royce C, Compton AA, Joshi RP, Weeks KA, et al. Lytic granule loading of CD8+ T cells is required for HIV-infected cell elimination associated with immune control. *Immunity*. (2008) 29:1009–1021. doi: 10.1016/j.immuni.2008.10.010

11

Multivariate Computational Analysis of Gamma Delta T Cell Inhibitory Receptor Signatures Reveals the Divergence of Healthy and ART-Suppressed HIV+ Aging

Anna C. Belkina[1,2], Alina Starchenko[3], Katherine A. Drake[4], Elizabeth A. Proctor[3], Riley M. F. Pihl[1], Alex Olson[5], Douglas A. Lauffenburger[3], Nina Lin[5†] and Jennifer E. Snyder-Cappione[1,6†]*

[1] Flow Cytometry Core Facility, Boston University School of Medicine, Boston, MA, United States, [2] Department of Pathology and Laboratory Medicine, Boston University School of Medicine, Boston, MA, United States, [3] Department of Biological Engineering, Massachusetts Institute of Technology, Cambridge, MA, United States, [4] Cytobank, Inc., Santa Clara, CA, United States, [5] Department of Medicine, Boston University School of Medicine, Boston, MA, United States, [6] Department of Microbiology, Boston University School of Medicine, Boston, MA, United States

***Correspondence:**
Jennifer E. Snyder-Cappione
cappione@bu.edu

†These authors have contributed equally to this work

Even with effective viral control, HIV-infected individuals are at a higher risk for morbidities associated with older age than the general population, and these serious non-AIDS events (SNAEs) track with plasma inflammatory and coagulation markers. The cell subsets driving inflammation in aviremic HIV infection are not yet elucidated. Also, whether ART-suppressed HIV infection causes premature induction of the inflammatory events found in uninfected elderly or if a novel inflammatory network ensues when HIV and older age co-exist is unclear. In this study we measured combinational expression of five inhibitory receptors (IRs) on seven immune cell subsets and 16 plasma markers from peripheral blood mononuclear cells (PBMC) and plasma samples, respectively, from a HIV and Aging cohort comprised of ART-suppressed HIV-infected and uninfected controls stratified by age ($\leq$35 or $\geq$50 years old). For data analysis, multiple multivariate computational algorithms [cluster identification, characterization, and regression (CITRUS), partial least squares regression (PLSR), and partial least squares-discriminant analysis (PLS-DA)] were used to determine if immune parameter disparities can distinguish the subject groups and to investigate if there is a cross-impact of aviremic HIV and age on immune signatures. IR expression on gamma delta ($\gamma\delta$) T cells exclusively separated HIV+ subjects from controls in CITRUS analyses and secretion of inflammatory cytokines and cytotoxic mediators from $\gamma\delta$ T cells tracked with TIGIT expression among HIV+ subjects. Also, plasma markers predicted the percentages of TIGIT+ $\gamma\delta$ T cells in subjects with and without HIV in PSLR models, and a PLS-DA model of γδ T cell IR signatures and plasma markers significantly stratified all four of the subject groups (uninfected younger, uninfected older, HIV+ younger, and HIV+ older). These data implicate γδ T cells as an inflammatory driver in ART-suppressed HIV infection and provide evidence of distinct "inflamm-aging" processes with and without ART-suppressed HIV infection.

Keywords: γδ T cell, TIGIT, HIV, aging, inflammation, citrus, immune exhaustion, checkpoint inhibition

INTRODUCTION

Although anti-retroviral therapy (ART) has dramatically reduced the rates of HIV-associated morbidity and mortality, HIV+ individuals have a shorter lifespan than uninfected counterparts (1–3) due in part to the onset and progression of co-morbidities associated with older age, including cardiovascular disease, stroke, neurocognitive impairment, diabetes mellitus, impaired renal function, non-AIDS malignancies, and osteoporosis (4–6). These conditions, sometimes referred to as serious non-AIDS events (SNAEs), afflict older HIV+ individuals more frequently than both younger counterparts (4, 6) and the uninfected elderly (6) and SNAE disease onset is reported to occur at younger ages in aviremic HIV+ individuals as compared with uninfected controls (5, 7), with the latter observations supporting the concept of HIV+ persons undergoing early or accelerated aging (8). Mortality and age-associated co-morbidities among HIV+ individuals track with plasma inflammatory and coagulation markers, such as C-reactive protein (CRP), IL-6, D-dimer, and fibrinogen (9–14), similar to the general population (15–21). These findings strongly implicate the general inflammation associated with aging, sometimes referred to as "inflamm-aging" (22, 23), as an integral link to SNAE occurrence in aviremic HIV infection.

Gamma delta (γδ) T cells are a unique T cell lineage that is typically <10% of T cells in the circulation yet are present in considerably higher proportions in the intestinal epithelium (24–27). With a limited T cell receptor repertoire and evidence indicating that a predominant mode of cell activation is in response to non-peptidic ligands, cytokines, and signaling via NKG2D and similar receptors (28–35), γδ T cells are implicated as early responders in immune responses and/or as innate-adaptive bridging cells, responding to innate signals to then direct the development of the adaptive immune response via secretion of cytokines and other factors. As a population, γδ T cells can exert inflammatory/cytotoxic (36, 37) or immuno-regulatory effector functions (38, 39), are integral to the control of infections (40, 41), and can exhibit potent anti-tumor activity (42–44). The role of γδ T cells in HIV viral pathogenesis is unclear to date; shifts in γδ T cell subsets defined by T cell receptor usage (Vδ1 and Vδ2) occur early in infection (45) due to a substantial loss of the Vγ2-Jγ1.2/Vδ2+ subset that is not always recovered with viral suppression (46). However, functional differences between γδ T cell subsets that differ in γ and δ chain usage are not well-established and therefore the significance of this subset shift in relation to disease pathogenesis is uncertain. Also, circulating γδ T cells serve as a reservoir for latent HIV infection (47) and thus may have relevance in cure strategies. To date, the role of γδ T cells in the inflammation observed in aviremic HIV infection is unknown.

To understand the cellular network that drives the onset and progression of age-associated morbidities in both ART-suppressed (aviremic) HIV and healthy aging, we conducted a study that measured a large number of immune parameters from a well-characterized HIV and Aging cohort, comprised of both ART-suppressed HIV+ and age-matched uninfected controls with similar exposures and demographics, stratified by age in younger and older groups. Our results from multivariate computational analyses of high parameter single cell cytometry, plasma markers, and *ex vivo* culture supernatant cytokine data identify γδ T cells as a putative key player in the immune cell network driving "inflamm-aging" in aviremic HIV infection. Also, our bioinformatic analyses revealed an novel combined impact of both virally suppressed HIV and aging on immune networks, thereby indicating that aviremic HIV+ persons do not simply prematurely age but undergo a novel inflammatory course when these two conditions collide.

RESULTS

Inhibitory Receptor (IR) Expression on γδ T Cells Distinguishes ART-Suppressed HIV+ Subjects From Uninfected Controls

Expression of IRs has been linked to altered functionality of immune cells (48–51). While increased IR expression on T cell populations has been reported with aging in mice and humans (52–56), and separately with HIV infection (49, 57–59), a more comprehensive investigation of IR signatures on circulating immune cells from matched younger and older subjects with and without ART-suppressed HIV infection had not been performed to our knowledge. Therefore, in this study we analyzed PBMC from our HIV and Aging Cohort, comprised of ART-suppressed HIV+ younger (≤35 yo), and older (≥50 yo) subjects age-matched with uninfected counterparts (**Table 1**). We measured five inhibitory receptors (PD-1, TIGIT, TIM-3, CD160, LAG-3) on seven immune cell subsets [CD4+ T, CD8+ T, T regulatory (Treg), $CD56^{bright}$ and $CD56^{dim}$ natural killer (NK), gamma delta T (γδ T), and invariant natural killer T (iNKT) cells] using the 16-color flow cytometry panel we developed and previously described (60). Using the CITRUS algorithm (61) we determined whether IR expression on any of the immune subsets (**Supplementary Figure 1**) could be used to distinguish ART-suppressed HIV+ subjects from uninfected controls. Using 10-fold cross-validation (CV) to select the model with the minimum number of features necessary to predict these two groups, only

TABLE 1 | Cohort characteristics.

	Uninfected controls		ART-suppressed HIV+[a]			
	Younger (≤35)	Older (≥50)	Younger (≤35)		Older (≥50)	
n	21	21	22		28	
Age (mean,range)	27 (22–35)	58 (50–72)	28 (22–33)		58 (50–76)	
Sex (%M/F)	100/0	100/0	100/0		86/14	
Ethnicity (C/B/A/O)[b]	15/3/3/0	11/6/3/2	17/3/1/0		18/10/0/0	
CD4 count (cells/mm^3, mean, range)[c]			611 (89–1,362)		719 (246–1,216)	
ART duration (years)			**Mean**	***n***	**Mean**	***n***
0–5	–	–	2.2	19	2.9	17
5–10	–	–	6.2	3	6.8	6
>10	–	–	–	0	16.5	5
Nadir CD4 count (cells/mm^3)			**Mean**	***n***	**Mean**	***n***
0–250	–	–	159	6	133	9
251–500	–	–	339	11	311	12
>501	–	–	649	5	680	6

[a]Undetectable HIV-1 viral loads for ≥ 6months; [b]Caucasian/Black/Asian/other; [c]Values within 1 year of enrollment.

TIGIT expression in four cellular clusters comprised of γδ T cells (**Figure 1A**, clusters 1–4 in red circles), was necessary to differentiate the two subject groups with 88.6% CV accuracy (**Supplementary Figure 1**). In all four clusters, TIGIT expression was higher in the ART-suppressed HIV+ subjects compared to the uninfected controls (**Figure 1B**). Expression of other surface antigens on the cells in clusters 1–4 was similar for CD4 and CD127 (all negative), CD56 (all clusters intermediate) and varied for other antigens, such as CD8 (low in cluster 1, intermediate in clusters 2–4), CD16 (intermediate in clusters 1, 2, and 4, and low in cluster 3), and CD3 (all four clusters positive, with cluster 3 intermediate) (**Figure 1C**). Next, a false discovery rate (FDR) threshold of 1% was used to identify all clusters that were significantly different between the two subject groups using IR expression differences. Using this method, seven clusters were significant and they all contained γδ T cells (**Figure 1D**); all seven clusters differed in TIGIT expression between the HIV+ subjects and uninfected controls, one (cluster 3) differed in CD160 expression, and one (cluster 4) differed in TIM-3 expression between the two subject groups. Six of the seven TIGIT expression clusters contain only or predominantly γδ T cells (**Supplementary Figure 1**, **Figure 1F**), with one cluster (cluster 5) containing both NK and γδ T cells; however, it is likely that γδ T cells are the sole driver of this finding given the γδ T predominance in all other clusters. Similar to the 10-fold CV results (**Figure 1B**), the expression of the defining IR for clusters 3–7 was consistently higher in the HIV+ subject group compared to uninfected controls (**Figure 1E**). Further phenotypic analysis of the three additional clusters that emerged from the FDR-constrained analysis (clusters 5, 6, and 7) show the presence of NK cells in cluster 5 (CD3-, CD16/56+), while clusters 6 and 7 are predominantly CD16-, CD56-, CD4-, CD8-, and γδ TcR^{lo} (**Figure 1F**). Together, these data demonstrate that the IR expression on circulating γδ T cells distinguishes ART-suppressed HIV+ subjects from uninfected controls. Also, the γδ T cell subsets that predict these two subject groups are diverse, including populations that differ in CD8, CD16, CD56, and CD127 expression.

γδ T Cell IR Expression Increases With Age and HIV Infection

We next investigated γδ T cells in more detail by performing traditional expert-driven gating and analysis. We first determined the frequencies and absolute counts of γδ T cells (gating strategy shown in **Supplementary Figure 2A**) and found overall similar γδ T cell levels within the HIV+ and uninfected control groups (**Supplementary Figures 2B–E**). We next measured Vδ1+ and Vδ2+ γδ T cell frequencies from a subset of samples and found an inversion of the Vδ1:Vδ2 ratio in the HIV+ subjects compared to the uninfected group, confirming that the findings in our cohort are consistent with previous reports (45, 62) (**Supplementary Figures 2F–I**). Next, we compared the percentages of IR+ γδ T cells between the ART-suppressed HIV+ and control groups and found that the HIV+ subjects expressed significantly higher frequencies of TIGIT+, CD160+, and TIM-3+ cells than age-matched controls (**Figure 2A**). As TIM-3 and LAG-3 are not bimodally expressed, setting flow cytometry gates to determine the percentage of positive cells is difficult; therefore, we also calculated the median expression of each IR and found significantly higher levels of TIM-3 but not LAG-3 on the γδ T cells from the HIV+ subjects compared with controls (**Figure 2B**). As expression of more than one IR on individual γδ T cells could reflect distinct states of activation or an advanced stage of immune exhaustion (63), we compared the expression of ≥2, ≥3, or ≥4 IRs per γδ T cell between our HIV+ and uninfected control subjects and found significantly higher levels in the HIV+ subjects for all comparisons (**Figure 2C**). To control for bias due to manual gating, γδ T cell events were extracted from the flow cytometry data using SPADE clustering

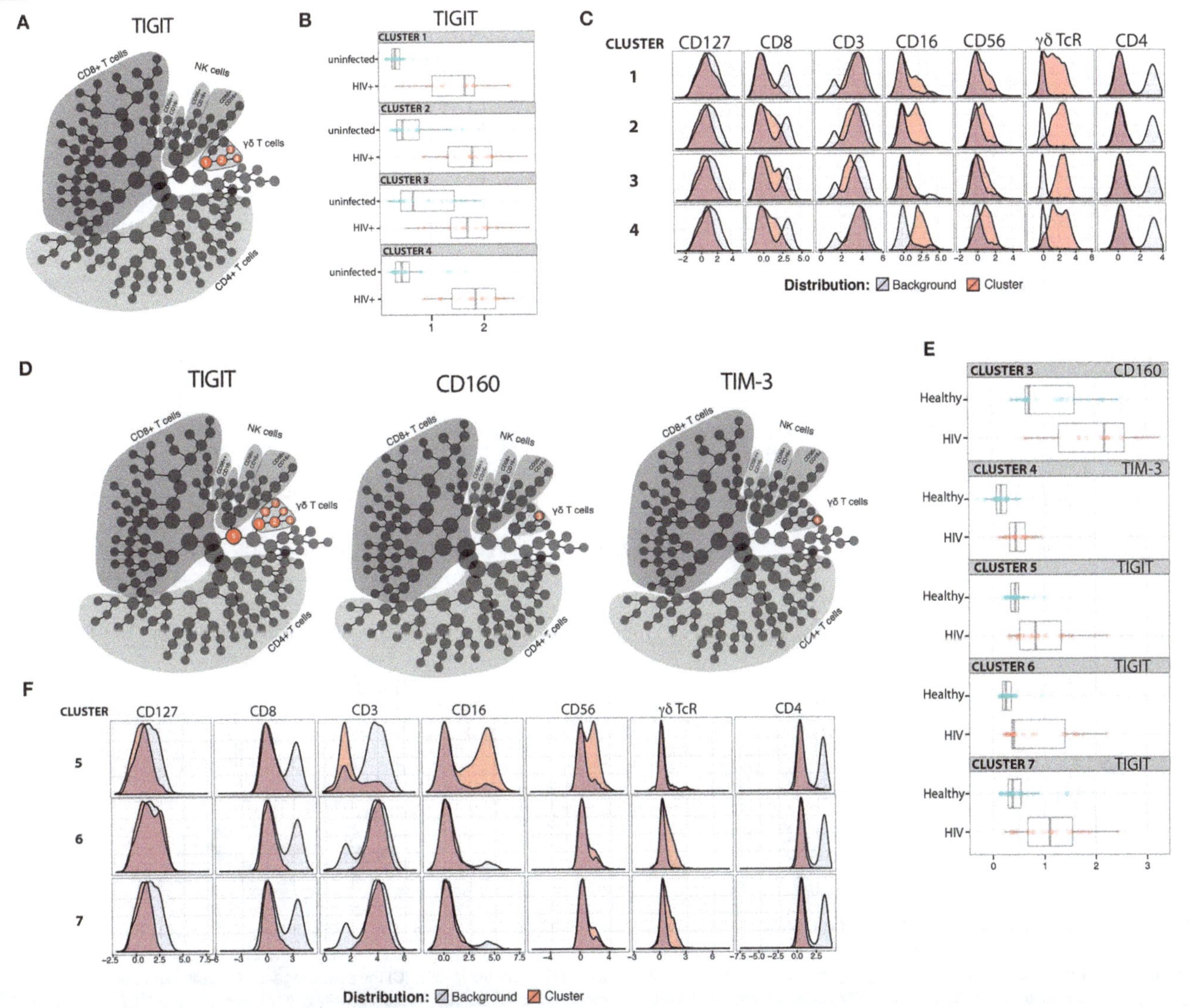

FIGURE 1 | TIGIT, CD160, and TIM-3 on γδ T cells distinguish ART-suppressed HIV+ subjects from uninfected controls. CITRUS analysis of a 16-parameter flow cytometry dataset from PBMC of ART-suppressed HIV+ subjects and uninfected controls. **(A)** Model selected by minimum cross-validated error rate yielded four clusters necessary to differentiate the groups, numbered 1–4 and highlighted in red. **(B)** TIGIT expression of cells in clusters 1–4 in the ART-suppressed HIV+ (red) and uninfected control (blue) groups, log-transformed Mean Fluorescence Intensity (MFI) is shown, and each dot represents one subject, **(C)** expression of other measured antigens on cells from clusters 1–4 as compared to all other (background) cells; **(D)** Model constrained to include all significant clusters below a FDR threshold of 1% reveals seven clusters with significantly different expression of TIGIT, CD160, and/or TIM-3 between the groups, **(E)** log-transformed MFI of CD160, TIM-3, and TIGIT expression per subject for clusters 3, 4, and 5–7, respectively, and **(F)** expression of other measured antigens on cells from clusters 5, 6, and 7. All scales in **(B,C,E,F)** are log-transformed. CITRUS clustering data per lineage channel are shown in **Supplementary Figure 1**.

(64) and γδ T cell IR median expression was assessed (LAG-3 not shown due to negligible results), confirming our manual gating findings (data not shown) and allowing visualization of IR expression from individual subjects (**Figure 2D**). Overall patterns indicate higher IR expression of the ART-suppressed HIV+ subjects compared with controls and also seemingly independent regulation of each of the four IRs within individual subjects. Next, subjects were further stratified into the younger and older groups as defined in **Table 1** and the percentages of IR+ γδ T cells were compared (**Figure 2E**). TIGIT+ γδ T cells were significantly higher in: (1) older vs. younger uninfected subjects, (2) HIV+ younger vs. uninfected younger subjects, (3) HIV+ older vs. uninfected older subjects, and (4) HIV older vs. uninfected younger subjects (**Figure 2E**). Analysis of the other IRs did not result in significant differences between the groups, with the exception of TIM-3 expression of the uninfected younger vs. HIV+ younger subjects (**Figure 2E**). Comparison of multi-IR expression with subjects stratified by both age and HIV status shows higher percentages of ≥2IR per cell with advancing age and with HIV infection. Notably, for all analyses in **Figures 2E,F**, no significant differences were found between the HIV+ younger and HIV+ older groups, indicating a lack of

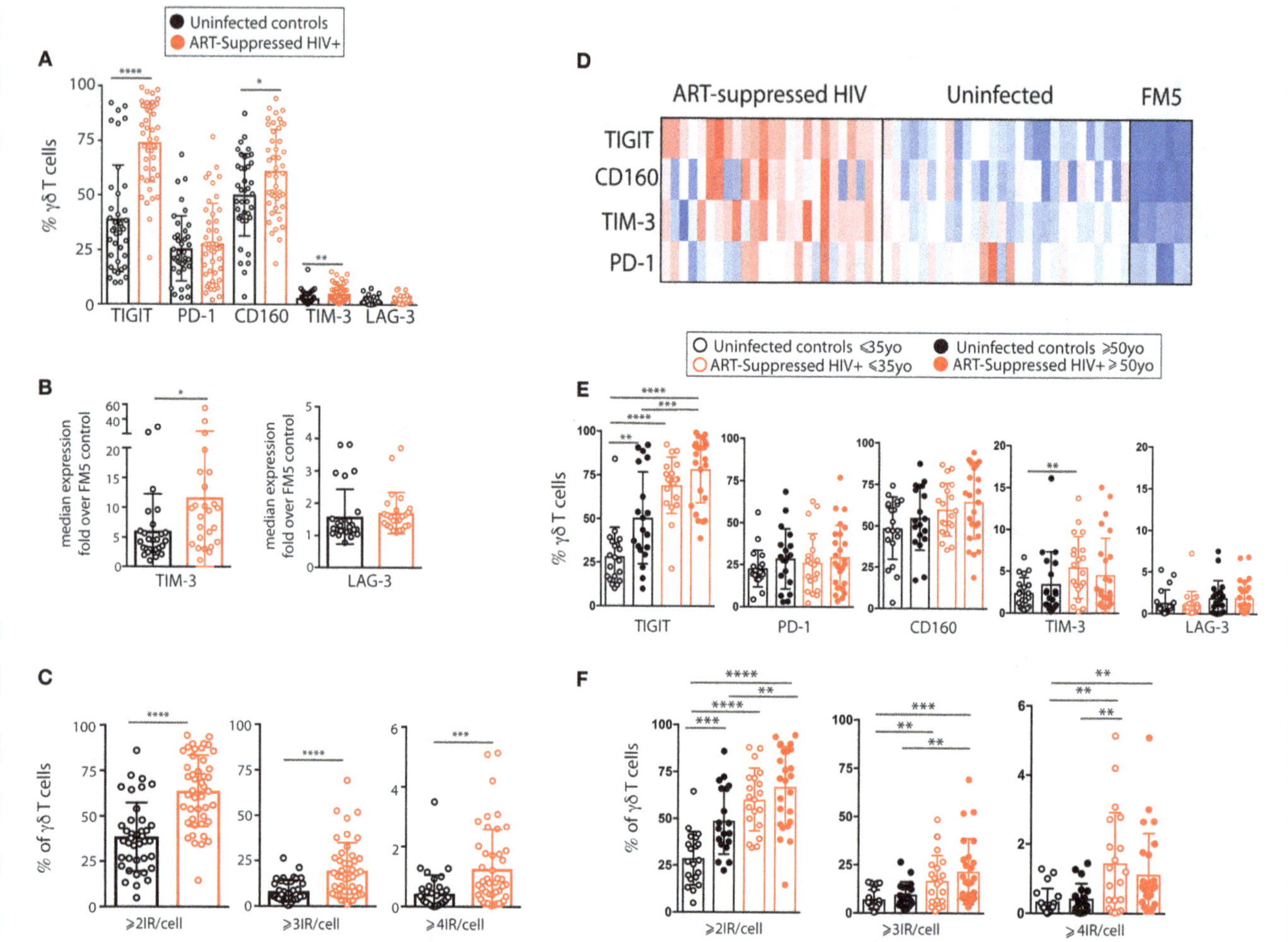

FIGURE 2 | IR expression on γδ T cells from ART-suppressed HIV+ subjects and uninfected controls stratified into younger and older groups. **(A)** The total percentages of IR+ γδ T cells in ART-suppressed HIV+ subjects and uninfected control groups; **(B)** the average fluorescence intensity of γδ T cell TIM-3 and LAG-3 expression for HIV+ and uninfected subjects, determined by median intensity divided by FM5 control results; **(C)** the percentage of γδ T cells expressing ≥2, ≥3, or ≥4 IRs, in any combination, of CD160, TIGIT, TIM-3, LAG-3, and PD-1 in HIV+ subjects and controls, **(D)** median intensity of IR expression on SPADE-identified γδ T cells per individual (one subject per column), including FM5 uninfected control samples from each batch run; **(E)** total percentages of IR+ γδ T cells and **(F)** percentages of γδ T cells expressing ≥2, ≥3, or ≥4 IRs, in any combination, of TIGIT, PD-1, CD160, TIM-3, and LAG-3, with subjects stratified by both HIV status and age. For **(A–C)**, two-tailed *t*-tests were performed for each comparison. For graphs with multiple comparisons **(E,F)** only significant results after Bonferroni correction ($p < 0.008$) are shown. *$p > 0.05$, **$p > 0.01$, ***$p > 0.001$, ****$p > 0.0001$.

a definitive additive or multiplicative effect of both age and HIV on γδ T cell IR expression found with univariate analysis. Also, HIV infection and not aging appears to drive γδ T cells to express ≥3 or ≥4 IR per cell (**Figure 2F**). Taken together, these results suggest that healthy aging and HIV infection independently drive TIGIT and multi-IR expression on γδ T cells, that IR expression does not change significantly as aviremic HIV+ individuals age, and HIV and not aging drives γδ T cells to a ≥3 or ≥4 IR per cell phenotype.

γδ T Cells Expressing Distinct Combinations of PD-1, TIGIT, and CD160 Vary With Aging and Aviremic HIV Infection

We next investigated how the combinational expression of PD-1, TIGIT, and CD160 on γδ T cells differed with healthy aging and ART-suppressed HIV infection. Due to the non-bimodal expression of TIM-3 and LAG-3 on the γδ T cells in our cohort, it was not possible to accurately define positive and negative cells for the multi-expression analysis shown in **Figure 3**. First, the percentage of γδ T cells expressing each of the eight possible combinations of these three IRs were compared across the four subject groups using beta regression of abundance on HIV status and age and correcting for multiple hypotheses testing with a family-wise error rate of 0.05. Both aging and HIV infection were significantly associated with lower percentages of PD-1- TIGIT- CD160- ("triple negative") and PD-1- TIGIT- CD160+ ("CD160 only") cells. HIV infection was also associated with a lower percentage of PD-1+ TIGIT- CD160- ("PD-1 only") cells and a higher percentage of three populations: PD-1- TIGIT+ CD160- ("TIGIT+ only"), PD1-, TIGIT+ CD160+ ("TIGIT and CD160 double positive") and

PD-1+ TIGIT+ CD160+ ("triple positive") cells (**Figure 3A**). Similar to the results for HIV infection, there were higher average frequencies of TIGIT only and TIGIT and CD160 double positive cells in older compared with younger uninfected subjects (albeit not statistically significant). To further assess the potential relationships between γδ T cells bearing different IR combinations, Pearson correlation coefficients were generated for the percentages of all eight possible IR combinations with one another in a pair-wise manner separately for the uninfected controls (**Figure 3B**) and ART-suppressed HIV+ subjects (**Figure 3C**). Within the uninfected group, strong inverse correlations were found that agree with the results in **Figure 3A**, specifically, the triple negative and CD160 only populations with the TIGIT single positive and the TIGIT CD160 double positive cells (**Figure 3B**, asterisks). Within the HIV+ group, there were also strong inverse correlations of the triple negative/CD160 only populations, in this case with the TIGIT CD160 double positive cells as well as the triple positive cells (**Figure 3C**, asterisks). These data suggest that both aging and HIV infection skew the circulating γδ T cell compartment from predominantly triple negative and CD160 only expressing cells to TIGIT only and CD160 TIGIT double positive cells (**Figure 3D**). The triple positive γδ T cell population, while inversely associated with no IR expressing cells in both uninfected controls and HIV+ subjects, is higher in frequency only of the HIV+ subjects compared with controls, and not between the uninfected younger and older groups. Taken together, these data suggest that the triple negative and CD160 only γδ T cell populations are a resting/precursor population to the subsets expressing TIGIT alone, TIGIT with CD160, and TIGIT, CD160, and PD-1, and such IR expression is suggestive of an activated or exhausted state (63, 65).

Spontaneous Secretion of Inflammatory Cytokines and Cytotoxic Mediators From γδ T Cells Differentially Tracks With TIGIT Expression During Aging +/- Aviremic HIV Infection

As an indirect measurement of the potential *in vivo* functional activity of the γδ T cells, cells were sorted and cultured overnight without stimulation and the secretion of 33 analytes was measured in the supernatants. The spontaneous release of sCD137, a marker of cell activation that correlates with circulating C-reactive protein (CRP) in plasma (66) and is positively associated with both acute coronary syndromes (66) and stroke (67), was significantly higher from the γδ T cells of HIV+ older subjects compared with the other three groups (**Figure 4A**, results from the other detected analytes are shown in **Supplementary Figure 4**). As each sample stained with the 16-color panel was run through the FACSARIA cell sorter, the percentages of TIGIT+ γδ T cells were determined and the γδ T cells were sorted for cell culture simultaneously. Ten analytes significantly correlated with percentages of defined IR-expressing γδ T cell subsets (**Figure 3D**) from either the HIV+ and/or the uninfected subject group (**Figure 4B**). Of the HIV+ data, 14 of the 15 significant results included negative correlations with "resting" and positive correlations with "activated/exhausted" populations as defined in **Figure 3D**; this suggests progression from a resting to an activated state with HIV infection. Next, we used linear regression to relate levels of eleven analytes detected in the supernatants of a substantial percentage (≥45%) of the subjects with the percentage of TIGIT+ γδ T cells (eight are shown in **Figure 4C**, three in **Supplementary Figure 4**). Of the analytes that were produced by <45% of the subjects, the average number of subjects whose γδ T cells produced the cytokine was only nine per cent. Therefore, we set 45% as the cutoff of "positive" responses by the cohort. All data where a detectable amount of analyte was found from at least one subject is included in **Supplementary Figure 4B**). Overall, of γδ T cells from the uninfected controls, the TIGIT+ percentages did not associate with cytokine release (**Figures 4B,C**), with the exception of MIP1-β, which showed a negative correlation. Conversely, the percentage of TIGIT+ γδ T cells from the ART-suppressed HIV+ subjects positively and significantly correlated with the secretion of five analytes: sCD137, Granzyme A, Granzyme B, MIP1-β, and CCL20/MIP3-α and showed a positive trend for others such as perforin, TNF-α, and IFN-γ (**Figures 4B,C**). Also, there is a notable trend of lower analyte release of γδ T cells from the older compared with younger uninfected subjects, and a converse trend of increased analyte secretion with older age within the HIV+ subject group. These data suggest unlike the uninfected controls, the γδ T cells from ART-suppressed HIV+ subjects are activated, secreting inflammatory factors *in vivo,* and possibly contributing to the inflammatory milieu linked to SNAEs in this population, and that TIGIT expression marks inflammatory activity of γδ T cells from aviremic HIV+ subjects. To further explore the relationships between TIGIT expression and *ex vivo* analyte production by γδ T cells in the HIV+ subjects vs. controls, two partial least square regression (PLSR) models (one for uninfected controls, one for HIV+ subjects) were generated to specifically ask if cytokine measurements in the supernatants can predict the percentage of TIGIT+ cells in the PBMC samples. In PLSR modeling, linear combinations of analytes are used to predict the variance in the dependent variables (68, 69), in this case the percentage of TIGIT+ cells. PLSR analysis is more potent than simple regression analyses when the behavior of multiple analytes of interest is known to be interdependent, since it enables determination of the combinations of analytes that maximally correlate with TIGIT expression. Analyte measurements were compressed in low-dimensional latent variable (LV) space; notably, the younger and older subjects separated into distinct groups for each model without the models being trained on age parameter (**Figures 4D,E** left panels). Both models significantly linked spontaneous analyte production with TIGIT expression by γδ T cells. VIP (variable importance of projection) calculation was then used to assess the importance of each analyte variable with values >1 considered influential above average in the model. Notably, the VIP (statistically significant) analytes within each model were different (**Figures 4D,E** right panels, light blue bars), confirming that there are distinct associations between TIGIT expression and the cytokines produced from γδ T cells of both HIV+ subjects and uninfected controls. These findings indicate that relationships between γδ T cell TIGIT expression

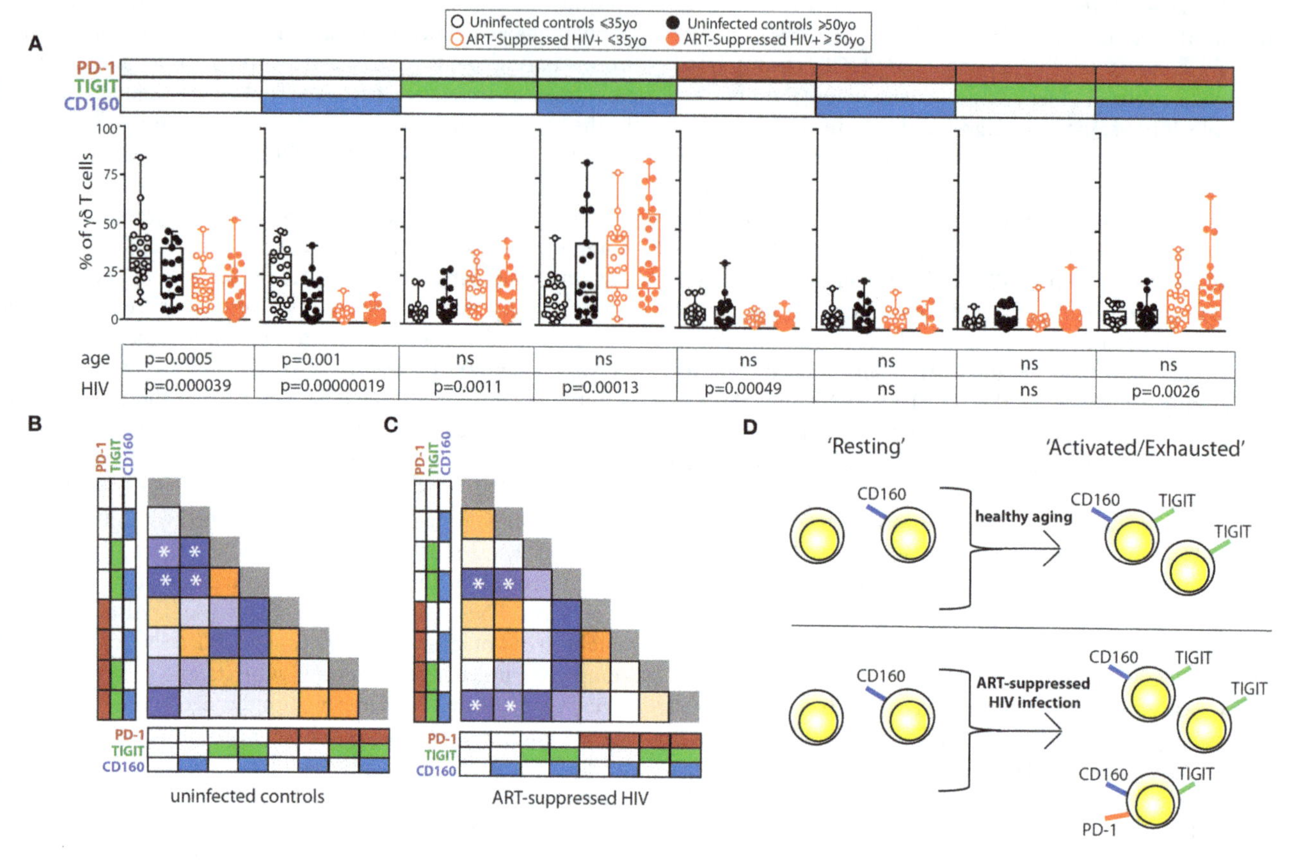

FIGURE 3 | Inhibitory receptor signatures of γδ T cells vary with aging, ART-suppressed HIV infection. **(A)** γδ T cell IR signature analysis of TIGIT, CD160, and PD-1 comparing younger and older subjects and ART-suppressed HIV+ and matched uninfected control groups. Positivity of PD-1, TIGIT, and CD160 is noted above each graph, with the white and colored boxes representing negative and positive expression, respectively. Abundance for each subset of γδ T cells expressing specific IRs was compared across the four groups using beta regression of abundance on HIV status and age group. Significance of age and HIV infection was determined after correcting for multiple hypotheses testing as described in the Materials and Methods section. **(B)** Correlation analysis of the abundances of each IR expressing subset of γδ T cells in uninfected controls and **(C)** ART-suppressed HIV+ subjects. Heatmaps are colored based on strength of the Pearson correlation coefficient between each IR subset (orange: positive, blue: negative). Both age groups are included in each heatmap. The Pearson correlation coefficients and *p*-values for these analyses are shown in **Supplementary Figure 3**. Asterisks indicate biologically interesting correlations used to inform **(D)** diagram depicting the hypothesized differential progression of IR expression due to healthy aging vs. ART-suppressed HIV infection.

and spontaneous cytokine release change with both normal aging and aging with aviremic HIV infection.

Plasma Markers of Inflammation and Coagulation Differentially Track With TIGIT Expression During Aging With and Without ART-Suppressed HIV Infection

We measured the concentrations of 16 analytes in plasma, many of which are well-defined markers of inflammation and have been strongly associated with the onset of co-morbid conditions and/or mortality in HIV-infected populations (10, 13, 70–73) as well as with disease in normal aging (15–21). We found significantly higher levels of sCD14, alpha-2 macroglobulin (A2M), fibrinogen, serum amyloid P (SAP), adipsin, and von Willebrand factor (vWF) in the plasma from HIV+ subjects compared to uninfected controls (**Supplementary Figure 5A**). When the subjects were further stratified by age, we found significant differences among subject groups for D-dimer, C-reactive protein (CRP), fibrinogen, SAP, adipsin, and vWF (**Supplementary Figure 5B**) that seem to be driven by age in uninfected subjects or by HIV infection, with no significant differences found between HIV+ younger and HIV+ older subjects. To determine if there are associations between IR expressing γδ T cell subsets and plasma marker levels, we performed linear regression analysis of the plasma marker data against the percentages of our "resting" or "activated/exhausted" γδ subsets (as defined in **Figure 3D**). Of the 16 analytes measured, nine were significantly associated with one or more γδ T cell IR-defined subset(s) in the uninfected controls and/or the ART-suppressed HIV+ groups (**Figure 5A**). For both the HIV+ and uninfected subject groups, there was a predominant trend of negative association with the "resting" and positive association with the "activated/exhausted" γδ T cell populations with plasma markers (**Figures 5A–E**). Also, it is notable that the younger and older age groups are clearly separated in these analyses among the

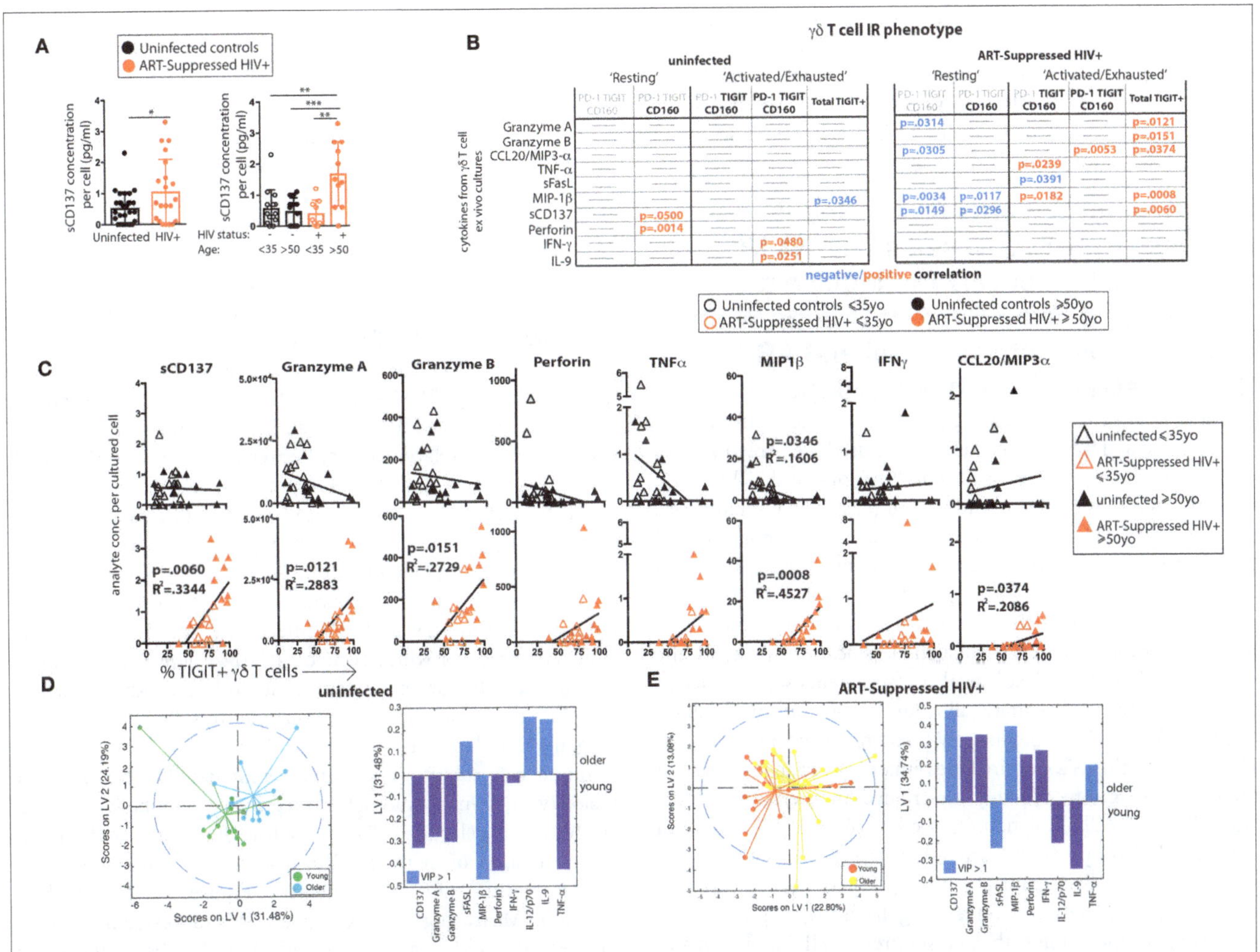

FIGURE 4 | γδ T cell *ex vivo* spontaneous cytokine secretion profiles reveal differential associations with IR expression and age in ART-suppressed HIV infection and uninfected controls. **(A)** sCD137 (pg) secreted per cultured γδ T cell from all HIV+ subjects compared with uninfected controls, and with data also stratified into younger and older sub-groups. **(B)** Tables showing the linear regression analysis results for the 10 analytes that significantly correlated with an IR signature-expressing γδ T cell subset in either subject group as defined in **Figure 3D**. Positive and negative expression of each IR is depicted with black bold and gray lettering, respectively, at the top of each table. **(C)** Linear regression plots of the percentage of TIGIT+ γδ T cells and cytokine concentration (average per cell) for uninfected controls and ART-suppressed HIV+ subjects for the 8 analytes that highlight the opposite trends between the subject groups (results from the other 3 analytes with >45% subject cells responding are shown in **Supplementary Figure 3**). Subjects within the younger and older groups are noted with open and solid triangles, respectively. Units for secreted analytes are as follows: sCD137, Granzyme A, Granzyme B, perforin, MIP-1β; pg/cell; TNF-α, IFN-γ, CCL20/MIP-3 α; pg × 10^4/cell. Scores plot and LV1 derived from a PLSR model of supernatant cytokines regressed against the percentage of TIGIT+ γδ T cells for each donor for uninfected controls **(D)** and ART-suppressed HIV+ subjects **(E)**. Dotted lines in **(D)** and **(E)** show the 95% confidence interval. *$p > 0.05$, **$p > 0.01$, ***$p > 0.001$, ****$p > 0.0001$.

controls but not the HIV-infected subjects (**Figures 5B–E**). These results indicate that TIGIT and multi-IR expression on γδ T cells is linked with the elevated general inflammation found in both healthy aging and ART-suppressed HIV infection, and that HIV appears to generate a new inflammatory status as defined by these plasma markers that is independent of aging. Next, we asked how the concentrations of plasma markers were connected to the percentage of TIGIT+ γδ T cells by training two orthogonalized PLSR models using plasma marker levels to predict the percentage of TIGIT positive cells in the uninfected and HIV+ subject groups (**Figures 5F,G**). We note that the models have differing contributions attributed to each marker (as determined by loadings on LV1), and that different markers emerged as the most important to the correlation of inflammatory state to percent TIGIT positive cells (as determined by VIP score); together, these results indicate that the connections between TIGIT+ γδ T cells and the immune network driving systemic inflammation are fundamentally different between aviremic HIV infection and healthy aging. Notably, this conclusion is based on the multivariate analysis of cytokine profiles that allow analysis of the co-varying multifactorial nature of the data that is characteristic of biological systems (74). Also, similar to the results in **Figures 4D,E**, subjects in the younger and older sub-groups for both uninfected and HIV+ subjects separated without age being added to either model; this indicates that the multivariate analyses (**Figures 5F,G**) reveal age-induced changes in the inflammatory network of ART-suppressed HIV+ subjects that are not apparent in the univariate (linear regression) dataset (**Figures 5A–E, Supplementary Figure 5B**). Overall, our data show that γδ T cells are integral components of distinct inflammatory processes that occur during aging both with and without ART-suppressed HIV infection.

Partial Least Squares Determinant Analysis (PLS-DA) Reveals That γδ IR Signatures Selectively Distinguish the Younger and Older Subject Groups Within Both the Uninfected Control and ART Suppressed HIV+ Subject Groups

To further confirm that the aging process is distinct in uninfected controls and aviremic HIV+ subjects, we used the percentages of γδ T cells expressing all possible combinations of the IRs PD-1, CD160, TIGIT, and TIM-3 and the 16 plasma marker datasets to train a PLS-DA model that determined if a combination of these variables can separate subjects into four groups based on age and HIV status. In the input data, PLS-DA finds which measurements from each subject would "fit" that subject into its clinical group and verifies if such classification is statistically significant. The chosen biological measurements were sufficient to significantly differentiate all four groups in our dataset (**Figure 6A**). In these models, LV1 separated mostly based on HIV status, while LV2 captured the remaining variance attributed mainly to age group. Notably, we trained an alternative model with CD8+ T cell IR signatures used in place of the γδ T cell data and the groups did not separate with significance (data not shown). This analysis indicates that γδ T cells are integral to the inflammatory networks underlying the divergent processes of healthy aging and aging with ART-suppressed HIV infection and we propose that IR expression marks different functional and/or activation/exhaustion states of the γδ T cells in these conditions.

DISCUSSION

In this study, we present evidence that γδ T cells are linked to and may help instigate and perpetuate the elevated inflammation found in aviremic HIV+ individuals, and our multivariate analyses indicate that a distinct inflammatory course occurs during ART-suppressed HIV+ aging. Currently, more than 50% of the HIV-infected population in the U.S. is older than 50 years (75) and the world population over the ages of 65 and 80 is predicted to double and nearly quadruple, respectively, by 2050 (76). Elucidating the cell populations and precise immune networks that drive "inflamm-aging" both with and without HIV infection is a preeminent global health priority.

There are multiple proposed triggers of the aberrant inflammation found in HIV+ persons with successful viral suppression, including the latent HIV viral reservoir itself (77), co-infections such as cytomegalovirus (CMV) (78), and translocation of microbial products across the epithelial barrier of the gastrointestinal tract into the systemic circulation (79). There is a reported connection between harboring latent HIV and IR expression on T cells: CD4+ T cells from virally suppressed HIV+ subjects that express at least one of the IRs TIGIT, PD-1, or LAG-3 contained the majority, on average, of CD4+ T cells with inducible HIV genomes, with multi-IR+ CD4+ T cells particularly enriched for integrated HIV DNA (80); also, TIGIT+ CD4+ T cell frequencies positively correlate with CD4+ T cell HIV DNA content (49), and TIGIT transcription is elevated in cells bearing replication competent latent HIV (81). Our recent studies indicate that sensing of HIV viral intron-containing RNA by infected macrophages leads to type I interferon secretion and induction of IRs on co-cultured T cells (82). Circulating γδ T cells are known to harbor latent virus at a high frequency (47), therefore it is worth investigating if IR+ γδ T cells, particularly TIGIT+ and multi-IR+ subsets, are selectively harboring inducible HIV genomes. Further studies investigating the mechanistic relationship(s) between intracellular HIV, γδ T cell IR expression, and the secretion of inflammatory cytokines and cytotoxic mediators could lead to novel targets for selective therapeutic γδ T cell ablation to help purge the latent HIV pool and reduce general inflammation.

The integrity of the gastrointestinal epithelial barrier is compromised in HIV and SIV infection (79, 83) and does not sufficiently recover with effective ART (84). This "gut leakiness" is connected to the movement of microbial products such as LPS into the systemic circulation and this likely contributes to general inflammation (85). γδ T cells are a predominant immune cell subset in intestinal epithelia (24, 25), and the majority of human mucosal intraepithelial lymphocytes (IELs) are Vδ1+ T cells (86, 87), the subset found to predominate the circulation of aviremic HIV+ subjects but not uninfected controls in this study (**Supplementary Figures 2G–I**) and others (45, 62). Measuring the IR signatures and resident memory markers on Vδ1+ and Vδ2+ γδ T cell subsets from our HIV and Aging cohort is an important next step to help elucidate if the IR differences noted between subject groups are impacted by Vδ1+ and Vδ2+ subset shifts in the circulation and if such shifts indicate emigration from the GI tract. Also, murine intestinal γδ T cells described as "activated yet resting" expressed very high levels of mRNA for Granzymes A and B (88). In light of our functional results showing that spontaneous production of cytolytic machinery tracked with TIGIT expression in HIV+ subjects, this is further evidence that the circulating TIGIT+ γδ T cells, activated and armed with cytolytic machinery, are from the GI tract. It should be noted that cytokine production in response to *in vitro* stimulation was not performed, due to the challenges of stimulating purified γδ T cell cultures efficiently. Functional profiles post-*ex vivo* re-stimulation would provide additional information about the γδ T cells activation/exhaustion status, as rested and not exhausted cells would likely produce higher numbers of analytes and at higher amounts than cells in an activated or exhausted state. Immune cell composition in the blood has reflected what is found in the GALT in aviremic HIV+ subjects (89). Future work examining mucosal resident γδ T cells in SIV-infected animals and HIV+ individuals could provide new insight into how immune

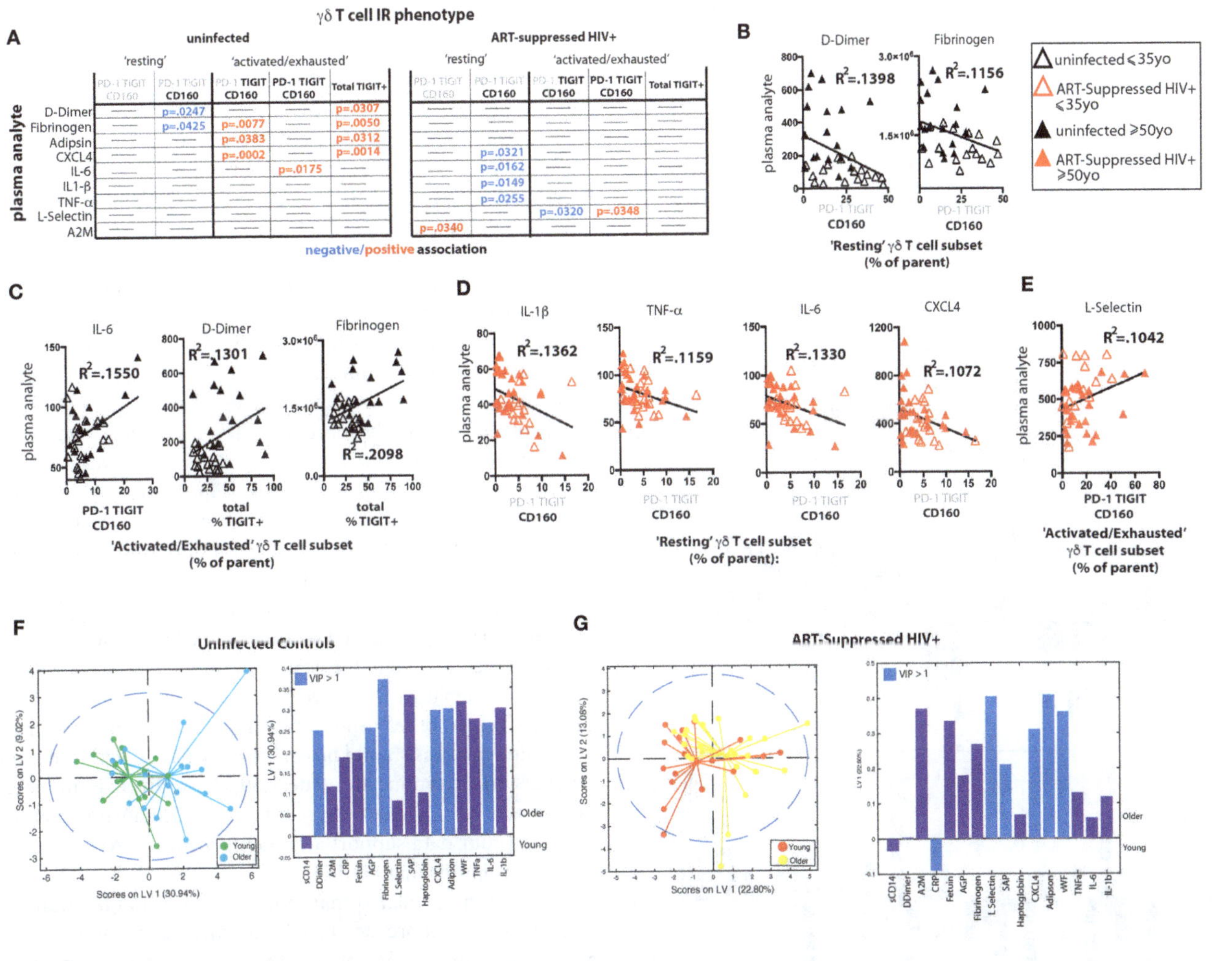

FIGURE 5 | γδ T cell IR signatures correlate with inflammatory plasma markers in both healthy aging and ART-suppressed HIV infection. Sixteen plasma analytes were measured and linear regression analysis was performed with the percentages of IR expressing γδ T cell subsets defined in **Figure 3D** (positive and negative expression of each IR is depicted with black bold and gray lettering, respectively, at the top of each table) and total percent TIGIT+; all statistically significant results ($p < 0.05$) are shown in the tables in **(A)** for uninfected controls and ART-suppressed HIV+ subjects. Examples of correlation plots with a fitted linear regression line comparing "Resting" or "Activated/Exhausted" γδ T cell subsets from uninfected controls with plasma inflammatory/coagulation markers **(B,C)** and analogous graphs for the ART-suppressed HIV+ subjects **(D,E)**. Subjects within the younger and older groups are noted with open and solid triangles, respectively, in **(B–E)**. Units for plasma analytes are as follows: D-Dimer, fibrinogen, CXCL4, L-selectin; ng/ml; IL-6, IL-1β, TNF-α; pg/ml. Scores plot and loadings on LV1 derived from a PLSR model of plasma markers vs. the percentage of TIGIT+ γδ T cells for uninfected controls **(F)** and ART-suppressed HIV+ subjects **(G)**.

changes in the gut direct general inflammation in aviremic HIV infection.

Unlike traditional (adaptive) T cells, a principal means of γδ T cell activation is via cytokine and NK receptors (34), mechanisms easily triggered by activated monocyte/macrophage populations, an immune cell subset strongly linked to inflammation in aviremic HIV+ infection. Markers of monocyte/macrophage activation in the circulation, such as sCD14, sCD163, and tissue factor (TF), have been linked with mortality, atherosclerosis, and other markers of inflammation and coagulation (90–92). Furthermore, TF-expressing monocytes, present with successful HIV viral suppression, produce multiple inflammatory cytokines upon exposure to LPS and induce a coagulation cascade and treatment of SIV-infected macaques with an anti-coagulant that blocks the TF pathway led to a decrease in circulating D-dimer levels as well as markers of immune activation (93). The effect of TF+ monocytes on γδ T cells is unknown to date. It is of interest to investigate the potential cross-activation of monocytes/macrophages and γδ T cells in aviremic HIV infection.

Inhibitory receptors, such as PD-1, TIM-3, and TIGIT, negatively regulate T cell activation and are believed to be critical for limiting immunopathology during immune responses. Expression of IRs is often associated with diminished functional capacity, frequently called immune exhaustion, in HIV, aging and other chronic diseases (50, 53, 59). TIGIT (T cell immunoreceptor with immunoglobulin and ITIM domains) is a more recently described inhibitory receptor that is a member of the

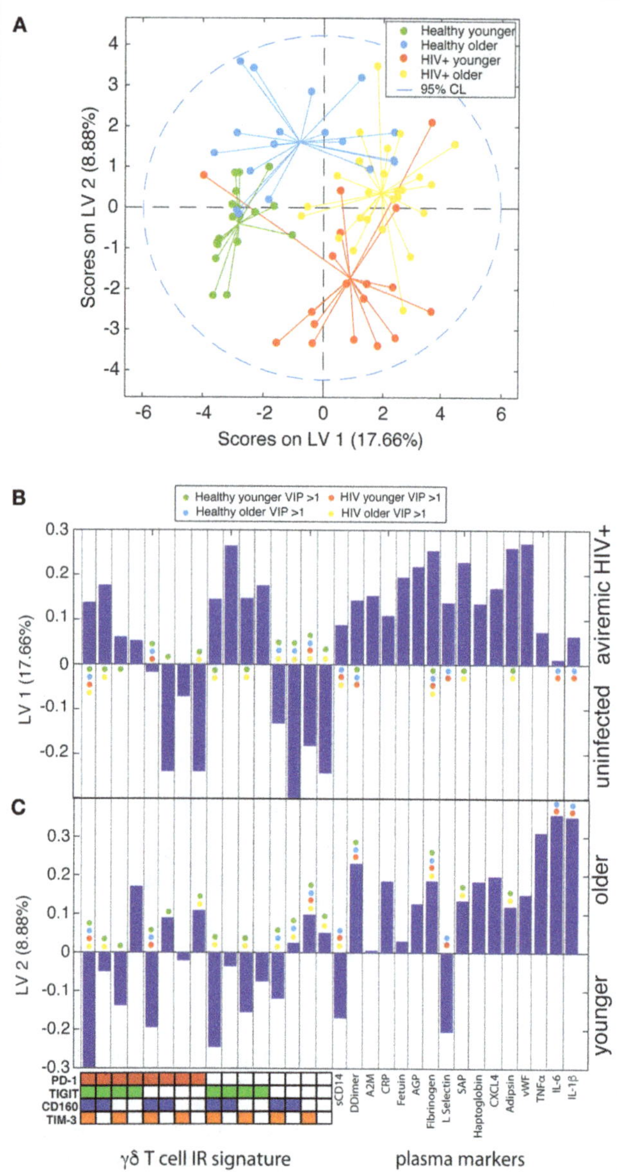

FIGURE 6 | γδ T cell IR signatures and plasma inflammatory cytokines define the divergent aging processes in ART-suppressed HIV+ individuals and uninfected controls. **(A)** A two-dimensional PLS-DA model constructed using the percentages of all possible combinations of the IRs PD-1, TIGIT, CD160, and TIM-3 and 16 markers of inflammation and coagulation in plasma. Each data point represents scores generated by the model, composed of all measurements for a given subject mapped onto the two-dimensional latent variable space. The percentages on the axes show the percent variance in the dataset captured by a particular LV. Dotted line shows the 95% confidence interval. **(B)** Bar plot showing the loadings on LV1 of all parameters used to train the PLS-DA model, which included all possible combinations of the IRs PD-1, TIGIT, CD160, and TIM-3 and the concentrations of all 16 plasma markers measured. LV1 is the latent variable that separated the scores predominantly based on presence or absence of HIV infection. The Y-axis quantifies the positive or negative contribution of a particular parameter to the indicated LV. **(C)** Bar plot as in **(B)**, showing the loadings on LV2, the latent variable that separates the scores affected by patient age, of all parameters used to train the model. The colored dots in **(B,C)** mark the parameters (IR signatures of γδ T cells and plasma markers) with a VIP score >1 (statistically significant) for each subject group in the model.

CD28 family of signaling molecules (94). It is expressed on NK cells, CD8+ T cells, and CD4+ T cells (94), is induced upon activation in multiple immune cell subsets (95–97), and its expression marks exhausted CD8+ T cells in HIV and SIV infection (49). Publications investigating IR expression on γδ T cells are scarce to date and include a report of PD-1 expression on $\gamma\delta^{lo}$ T cells in mouse skin (98) another of TIGIT expression on γδ T cells in the epidermis of stem cell transplant recipients (99), and a recent study reporting higher percentages of IR+ γδ T cells with Plasmodium vivax infection (100). γδ T cells are also implicated as pro-tumorigenic with the PD-1:PDL-1 pathway one proposed mechanism of action (101). Here, TIGIT expression tracked with *ex vivo* secretion of inflammatory cytokines and cytotoxic mediators without re-stimulation from the γδ T cells of aviremic HIV+ subjects. These findings suggest that TIGIT+ γδ T cells are activated in ART-suppressed HIV+ subjects and secrete inflammatory mediators *in vivo*. This association was not found in the uninfected control subjects (**Figure 4**). However, it is important to note that while the percentage of TIGIT+ γδ T cells sorted into the individual culture wells significantly correlates with the amount of inflammatory analyte measured, the functional profiles of actual TIGIT+ vs. TIGIT- γδ T cells were not directly measured in this study. From these results it can be concluded that the same immune cell subset with an identical IR signature may have different functionality in different disease states or other conditions. Therefore, we contend that IR expression analysis should be consistently paired with functional readouts to determine the true status of a given immune cell population. As IRs have been referred to as "exhaustion markers" (102, 103) our data support arguments by others to not limit IR definitions in this manner (65).

It has been postulated that multi-IR expression by individual T cells reflects more advanced immune exhaustion (104) in agreement with reports of T cells in virally infected mice (63, 105). In our study, the percentages of γδ T cells expressing ≥2IR per cell were higher with both healthy aging and HIV infection, yet the ≥3IR and ≥4IR per cell levels were elevated only with HIV infection (**Figures 2C,F**) possibly suggesting a more progressed immune exhaustion status of these cells. However, our measurements of analyte secretion indicate that the HIV+ subjects' γδ T cells expressing IRs are activated and not exhausted (**Figure 4B**). When we performed more detailed IR signature analysis to parse out potential lineage trajectories of γδ T cell subsets bearing combinations of PD-1, TIGIT, and CD160 in ART-suppressed HIV infection and/or aging, interesting findings emerged; firstly, our results show that a substantial proportion of the circulating γδ T cell compartment in healthy younger subjects express CD160 (**Figure 3A**) that is not elevated with HIV- or age-associated activation or exhaustion (**Figures 3A–C**). CD160 recognizes class 1a and 1b molecules (106) and serves as a co-receptor for activation of γδ T cells (107) yet its expression has been linked to immune exhaustion on CD8+ T cells in HIV and other chronic diseases (108, 109). These results underscore the importance of evaluating IR expression in a cell type and disease-specific manner. Also, our data indicate that TIGIT and PD-1 are up-regulated on what we cautiously define as "activated/exhausted" cell subsets, and the PD-1+ TIGIT+ CD160+ (triple positive) T cells are elevated with aviremic HIV infection and not healthy aging, suggesting that HIV drives further progression of γδ T cell populations along activation/exhaustion routes. Taken together, our data suggest that multi-IR expression per cell may not always signify advanced immune exhaustion and that combinational IR signature analysis could provide new insight into the progression of changes in immune cell functional activity and capacity (activation vs. exhaustion) in chronic conditions. Future work measuring the functional profiles of sorted γδ T populations with distinct IR signatures from our cohort will help elucidate how functions change with IR expression during aging with and without aviremic HIV infection.

There is debate in the literature as to whether aviremic HIV infection leads to a distinct inflammatory signature that exists regardless of age (110–112). If so, we would expect similarities in immune signatures between the younger HIV+ and healthy older subjects, as well as between the HIV+ younger and HIV+ older individuals. Our univariate analyses agree with this concept, for comparisons of γδ T cell IR expression, spontaneous *ex vivo* cytokine production, and γδ T cell links with and the total levels of inflammatory plasma analytes are not significantly different between HIV+ younger and older subject groups (**Figures 2E,F**, **3A**, **4C**, **5D,E**, and **Supplementary Figure 5B**). Therefore, this data suggests that aviremic HIV infection and aging are not impacting immune cell phenotypes in an additive or multiplicative manner, consistent with a report of CD8+ T cells (113). However, γδ T cell secretion of sCD137 is significantly higher from the cells from the HIV older group compared to all other three subject groups (HIV younger, uninfected younger, and uninfected older) (**Figure 4A**), indicating a synergistic impact of age and HIV on the activation of γδ T cells. sCD137 is a pro-inflammatory molecule that can be produced as an alternatively spliced variant or by proteolytic cleavage of CD137 (4-1BB) (114), a member of TNF superfamily, and a marker associated with multiple inflammatory diseases. sCD137 plasma levels positively associate with acute coronary syndromes (66) and atherothrombotic stroke (67), and we hypothesize that *in vivo*, γδ T cells produce sCD137 which is also known to trigger pro-inflammatory networks that involve macrophages and DCs (115) Also, our multivariate PSLR results (**Figures 4D,E**, and **Figures 5F,G**) show that the relationships between γδ IR signatures and both the cytokines they produce and plasma markers with which they co-vary are different in the younger vs. older subjects in both the uninfected control and HIV+ groups, since the younger and older subjects separated in all four PLSR models without age being added as a variable. These results show that there are distinct aging courses in relation to immune network changes with and without HIV infection. Finally and perhaps most importantly, in our PLS-DA model all four subject groups separated with significance (**Figure 6**) demonstrating separate aging processes with and without HIV infection. Our multivariate results underscore the importance of performing this type of analyses to gain novel insights into immune networks in relation to inflammation and other states.

Altogether, our findings indicate that γδ T cells are a possible source of inflammation in aviremic HIV infection and potentially other inflammatory diseases. IR expression on circulating γδ T cells, and TIGIT in particular, should be investigated for biomarker utility to effectively diagnose, predict, and/or treat both general inflammation and propensity to age-associated morbidities and mortality with and without HIV infection.

MATERIALS AND METHODS

Participants

The subjects were part of the HIV and aging cohort which enrolled HIV+ subjects with ART effective viral suppression (undetectable HIV-1 RNA <50 copies/ml) for a minimum of 6 months and were age-stratified into≤35 years and ≥50 years age groups from the infectious disease clinics at Brigham and Women's Hospital, Beth Israel Deaconess Hospital, Massachusetts General Hospital, and Boston Medical Center, all located in Boston, MA. Study protocols were approved by the institutional review boards at each institution and all subjects provided written informed consent. The committee that approved the research protocol was the Boston University Institutional Review Board, IRB# H-33095. Uninfected controls were recruited from the same clinics in Boston and had similar demographic and socioeconomic status as HIV+ subjects. HIV negative status was verified with both a negative HIV antibody test and HIV-1 viral load test. Exclusion criteria included active hepatitis B or C, recent active infection within past 6 months, recent immunomodulatory therapy, and receipt of an HIV vaccine. HIV+ subjects in different age groups are matched by duration of ART (**Table 1**). Detailed information about the study subject characteristics can be found in **Table 1** and **Supplemental Table 2**. All subjects were recruited with detailed clinical history and socio-demographic data, and information of other common confounders, such as gender, co-infections, and other pro-inflammatory exposures (i.e., STDs, obesity, and drug/tobacco use).

Peripheral Blood Processing

Peripheral blood mononuclear cells (PBMC) were isolated from blood originally drawn into EDTA tubes by Ficoll-Hypaque and cryopreserved in liquid nitrogen until use. Plasma was acquired from whole blood and stored at −80°C until use. All paired plasma and PBMC samples used in this study are from the same blood draw.

Flow Cytometry Panels and Reagents

Two flow cytometry panels were used in the study. Panel 1 was a modified version of the previously published panel (60) where 3 markers were moved to different detection channels and one replaced. Panel 2 was a modification of Panel 1 constructed to allow detection of γδ T cell Vδ1 and Vδ2 subsets. All reagents used in both panels are listed in **Supplementary Table 1**. Buffers and blocking reagents were used as described (60). All fluorescent reagents were titrated and Fluorescence Minus One (FMO) controls were performed to verify the validity of the modified panels. Ultracomp capture beads (Thermo Fisher) were used to establish the compensation matrix. Ultra Rainbow Beads (Spherotech) were used to establish target values for running the instrument. CS&T beads (BD) were used for daily QC of the instruments.

Flow Cytometry Protocol

1×10^7 PBMC per donor were thawed and immediately stained with a 16-color antibody/reagent cocktail developed for the BUMC FACSARIA (BD Biosciences) cell sorter as previously described (60). Briefly, cells were washed, stained with live/dead reagent (Biolegend's Zombie NIR) in DPBS for 20 min, washed again with FACS buffer (DPBS/0.5% BSA/2 mM EDTA), and pre-blocked with human Fc-blocking reagent (Biolegend) for 10 min. The antibody cocktail was prepared by combining antibody stocks with BD Brilliant Buffer and adding the master mixes to the pre-blocked cells that were then incubated for 20 min at room temperature. After staining, cells were washed twice with FACS buffer (PBS 0.5% BSA 2 mM EDTA), resuspended in FACS buffer and run on the BUMC FACSARIA cell sorter (BD Biosciences). Samples were divided into 11 different runs and a mix of subjects from the four groups (uninfected younger, uninfected older, ART Suppressed HIV+ younger, ART-suppressed HIV+ older) were included in each run to control for potential alterations in machine performance and batch effects. For each run, a mixture containing 5% of each individual sample was prepared and stained with the reagent mix that did not include IR-specific fluorescent antibodies (Fluorescence Minus Five, or FM5). For Panel 2, anti-Vδ2-biotin and anti-Vδ1-PE added were added to cells for 20 min then cells were washed prior to the addition of other reagents that were then added and incubated for 20 min. For each batch run, Ultracomp capture beads (Thermo Fisher) were stained with same reagents and acquired prior to the samples. PDGFRα-APC antibody (Biolegend) was used for the APC single stain.

γδ T cell cultures: During data acquisition and sample running on the BD FACSARIA, γδ T cells (LIVE/DEAD–, CD14–, CD19–, CD3+, γδTCR+) were sorted into tubes and cultured in 25 μl of RPMI1640 10% FBS/1% pen-strep in half-area 96-well flat-bottom plates (Greiner) for 20 h. The number of cells cultured per well-varied from 2,000 to 26,000, with a comparable range in numbers across each of the four subject groups. At the end of the culture period, supernatants were frozen into multiple aliquots and later thawed to perform analyte measurements.

Milliplex Bead Assays of Culture Supernatants

Supernatant samples were thawed, centrifuged for 30 seconds to remove debris, and added to a 384-well plate for analyte measurement via use of the Milliplex human Th17 25-plex kit (Millipore Sigma) and a modified Milliplex human CD8 9-plex kit (Millipore Sigma). Antibodies and magnetic beads were diluted 1:1 with assay buffer and utilized at half-volume to adjust the manufacturer's protocol to the 384-well plate format. Plates were washed in between incubations using a BioTek 406 Touch plate washer (BioTek) and read using the Luminex FlexMap 3D system (Luminex). Observed concentration values were adjusted to cell counts per well.

Milliplex and ELISA Assays of Plasma Samples

Frozen plasma samples were thawed and analyzed using (1) the 11-plex Human Cardiovascular Disease (Acute Phase) Milliplex kit (MilliporeSigma, HCVD3MAG-67K), (2) a custom 3-plex Milliplex kit for TNF-α, IL-6, and IL-1β (HCYTOMAG-3K) sCD14 and D-dimer ELISA kits (from RD Systems and Abcam, respectively). For (1), samples were pre-diluted 1:40,000 and the kit was run according to manufacturer's instructions and similar to the culture supernatants described above.

Flow Cytometry Data Analysis

Data were recorded with BD FACSDIVA 6.1.2 and automatically compensated with compensation matrix recorded within the sample files according to FCS 3.0 standards. Manual gating (expert-guided analysis) was performed in FlowJo v.10.2-10.3 (FlowJo, Inc) while blinded to sample identifier. Inhibitory receptor (IR) gating was guided using the FM5 sample from each run as described above. Numeric values from FlowJo data analysis were exported to Prism 7.0 (Graphpad) for statistical analysis. Flow cytometry data files were also uploaded to Cytobank, a cloud-based computational platform, and arcsin-transformed. Doublets, dead cells, debris, CD14+ cells, and CD19+ cells were excluded by manual gating and remaining live single non-CD14, non-CD19 events (downsampled to 10,000 events/subject) were input into the CITRUS algorithm (61). After hierarchical clustering based on lineage markers (CD3, CD4, CD8, γδ TCR, CD127, CD16, CD56) shown in **Supplementary Figure 1**, median fluorescence of TIGIT, TIM-3, PD-1, CD160, and LAG-3 expression was measured and a supervised comparison between HIV- and HIV+ individuals was carried out and assessed via Nearest Shrunken Centroid (PAMR) association modeling (**Supplementary Figure 1**). Additionally, live, single, non-CD14, non-CD19 events were input to the SPADE clustering algorithm, and the nodes containing cells with higher γδ TCR expression were exported from each sample file and used for IR median fluorescence intensity representation (**Figure 2D**). Beta regression of abundance on HIV status and age group was performed in **Figure 3A**. To correct for multiple hypothesis testing, a significance threshold was set for each regression term using a family-wise error rate of 0.05. The significance threshold was established in the following manner. First, 100 permuted abundance datasets were created by randomly resampling without replacement the abundance of each of the eight IR subsets within each subject, so that the inter-dependency of the IR subset abundances for an individual was maintained. Then, for each of the 100 permuted abundances, the beta regression for each IR subset was performed and the minimum p-value across all IR subsets was recorded for each model term. Finally, the 5th percentile of this distribution of minimum p-values was set as the significance threshold for each model term (HIV threshold: 0.0047; age group threshold: 0.0068).

PLS Analysis

Partial least squares discriminant analysis (PLSDA) and partial least squares regression (PLSR) were performed using the

MATLAB PLS Toolbox (Eigenvector Research, Inc.). Data were normalized along each X and Y parameter by Z-score before application of the algorithm. Cross-validation was performed with one-third of the relevant dataset. The number of latent variables (LVs) was chosen so as to minimize cumulative error over all predictions. We orthogonally rotated the models so that maximal separation was achieved across LV1 where noted. We calculated model confidence by randomly permuting Y 100 times and rebuilding the model to form a distribution of error for these randomly generated models. We compared our model to this distribution with the Mann–Whitney *U*-test to determine the significance of our model. The importance of each parameter to the overall model prediction was quantified using variable importance in projection (VIP) score. A VIP score >1 (above average contribution) was considered important for model performance and prediction.

ETHICS STATEMENT

The study protocol was approved by the Boston University School of Medicine, Partners Healthcare, and Beth Israel Deaconess Medical Center institutional review boards. All participants provided written informed consent to participate in the study.

AUTHOR CONTRIBUTIONS

AB, AO, NL, and JS-C conceived and designed the experiments. KD, DL, NL, and JS-C contributed to reagents, materials, and funding. AB, RP, and JS-C performed experiments. AB, AS, KD, EP, RP, and JS-C analyzed data and JS-C wrote the manuscript. All authors read and approved the final version of the manuscript.

ACKNOWLEDGMENTS

We thank Drs. Jeffrey Browning, Amedeo Cappione, Andrew Henderson, and Barbara Nikolajczyk for their critical reading of the manuscript, Drs. Suryaram Gummuluru and Manish Sagar for their helpful discussions regarding data interpretation, and Dr. Barbara Nikolajczyk and Dr. Madhur Agrawal for their assistance with the multiplex assays. All flow cytometry data were collected at the Boston University School of Medicine Flow Cytometry Core Facility.

REFERENCES

1. Wada N, Jacobson LP, Cohen M, French A, Phair J, Muñoz A. Cause-specific life expectancies after 35 years of age for human immunodeficiency syndrome-infected and human immunodeficiency syndrome-negative individuals followed simultaneously in long-term cohort studies, 1984-2008. *Am J Epidemiol.* (2013) 177:116–25. doi: 10.1093/aje/kws321
2. Marcus JL, Chao CR, Leyden WA, Xu L, Quesenberry CP, Klein DB, et al. Narrowing the gap in life expectancy between HIV-infected and HIV-uninfected individuals with access to care. *J Acquir Immune Defic Syndr.* (2016) 73:39–46. doi: 10.1097/QAI.0000000000001014
3. Antiretroviral Therapy Cohort Collaboration. Life expectancy of individuals on combination antiretroviral therapy in high-income countries: a collaborative analysis of 14 cohort studies. *Lancet* (2008) 372:293–9. doi: 10.1016/S0140-6736(08)61113-7
4. Hasse B, Ledergerber B, Furrer H, Battegay M, Hirschel B, Cavassini M, et al. Morbidity and aging in HIV-infected persons: the Swiss HIV cohort study. *Clin Infect Dis.* (2011) 53:1130–9. doi: 10.1093/cid/cir626
5. Schouten J, Wit FW, Stolte IG, Kootstra NA, van der Valk M, Geerlings SE, et al. Cross-sectional comparison of the prevalence of age-associated comorbidities and their risk factors between HIV-infected and uninfected individuals: the AGEhIV cohort study. *Clin Infect Dis.* (2014) 59:1787–97. doi: 10.1093/cid/ciu701
6. Rodriguez-Penney AT, Iudicello JE, Riggs PK, Doyle K, Ellis RJ, Letendre SL, et al. Co-morbidities in persons infected with HIV: increased burden with older age and negative effects on health-related quality of life. *AIDS Patient Care STDS* (2013) 27:5–16. doi: 10.1089/apc.2012.0329
7. Guaraldi G, Orlando G, Zona S, Menozzi M, Carli F, Garlassi E, et al. Premature age-related comorbidities among HIV-infected persons compared with the general population. *Clin Infect Dis.* (2011) 53:1120–6. doi: 10.1093/cid/cir627
8. Capeau J. Premature aging and premature age-related comorbidities in HIV-infected patients: facts and hypotheses. *Clin Infect Dis.* (2011) 53:1127–9. doi: 10.1093/cid/cir628
9. So-Armah KA, Tate JP, Chang CH, Butt AA, Gerschenson M, Gibert CL, et al. Do biomarkers of inflammation, monocyte activation, and altered coagulation explain excess mortality between HIV infected and uninfected people? *J Acquir Immune Defic Syndr.* (2016) 72:206–213. doi: 10.1097/QAI.0000000000000954
10. Kuller LH, Tracy R, Belloso W, De Wit S, Drummond F, Lane HC, et al. Inflammatory and coagulation biomarkers and mortality in patients with HIV infection. *PLoS Med.* (2008) 5:e203. doi: 10.1371/journal.pmed.0050203
11. Duprez DA, Neuhaus J, Kuller LH, Tracy R, Belloso W, De Wit S, et al. Inflammation, coagulation and cardiovascular disease in HIV-infected individuals. *PLoS ONE* (2012) 7:e44454. doi: 10.1371/journal.pone.0044454
12. Montoya JL, Iudicello J, Oppenheim HA, Fazeli PL, Potter M, Ma Q, et al. Coagulation imbalance and neurocognitive functioning in older HIV-positive adults on suppressive antiretroviral therapy. *AIDS* (2017) 31:787–95. doi: 10.1097/QAD.0000000000001404
13. Tenorio AR, Zheng Y, Bosch RJ, Krishnan S, Rodriguez B, Hunt PW, et al. Soluble markers of inflammation and coagulation but not T-cell activation predict non-AIDS-defining morbid events during suppressive antiretroviral treatment. *J Infect Dis.* (2014) 210:1248–59. doi: 10.1093/infdis/jiu254
14. Hart BB, Nordell AD, Okulicz JF, Palfreeman A, Horban A, Kedem E, et al. Inflammation-related morbidity and mortality among HIV-positive adults: how extensive is it? *J Acquir Immune Defic Syndr.* (2018) 77:1–7. doi: 10.1097/QAI.0000000000001554
15. Folsom AR, Alonso A, George KM, Roetker NS, Tang W, Cushman M. Prospective study of plasma D-dimer and incident venous thromboembolism: the atherosclerosis risk in communities (ARIC) study. *Thromb Res.* (2015) 136:781–5. doi: 10.1016/j.thromres.2015.08.013
16. Folsom AR, Delaney JA, Lutsey PL, Zakai NA, Jenny NS, Polak JF, et al. Associations of factor VIIIc, D-dimer, and plasmin-antiplasmin with incident cardiovascular disease and all-cause mortality. *Am J Hematol.* (2009) 84:349–53. doi: 10.1002/ajh.21429
17. Folsom AR, Gottesman RF, Appiah D, Shahar E, Mosley TH. Plasma d-Dimer and incident ischemic stroke and coronary heart disease: the atherosclerosis risk in communities study. *Stroke* (2016) 47:18–23. doi: 10.1161/STROKEAHA.115.011035
18. Danesh J, Kaptoge S, Mann AG, Sarwar N, Wood A, Angleman SB, et al. Long-term interleukin-6 levels and subsequent risk of coronary heart disease: two new prospective studies and a systematic review. *PLoS Med.* (2008) 5:e78. doi: 10.1371/journal.pmed.0050078

19. Ridker PM, Rifai N, Stampfer MJ, Hennekens CH. Plasma concentration of interleukin-6 and the risk of future myocardial infarction among apparently healthy men. *Circulation* (2000) 101:1767–72. doi: 10.1161/01.CIR.101.15.1767
20. Stack AG, Donigiewicz U, Abdalla AA, Weiland A, Casserly LF, Cronin CJ, et al. Plasma fibrinogen associates independently with total and cardiovascular mortality among subjects with normal and reduced kidney function in the general population. *QJM* (2014) 107:701–13. doi: 10.1093/qjmed/hcu057
21. Kuller LH, Tracy RP, Shaten J, Meilahn EN. Relation of C-reactive protein and coronary heart disease in the MRFIT nested case-control study. Multiple risk factor intervention trial. *Am J Epidemiol.* (1996) 144:537–47. doi: 10.1093/oxfordjournals.aje.a008963
22. Nasi M, De Biasi S, Gibellini L, Bianchini E, Pecorini S, Bacca V, et al. Ageing and inflammation in patients with HIV infection. *Clin Exp Immunol.* (2017) 187:44–52. doi: 10.1111/cei.12814
23. Franceschi C. Inflammaging as a major characteristic of old people: can it be prevented or cured? *Nutr Rev.* (2007) 65(12 Pt 2):S173–6.
24. Goodman T, Lefrançois L. Expression of the gamma-delta T-cell receptor on intestinal CD8+ intraepithelial lymphocytes. *Nature* (1988) 333:855–8. doi: 10.1038/333855a0
25. Bonneville M, Janeway CA, Ito K, Haser W, Ishida I, Nakanishi N, et al. Intestinal intraepithelial lymphocytes are a distinct set of gamma delta T cells. *Nature* (1988) 336:479–81. doi: 10.1038/336479a0
26. Kyes S, Carew E, Carding SR, Janeway CA, Hayday A. Diversity in T-cell receptor gamma gene usage in intestinal epithelium. *Proc Natl Acad Sci USA.* (1989) 86:5527–31. doi: 10.1073/pnas.86.14.5527
27. Bucy RP, Chen CL, Cooper MD. Tissue localization and CD8 accessory molecule expression of T gamma delta cells in humans. *J Immunol.* (1989) 142:3045–9.
28. Constant P, Davodeau F, Peyrat MA, Poquet Y, Puzo G, Bonneville M, et al. Stimulation of human gamma delta T cells by nonpeptidic mycobacterial ligands. *Science* (1994) 264:267–70. doi: 10.1126/science.8146660
29. Girardi M, Oppenheim DE, Steele CR, Lewis JM, Glusac E, Filler R, et al. Regulation of cutaneous malignancy by gammadelta T cells. *Science* (2001) 294:605–9. doi: 10.1126/science.1063916
30. Hintz M, Reichenberg A, Altincicek B, Bahr U, Gschwind RM, Kollas AK, et al. Identification of (E)-4-hydroxy-3-methyl-but-2-enyl pyrophosphate as a major activator for human gammadelta T cells in Escherichia coli. *FEBS Lett.* (2001) 509:317–22. doi: 10.1016/S0014-5793(01)03191-X
31. Martin B, Hirota K, Cua DJ, Stockinger B, Veldhoen M. Interleukin-17-producing gammadelta T cells selectively expand in response to pathogen products and environmental signals. *Immunity* (2009) 31:321–30. doi: 10.1016/j.immuni.2009.06.020
32. Qin G, Mao H, Zheng J, Sia SF, Liu Y, Chan PL, et al. Phosphoantigen-expanded human gammadelta T cells display potent cytotoxicity against monocyte-derived macrophages infected with human and avian influenza viruses. *J Infect Dis.* (2009) 200:858–65. doi: 10.1086/605413
33. Shibata K, Yamada H, Hara H, Kishihara K, Yoshikai Y. Resident Vdelta1+ gammadelta T cells control early infiltration of neutrophils after *Escherichia coli* infection via IL-17 production. *J Immunol.* (2007) 178:4466–72. doi: 10.4049/jimmunol.178.7.4466
34. Silva-Santos B, Strid J. Working in "NK Mode": Natural killer group 2 member D and natural cytotoxicity receptors in stress-surveillance by gammadelta T cells. *Front Immunol.* (2018) 9:851. doi: 10.3389/fimmu.2018.00851
35. Tanaka Y, Morita CT, Tanaka Y, Nieves E, Brenner MB, Bloom BR. Natural and synthetic non-peptide antigens recognized by human gamma delta T cells. *Nature* (1995) 375:155–8. doi: 10.1038/375155a0
36. Biswas P, Ferrarini M, Mantelli B, Fortis C, Poli G, Lazzarin A, et al. Double-edged effect of Vgamma9/Vdelta2 T lymphocytes on viral expression in an *in vitro* model of HIV-1/mycobacteria co-infection. *Eur J Immunol.* (2003) 33:252–63. doi: 10.1002/immu.200390028
37. Wallace M, Gan YH, Pauza CD, Malkovsky M. Antiviral activity of primate gamma delta T lymphocytes isolated by magnetic cell sorting. *J Med Primatol.* (1994) 23:131–5. doi: 10.1111/j.1600-0684.1994.tb00113.x
38. Ye J, Ma C, Hsueh EC, Eickhoff CS, Zhang Y, Varvares MA, et al. Tumor-derived gammadelta regulatory T cells suppress innate and adaptive immunity through the induction of immunosenescence. *J Immunol.* (2013) 190:2403–14. doi: 10.4049/jimmunol.1202369
39. Ye J, Ma C, Wang F, Hsueh EC, Toth K, Huang Y, et al. Specific recruitment of gammadelta regulatory T cells in human breast cancer. *Cancer Res.* (2013) 73:6137–48. doi: 10.1158/0008-5472.CAN-13-0348
40. Qaqish A, Huang D, Chen CY, Zhang Z, Wang R, Li S, et al. Adoptive transfer of phosphoantigen-specific gammadelta T Cell Subset Attenuates Mycobacterium tuberculosis Infection in Nonhuman Primates. *J Immunol.* (2017) 198:4753–63. doi: 10.4049/jimmunol.1602019
41. Dillen CA, Pinsker BL, Marusina AI, Merleev AA, Farber ON, Liu H, et al. Clonally expanded gammadelta T cells protect against Staphylococcus aureus skin reinfection. *J Clin Invest.* (2018) 128:1026–42. doi: 10.1172/JCI 96481
42. Cordova A, Toia F, La Mendola C, Orlando V, Meraviglia S, Rinaldi G, et al. Characterization of human gammadelta T lymphocytes infiltrating primary malignant melanomas. *PLoS ONE* (2012) 7:e49878. doi: 10.1371/journal.pone.0049878
43. Zocchi MR, Ferrarini M, Rugarli C. Selective lysis of the autologous tumor by delta TCS1+ gamma/delta+ tumor-infiltrating lymphocytes from human lung carcinomas. *Eur J Immunol.* (1990) 20:2685–9. doi: 10.1002/eji.1830201224
44. Meraviglia S, Lo Presti E, Tosolini M, La Mendola C, Orlando V, Todaro M, et al. Distinctive features of tumor-infiltrating gammadelta T lymphocytes in human colorectal cancer. *Oncoimmunology* (2017) 6:e1347742. doi: 10.1080/2162402X.2017.1347742
45. Autran B, Triebel F, Katlama C, Rozenbaum W, Hercend T, Debre P. T cell receptor gamma/delta+ lymphocyte subsets during HIV infection. *Clin Exp Immunol.* (1989) 75:206–10.
46. Bordon J, Evans PS, Propp N, Davis CE, Redfield RR, Pauza CD. Association between longer duration of HIV-suppressive therapy and partial recovery of the V gamma 2 T cell receptor repertoire. *J Infect Dis.* (2004) 189:1482–6. doi: 10.1086/382961
47. Soriano-Sarabia N, Archin NM, Bateson R, Dahl NP, Crooks AM, Kuruc JD, et al. Peripheral Vgamma9Vdelta2 T cells are a novel reservoir of latent HIV infection. *PLoS Pathog.* (2015) 11:e1005201. doi: 10.1371/journal.ppat.1005201
48. Snyder-Cappione JE, Nixon DF, Chi JC, Nguyen ML, Kirby CK, Milush JM, et al. Invariant natural killer T (iNKT) cell exhaustion in sarcoidosis. *Eur J Immunol.* (2013) 43:2194–205. doi: 10.1002/eji.201243185
49. Chew GM, Fujita T, Webb GM, Burwitz BJ, Wu HL, Reed JS, et al. TIGIT marks exhausted T cells, correlates with disease progression, and serves as a target for immune restoration in HIV and SIV Infection. *PLoS Pathog.* (2016) 12:e1005349. doi: 10.1371/journal.ppat.1005349
50. Wherry EJ, Ha SJ, Kaech SM, Haining WN, Sarkar S, Kalia V, et al. Molecular signature of CD8+ T cell exhaustion during chronic viral infection. *Immunity* (2007) 27:670–84. doi: 10.1016/j.immuni.2007.09.006
51. Horne-Debets JM, Faleiro R, Karunarathne DS, Liu XQ, Lineburg KE, Poh CM, et al. PD-1 dependent exhaustion of CD8+ T cells drives chronic malaria. *Cell Rep.* (2013) 5:1204–13. doi: 10.1016/j.celrep.2013.11.002
52. Channappanavar R, Twardy BS, Krishna P, Suvas S. Advancing age leads to predominance of inhibitory receptor expressing CD4 T cells. *Mech Ageing Dev.* (2009) 130:709–12. doi: 10.1016/j.mad.2009.08.006
53. Decman V, Laidlaw BJ, Doering TA, Leng J, Ertl HC, Goldstein DR, et al. Defective CD8 T cell responses in aged mice are due to quantitative and qualitative changes in virus-specific precursors. *J Immunol.* (2012) 188:1933–41. doi: 10.4049/jimmunol.1101098
54. Lee KA, Shin KS, Kim GY, Song YC, Bae EA, Kim IK, et al. Characterization of age-associated exhausted CD8(+) T cells defined by increased expression of Tim-3 and PD-1. *Aging Cell* (2016) 15:291–300. doi: 10.1111/acel.12435
55. Shimada Y, Hayashi M, Nagasaka Y, Ohno-Iwashita Y, Inomata M. Age-associated up-regulation of a negative co-stimulatory receptor PD-1 in mouse CD4+ T cells. *Exp Gerontol.* (2009) 44:517–22. doi: 10.1016/j.exger.2009.05.003
56. Song Y, Wang B, Song R, Hao Y, Wang D, Li Y, et al. T-cell Immunoglobulin and ITIM Domain Contributes to CD8(+) T-cell Immunosenescence. *Aging Cell* (2018) 17:e12716. doi: 10.1111/acel. 12716

57. Jones RB, Ndhlovu LC, Barbour JD, Sheth PM, Jha AR, Long BR, et al. Tim-3 expression defines a novel population of dysfunctional T cells with highly elevated frequencies in progressive HIV-1 infection. *J Exp Med.* (2008) 205:2763–79. doi: 10.1084/jem.20081398
58. Trautmann L, Janbazian L, Chomont N, Said EA, Gimmig S, Bessette B, et al. Upregulation of PD-1 expression on HIV-specific CD8+ T cells leads to reversible immune dysfunction. *Nat Med.* (2006) 12:1198–202. doi: 10.1038/nm1482
59. Day CL, Kaufmann DE, Kiepiela P, Brown JA, Moodley ES, Reddy S, et al. PD-1 expression on HIV-specific T cells is associated with T-cell exhaustion and disease progression. *Nature* (2006) 443:350–4. doi: 10.1038/nature05115
60. Belkina AC, Snyder-Cappione JE. OMIP-037: 16-color panel to measure inhibitory receptor signatures from mulitple immune cell subsets. *Cytometry A* (2016) 91:175–9. doi: 10.1002/cyto.a.22983
61. Bruggner RV, Bodenmiller B, Dill DL, Tibshirani RJ, Nolan GP. Automated identification of stratifying signatures in cellular subpopulations. *Proc Natl Acad Sci USA.* (2014) 111:E2770–7. doi: 10.1073/pnas.1408792111
62. De Paoli P, Gennari D, Martelli P, Basaglia G, Crovatto M, Battistin S, et al. A subset of gamma delta lymphocytes is increased during HIV-1 infection. *Clin Exp Immunol.* (1991) 83:187–91. doi: 10.1111/j.1365-2249.1991.tb05612.x
63. Blackburn SD, Shin H, Haining WN, Zou T, Workman CJ, Polley A, et al. Coregulation of CD8+ T cell exhaustion by multiple inhibitory receptors during chronic viral infection. *Nat Immunol.* (2009) 10:29–37. doi: 10.1038/ni.1679
64. Qiu P, Simonds EF, Bendall SC, Gibbs KD, Bruggner, RV, Linderman MD, et al. Extracting a cellular hierarchy from high-dimensional cytometry data with SPADE. *Nat Biotechnol.* (2011) 29:886–91. doi: 10.1038/nbt.1991
65. Fuertes Marraco SA, Neubert NJ, Verdeil G, Speiser DE. Inhibitory receptors beyond T cell exhaustion. *Front Immunol.* (2015) 6:310. doi: 10.3389/fimmu.2015.00310
66. Dongming L, Zuxun L, Liangjie X, Biao W, Ping Y. Enhanced levels of soluble and membrane-bound CD137 levels in patients with acute coronary syndromes. *Clin Chim Acta* (2010) 411:406–10. doi: 10.1016/j.cca.2009.12.011
67. He Y, Ao DH, Li XQ, Zhong SS, A R, Wang YY, et al. Increased Soluble CD137 Levels and CD4+ T-cell-associated expression of CD137 in acute atherothrombotic stroke. *Clin Transl Sci.* (2018). 11:428–34. doi: 10.1111/cts.12553
68. Lau KS, Juchheim AM, Cavaliere KR, Philips SR, Lauffenburger DA, Haigis KM. *In vivo* systems analysis identifies spatial and temporal aspects of the modulation of TNF-alpha-induced apoptosis and proliferation by MAPKs. *Sci Signal.* (2011) 4:ra16. doi: 10.1126/scisignal.2001338
69. Simmons RP, Scully EP, Groden EE, Arnold KB, Chang JJ, Lane K, et al. HIV-1 infection induces strong production of IP-10 through TLR7/9-dependent pathways. *AIDS* (2013) 27:2505–17. doi: 10.1097/01.aids.0000432455.06476.bc
70. Tien PC, Choi AI, Zolopa AR, Benson C, Tracy R, Scherzer R, et al. Inflammation and mortality in HIV-infected adults: analysis of the FRAM study cohort. *J Acquir Immune Defic Syndr.* (2010) 55:316–22. doi: 10.1097/QAI.0b013e3181e66216
71. Triant VA, Meigs JB, Grinspoon, SK. Association of C-reactive protein and HIV infection with acute myocardial infarction. *J Acquir Immune Defic Syndr.* (2009) 51:268–73. doi: 10.1097/QAI.0b013e3181a9992c
72. Ford ES, Greenwald JH, Richterman AG, Rupert A, Dutcher L, Badralmaa Y, et al. Traditional risk factors and D-dimer predict incident cardiovascular disease events in chronic HIV infection. *AIDS* (2010) 24:1509–17. doi: 10.1097/QAD.0b013e32833ad914
73. Nordell AD, McKenna M, Borges ÁH, Duprez D, Neuhaus J, Neaton JD, et al. Severity of cardiovascular disease outcomes among patients with HIV is related to markers of inflammation and coagulation. *J Am Heart Assoc.* (2014) 3:e000844. doi: 10.1161/JAHA.114.000844
74. Benedict KF, Lauffenburger DA. Insights into proteomic immune cell signaling and communication via data-driven modeling. *Curr Top Microbiol Immunol.* (2013) 363:201–33. doi: 10.1007/82_2012_249
75. Effros RB, Fletcher CV, Gebo K, Halter JB, Hazzard WR, Horne FM, et al. Aging and infectious diseases: workshop on HIV infection and aging: what is known and future research directions. *Clin Infect Dis.* (2008) 47:542–53. doi: 10.1086/590150
76. He W, Goodkind D, Kowal P. *An Aging World: 2015.* United States Census Bureau (2016).
77. Hatano H. Immune activation and HIV persistence: considerations for novel therapeutic interventions. *Curr Opin HIV AIDS* (2013) 8:211–6. doi: 10.1097/COH.0b013e32835f9788
78. Hunt PW, Martin JN, Sinclair E, Epling L, Teague J, Jacobson MA, et al. Valganciclovir reduces T cell activation in HIV-infected individuals with incomplete CD4+ T cell recovery on antiretroviral therapy. *J Infect Dis.* (2011) 203:1474–83. doi: 10.1093/infdis/jir060
79. Brenchley JM, Price DA, Schacker TW, Asher TE, Silvestri G, Rao S, et al. Microbial translocation is a cause of systemic immune activation in chronic HIV infection. *Nat Med.* (2006) 12:1365–71. doi: 10.1038/nm1511
80. Fromentin R, Bakeman W, Lawani MB, Khoury G, Hartogensis W, DaFonseca S, et al. CD4+ T cells expressing PD-1, TIGIT and LAG-3 contribute to HIV persistence during ART. *PLoS Pathog.* (2016) 12:e1005761. doi: 10.1371/journal.ppat.1005761
81. Cohn LB, da Silva IT, Valieris R, Huang AS, Lorenzi JCC, Cohen YZ, et al. Clonal CD4(+) T cells in the HIV-1 latent reservoir display a distinct gene profile upon reactivation. *Nat Med.* (2018) 24:604–9. doi: 10.1038/s41591-018-0017-7
82. Akiyama H, Miller CM, Ettinger CR, Belkina AC, Snyder-Cappione JE, Gummuluru S. HIV-1 intron-containing RNA expression induces innate immune activation and T cell dysfunction. *Nat Commun.* (2018) 9:3450. doi: 10.1038/s41467-018-05899-7
83. George MD, Reay E, Sankaran S, Dandekar S. Early antiretroviral therapy for simian immunodeficiency virus infection leads to mucosal CD4+ T cell restoration and enhanced gene expression regulating mucosal repair and regeneration. *J Virol.* (2005) 79:2709–19. doi: 10.1128/JVI.79.5.2709-2719.2005
84. Wojcik-Cichy K, Piekarska A, Jablonowska, E. Intestinal barrier impairment and immune activation in HIV-infected advanced late presenters are not dependent on CD4 Recovery. *Arch Immunol Ther Exp.* (2018) 66:321–7. doi: 10.1007/s00005-018-0508-8
85. Ortiz AM, Brenchley JM. Microbial translocation: translating simian immunodeficiency virus to HIV. *Curr Opin HIV AIDS* (2018) 13:15–21. doi: 10.1097/COH.0000000000000424
86. Bucht A, Söderström K, Esin S, Grunewald J, Hagelberg S, Magnusson I, et al. Analysis of gamma delta V region usage in normal and diseased human intestinal biopsies and peripheral blood by polymerase chain reaction (PCR) and flow cytometry. *Clin Exp Immunol.* (1995) 99:57–64. doi: 10.1111/j.1365-2249.1995.tb03472.x
87. Holtmeier W, Chowers Y, Lumeng A, Morzycka-Wroblewska E, Kagnoff MF. The delta T cell receptor repertoire in human colon and peripheral blood is oligoclonal irrespective of V region usage. *J Clin Invest.* (1995) 96:1108–17. doi: 10.1172/JCI118097
88. Shires J, Theodoridis E, Hayday AC. Biological insights into TCRgammadelta+ and TCRalphabeta+ intraepithelial lymphocytes provided by serial analysis of gene expression (SAGE). *Immunity* (2001) 15:419–34.
89. Serrano-Villar S, Sainz T, Lee SA, Hunt PW, Sinclair E, Shacklett BL, et al. HIV-infected individuals with low CD4/CD8 ratio despite effective antiretroviral therapy exhibit altered T cell subsets, heightened CD8+ T cell activation, and increased risk of non-AIDS morbidity and mortality. *PLoS Pathog.* (2014) 10:e1004078. doi: 10.1371/journal.ppat.1004078
90. Wilson EM, Singh A, Hullsiek KH, Gibson D, Henry WK, Lichtenstein K, et al. Monocyte-activation phenotypes are associated with biomarkers of inflammation and coagulation in chronic HIV infection. *J Infect Dis.* (2014) 210:1396–406. doi: 10.1093/infdis/jiu275
91. Sandler NG, Wand H, Roque A, Law M, Nason MC, Nixon DE, et al. Plasma levels of soluble CD14 independently predict mortality in HIV infection. *J Infect Dis.* (2011) 203:780–90. doi: 10.1093/infdis/jiq118
92. McKibben RA, Margolick JB, Grinspoon S, Li X, Palella FJ, Kingsley LA, et al. Elevated levels of monocyte activation markers are associated with subclinical atherosclerosis in men with and those without HIV infection. *J Infect Dis.* (2015) 211:1219–28. doi: 10.1093/infdis/jiu594

93. Schechter ME, Andrade BB, He T, Richter GH, Tosh KW, Policicchio BB, et al. Inflammatory monocytes expressing tissue factor drive SIV and HIV coagulopathy. *Sci Transl Med.* (2017) 9:eaam5441. doi: 10.1126/scitranslmed.aam5441
94. Yu X, Harden K, Gonzalez LC, Francesco M, Chiang E, Irving B, et al. The surface protein TIGIT suppresses T cell activation by promoting the generation of mature immunoregulatory dendritic cells. *Nat Immunol.* (2009) 10:48–57. doi: 10.1038/ni.1674
95. Stengel KF, Harden-Bowles K, Yu X, Rouge L, Yin J, Comps-Agrar L, et al. Structure of TIGIT immunoreceptor bound to poliovirus receptor reveals a cell-cell adhesion and signaling mechanism that requires cis-trans receptor clustering. *Proc Natl Acad Sci USA.* (2012) 109:5399–404. doi: 10.1073/pnas.1120606109
96. Joller N, Hafler JP, Brynedal B, Kassam N, Spoerl S, Levin SD, et al. Cutting edge: TIGIT has T cell-intrinsic inhibitory functions. *J Immunol.* (2011) 186:1338–42. doi: 10.4049/jimmunol.1003081
97. Stanietsky N, Simic H, Arapovic J, Toporik A, Levy O, Novik A, et al. The interaction of TIGIT with PVR and PVRL2 inhibits human NK cell cytotoxicity. *Proc Natl Acad Sci USA.* (2009) 106:17858–63. doi: 10.1073/pnas.0903474106
98. Imai Y, Ayithan N, Wu X, Yuan Y, Wang L, Hwang ST. Cutting Edge: PD-1 Regulates Imiquimod-Induced Psoriasiform Dermatitis through Inhibition of IL−17A Expression by Innate gammadelta-Low T Cells. *J Immunol.* (2015) 195:421–5. doi: 10.4049/jimmunol.1500448
99. de Witte MA, Sarhan D, Davis Z, Felices M, Vallera DA, Hinderlie P, et al. Early Reconstitution of NK and gammadelta T Cells and Its Implication for the Design of Post-Transplant Immunotherapy. *Biol Blood Marrow Transplant.* (2018) 24:1152–62. doi: 10.1016/j.bbmt.2018.02.023
100. Gogoi D, Biswas D, Borkakoty B, Mahanta J. Exposure to Plasmodium vivax is associated with the increased expression of exhaustion markers on gammadelta T lymphocytes. *Parasite Immunol.* 2018:e12594. doi: 10.1111/pim.12594
101. Fleming C, Morrissey S, Cai Y, Yan J. gammadelta T Cells: unexpected regulators of cancer development and progression. *Trends Cancer* (2017) 3:561–570. doi: 10.1016/j.trecan.2017.06.003
102. Henao-Tamayo M, Irwin SM, Shang S, Ordway D, Orme IM. T lymphocyte surface expression of exhaustion markers as biomarkers of the efficacy of chemotherapy for tuberculosis. *Tuberculosis* (2011) 91:308–13. doi: 10.1016/j.tube.2011.04.001
103. Shin EC, Park SH, Nascimbeni M, Major M, Caggiari L, de Re V, et al. The frequency of CD127(+) hepatitis C virus (HCV)-specific T cells but not the expression of exhaustion markers predicts the outcome of acute HCV infection. *J Virol.* (2013) 87:4772–7. doi: 10.1128/JVI.03122-12
104. Wherry EJ. T cell exhaustion. *Nat Immunol.* (2011) 12:492–9.
105. Jin HT, Anderson AC, Tan WG, West EE, Ha SJ, Araki K, et al. Cooperation of Tim-3 and PD-1 in CD8 T-cell exhaustion during chronic viral infection. *Proc Natl Acad Sci USA.* (2010) 107:14733–8. doi: 10.1073/pnas.1009731107
106. Le Bouteiller P, Tabiasco J, Polgar B, Kozma N, Giustiniani J, Siewiera J, et al. CD160: a unique activating NK cell receptor. *Immunol Lett.* (2011) 138:93–6. doi: 10.1016/j.imlet.2011.02.003
107. Nikolova M, Marie-Cardine A, Boumsell L, Bensussan A. BY55/CD160 acts as a co-receptor in TCR signal transduction of a human circulating cytotoxic effector T lymphocyte subset lacking CD28 expression. *Int Immunol.* (2002) 14:445–51. doi: 10.1093/intimm/14.5.445
108. Wentink MWJ, Mueller YM, Dalm VASH, Driessen GJ, van Hagen PM, van Montfrans JM, et al. Exhaustion of the CD8(+) T cell compartment in patients with mutations in phosphoinositide 3-kinase delta. *Front Immunol.* (2018) 9:446. doi: 10.3389/fimmu.2018.00446
109. Peretz Y, He Z, Shi Y, Yassine-Diab B, Goulet JP, Bordi R, et al. CD160 and PD-1 co-expression on HIV-specific CD8 T cells defines a subset with advanced dysfunction. *PLoS Pathog.* (2012) 8:e1002840. doi: 10.1371/journal.ppat.1002840
110. Althoff KN, McGinnis KA, Wyatt CM, Freiberg MS, Gilbert C, Oursler KK, et al. Comparison of risk and age at diagnosis of myocardial infarction, end-stage renal disease, and non-AIDS-defining cancer in HIV-infected versus uninfected adults. *Clin Infect Dis.* (2015) 60:627–38. doi: 10.1093/cid/ciu869
111. Scully E, Lockhart A, Huang L, Robles Y, Becerril C, Romero-Tejeda M, et al. Elevated levels of microbial translocation markers and CCL2 among older HIV-1-infected men. *J Infect Dis.* (2015) 213:771–5. doi: 10.1093/infdis/jiv501
112. Shiels MS, Althoff KN, Pfeiffer RM, Achenbach CJ, Abraham AG, Castilho J, et al. HIV infection, immunosuppression, and age at diagnosis of non-AIDS-defining cancers. *Clin Infect Dis.* (2017) 64:468–75. doi: 10.1093/cid/ciw764
113. Remacha AF, Cadafalch J, Sardà P, Barceló M, Fuster M. HIV and age do not synergistically affect age-related T-cell markers. *J Acquir Immune Defic Syndr.* (2018) 77:337–44. doi: 10.1097/QAI.0000000000001595
114. Setareh M, Schwarz H, Lotz M. A mRNA variant encoding a soluble form of 4-1BB, a member of the murine NGF/TNF receptor family. *Gene* (1995) 164:311–5.
115. Croft M. The role of TNF superfamily members in T-cell function and diseases. *Nat Rev Immunol.* (2009) 9:271–85. doi: 10.1038/nri2526

12

Galectin-9 Mediates HIV Transcription by Inducing TCR-Dependent ERK Signaling

*Florent Colomb[1], Leila B. Giron[1], Thomas A. Premeaux[2], Brooks I. Mitchell[2], Toshiro Niki[3,4], Emmanouil Papasavvas[1], Luis J. Montaner[1], Lishomwa C. Ndhlovu[2] and Mohamed Abdel-Mohsen[1]**

[1] *Vaccine and Immunotherapy Center, The Wistar Institute, Philadelphia, PA, United States,* [2] *Department of Tropical Medicine, Hawaii Center for AIDS, John A. Burns School of Medicine, University of Hawaii, Honolulu, HI, United States,* [3] *GalPharma Co., Ltd., Takamatsu-shi, Takamatsu, Japan,* [4] *Department of Immunology and Immunopathology, Kagawa University, Takamatsu, Japan*

***Correspondence:**
Mohamed Abdel-Mohsen
mmohsen@wistar.org

Endogenous plasma levels of the immunomodulatory carbohydrate-binding protein galectin-9 (Gal-9) are elevated during HIV infection and remain elevated after antiretroviral therapy (ART) suppression. We recently reported that Gal-9 regulates HIV transcription and potently reactivates latent HIV. However, the signaling mechanisms underlying Gal-9-mediated viral transcription remain unclear. Given that galectins are known to modulate T cell receptor (TCR)-signaling, we hypothesized that Gal-9 modulates HIV transcriptional activity, at least in part, through inducing TCR signaling pathways. Gal-9 induced T cell receptor ζ chain (CD3ζ) phosphorylation (11.2 to 32.1%; $P = 0.008$) in the J-Lat HIV latency model. Lck inhibition reduced Gal-9-mediated viral reactivation in the J-Lat HIV latency model (16.8–0.9%; $P < 0.0001$) and reduced both Gal-9-mediated CD4$^+$ T cell activation (10.3 to 1.65% CD69 and CD25 co-expression; $P = 0.0006$), and IL-2/TNFα secretion ($P < 0.004$) in primary CD4$^+$ T cells from HIV-infected individuals on suppressive ART. Using phospho-kinase antibody arrays, we found that Gal-9 increased the phosphorylation of the TCR-downstream signaling molecules ERK1/2 (26.7-fold) and CREB (6.6-fold). ERK and CREB inhibitors significantly reduced Gal-9-mediated viral reactivation (16.8 to 2.6 or 12.6%, respectively; $P < 0.0007$). Given that the immunosuppressive rapamycin uncouples HIV latency reversal from cytokine-associated toxicity, we also investigated whether rapamycin could uncouple Gal-9-mediated latency reactivation from its concurrent pro-inflammatory cytokine production. Rapamycin reduced Gal-9-mediated secretion of IL-2 (4.4-fold, $P = 0.001$) and TNF (4-fold, $P = 0.02$) without impacting viral reactivation (16.8% compared to 16.1%; $P = 0.2$). In conclusion, Gal-9 modulates HIV transcription by activating the TCR-downstream ERK and CREB signaling pathways in an Lck-dependent manner. Our findings could have implications for understanding the role of endogenous galectin interactions in modulating TCR signaling and maintaining chronic immune activation during ART-suppressed HIV infection. In addition, uncoupling Gal-9-mediated viral reactivation from undesirable pro-inflammatory effects, using rapamycin, may increase the potential utility of recombinant Gal-9 within the reversal of HIV latency eradication framework.

Keywords: HIV, lectins, galectin-9, T cell receptor, TCR signaling, rapamycin, HIV latency, HIV persistence

INTRODUCTION

Antiretroviral therapy (ART) effectively suppresses HIV replication but does not achieve viral eradication due to the persistence of latently-infected, long-lived CD4$^+$ T cells (1, 2). This persistent infection leads to continued immune activation, chronic inflammation, and ongoing damage to multiple organ systems (3, 4). Many studies indicate that HIV persistence is regulated, at least in part, by the immune system (5–8). Thus, understanding the host immune factors driving and maintaining HIV persistence is needed to develop new strategies to cure HIV and/or prevent the development of HIV-associated co-morbidities, which remain prevalent despite suppressive therapy.

One key regulator of immunological functions, and several cellular processes, is interactions between cell-surface glycans and glycan-binding proteins (lectins) (9–12). One class of lectins that play critical roles in T cell function are galectins, a family of β-galactoside-binding, soluble lectins (13–17). Among galectins, galectin-9 (Gal-9) has recently been recognized to play an essential role in regulating both adaptive and innate defense mechanisms and thus may be involved in HIV pathogenesis (18–20). Our prior work showed that endogenous secretion of Gal-9 is rapidly increased after HIV infection, and that elevated levels of Gal-9 do not return to normal after suppressive ART (20). More recently, we reported that the endogenous levels of Gal-9 are associated with HIV transcription *in vivo,* in plasma of HIV-infected, ART-suppressed individuals (8). We also demonstrated that treating CD4$^+$ T cells with recombinant Gal-9 (rGal-9) induces HIV transcription and reverses HIV latency *in vitro* and *ex vivo* (8). However, the signaling pathways by which Gal-9 modulates HIV transcriptional activity remain unclear.

The goal of this work was to identify the signaling mechanisms underlying Gal-9-mediated HIV transcription. We hypothesized that Gal-9 modulates HIV transcriptional activity through T cell receptor (TCR) signaling transduction, based on results in non-HIV contexts showing that galectins, including Gal-9, modulate TCR-signaling (21–23), and that Gal-9 interacts with various cell-surface proteins known to induce TCR signaling, including CD44 (24) and 41-BB (25–27). We show that Gal-9 modulates HIV transcription through activating the TCR-downstream ERK and CREB signaling pathways in a lymphocyte-specific protein tyrosine kinase (Lck)-dependent manner. This signaling pathway also induces an undesirable, pro-inflammatory response, namely secretion of IL-2 and TNF-α, and activating CD4$^+$ T cells. This pro-inflammatory response can be inhibited using the mTOR pathway inhibitor, rapamycin, without impacting Gal-9-mediated viral reactivation. Our results could have implications for understanding the role of endogenous galectin-9 in modulating TCR signaling *in vivo* and maintaining chronic immune activation during ART-suppressed HIV infection. In addition, uncoupling Gal-9-mediated viral reactivation from undesirable pro-inflammatory effects, using rapamycin, may increase the potential utility of rGal-9 within the reversal of HIV latency eradication framework.

MATERIALS AND METHODS

Cell Lines

As a model of HIV latency, we used "J-Lat" cells, which harbor latent, transcriptionally competent HIV provirus that encodes green fluorescent protein (GFP) as an indicator of viral reactivation (28, 29). We have shown in our previous work (8) that this latency model mimics the impact of Gal-9 on HIV transcription *ex vivo* using CD4$^+$ T cells from HIV-infected ART-suppressed individuals. Therefore, it can be used to investigate the signaling mechanisms underlying Gal-9-mediated viral transcription. J-Lat 5A8 clone was kindly provided by Dr. Warner Greene (The Gladstone Institute of Virology and Immunology). J-Lat 15.4 (catalog number 9850), 10.6 (catalog number 9849), and Jurkat E6-1 (catalog number 177) clones were provided by the NIH AIDS Reagent Program (Germantown, MD). J.CaM1.6 clone, a derivative mutant of Jurkat cells, which is deficient in Lck activity (30), was purchased from American Type Culture Collection (ATCC; Manassas, VA; catalog number CRL-2063). Cell lines were maintained in Roswell Park Memorial Institute (RPMI) medium with L-glutamine (Corning Cellgro, Tewksbury, MA, United States), supplemented with 10% Fetal Bovine Serum (Gibco, Thermo Fisher Scientific, Waltham, MA, United States), and 1% Penicillin/Streptomycin (Thermo Fisher Scientific, Waltham, MA, United States).

Primary Cells

Cryopreserved peripheral blood mononuclear cells (PBMCs) were retrospectively collected from five HIV-infected individuals on suppressive ART, enrolled in the Philadelphia FIGHT cohort. Research protocols were approved by Wistar Institute and Philadelphia FIGHT Committees on Human Research. Written informed consent was obtained for all participants, and all data and specimens were coded to protect confidentiality. Subject characteristics are documented in **Supplementary Table 1.**

Reagents

A stable form of recombinant galectin-9 was obtained through our collaborators at GalPharma Co., Ltd. (Kagawa, Japan). A natural form of recombinant galectin-9 was purchased from R&D Systems (Minneapolis, MN; catalog # 2045-GA-050). Lck inhibitor A770041 was purchased from Axon Med Chem (Reston, VA). ERK inhibitor LY3214996 was purchased from Selleck Chemicals (Houston, TX). CREB inhibitor 666-15 and InSolution Rapamycin were purchased from Millipore Sigma (Burlington, MA). SMARTpool Accell Lck siRNA was purchased from Dharmacon (Lafayette, CO; cat # E-003151-00-0005) and Silencer™ Select Negative Control No. 1 siRNA was purchased from Thermo Fisher (Waltham, MA; cat# 4390843). ImmunoCult Human CD3/CD28 T Cell Activator was purchased from STEMCELL (Vancouver, BC, Canada).

Phosphorylated CD3ζ-Chain Quantification

J-Lat 5A8, Jurkat, or J.CaM1.6 cells were cultured at 1×10^6 cells/ml and treated with stable form of rGal-9 (200 nM), natural form of rGal-9 (200 nM), or an equivalent volume of phosphate buffered saline (PBS), in the presence of Lck inhibitor (1 μM) or an equivalent volume of dimethyl sulfoxide (DMSO). After 15 min, cells were collected, washed twice in ice-cold PBS, fixed, and permeabilized using the BD Cytofix/Cytoperm kit according to the manufacturer's instructions. Fixed cells were stained with PE anti-CD247 (TCRζ, CD3ζ) antibody (Clone 6B10.2, Biolegend), washed, and analyzed for PE fluorescence using LSR II flow cytometer and FACSDiva software (Becton Dickinson, Mountain View, CA, United States). Data were analyzed using FlowJo (TreeStar Inc., Ashland, OR, United States).

Human Phospho-Kinase Antibody Array

Proteome profiler human phospho-kinase arrays were purchased from R&D Systems, Inc. (Minneapolis, MN, United States). Ten million J-Lat 5A8 cells were treated for 30 min with 200 nM rGal-9 or an equivalent volume of PBS. Cells were washed twice in cold PBS and processed according to the manufacturer's instructions. Briefly, the cells were lysed for 30 min on a rotating shaker at 4°C. Lysates were centrifuged at 14,000 g for 5 min, and supernatants were incubated on the array membrane overnight on an orbital shaker at 4°C. Membranes were washed three times and incubated for 2 h at room temperature with anti-horseradish peroxidase antibody. After another three washes, membranes were incubated for 1 min with Chemi Reagent. Membrane images were captured using ImageQuant LAS 4010 (GE Healthcare Bio-Sciences, Pittsburg, PA, United States) and densitometry analysis was performed with Image Studio Lite Version 5.2 (LI-COR Biotechnology, Lincoln, NE, United States).

Measurement of HIV Latency Reversal

J-Lat 5A8, 10.6, and 15.4 cells were pre-incubated for 1 h with 1 μM for Lck inhibitor, 1 μM for ERK1/2 inhibitor, 1 μM for CREB inhibitor, 5 μM for rapamycin, or an equivalent volume of PBS. Cells were then treated with rGal-9 (multiple concentrations), 25 μl of ImmunoCult human CD3/CD28 T Cell Activator, or an equivalent volume of PBS, for 24 h. Mean fluorescence intensity of HIV-encoded GFP expression was assessed using LSR II flow cytometer and FACSDiva software. Data were analyzed with FlowJo.

Lck Silencing Using Small Interfering RNA (siRNA)

J-Lat 5A8 were resuspended in Nucleofector solution (Lonza) at 1×10^6 cells/100 μL, in the presence of 1.5 μM of Silencer™ Select (non-target) negative control No. 1 siRNA (Thermo Fisher, Cat# 4390843) or SMARTpool Accell Lck siRNA (Dharmacon, Cat # E-003151-00-0005). Cells were nucleofected using Amaxa Nucleofector4D (Lonza), according to manufacturer protocol for Jurkat clone E6.1 nucleofection. Cells were then plated in 1 ml of RPMI supplemented with 10% FBS. After 48 h, cells were resuspended in fresh medium at 1×10^6 cells/ml, plated in 96-well plates, and treated with rGal-9 (200 nM), or an equivalent volume of PBS, for 24 h. Mean fluorescence intensity of HIV-encoded GFP expression was assessed using LSR II flow cytometer and FACSDiva software. Data were analyzed with FlowJo.

Isolation and Treatment of Primary CD4+ T Cells

CD4+ T cells were enriched from the cryopreserved PBMCs by negative selection using the EasySep Human CD4+ T Cell Enrichment Kit (Stemcell Technologies), according to the manufacturer's instructions. Primary CD4+ T cells were maintained in RPMI with L-glutamine supplemented with 20% FBS. Primary CD4+ T cells were pre-incubated with 1 μM for Lck inhibitor or 5 μM for rapamycin. Cells were then treated with 500 nM of rGal-9, ImmunoCult human CD3/CD28 T Cell Activator, or an equivalent volume of PBS, for 24 h. Cells were centrifuged for 5 min at 250 g, and cells and supernatants were collected separately.

Measurement of CD4+ T Cells Viability and Activation

The surface expression of CD69 and CD25 markers of T-cell activation were measured using flow cytometry. Cells were stained with Zombie Aqua Fixable Viability Kit (Biolegend) and then stained with the following fluorescently-conjugated monoclonal antibodies: APC mouse anti-human CD3 (Clone UCHT1, Biolegend), V450 mouse anti-human CD4 (Clone RPA-T4, Biolegend), PE mouse anti-human CD69 (Clone FN50, Biolegend), PerCP-Cy5.5 mouse anti-human CD25 (Clone M-A251, Biolegend). Apoptosis was determined using Propidium iodide and Annexin V Pacific blue (Biolegend). anti-CD95 (1 ug/ml; clone E0S9.1; Biolegend) stimulation for 6 h was used as positive control for apoptosis. Cells were analyzed using LSR II flow cytometer and FACSDiva software. Data were analyzed with FlowJo software.

Measurement of TNF-α and IL-2 Levels Using ELISA

Supernatants from J-Lat 5A8 and primary CD4+ T cells cultures treated or not with rGal-9, αCD3/αCD28, and inhibitors were collected. Levels of TNFα and IL-2 cytokines were quantified using human TNF and IL-2 DuoSet Elisa kits (R&D Systems, Inc., Minneapolis, MN) according to the manufacturer's instructions. Optical density was measured at 450 and 540 nm using Versa Max microplate reader. Data were analyzed using GraphPad Prism.

Measurement of Cytokine Secretion Using Multiplex Luminex

Isolated CD4+ T cells from three HIV-infected ART-suppressed individuals were treated with 200 nM Gal-9, 500 nM Gal-9, or 0.5% DMSO as control for 4 h, 24 h, or 3 days. Culture supernatants were collected after 3 days and were processed according to recommended manufacture procedure with a Milliplex MAP Human High Sensitivity T Cell Panel (EMD Millipore, Billerica, Massachusetts) for GM-CSF, TNF-α, IL-13, IL-12 (p70), IL-10, IL-8, IL-7, IL-6, IL-5, IL-4, IL-2, IL-1b, and IFN-γ. Samples were acquired on a Luminex 200 (EMD Millipore). Samples were run in duplicate. The intra-assay CV% for analytes measured was <7%. The inter-assay CV% was <11%.

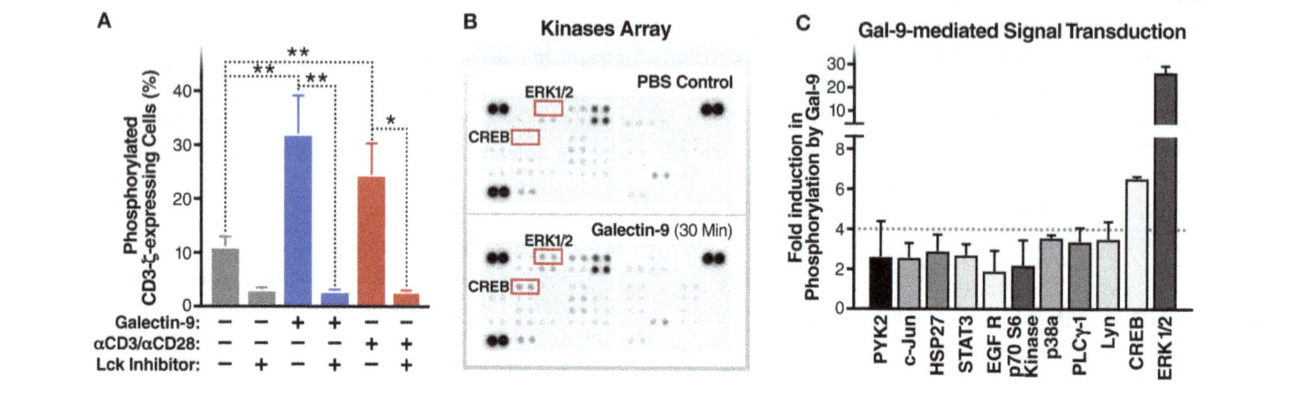

FIGURE 1 | Gal-9 induces the phosphorylation of TCR complex CD3ζ chain, ERK, and CREB. **(A)** J-Lat 5A8 cells were treated with Gal-9 (200 nM, blue bars) or αCD3/αCD28 antibodies (red bars) for 15 min in the presence or absence of Lck inhibitor (1 μM) and stained with PE-conjugated anti-phospho-CD3ζ antibody. Cell staining/phosphorylation was quantified by flow cytometry. Mean ± SD is displayed, and statistical comparisons were performed using two-tailed unpaired *t*-tests. **p* < 0.05, and ***p* < 0.01. **(B,C)** J-Lat 5A8 cells were treated with Gal-9 (200 nM) or an equivalent volume of PBS for 30 min and analyzed using Proteome Profiler Human Phospho-Kinase Array Kit. **(B)** Array images were captured using ImageQuant^{TM} LAS 4,000 and **(C)** phosphorylation signal intensity was analyzed by pixel density quantification using Image Studio Lite.

Statistical Analysis

Two-tailed paired and unpaired *t*-tests were used for comparisons. All statistical analyses were conducted using GraphPad Prism release 7.0 (GraphPad Software, San Diego, CA, United States) and statistical significance was set at a *p*-value of 0.05.

RESULTS

Gal-9 Induces Lck-Dependent T Cell Receptor ζ Chain (CD3ζ) Phosphorylation

The T cell receptor ζ chain (CD3ζ) is the principal signal transduction component of TCR signaling (31–33). Lck activity is required for the phosphorylation of signaling motifs in CD3-ζ and this phosphorylation is the initial step in the TCR signaling cascade (34, 35). To begin to test our hypothesis that Gal-9-mediates HIV transcriptional activity by activating TCR signaling, we examined the impact of rGal-9 on the phosphorylation of CD3ζ in the J-Lat 5A8 latency model. rGal-9 significantly induced the percentage of cells expressing phosphorylated CD3ζ [from 11.2 ± 1.8% to 32.1 ± 7.0% (mean ± SD); $P = 0.0076$] (**Figure 1A**). This induction was completely inhibited by preincubation with an Lck inhibitor (from 32.1 ± 7.0% to 2.8 ± 0.2%; $P = 0.002$) (**Figure 1A**). To confirm that Gal-9-mediated CD3ζ phosphorylation is Lck-dependent, we used the J.CaM1.6 clone (a derivative mutant of Jurkat cells, which is deficient in Lck activity). rGal-9 induced CD3ζ phosphorylation in wild type Jurkat cells [from 8.2 ± 2.2% to 44.4 ± 6.2% (mean ± SD); $P = 0.0007$], but had no effect on J.CaM1.6 (from 2.1 ± 0.6% to 1.6 ± 0.02%; $P = 0.23$) (**Supplementary Figure 1**). Confirming dose-dependent relationship, we found that rGal-9 is able to phosphorylate CD3ζ starting from 25 nM in the J-Lat 5A8 HIV latency model (**Supplementary Figure 2**). These data demonstrate that Gal-9 induces TCR-signaling in HIV latently-infected cells through Lck-mediated CD3ζ phosphorylation.

Gal-9 Induces Phosphorylation of ERK and CREB Signaling Molecules

To identify components of the TCR signaling cascade that are induced by Gal-9 downstream of CD3ζ phosphorylation, we used Proteome Profiler Human Phospho-Kinase arrays to assess the phosphorylation levels of 43 kinases and related transcription factors. rGal-9 treatment of J-Lat 5A8 cells induced the phosphorylation of several downstream effectors of TCR signaling, including ERK1/2 (26.7-fold) and CREB (6.6-fold) (**Figures 1B,C**). These data demonstrate that Gal-9-mediated induction of CD3ζ phosphorylation results in activation of ERK1/2 and CREB signaling pathways.

Gal-9 Modulates HIV Transcription Through Activating the TCR Downstream Signaling, ERK and CREB, in an Lck Dependent Manner

To evaluate whether TCR/Lck-dependent ERK1/2-CREB phosphorylation modulate the reactivation of latent HIV by Gal-9, we assessed the impact of Lck, ERK, and CREB inhibitors on rGal-9-mediated HIV latency reactivation in three J-Lat HIV latency model clones, 5A8, 10.6, and 15.4. Lck inhibition strongly reduced rGal-9-mediated HIV latency reactivation in the J-Lat 5A8 clone [from 16.8 ± 0.7% to 0.9 ± 0.03% (mean ± SD); $P < 0.0001$], the J-Lat 10.6 clone (from 41.9 ± 4.9% to 9.9 ± 0.44%; $P = 0.0004$), and the J-Lat 15.4 clone (from 2.5 ± 0.64% to 0.1 ± 0.06%; $P = 0.0027$). ERK inhibition showed a similar strong reduction of rGal-9-mediated HIV latency reactivation in the J-Lat 5A8 clone [from 16.8 ± 0.7% to 2.6 ± 0.3% (mean ± SD); $P < 0.0001$], the J-Lat 10.6 clone (from 41.9 ± 4.9% to 21.23 ± 1.29%; $P = 0.002$), and the J-Lat 15.4 clone (from 2.5 ± 0.64% to 0.1 ± 0.1%; $P = 0.0029$). Last, CREB inhibition showed a modest, yet significant, reduction in rGal-9-mediated HIV latency reactivation in the J-Lat 5A8 clone [from 16.8 ± 0.7% to 12.6 ± 0.3% (mean ± SD); $P =$

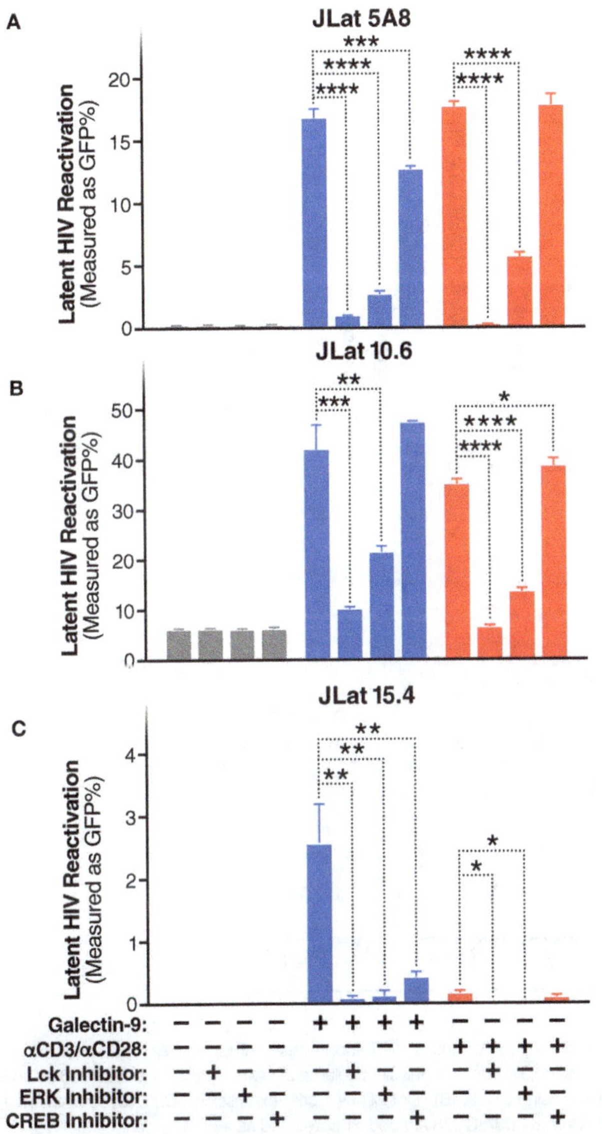

FIGURE 2 | Gal-9 induces HIV transcription through TCR-dependent ERK/CREB signaling. Levels of latent HIV reactivation in three J-Lat clones 24 h after *in vitro* stimulation with Gal-9 (200 nM) in the presence or absence of 1 μM of Lck inhibitor, ERK inhibitor, or CREB inhibitor. HIV-encoded GFP expression was detected by flow cytometry. **(A)** J-Lat 5A8, **(B)** J-Lat 10.6, **(C)** J-Lat 15.4 cells. αCD3 /αCD28 antibodies (red bars) were used as a positive control. Mean ± SD is displayed, and statistical comparisons were performed using two-tailed unpaired *t*-tests. $^{*}p < 0.05$; $^{**}p < 0.01$, $^{***}p < 0.001$, and $^{****}p < 0.0001$.

0.0007], and the J-Lat 15.4 clone (from 2.5 ± 0.64% to 0.4 ± 0.1%; $P = 0.0047$) (**Figures 2A–C**). As expected, Lck/ERK/CREB inhibition had a similar impact on αCD3/αCD28-mediated HIV latency reactivation (**Figures 2A–C**). To confirm the role of Lck in Gal-9-mediated HIV latency reactivation, we used siRNA to silence Lck in the J-Lat 5A8 HIV latency model. Lck siRNA significantly reduced Gal-9-mediated HIV latency reactivation compared to non-target siRNA control [from 13.4 ± 0.3% to 6.8 ± 0.2% (mean ± SD); $P < 0.0001$] (**Supplementary Figure 3**). Confirming a dose-dependent relationship, we found that rGal-9 is able to reactivate a fraction of latent HIV at 10 nM in the J-Lat 5A8 HIV latency model (**Supplementary Figure 4**). Together, these data indicate that Gal-9 modulates HIV transcriptional activity through induction of TCR/Lck-mediated ERK1/2 signaling and to a lesser extent CREB signaling.

Throughout this study, we are using a stable form of galectin-9 (8, 22, 26, 36–39). To confirm that the natural form of Gal-9 functions in a similar way as the stable form in phosphorylating CD3ζ and reactivating HIV latency, we repeated some of the above experiments using a natural form of recombinant Gal-9 (R&D systems). The natural form of recombinant Gal-9 induced CD3ζ phosphorylation [from 8.2 ± 2.2% to 44.4 ± 6.2% (mean ± SD); $P = 0.0007$], and HIV latency reactivation [from 0.1 ± 00.6% to 20.2 ± 0.8% (mean ± SD); $P < 0.0001$] in the J-Lat 5A8 HIV latency model, and these effects were significantly inhibited by Lck inhibitor (**Supplementary Figures 5A,B**).

Gal-9-Mediated CD4^{+} T Cell Activation Is Lck-Dependent

Next, to determine whether Gal-9-mediated T cell activation is dependent on the same mechanism as Gal-9-mediated viral activation, we examined the impact of Lck inhibition of Gal-9-mediated CD4^{+} T cell activation in primary cells from HIV-infected ART-suppressed individuals. Cell viability was determined using Zombie Aqua Fixable Viability and apoptosis was determined using Propidium iodide and Annexin V staining (**Supplementary Figure 6**). T cell activation was measured by co-expression of the T cell-surface activation markers CD69 and CD25. rGal-9 induced CD4^{+} T cell activation [from 0.14 ± 0.03% to 10.34 ± 1.1% (mean ± SEM)]. This effect was significantly reduced by Lck inhibition (from 10.34 ± 1.1% to 1.65 ± 0.5%; $P = 0.0006$) (**Figure 3**). Lck inhibition did not fully inhibit Gal-9-mediated T cell activation, suggesting that while TCR signaling plays a major role in Gal-9-mediated T cell activation, other signaling pathways may contribute to this effect.

Gal-9 Induces IL2 and TNF-α Secretion by Inducing Lck-Dependent ERK and CREB Signaling

Given that Gal-9 induces TCR signaling and activates T cells, we posited that the Gal-9-mediated reactivation of HIV latency would be accompanied by secretion of pro-inflammatory cytokines. Indeed, rGal-9 treatment of J-Lat 5A8 cells was associated with a significant induction of IL2 [from < 15.6 pg/ml to 375.6 ± 28.1 pg/ml (mean ± SD)] and TNFα (from <15.6 pg/ml to 208.8 ± 9.7 pg/ml). This effect was significantly reduced by inhibiting Lck, ERK, or CREB activity ($P < 0.001$; **Figures 4A,B**). Similar results were obtained using primary CD4^{+} T cells from HIV-infected, ART-suppressed individuals: rGal-9 significantly induced the production of IL2 (from < 15.6 pg/ml to 700.2 ± 93.1 pg/ml (mean ± SEM)] and TNFα (from <15.6 pg/ml to 1372.68 ± 240.75 pg/ml); Lck inhibition significantly reduced IL2 (from 700.2 ± 93.1 pg/ml to 47.9 ± 47.9

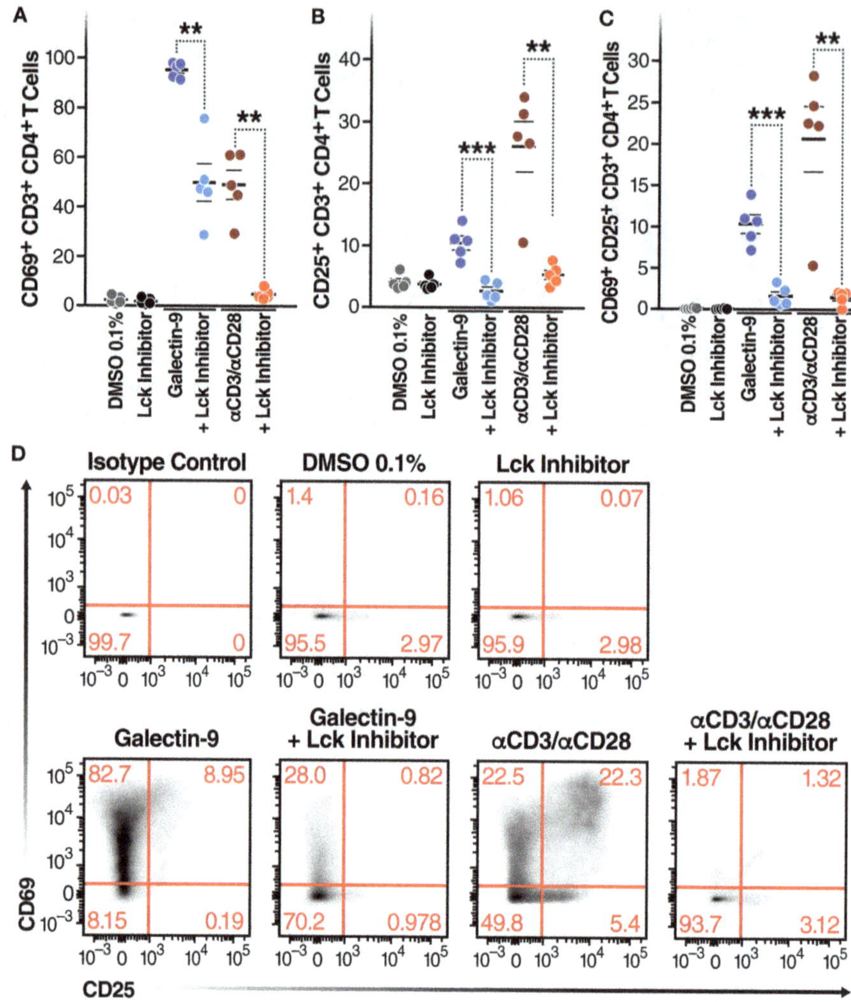

FIGURE 3 | Gal-9-mediated CD4+ T cell activation is Lck-dependent. CD4+ T cells isolated from 5 HIV-infected ART-suppressed individuals were treated for 24 h with Gal-9 (500 nM) or the equivalent volume of PBS (Control) in the presence of 1 μM of Lck inhibitor or the equivalent volume of DMSO. Cells were analyzed by flow cytometry for expression of CD69 and CD25 activation markers. **(A)** % of CD4+ T cells expressing CD69, **(B)** % of CD4+ T cells expressing CD25, **(C)** % of CD4+ T cells co-expressing CD69 and CD25. **(D)** A representative flow cytometry plot of one individual. αCD3/αCD28 antibodies were used as a positive control. Mean ± SEM is displayed, and statistical comparisons were performed using two-tailed paired *t*-tests. $^{**}p < 0.01$, and $^{***}p < 0.001$.

pg/ml; $P = 0.0006$) and TNFα secretion (from 1372.68 ± 240.75 pg/ml to 37.8 ± 37.8 pg/ml; $P = 0.0035$) (**Figures 4C,D**). Further, we examined the impact of rGal-9 on the secretion of a panel of pro and anti-inflammatory cytokines. **Supplementary Figure 7** shows that rGal-9 induces the secretion of several pro- and anti- inflammatory cytokines. Together the data in **Figures 3, 4** demonstrate that Gal-9-mediated T cell activation and pro-inflammatory cytokine secretion are dependent on the same mechanism that induces HIV transcriptional activity, namely Lck-mediated induction of the TCR downstream ERK/CREB signaling. These undesirable, pro-inflammatory effects of Gal-9 limit its potential to be used as an HIV latency reversal agent. Thus, we asked whether it would be possible to separate the desirable (HIV latency reversal) from the undesirable (T cell activation and cytokine secretion) effects of Gal-9.

Rapamycin Reduces Gal-9-Mediated Cytokine-Secretion Without Impacting the Ability of Gal-9 to Reactivate HIV

A recent study demonstrated that the immunosuppressive mTOR inhibitor rapamycin can uncouple HIV latency reversal from cytokine-associated toxicity (40). Furthermore, it has been shown that rapamycin can inhibit the proinflammatory effects of Gal-9 (41). We, therefore, investigated whether rapamycin could uncouple Gal-9-mediated latency reactivation from its concurrent effect on pro-inflammatory cytokine production. Co-treatment with rapamycin (5 μM) did not reduce the ability of Gal-9 to reactivate latent HIV (5 μM) [16.8 ± 0.7% compared to 16.1 ± 0.3% (mean ± SD); $P = 0.2$] (**Figure 5A**). However, rapamycin did significantly reduce Gal-9-mediated secretion of IL-2 [from 375.6 ± 28.13 pg/ml to 194.8 ± 12.43 pg/ml

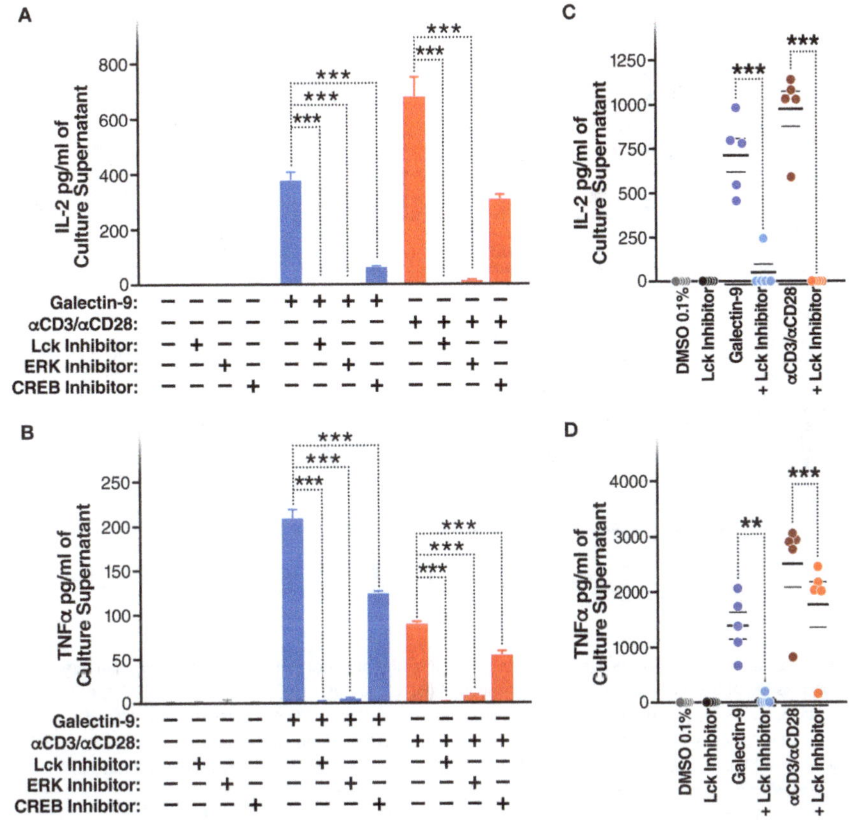

FIGURE 4 | Gal-9 induces IL2 and TNF-α secretion by the same mechanism as viral reactivation. **(A)** IL2 and **(B)** TNF-α concentrations quantified by ELISA, in J-LAT 5A8 cell culture supernatants, after 24 h of Gal-9 treatment (200 mM) in presence or absence of 1 μM of Lck inhibitor, ERK inhibitor, or CREB inhibitor. Mean ± SD is displayed, and statistical comparisons were performed using two-tailed unpaired *t*-tests. ***$p < 0.001$. **(C)** IL2 and **(D)** TNF concentrations quantified by ELISA, in supernatants from CD4+ T cells from five HIV-infected, ART-suppressed individuals, after 24 h treatment with Gal-9 (500 nM) or the equivalent volume of PBS (Control) in the presence of 1 μM of Lck inhibitor or the equivalent volume of DMSO. αCD3/αCD28 antibodies were used as a positive control. Mean ± SEM is displayed, and statistical comparisons were performed using two-tailed paired *t*-tests. **$p < 0.01$, and ***$p < 0.001$.

(mean ± SD); $P < 0.001$] and TNF (from 208.8 ± 9.7 pg/ml to 107.2 ± 5 pg/ml; $P < 0.001$) in the J-Lat 5A8 latency model (**Figures 5B,C**). Similarly, Rapamycin reduced Gal-9-mediated secretion of IL-2 [from 700.23 ± 91.1 pg/ml to 160.36 ± 105.9 pg/ml (mean ± SEM); $P = 0.0006$] and TNF (from 1372.68 ± 240.75 pg/ml to 340.13 ± 120.6 pg/ml; $P = 0.0015$) in primary $CD4^+$ T cells from HIV-infected individuals on suppressive ART (**Figures 5D,E**). These data demonstrate that mTOR signaling inhibition may be used to uncouple Gal-9-mediated viral reactivation from undesirable pro-inflammatory effects.

DISCUSSION

Gal-9 promotes HIV transcription by a previously unidentified mechanism (8). Given that Gal-9 is known to cross-link several surface proteins, some of which are involved in TCR signaling and that Gal-9 can induce TCR signaling (22), we hypothesized that Gal-9 promotes HIV transcriptional activity through TCR signaling transduction. In this study, we demonstrate that Gal-9 modulates HIV transcription through activating the TCR-downstream ERK and CREB signaling pathways, in an Lck-dependent manner. We also show that this same signaling pathway that induces HIV transcription also induces an undesirable pro-inflammatory response, namely secretion of IL-2 and TNFα as a consequence of T cell activation. These undesirable, Gal-9-mediated pro-inflammatory responses can be inhibited using the mTOR pathway inhibitor, rapamycin, without blunting Gal-9-mediated viral reactivation.

Gal-9 has several effects on T cells during HIV infection. It renders $CD4^+$ T cells less susceptible to HIV infection via induction of the host restriction factor cyclin-dependent kinase inhibitor 1 (p 21) (42). It can also increase HIV entry by inducing the $CD4^+$ T cell-surface concentration of protein disulfide isomerase (PDI) (43). We have previously shown that the endogenous levels of Gal-9 are induced after HIV infection and that these levels do not return to normal levels after ART suppression (20). We also found a positive correlation between endogenous levels of Gal-9 and levels of HIV transcription in $CD4^+$ T cells during ART suppression (8). The impact of this chronically elevated levels of Gal-9 on immune functions during ART-suppressed HIV infection is not

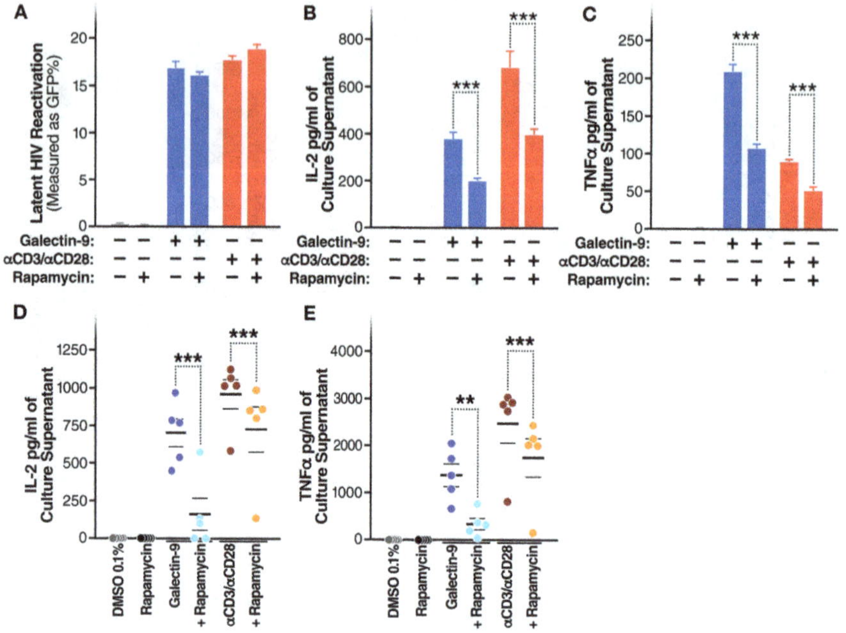

FIGURE 5 | Rapamycin reduces Gal-9-mediated cytokine-secretion without impacting the ability of Gal-9 to reactivate HIV. **(A)** Viral reactivation in J-Lat 5A8 cells by Gal-9 (200 nM) in the presence or absence of 5 μM of rapamycin. Concentration of **(B)** IL2, and **(C)** TNF-α quantified by ELISA in cell culture supernatants. Mean ± SD is displayed, and statistical comparisons were performed using two-tailed unpaired *t*-tests. $^{***}p < 0.001$. Concentration of IL2 **(D)** and TNF-α **(E)** secretion quantified by ELISA in culture supernatants of CD4^{+} T cells isolated from five HIV+ ART-suppressed individuals after 24 h of Gal-9 stimulation (500 mM) in the presence of absence of 5 μM rapamycin. Mean ± SEM are displayed, and statistical comparisons were performed using two-tailed paired *t*-tests. $^{**}p < 0.01$, and $^{***}p < 0.001$.

clear. Our current study demonstrates that Gal-9 induces Lck-dependent ERK/CREB signaling in HIV-infected latently infected cells, which may explain the correlation between Gal-9 and HIV transcriptional activity *in vivo*. However, this induction of TCR signaling by Gal-9 raises an important question of whether elevated endogenous Gal-9 levels contribute to the state of chronic inflammation and chronic immune activation during suppressive ART. Elevated T cell activation persists during suppressive ART (44) and is associated with the development of HIV-associated co-morbidities and premature mortality (44–47); it may also contribute to HIV persistence (48–51). This chronic immune activation involves multifactorial mechanisms (52–59), and the persistent induction of TCR signaling by the elevated levels of endogenous Gal-9 may be playing an important, unrecognized, role in sustaining it. Interventions that target Gal-9 may prove useful in inhibiting chronic immune activation, which might ultimately reduce the development of HIV-associated co-morbidities and levels of HIV persistence during suppressive ART.

Gal-9 is a multifaceted lectin, with opposing roles in modulating innate and adaptive immune responses. Gal-9 was mainly described to exhibit immunosuppressive activities (24, 60–67). Gal-9 can also increase the function of regulatory T cells (T-regs) through interaction with CD44 (24) and may impair Natural Killer cells (NK) cytotoxicity and cytokine production through a Tim-3 independent mechanism (68). Along the same line, two recent studies demonstrated that Gal-9 suppresses B cell receptor signaling and B cell activation through interaction with CD45 and IgM-BCR complex (69, 70). However, other studies showed that Gal-9 exhibits immunopotentiating activity in the setting of immunosuppression (71) and induces TCR signaling (22), similar to our current study. Also, the endogenous levels of Gal-9 are induced during many inflammatory conditions (66, 72–74). Together, it is likely that Gal-9 effects are context-dependent and cell-type-dependent. The effect of Gal-9 on cell-mediated immunity in different subsets of T cells and other immune cells, during ART-suppressed HIV infection, warrants a broader investigation. Clarifying the signaling pathways induced or inhibited by Gal-9 in different cell-population, during HIV infection, may provide insights that may lead to the development of novel therapies to improve immune functionality, and reduce inflammation-associated co-morbidities, in the setting of viral suppression by ART.

The ability of Gal-9 to potently induce latent HIV transcription suggested that it could be considered within the "shock and kill" HIV eradication framework (8). However, the adverse Gal-9-mediated induction of pro-inflammatory cytokines, by the same pathway, limits the potential use of Gal-9 as a shock and kill agent. The recent study by Martin et al. (40) raised the possibility of using rapamycin, an immunosuppressive agent that does not affect TCR signaling, to prevent the adverse effects of T cell activation without impacting HIV transcription. Unlike several immunosuppressive agents that impact TCR signaling, rapamycin suppresses IL-2 downstream signaling (75, 76). Our data show that rapamycin is able to inhibit the pro-inflammatory impact of Gal-9 without affecting its ability to reactivate latent infection. That is in agreement with a previous study that used rapamycin to inhibit the proinflammatory effects of galectin-9 on dendritic cells and promote allograft tolerance in mice (41). Uncoupling Gal-9-mediated viral reactivation from undesirable pro-inflammatory effects, using rapamycin, may increase the potential utility of recombinant Gal-9 within the "reversal of HIV latency" eradication framework.

In summary, we identified TCR/Lck-dependent ERK1/2-CREB as the signaling pathways underlying Gal-9 modulation of HIV transcriptional activity. We also found that rapamycin can uncouple the Gal-9 impact on HIV transcription from the undesirable, pro-inflammatory secretions associated with inducing TCR signaling. Our data highlight the further investigations needed to comprehensively understand the immunologic consequences of Gal-9 *in vivo*, during ART-suppressed HIV infection. Our findings could have implications for understanding the role of endogenous galectin interactions in modulating TCR signaling and maintaining chronic immune activation, that persists during ART-suppressed HIV infection. Finally, uncoupling Gal-9-mediated viral reactivation from undesirable pro-inflammatory effects, using rapamycin, may increase the potential utility of recombinant Gal-9 within the reversal of HIV latency eradication framework.

AUTHOR CONTRIBUTIONS

FC, LG, TP, BM, EP, LM, LN, and MA M designed and carried out experiments. EP and LM selected study subjects and provided samples. TN contributed reagents. FC, LG, TP, EP, TN, LM, LN, and MA-M analyzed and interpreted data. FC and MA-M wrote the manuscript, and all authors edited it.

FUNDING

This work was supported by NIH (R21 AI129636, R21 NS106970, and P30CA010815-49S2), W.W. Smith Charitable Trust (grant # A1701), Campbell Foundation award, Penn Center for AIDS Research (P30 AI 045008), and The Foundation for AIDS Research (amfAR) Impact Grant # 109840-65-RGRL. Additional support was provided by the NIH-funded BEAT-HIV Martin Delaney Collaboratory to cure HIV-1 infection (1UM1Al126620) and the Philadelphia Foundation.

ACKNOWLEDGMENTS

We would like to thank Rachel E. Locke, Ph.D. for providing comments and editing.

SUPPLEMENTARY MATERIAL

Supplementary Figure 1 | Gal-9-mediated CD3ζ phosphorylation is Lck-dependent. Jurkat E6-1 and J.CaM1.6 (a derivative mutant of Jurkat cells, which are deficient in Lck activity) cells were treated with Gal-9 (200 nM), or an equivalent volume of PBS, for 15 min and stained with PE-conjugated anti-phospho-CD3ζ antibody. Cell staining/phosphorylation was quantified by flow cytometry. Mean ± SD is displayed, and statistical comparisons were performed using two-tailed unpaired *t*-tests. $^{***}p < 0.001$.

Supplementary Figure 2 | Low concentrations of Gal-9 induce CD3ζ phosphorylation. J-Lat 5A8 cells were treated with escalating doses of Gal-9 (0–200 nM) for 15 min and stained with PE-conjugated anti-phospho-CD3ζ antibody. Cell staining/phosphorylation was quantified by flow cytometry. Mean ± SD is displayed, and statistical comparisons were performed using two-tailed unpaired *t*-tests comparing each concentration to the 0 nM control. $^{*}p < 0.05$, and $^{**}p < 0.01$.

Supplementary Figure 3 | Gal-9-mediated HIV latency reactivation is Lck-dependent. J-Lat 5A8 were transfected with Lck siRNA or non-target siRNA control using Amaxa Nucleofector4D. After 48 h, cells were treated with rGal-9 (200 nM), or an equivalent volume of PBS, for 24 h. HIV-encoded GFP expression was detected by flow cytometry. Mean ± SD is displayed, and statistical comparisons were performed using two-tailed unpaired *t*-tests. $^{***}p < 0.001$, and $^{****}p < 0.0001$.

Supplementary Figure 4 | Low concentrations of Gal-9 reactivate latent HIV in the J-Lat HIV latency model. J-Lat 5A8 cells were treated with escalating doses of Gal-9 (0–200 nM) for 24 h. HIV-encoded GFP expression was detected by flow cytometry. Mean ± SD is displayed, and statistical comparisons were performed using two-tailed unpaired *t*-tests comparing each concentration to the 0 nM control. $^{*}p < 0.05$, $^{***}p < 0.001$, and $^{****}p < 0.0001$.

Supplementary Figure 5 | The natural form of Gal-9 phosphorylates CD3ζ and reactivates latent HIV in Lck dependent. **(A)** J-Lat 5A8 cells were treated with the natural form of Gal-9 (200 nM) or an equivalent volume of PBS for 15 min and stained with PE-conjugated anti-phospho-CD3ζ antibody. Cell staining/phosphorylation was quantified by flow cytometry. **(B)** J-Lat 5A8 cells were treated with the natural form of Gal-9 (200 nM) or an equavelent volume of PBS for 24 h. HIV-encoded GFP expression was detected by flow cytometry. Mean ± SD is displayed, and statistical comparisons were performed using two-tailed unpaired *t*-tests. $^{****}p < 0.0001$.

Supplementary Figure 6 | Impact of Gal-9 on CD4+ T cell viability and apoptosis. **(A)** CD4^{+} T cells isolated from 5 HIV-infected ART-suppressed individuals were treated for 24 h with Gal-9 (500 nM) or DMSO Control in the presence of 1 μM of Lck inhibitor or the equivalent volume of DMSO. Cell viability was determined using Zombie Aqua Fixable Viability staining. **(B)** A representative flow cytometry plot from one individual. **(C)** CD4^{+} T cells isolated from one HIV-infected ART-suppressed individual were treated for 24 h with Gal-9 (500 nM) or DMSO Control. Apoptosis was determined using Propidium iodide and Annexin V Pacific blue (Biolegend). anti-CD95 (1 ug/ml) stimulation for 6 h was used as positive control. Experiment was performed in duplicates. Mean ± SD is displayed **(D)** A representative flow cytometry plot of one replicate.

Supplementary Figure 7 | Gal-9 induces the secretion of several pro- and anti-inflammatory cytokines. CD4^{+} T cells isolated from 3 HIV-infected ART-suppressed individuals were treated for 24 h with Gal-9 (200 nM), rGal-9 (500 nM), or DMSO Control for 4 h, 24 h, or 3 days. Culture supernatants were collected on day 3 and levels the 13 indicated pro- and anti-inflammatory cytokines were determined using Luminex assay.

Supplementary Table 1 | Subject characteristics.

REFERENCES

1. Finzi D, Hermankova M, Pierson T, Carruth LM, Buck C, Chaisson RE, et al. Identification of a reservoir for HIV-1 in patients on highly active antiretroviral therapy. *Science* (1997) 278:1295–300. doi: 10.1126/science.278.5341.1295
2. Wong JK, Hezareh M, Gunthard HF, Havlir DV, Ignacio CC, Spina CA, et al. Recovery of replication-competent HIV despite prolonged suppression of plasma viremia. *Science* (1997) 278:1291–5. doi: 10.1126/science.278.5341.1291
3. Rodger AJ, Lodwick R, Schechter M, Deeks S, Amin J, Gilson R, et al. Mortality in well controlled HIV in the continuous antiretroviral therapy arms of the

SMART and ESPRIT trials compared with the general population. *AIDS* (2013) 27:973–9. doi: 10.1097/QAD.0b013e32835cae9c

4. Wandeler G, Johnson LF, Egger M. Trends in life expectancy of HIV-positive adults on antiretroviral therapy across the globe: comparisons with general population. *Curr Opin HIV AIDS* (2016) 11:492–500. doi: 10.1097/COH.0000000000000298
5. Shan L, Deng K, Shroff NS, Durand CM, Rabi SA, Yang HC, et al. Stimulation of HIV-1-specific cytolytic T lymphocytes facilitates elimination of latent viral reservoir after virus reactivation. *Immunity* (2012) 36:491–501. doi: 10.1016/j.immuni.2012.01.014
6. Graf EH, Pace MJ, Peterson BA, Lynch LJ, Chukwulebe SB, Mexas AM, et al. Gag-positive reservoir cells are susceptible to HIV-specific cytotoxic T lymphocyte mediated clearance. *PLoS ONE* (2013) 8:e71879. doi: 10.1371/annotation/3aa92c3d-b6dd-4c6e-8cee-9587ce80a9c9
7. Abdel-Mohsen M, Wang C, Strain MC, Lada SM, Deng X, Cockerham LR, et al. Select host restriction factors are associated with HIV persistence during antiretroviral therapy. *AIDS* (2015) 29:411–20. doi: 10.1097/QAD.0000000000000572
8. Abdel-Mohsen M, Chavez L, Tandon R, Chew GM, Deng X, Danesh A, et al. Human galectin-9 is a potent mediator of HIV transcription and reactivation. *PLoS Pathog.* (2016) 12:e1005677. doi: 10.1371/journal.ppat.1005677
9. Barrera C, Espejo R, Reyes VE. Differential glycosylation of MHC class II molecules on gastric epithelial cells: implications in local immune responses. *Hum Immunol.* (2002) 63:384–93. doi: 10.1016/S0198-8859(02)00386-5
10. Dwek RA, Butters TD, Platt FM, Zitzmann N. Targeting glycosylation as a therapeutic approach. *Nat Rev Drug Discov.* (2002) 1:65–75. doi: 10.1038/nrd708
11. De Freitas Junior JC, Silva Bdu R, De Souza WF, De Araujo WM, Abdelhay ES, Morgado-Diaz JA. Inhibition of N-linked glycosylation by tunicamycin induces E-cadherin-mediated cell-cell adhesion and inhibits cell proliferation in undifferentiated human colon cancer cells. *Cancer Chemother Pharmacol.* (2011) 68:227–38. doi: 10.1007/s00280-010-1477-8
12. Walt D, Aoki-Kinoshita KF, Bendiak B, Bertozzi CR, Boons GJ, Darvill A, et al. *Transforming Glycoscience: A Roadmap for the Future.* Washington, DC: Nacional Academies Press (2012).
13. Barondes SH, Cooper DN, Gitt MA, Leffler H. Galectins. Structure and function of a large family of animal lectins *J Biol Chem.* (1994) 269:20807–10.
14. Zhuo Y, Bellis SL. Emerging role of alpha2,6-sialic acid as a negative regulator of galectin binding and function. *J Biol Chem.* (2011) 286:5935–41. doi: 10.1074/jbc.R110.191429
15. Gordon-Alonso M, Hirsch T, Wildmann C, Van Der Bruggen P. Galectin-3 captures interferon-gamma in the tumor matrix reducing chemokine gradient production and T-cell tumor infiltration. *Nat Commun.* (2017) 8:793. doi: 10.1038/s41467-017-00925-6
16. Mendez-Huergo SP, Blidner AG, Rabinovich GA. Galectins: emerging regulatory checkpoints linking tumor immunity and angiogenesis. *Curr Opin Immunol.* (2017) 45:8–15. doi: 10.1016/j.coi.2016.12.003
17. Smith LK, Boukhaled GM, Condotta SA, Mazouz S, Guthmiller JJ, Vijay R, et al. Interleukin-10 directly inhibits CD8(+) T cell function by enhancing N-glycan branching to decrease antigen sensitivity. *Immunity* (2018) 48:299–312 e295. doi: 10.1016/j.immuni.2018.01.006
18. Sehrawat S, Reddy PB, Rajasagi N, Suryawanshi A, Hirashima M, Rouse BT. Galectin-9/TIM-3 interaction regulates virus-specific primary and memory CD8 T cell response. *PLoS Pathog.* (2010) 6:e1000882. doi: 10.1371/journal.ppat.1000882
19. Jost S, Moreno-Nieves UY, Garcia-Beltran WF, Rands K, Reardon J, Toth I, et al. Dysregulated Tim-3 expression on natural killer cells is associated with increased Galectin-9 levels in HIV-1 infection. *Retrovirology* (2013) 10:74. doi: 10.1186/1742-4690-10-74
20. Tandon R, Chew GM, Byron MM, Borrow P, Niki T, Hirashima M, et al. Galectin-9 is rapidly released during acute HIV-1 infection and remains sustained at high levels despite viral suppression even in elite controllers. *AIDS Res Hum Retroviruses* (2014) 30:654–64. doi: 10.1089/aid.2014.0004
21. Chen HY, Fermin A, Vardhana S, Weng IC, Lo KF, Chang EY, et al. Galectin-3 negatively regulates TCR-mediated CD4+ T-cell activation at the immunological synapse. *Proc Natl Acad Sci USA.* (2009) 106:14496–501. doi: 10.1073/pnas.0903497106
22. Lhuillier C, Barjon C, Niki T, Gelin A, Praz F, Morales O, et al. Impact of exogenous galectin-9 on Human T Cells: contribution of the t cell receptor complex to antigen-independent activation but not to apoptosis induction. *J Biol Chem.* (2015) 290:16797–811. doi: 10.1074/jbc.M115.661272
23. Gordon-Alonso M, Bruger AM, Van Der Bruggen P. Extracellular galectins as controllers of cytokines in hematological cancer. *Blood* (2018) 132:484–91. doi: 10.1182/blood-2018-04-846014
24. Wu C, Thalhamer T, Franca RF, Xiao S, Wang C, Hotta C, et al. Galectin-9-CD44 interaction enhances stability and function of adaptive regulatory T cells. *Immunity* (2014) 41:270–82. doi: 10.1016/j.immuni.2014.06.011
25. Nam KO, Kang H, Shin SM, Cho KH, Kwon B, Kwon BS, et al. Cross-linking of 4-1BB activates TCR-signaling pathways in CD8+ T lymphocytes. *J Immunol.* (2005) 174:1898–905. doi: 10.4049/jimmunol.174.4.1898
26. Madireddi S, Eun SY, Lee SW, Nemcovicova I, Mehta AK, Zajonc DM, et al. Galectin-9 controls the therapeutic activity of 4-1BB-targeting antibodies. *J Exp Med.* (2014) 211:1433–48. doi: 10.1084/jem.20132687
27. Bitra A, Doukov T, Wang J, Picarda G, Benedict CA, Croft M, et al. Crystal structure of murine 4-1BB and its interaction with 4-1BBL support a role for galectin-9 in 4-1BB signaling. *J Biol Chem.* (2018) 293:1317–29. doi: 10.1074/jbc.M117.814905
28. Jordan A, Bisgrove D, Verdin E. HIV reproducibly establishes a latent infection after acute infection of T cells *in vitro*. *EMBO J.* (2003) 22:1868–77. doi: 10.1093/emboj/cdg188
29. Chavez L, Kauder S, Verdin E. *In vivo, in vitro*, and *in silico* analysis of methylation of the HIV-1 provirus. *Methods* (2011) 53:47–53. doi: 10.1016/j.ymeth.2010.05.009
30. Jiang Y, Cheng H. Evidence of LAT as a dual substrate for Lck and Syk in T lymphocytes. *Leuk Res.* (2007) 31:541–5. doi: 10.1016/j.leukres.2006.07.010
31. Minami Y, Weissman AM, Samelson LE, Klausner RD. Building a multichain receptor: synthesis, degradation, and assembly of the T-cell antigen receptor. *Proc Natl Acad Sci USA.* (1987) 84:2688–92. doi: 10.1073/pnas.84.9.2688
32. Weissman AM, Ross P, Luong ET, Garcia-Morales P, Jelachich ML, Biddison WE, et al. Tyrosine phosphorylation of the human T cell antigen receptor zeta-chain: activation via CD3 but not CD2. *J Immunol.* (1988) 141:3532–6.
33. Irving BA, Weiss A. The cytoplasmic domain of the T cell receptor zeta chain is sufficient to couple to receptor-associated signal transduction pathways. *Cell* (1991) 64:891–901. doi: 10.1016/0092-8674(91)90314-O
34. Iwashima M, Irving BA, Van Oers NS, Chan AC, Weiss A. Sequential interactions of the TCR with two distinct cytoplasmic tyrosine kinases. *Science* (1994) 263:1136–9. doi: 10.1126/science.7509083
35. Thome M, Duplay P, Guttinger M, Acuto O. Syk and ZAP-70 mediate recruitment of p56lck/CD4 to the activated T cell receptor/CD3/zeta complex. *J Exp Med.* (1995) 181:1997–2006. doi: 10.1084/jem.181.6.1997
36. Mishra R, Grzybek M, Niki T, Hirashima M, Simons K. Galectin-9 trafficking regulates apical-basal polarity in Madin-Darby canine kidney epithelial cells. *Proc Natl Acad Sci USA.* (2010) 107:17633–8. doi: 10.1073/pnas.1012424107
37. Gleason MK, Lenvik TR, Mccullar V, Felices M, O'brien MS, Cooley SA, et al. Tim-3 is an inducible human natural killer cell receptor that enhances interferon gamma production in response to galectin-9. *Blood* (2012) 119:3064–72. doi: 10.1182/blood-2011-06-360321
38. Wiersma VR, De Bruyn M, Wei Y, Van Ginkel RJ, Hirashima M, Niki T, et al. The epithelial polarity regulator LGALS9/galectin-9 induces fatal frustrated autophagy in KRAS mutant colon carcinoma that depends on elevated basal autophagic flux. *Autophagy* (2015) 11:1373–88. doi: 10.1080/15548627.2015.1063767
39. Madireddi S, Eun SY, Mehta AK, Birta A, Zajonc DM, Niki T, et al. Regulatory T cell-mediated suppression of inflammation induced by DR3 signaling is dependent on galectin-9. *J Immunol.* (2017) 199:2721–8. doi: 10.4049/jimmunol.1700575
40. Martin AR, Pollack RA, Capoferri A, Ambinder RF, Durand CM, Siliciano RF. Rapamycin-mediated mTOR inhibition uncouples HIV-1 latency reversal from cytokine-associated toxicity. *J Clin Invest.* (2017) 127:651–6. doi: 10.1172/JCI89552
41. Cai L, Zhou H, Fang Z, Yuan J, Niki T, Hirashima M, et al. Galectin-9 in combination with rapamycin induces cardiac allograft tolerance in mice. *Transplantation* (2013) 96:379–86. doi: 10.1097/TP.0b013e31829b07b5
42. Elahi S, Niki T, Hirashima M, Horton H. Galectin-9 binding to Tim-3 renders activated human CD4+ T cells less susceptible to HIV-1 infection. *Blood* (2012) 119:4192–204. doi: 10.1182/blood-2011-11-389585

43. Schaefer K, Webb NE, Pang M, Hernandez-Davies JE, Lee KP, Gonzalez P, et al. Galectin-9 binds to O-glycans on protein disulfide isomerase. *Glycobiology* (2017) 27:878–87. doi: 10.1093/glycob/cwx065
44. Hunt PW, Martin JN, Sinclair E, Bredt B, Hagos E, Lampiris H, et al. T cell activation is associated with lower CD4+ T cell gains in human immunodeficiency virus-infected patients with sustained viral suppression during antiretroviral therapy. *J Infect Dis.* (2003) 187:1534–43. doi: 10.1086/374786
45. Hunt PW, Cao HL, Muzoora C, Ssewanyana I, Bennett J, Emenyonu N, et al. Impact of CD8+ T-cell activation on CD4+ T-cell recovery and mortality in HIV-infected Ugandans initiating antiretroviral therapy. *AIDS* (2011) 25:2123–31. doi: 10.1097/QAD.0b013e32834c4ac1
46. Kaplan RC, Sinclair E, Landay AL, Lurain N, Sharrett AR, Gange SJ, et al. T cell activation and senescence predict subclinical carotid artery disease in HIV-infected women. *J Infect Dis.* (2011a) 203:452–63. doi: 10.1093/infdis/jiq071
47. Kaplan RC, Sinclair E, Landay AL, Lurain N, Sharrett AR, Gange SJ, et al. T cell activation predicts carotid artery stiffness among HIV-infected women. *Atherosclerosis* (2011b) 217:207–13. doi: 10.1016/j.atherosclerosis.2011.03.011
48. Chun TW, Justement JS, Pandya P, Hallahan CW, Mclaughlin M, Liu S, et al. Relationship between the size of the human immunodeficiency virus type 1 (HIV-1) reservoir in peripheral blood CD4+ T cells and CD4+:CD8+ T cell ratios in aviremic HIV-1-infected individuals receiving long-term highly active antiretroviral therapy. *J Infect Dis.* (2002) 185:1672–6. doi: 10.1086/340521
49. Chomont N, El-Far M, Ancuta P, Trautmann L, Procopio FA, Yassine-Diab B, et al. HIV reservoir size and persistence are driven by T cell survival and homeostatic proliferation. *Nat Med.* (2009) 15:893–900. doi: 10.1038/nm.1972
50. Hatano H, Jain V, Hunt PW, Lee TH, Sinclair E, Do TD, et al. Cell-based measures of viral persistence are associated with immune activation and programmed cell death protein 1 (PD-1)-expressing CD4+ T cells. *J Infect Dis.* (2013) 208:50–6. doi: 10.1093/infdis/jis630
51. Khoury G, Fromentin R, Solomon A, Hartogensis W, Killian M, Hoh R, et al. Human immunodeficiency virus persistence and T-cell activation in blood, rectal, and lymph node tissue in human immunodeficiency virus-infected individuals receiving suppressive antiretroviral therapy. *J Infect Dis.* (2017) 215:911–9. doi: 10.1093/infdis/jix039
52. Schacker TW, Nguyen PL, Beilman GJ, Wolinsky S, Larson M, Reilly C, et al. Collagen deposition in HIV-1 infected lymphatic tissues and T cell homeostasis. *J Clin Invest.* (2002) 110:1133–9. doi: 10.1172/JCI0216413
53. Naeger DM, Martin JN, Sinclair E, Hunt PW, Bangsberg DR, Hecht F, et al. Cytomegalovirus-specific T cells persist at very high levels during long-term antiretroviral treatment of HIV disease. *PLoS ONE* (2010) 5:e8886. doi: 10.1371/journal.pone.0008886
54. Nixon DE, Landay AL. Biomarkers of immune dysfunction in HIV. *Curr Opin HIV AIDS* (2010) 5:498–503. doi: 10.1097/COH.0b013e32833ed6f4
55. Kamat A, Misra V, Cassol E, Ancuta P, Yan Z, Li C, et al. A plasma biomarker signature of immune activation in HIV patients on antiretroviral therapy. *PLoS ONE* (2012) 7:e30881. doi: 10.1371/journal.pone.0030881
56. Weber R, Ruppik M, Rickenbach M, Spoerri A, Furrer H, Battegay M, et al. Decreasing mortality and changing patterns of causes of death in the Swiss HIV Cohort Study. *HIV Med.* (2013) 14:195–207. doi: 10.1111/j.1468-1293.2012.01051.x
57. Borges AH, O'connor JL, Phillips AN, Ronsholt FF, Pett S, Vjecha MJ, et al. Factors associated with plasma IL-6 levels during HIV infection. *J Infect Dis.* (2015) 212:585–95. doi: 10.1093/infdis/jiv123
58. Freiberg MS, Bebu I, Tracy R, So-Armah K, Okulicz J, Ganesan A, et al. D-Dimer levels before HIV seroconversion remain elevated even after viral suppression and are associated with an increased risk of non-AIDS events. *PLoS ONE* (2016) 11:e0152588. doi: 10.1371/journal.pone.0152588
59. So-Armah KA, Tate JP, Chang CH, Butt AA, Gerschenson M, Gibert CL, et al. Do biomarkers of inflammation, monocyte activation, and altered coagulation explain excess mortality between HIV infected and uninfected people? *J Acquir Immune Defic Syndr.* (2016) 72:206–13. doi: 10.1097/QAI.0000000000000954
60. Zhu C, Anderson AC, Schubart A, Xiong H, Imitola J, Khoury SJ, et al. The Tim-3 ligand galectin-9 negatively regulates T helper type 1 immunity. *Nat Immunol.* (2005) 6:1245–52. doi: 10.1038/ni1271
61. Wang F, He W, Zhou H, Yuan J, Wu K, Xu L, et al. The Tim-3 ligand galectin-9 negatively regulates CD8+ alloreactive T cell and prolongs survival of skin graft. *Cell Immunol.* (2007) 250:68–74. doi: 10.1016/j.cellimm.2008.01.006
62. Seki M, Oomizu S, Sakata KM, Sakata A, Arikawa T, Watanabe K, et al. Galectin-9 suppresses the generation of Th17, promotes the induction of regulatory T cells, and regulates experimental autoimmune arthritis. *Clin Immunol.* (2008) 127:78–88. doi: 10.1016/j.clim.2008.01.006
63. Lv K, Zhang Y, Zhang M, Zhong M, Suo Q. Galectin-9 promotes TGF-beta1-dependent induction of regulatory T cells via the TGF-beta/Smad signaling pathway. *Mol Med Rep.* (2013) 7:205–10. doi: 10.3892/mmr.2012.1125
64. Ungerer C, Quade-Lyssy P, Radeke HH, Henschler R, Konigs C, Kohl U, et al. Galectin-9 is a suppressor of T and B cells and predicts the immune modulatory potential of mesenchymal stromal cell preparations. *Stem Cells Dev.* (2014) 23:755–66. doi: 10.1089/scd.2013.0335
65. Kim SN, Lee HJ, Jeon MS, Yi T, Song SU. Galectin-9 is involved in immunosuppression mediated by human bone marrow-derived clonal mesenchymal stem cells. *Immune Netw.* (2015) 15:241–51. doi: 10.4110/in.2015.15.5.241
66. Yang S, Wang J, Chen F, Liu G, Weng Z, Chen J. Elevated galectin-9 suppresses Th1 effector function and induces apoptosis of activated CD4(+) T cells in osteoarthritis. *Inflammation* (2017) 40:1062–71. doi: 10.1007/s10753-017-0549-x
67. Panda SK, Facchinetti V, Voynova E, Hanabuchi S, Karnell JL, Hanna RN, et al. Galectin-9 inhibits TLR7-mediated autoimmunity in murine lupus models. *J Clin Invest.* (2018) 128:1873–87. doi: 10.1172/JCI97333
68. Golden-Mason L, Mcmahan RH, Strong M, Reisdorph R, Mahaffey S, Palmer BE, et al. Galectin-9 functionally impairs natural killer cells in humans and mice. *J Virol.* (2013) 87:4835–45. doi: 10.1128/JVI.01085-12
69. Cao A, Alluqmani N, Buhari FHM, Wasim L, Smith LK, Quaile AT, et al. Galectin-9 binds IgM-BCR to regulate B cell signaling. *Nat Commun.* (2018) 9:3288. doi: 10.1038/s41467-018-05771-8
70. Giovannone N, Liang J, Antonopoulos A, Geddes Sweeney J, King SL, Pochebit SM, et al. Galectin-9 suppresses B cell receptor signaling and is regulated by I-branching of N-glycans. *Nat Commun.* (2018) 9:3287. doi: 10.1038/s41467-018-05770-9
71. Nagahara K, Arikawa T, Oomizu S, Kontani K, Nobumoto A, Tateno H, et al. Galectin-9 increases Tim-3+ dendritic cells and CD8+ T cells and enhances antitumor immunity via galectin-9-Tim-3 interactions. *J Immunol.* (2008) 181:7660–9. doi: 10.4049/jimmunol.181.11.7660
72. He XW, Li WL, Li C, Liu P, Shen YG, Zhu M, et al. Serum levels of galectin-1, galectin-3, and galectin-9 are associated with large artery atherosclerotic stroke. *Sci Rep.* (2017) 7:40994. doi: 10.1038/srep40994
73. Liu Y, Liu Z, Fu Q, Wang Z, Fu H, Liu W, et al. Galectin-9 as a prognostic and predictive biomarker in bladder urothelial carcinoma. *Urol Oncol.* (2017) 35:349–55. doi: 10.1016/j.urolonc.2017.02.008
74. Enninga EAL, Harrington SM, Creedon DJ, Ruano R, Markovic SN, et al. and Dronca RS. Immune checkpoint molecules soluble program death ligand 1 and galectin-9 are increased in pregnancy. *Am J Reprod Immunol.* (2018) 79:e12795. doi: 10.1111/aji.12795
75. Sehgal SN. Rapamune (RAPA, rapamycin, sirolimus): mechanism of action immunosuppressive effect results from blockade of signal transduction and inhibition of cell cycle progression. *Clin Biochem.* (1998) 31:335–40. doi: 10.1016/S0009-9120(98)00045-9
76. Powell JD, Pollizzi KN, Heikamp EB, Horton MR. Regulation of immune responses by mTOR. *Annu Rev Immunol.* (2012) 30:39–68. doi: 10.1146/annurev-immunol-020711-075024

13

The Use of Toll-Like Receptor Agonists in HIV-1 Cure Strategies

*Janne Tegder Martinsen, Jesper Damsgaard Gunst, Jesper Falkesgaard Højen, Martin Tolstrup and Ole Schmeltz Søgaard**

Department of Infectious Diseases, Aarhus University Hospital, Aarhus, Denmark

***Correspondence:**
Ole Schmeltz Søgaard
olesoega@rm.dk

Toll-like receptors (TLRs) are a family of pattern recognition receptors and part of the first line of defense against invading microbes. In humans, we know of 10 different TLRs, which are expressed to varying degrees in immune cell subsets. Engaging TLRs through their specific ligands leads to activation of the innate immune system and secondarily priming of the adaptive immune system. Because of these unique properties, TLR agonists have been investigated as immunotherapy in cancer treatment for many years, but in recent years there has also been growing interest in the use of TLR agonists in the context of human immunodeficiency virus type 1 (HIV-1) cure research. The primary obstacle to curing HIV-1 is the presence of a latent viral reservoir in transcriptionally silent immune cells. Due to the very limited transcription of the integrated HIV-1 proviruses, latently infected cells cannot be targeted and cleared by immune effector mechanisms. TLR agonists are very interesting in this context because of their potential dual effects as latency reverting agents (LRAs) and immune modulatory compounds. Here, we review preclinical and clinical data on the impact of TLR stimulation on HIV-1 latency as well as antiviral and HIV-1-specific immunity. We also focus on the promising role of TLR agonists in combination strategies in HIV-1 cure research. Different combinations of TLR agonists and broadly neutralizing antibodies or TLRs agonists as adjuvants in HIV-1 vaccines have shown very encouraging results in non-human primate experiments and these concepts are now moving into clinical testing.

Keywords: HIV-1, TLR, innate immunity, HIV-1 cure, HIV-1 vaccine, latency reversing agents, immune modulation

INTRODUCTION

Human immunodeficiency virus type 1 (HIV-1) infection can today be completely suppressed by antiretroviral therapy (ART). However, during the early phase of primary HIV-1 infection, the virus establishes a reservoir in infected long-lived immune cells, which necessitates life-long ART in order to prevent disease progression (1, 2). This latent HIV-1 reservoir is predominantly found in long-lived memory CD4+ T cells in which the provirus is transcriptionally silent and thus go undetected by the host immune system (3, 4). These proviruses can be (re)activated and go on to transcribe and form infectious particles, leading to re-emergence of active infection if ART is stopped. The HIV-1 reservoir is believed to be maintained through the long-lived nature and homeostatic proliferative capabilities of the latently infected memory T cells (5, 6).

The innate immune system constitutes a vital part of the early defense against infections and in controlling established HIV-1 infection. Therefore, strategies aimed at boosting innate immunity have gained great interest in HIV-1 cure research. Endogenous interferon production induced by activation of Toll-like receptors (TLRs) is one of the innate immune'system's first antiviral responses upon infection. TLRs are in the family of pattern recognition receptors (PRRs) which detect pathogen-associated molecular patterns (PAMPs) (7, 8). TLRs also respond to signs of host cell damage through ligands called damage-associated molecular patterns (DAMPs) (9).

TLRs are expressed on many different immune cells including natural killer (NK) cells, macrophages, B cells, and to a high degree on dendritic cells (DCs) (10) (**Table 1**). TLR1, TLR2, TLR4, TLR5, TLR6, and TLR10 are expressed on the cell surface, whereas TLR3, TLR7, TLR8, and TLR9 are located in the membrane of the intracellular endosomes (8, 14, 20). This partition in localization reflects the disparate pathogen-sensing function of these two groups. The cell surface-associated TLRs are mainly responsible for detecting components from extracellular microbes such as bacteria and fungi, whereas the TLRs in the endosomal compartment mainly detect virus and intracellular bacteria (18, 22, 23) (**Table 1**). TLRs are transmembrane proteins consisting of three different domains: an ectodomain consisting of leucine-rich-repeats (LRR) mediating ligand recognition, a transmembrane domain, and the cytosolic domain Toll/IL-1R (TIR), which mediates downstream signaling (18). The cytosolic domain can, upon activation of the TLR, recruit different domain-containing adaptor molecules such as myeloid differentiation primary-response protein 88 (MyD88), TIR-domain containing adaptor protein (TIRAP)] also called MyD88 adaptor-like (MAL), TIR-domain containing adaptor protein inducing IFN-β (TRIF), and TRIF-related adaptor molecule (TRAM) (23–25). The MyD88 signaling pathway used by all of the TLRs, except for TLR3, activates nuclear factor-κB (NF-κB) and mitogen-activated protein kinases (MAPKs) leading to the production of pro-inflammatory cytokines. The TRIF-dependent pathway used by TLR3 and TLR4 leads to induction of type 1 interferons (IFNs) in addition to pro-inflammatory cytokines (18, 20, 23). The cytokine induction initiated by TLR activation not only triggers an innate immune response, but also takes part in initiating and shaping the adaptive immune response (22, 26).

The present review focuses on the emerging potential of synthetic TLR agonist treatment in HIV-1 cure research both alone and in combination with other interventions.

TABLE 1 | A schematic outline of TLR localization, expression on immune cells, receptor complex formations, ligands, recruited TIR domain-containing adaptor molecules, and cytokine outcomes.

TLR type	Cell type	Receptor-complex	Ligand	TIR-adaptor	Outcome
(A) TLRs on cell surface					
TLR1	Monocytes DCs T cells	1–2	- Lipopeptides from bacteria and mycobacteria	MyD88	Pro-inflammatory cytokines
TLR2	Monocytes Macrophages DCs	2–1 2–2 2–6 2–10	- Components from the cell wall of gram-positive bacteria - Glycoprotein from virus - Zymosan from fungi	MyD88	Pro-inflammatory cytokines
TLR4	Monocytes DCs	4-MD2	- Lipopolysaccharides from gram-negative bacteria - Envelope components of respiratory syncytial virus	MyD88 TRIF TRAM TIRAP/MAL	Pro-inflammatory cytokines IFNs
TLR5	Monocytes T cells	5–5	- Flagellin from flagellated bacteria	MyD88	Pro-inflammatory cytokines
TLR6	Monocytes Macrophages B cells	6–2	- Lipopeptides from Mycoplasma	MyD88	Pro-inflammatory cytokines
TLR10	B-cells	10–2	- Ligands from Listeria - Ligands from Influenza A		
(B) TLRs in endosomal compartments					
TLR3	DCs	3-3	- Viral double-stranded RNA - Self-RNA from damaged cells	TRIF	Pro-inflammatory cytokines IFNs
TLR7	pDCs B cells	7-7	- Viral single-stranded RNA	MyD88	Pro-inflammatory cytokines IFNs*
TLR8	Monocytes DCs	8-8	- Viral single-stranded RNA - Bacterial RNA	MyD88	Pro-inflammatory cytokines
TLR9	pDCs B cells	9-9	- CpG containing DNA from bacteria and virus - Self-DNA from damaged cells - Hemozoin from Plasmodium Falciparum	MyD88	Pro-inflammatory cytokines IFNs*

**IFNs through MyD88.*

*The table is a summary of TLR properties described previously (11–20). It should be noted that some immune cells subsets and ligands have been left out for the sake of overview and relevance to the subjects at hand. TLR expression on epithelial cells have been left out of **Table 1** as well, but have been reviewed elsewhere (21).*

TLR AGONISTS AS LATENCY REVERSING AGENTS (LRA)

The latent HIV-1 reservoir constitutes the main barrier to a cure for HIV-1 infection (27, 28). One of the proposed strategies toward overcoming this obstacle is the "shock and kill" approach (28, 29). The hypothesis behind this strategy is that LRA administration will (re)activate HIV-1 transcription in latently infected cells, leading to expression of viral antigens on their surface. This will in turn expose infected cells to immune-mediated killing and/or apoptosis due to viral-cytopathic effects while concurrent ART prevents released virions from infecting other immune cells (30).

A widely investigated group of LRAs is the histone deacetylase inhibitors (HDACi) including romidepsin, vorinostat, panobinostat, and chidamide (31–33). Inhibition of the histone deacetylase enzymes leads to a more accessible chromatin structure, thus enabling transcription of the latent proviral HIV-1 DNA (34, 35). While HDACi are now being investigated in combination with HIV-1 vaccines (36), broadly neutralizing antibodies (bNAbs) (www.clinicaltrials.gov: NCT03041012), and other LRAs, none of these HDACi alone have so far been capable of inducing a substantial reduction of the HIV-1 reservoir in clinical trials (37).

Protein kinase C (PKC) agonists such as bryostatin and prostratin (38) have shown significant latency reversal activity *ex vivo* but may be too toxic to be dosed at active concentrations in humans (39). However, the latency reverting effects of a natural plant extract containing ingenols, yet another group of PKC agonist, is currently under being tested in a clinical trial in HIV-1 infected individuals (NCT02531295). Disulfiram, a drug used for alcohol cessation, has also been tested in clinical trials as a potential LRA (40). Disulfiram induced increased levels of cell-associated unspliced HIV-1 RNA (usRNA) in study participants of three different dosing groups, but it did not lead to significant changes in either total HIV-1 DNA or plasma levels of HIV-1 RNA. The latency reversing properties of other compounds such as cytokines and other epigenetic modifiers have similarly been investigated (41, 42). However, the discovery of a single therapeutic capable of inducing significant HIV-1 reservoir alterations is still to be made.

The first TLR agonist to draw attention to the potential utilization of TLR agonists as LRAs was that of the antisense oligodeoxynucleotide (ODN) phosphorothioate Gene-Expression Modulator 91 (GEM91). GEM91 was initially shown to inhibit HIV-1 replication *ex vivo* in human peripheral blood mononuclear cells (PBMCs) from HIV-1 infected donors (43). Unexpectedly, a subsequent GEM91 dose-escalation study showed increased viremia following administration in HIV-1 infected individuals contradictory of the *ex vivo* findings (44). It was later discovered that this potential induction of viremia was due to a CpG motif in GEM91 leading to TLR9 stimulation. Thus, it was proposed that the increased viremia was caused by innate immune activation and concomitant HIV-1 (re)activation (45–47).

Several TLR agonists have since been investigated as LRAs because of their ability to induce immune activation, and in doing so, causing (re)activation of silent HIV-1 in latently infected cells and boosting the antiviral immune response. These mechanisms are elaborated in the section "Immunomodulatory properties of TLR agonists."

Ex vivo Experiments

Utilizing the optimal cell model for assessment of latency reversal is of great importance and should consider the type of LRA investigated. The majority of *in vitro/ex vivo* LRA experiments focuses on latently infected T cell lines or primary T cells. These cell models work well when investigating LRAs such as HDACi which (re)activate HIV-1 transcription by a direct impact on the target cell. Yet, most TLRs are not expressed at physiological levels on CD4+ T cells, which is why this lymphocyte subset is often unresponsive to direct TLR stimulation (e.g., by TLR7 or TLR9 agonists) (**Table 1**). Instead, these TLR agonists induce HIV-1 transcription indirectly through activation of innate immune cells such as DCs (**Table 2**) (18, 22, 23, 54).

This issue was highlighted in a study by Novis et al. who tested a broad panel of TLR agonists as LRAs (48). In a central memory CD4+ T cell (T_{CM}) model, they found that only the TLR1/2 agonist Pam3CSK4 was able to significantly increase HIV-1 transcription, measured by intracellular p24 Gag protein expression, after stimulating the cells for 3 days (48). Subsequently, the latency reversing properties of Pam3CSK4 were tested *ex vivo* utilizing T_{CM} isolated from aviremic HIV-1 infected donors. They found that HIV-1 transcription increased in two out of seven donors after Pam3CSK4 stimulation compared to five out of seven after panobinostat stimulation, measured by the level of usRNA. Pam3CSK4 was demonstrated to (re)activate HIV-1 transcription via an NF-κB and NFAT-dependent pathway, but without induction of IFNs, thereby avoiding T cell activation (CD69+ and CD25+) and proliferation (cell proliferation dye assessment). However, the degree of HIV-1 (re)activation induced by Pam3CSK4 was lower than that of panobinostat.

In 2018, Kaur et al. conducted a comprehensive investigation of the LRA properties of agonists of 6 different TLRs(1/2, 3, 4, 5, 7, and 8) on both PBMCs and isolated CD4+ T cells from HIV-1 infected donors on long term ART (49). All TLR agonists were able to induce a modest but statistically significant fold-increase of supernatant HIV-1 RNA from PBMCs compared to vehicle controls. In isolated CD4+ T cells however, only the TLR1/2 agonist Pam3CSK4 was able to significantly increase the supernatant HIV-1 RNA level. These findings are in line with the findings of Novis et al. and indicate TLR1/2 expression on CD4+ T cells.

Thibault et al. tested the direct HIV-1 latency reversing properties of the TLR5 agonist flagellin on T_{CM} (50), which in a previous study showed indications of TLR5 expression (55) (**Table 1**). Resting T_{CM} isolated from healthy donor PBMCs were infected with luciferease-encoding pseudotyped HIV-1 particles. When treated with flagellin, the isolated T_{CM} showed enhanced HIV-1 gene expression compared to mock-treated controls, assessed by fold increase of HIV-1 long terminal repeat-driven luciferase activity. However, when flagellin stimulation

TABLE 2 | Schematic overview of *ex vivo* experiments investigating the utility of TLR agonists as LRAs included in the manuscript.

References	TLR agonist	Cell type	Study design	Endpoint	Results
Novis et al. (48)	1) 1/2, 2/6, 3, 4, 5, 7, 7/8, 9	1) T_{CM} cell model	1) *In vitro* stimulation	1) Intracellular p24 Gag protein expression	1) Only the TLR1/2 agonist induced significant increase (but the T_{CM} cell model does not express most TLRs)
	2) 1/2	2) T_{CM} from aviremic HIV-1 infected donors	2) *Ex vivo* stimulation	2) Intracellular level of usRNA	2) Significant increase in 2 of 7 donor samples (5 of 7 for panobinostat)
Kaur et al. (49)	1) 1/2, 3, 4, 5, 7, 8	1) PBMCs from aviremic HIV-1 infected donors	1) *Ex vivo* stimulation	1) Supernatant HIV-1 RNA level	1) All TLR agonists induced significant increase
	2) 1/2, 3, 4, 5, 7, 8	2) CD4+ T cells from aviremic HIV-1 infected donors	2) *Ex vivo* stimulation	2) Supernatant HIV-1 RNA level	2) Only TLR ½ agonist Pam3CSK4 induced significant increase
Thibailt et al. (50)	1) 5	1) Resting T_{CM} from healthy donor PBMCs, infected with luciferase-encoding pseudotyped HIV-1	1) *Ex vivo* stimulation	1) HIV-1 long terminal repeat-driven luciferase activity	1) Increase
	2) 5	2) resting CD4+ T cells from aviremic HIV-1 infected donors	2) *Ex vivo* stimulation	2) Intracellular p24 Gag protein level	2) No increase
Tsai et al. (51)	1) 7	1) PBMCs from aviremic HIV-1 infected donors	1) *Ex vivo* stimulation	1) Supernatant mean HIV-1 RNA levels	1) Increase
	2) 7	2) PBMCs from aviremic HIV-1 infected donors, treated with antibodies against IFNAR on T cells	2) *Ex vivo* stimulation	2) Supernatant mean HIV-1 RNA levels	2) No increase
	3) 7	3) CD4+ T cells from aviremic HIV-1 infected donors	3) *Ex vivo* stimulation	3) Supernatant mean HIV-1 RNA levels	3) No increase
Bam et al. (52)	1) 7	1) PBMCs from healthy donors	1) Pre-stimulating with GS-9620 for 2 days prior to infection with a luciferase reporter virus containing HIV-1	1) HIV-1 replication	1) Inhibition
	2) 7	2) CD4+ T cells from healthy donors	2) Pre-stimulating with GS-9620 for 2 days prior to infection with a luciferase reporter virus containing HIV-1	2) HIV-1 replication	2) No inhibition
Offersen et al. (53)	1) 9	1) PBMCs from aviremic HIV-1 infected donors	1) *Ex vivo* stimulation	1a) Level of usRNA in CD4+ T-cells extracted from PBMCs post stimulation	1a) Increase
				1b) Level of IFN-α in cell supernatant	1b) Increase

The studies all have several endpoints in their study setup. The most relevant endpoints in the setting of this review have been outlined as (1), (2), and (3) for overview.

was tested on resting CD4+ T-cells from virally suppressed HIV-1 infected donors, no induction of intracellular p24 Gag protein was detectable. The results of Thibault et al. are in accordance with those of Novis et al. and Kaur et al., but raise uncertainty regarding the physiological effects of the previously indicated TLR5 expression on T cells.

Tsai et al. demonstrated that GS-9620, a TLR7 agonist, was capable of (re)activating latent HIV-1 in PBMCs from HIV-1 infected donors after 4 days of stimulation, measured as a 1.6-fold increase in mean HIV-1 RNA levels in the cell supernatant compared to vehicle-treated controls (51). This effect was mediated by activation of plasmacytoid dendritic cells (pDCs) leading to an IFN-driven CD4+ T cell activation (CD69+), which was demonstrated by the lack of HIV-1 RNA production when PBMCs were treated with antibodies against interferon-α receptors (IFNAR) on T cells. No changes in supernatant HIV-1 RNA was found when performing direct stimulating of pure CD4+ T-cells, which is consistent with the above-mentioned inconsiderable TLR7 expression on human T-cells. In corroboration with these findings, Bam et al. demonstrated inhibition of HIV-1 replication in PMBCs pre-stimulated with GS-9620 for 2 days prior to infection with a luciferase reporter virus containing HIV-1 (52). This antiviral effect was not observed when isolated CD4+ T cells or macrophages were equivalently pre-stimulated.

As briefly described above, synthetic ODNs containing CpG motifs were the first version of the TLR9 agonists and were mainly investigated in the context of cancer treatment (56). The structurally different TLR9 agonists such as MGN1703 were later developed to improve the tolerability of the drug class (57). Our group investigated the "shock and kill" properties of the TLR9 agonist MGN1703 on PBMCs from HIV-1 infected individuals on ART (53). MGN1703 stimulation led to increased levels of usRNA in CD4+ T-cells after 16 h. This effect was mediated indirectly by activated pDCs secreting IFNs, inducing T-cell activation (CD69+). MGN1703 did however not increase the usRNA levels to the same extent as panobinostat.

Lastly, other studies have also suggested that agonists of TLR2/7 and TLR8 possess latency reversing properties *ex vivo* and *in vivo* (58, 59). Extensional investigation of latency reversing properties of TLR agonists utilizing cell lines and mouse models have been reviewed elsewhere (25, 60, 61).

The findings of the preclinical studies presented here suggest that while some TLRs are present on T cells, the physiological effect of TLR-mediated (re)activation of latent HIV-1 in transcriptionally quiescent memory T cells occur in large by means of DC activation and subsequent IFN-α stimulation of T cells. Therefore, the full immune stimulating or latency reversing effect of synthetic TLR agonists can often not be evaluated by utilizing single immune cell models (**Table 2**).

Non-Human Primate (NHP) Studies

Evaluating pre-clinical *in vivo* studies investigating the therapeutic potential of TLR agonists in HIV-1 cure research, the present review will be focusing on NHP studies, as the TLR expression on immune cells of NHPs bare the closest resemblance to that of human immune cells, compared to smaller animal models (62, 63).

Of the TLR agonists investigated *ex vivo* as described above, only agonists of TLR3, TLR7, and TLR9 have progressed into clinical testing as potential LRAs in the field of HIV-1 cure research. However, TLR3 agonist testing quickly progressed from small animal models into clinical trials in advanced cancer disease and its LRA potential has not been assessed in NHPs (64–67). The majority of the preclinical work concerning TLR9 agonists have similarly been conducted in the field of cancer treatment and is thus beyond the scope of this review but has been described elsewhere (68).

Two different groups have investigated the potential of TLR7 agonists as LRAs *in vivo* in NHP. Lim et al. showed that the TLR7 agonist GS-986, was capable of inducing transient simian immunodeficiency virus (SIV) plasma RNA blips of up to 1,000 copies/mL, after 24 to 48 h (69). GS-986 was administered in escalating doses (0.1–0.3 mg/kg) by oral gavage and led to SIV RNA blips in 4 out of 4 virally suppressed rhesus macaques on ART, compared to 0 of 6 vehicle-treated controls. The blips were seen after dose 4, 5, 6, and 7, but not after the first 3 doses, which could indicate a priming effect of the TLR agonist. T, NK, and B cells were transiently activated within 24 to 48 h following stimulation and then returned to baseline. In the TLR7 agonist treated NHPs, the viral reservoir was reduced by an average of 75% as measured by total SIV DNA in memory CD4+ T cells [isolated from PBMCs, mononuclear cells from lymph node (LNMCs) and gastrointestinal mucosa (GMMCs)] compared to no change in total SIV DNA among control animals. However, there was no difference in time to viral rebound between the GS-986-treated group and the control group following ART cessation.

In a subsequent experiment, 9 NHPs, received 10 administrations of either GS-986 (0.1 mg/kg) or GS-9620 (0.05 or 0.15 mg/kg) followed by a 3-months resting period and then another 9 doses. 2 NHPs constituted a vehicle-control group. All TLR7 agonist-treated NHPs experienced blips in plasma SIV RNA levels during the first interventional period, but during the second interventional period, only 1 viral blip was measured, even though the activation level of T, NK and B cells was comparable between the two dosing periods. The reason for this variation is not clear but it could indicate increasing immune tolerance to TLR7 activation following repeated stimulation. Total SIV DNA was however again significantly reduced in both PBMCs and GMMCs in a combined analysis of all TLR7-agonists-treated groups compared to controls. In a modified viral outgrowth assay, the majority of TLR7-treated NHPs displayed a reduction in the inducible SIV reservoir. Two of the NHPs had no inducible SIV reservoir and showed durable control for more than 700 days after interruption of ART. Subsequent CD8+ T-cell depletion did not lead to emergence of virus, and neither did adoptive transfer of PBMCs and LMMCs to naïve macaques, suggesting a complete eradication of the viral reservoir.

Surprisingly, Del Prete et al. were unable to reproduce the findings of Lim et al. (70). Their study also included SIV-infected rhesus macaques that received 12 doses (0.15 or 0.5 mg/kg) of GS-9620, administered by oral gavage. No spikes in plasma SIV RNA levels were observed and no significant changes in transcriptional RNA/DNA ratios in PBMCs, LNMCs, or GMMCs were detected at 24 and 48 h post-dosing. All NHPs rebounded within 4 weeks upon ART cessation. CD4+ T cells showed no increased activation but at 24 h post-dosing CD8+ T cells had increased co-expression of CD38 and HLA-DR.

The cause of the difference in LRA effect and outcome in the two comparable NHP studies is unclear. In the study by Lim et al., ART was initiated on day 65 of infection and continued for around 437 days before the intervention, whereas Del Prete et al. initiated ART on day 13 and waited 525 days before intervening. The timing of ART initiation and/or of intervention might affect the viral reservoirs differently which could contribute to the discrepant findings. NHPs were infected intrarectally with SIVmac251 in the study of Lim et al., and intravenously with SIVmac239X in the study of Del Prete et al., which could also lead to varying reservoir properties.

Collectively, these findings indicate that the latency reversing effect of TLR7 agonists in NHPs might be very sensitive to alterations in model conditions such as timing of treatment initiation in relation to the course of infection, immune status, and SIV/SHIV challenge strain. The measured effects of the treatment may also depend greatly on the administered dose, dosing intervals, and timing of sampling.

Clinical Trials

The first clinical trial investigating the effects of a TLR3 agonist in HIV-1 infected individuals on long-term ART was recently published by Saxena et al. (71). The synthetic double-stranded RNA polyinosinic:polycytidylic acid (poly-I:C) and its more stabilized form containing poly-L-lysine (poly-ICLC) have previously been tested in human cancer studies (67, 72). Saxena et al. tested poly-ICLC on 12 HIV-1 infected donors in doses of 1.4 mg administered subcutaneously once daily on two consecutive days. Follow-up measurements were obtained on day 4 and 8 and at week 4, 16, and 48. During the study period, poly-ICLC treatment did not affect the level of usRNA or total HIV-1 DNA in CD4+ T-cells. In addition, no significant changes in activation of DCs (CD40+CD83+CD86^{+}) or T cells (HLA-DR+CD38+) were observed, except for a significant upregulation of CD38 expression on CD8+ T-cells at day 4, which normalized at day 8. The authors speculated that higher poly-ICLC doses, more frequent administration, or combinations with other therapeutics might be needed to achieve a robust immunological impact.

Assessing the safety of the TLR7 agonist GS-9620, Riddler et al. recently reported findings from a phase I dose escalation placebo-controlled study including 48 HIV-1 infected individuals on ART (NCT02858401) (73). In 6 treatment groups, GS-9620 doses ranging from 1 to 12 mg GS-9620 were administered every other week for up to 19 weeks. GS-9620 was generally well-tolerated, even in the 12 mg group, and there were no discontinuations due to adverse events. There was however no evidence of GS-9620 effectively impacting the latent HIV-1 reservoir as no consistent changes were observed in levels of plasma HIV-1 RNA, usRNA or total HIV-1 DNA in CD4+ T cells between the different groups. Another ongoing study with this compound is assessing the safety and efficacy of GS-9620 in ART-treated HIV-1 infected controllers, defined as individuals having a pre-ART viral load between 50 and 5,000 copies/mL (NCT03060447).

Since 2007, our group has been working with TLR9 agonists both as vaccine adjuvant and immune stimulator in HIV-1 infection. We conducted a pilot study in HIV-1 infected individuals whom received 60 mg of TLR9 agonist MGN1703, administered subcutaneously twice weekly over 4 weeks (74). During the 4-week intervention period, 6 of the 15 participants had detectable plasma HIV-1 RNA levels in the range of 21–1,571 copies/mL. This suggested a moderate latency reversing effect of MGN1703, but no reduction was observed in the proviral reservoir size assessed by total and integrated HIV-1 DNA in CD4+ T cells. No changes in levels of replication-competent proviruses were detected either. Both pDCs and T cells were activated as demonstrated by increased expression of the co-stimulatory markers CD40 and CD86 on pDCs and CD38 and HLA-DR on T cells. Surprisingly, the level of transcriptionally active CD4+ T cells, measured as cell-associated usRNA levels, decreased significantly during the 80-days follow-up period.

Based on these favorable immunological findings, an extension of the this study was conducted during which MGN1703 was administered twice weekly for 24 weeks to 12 HIV-1 infected participants (75). The prolonged intervention did, however, not reduce the size of the viral reservoir, assessed by measurements of total HIV-1 DNA or replication competent virus in a viral outgrowth assay. One participant (ID113) was able to control viral replication to undetectable levels for 150 days upon ART cessation. Immunological control in this individual was shown to be mediated in part by a superior level of HIV-1-specific CD8+ effector memory T cells, compared to the other study individuals. Of note, the IgG neutralization capacity of ID113 had increased during the MGN1703 treatment, supporting beneficial effect of the TLR agonist on adaptive immunity and in particular on B cell maturation (76).

Although several *ex vivo* and some *in vivo* studies have demonstrated encouraging results regarding the latency reversing effect of TLR agonists, there are no reproduceable data showing significant impact on the HIV-1 reservoir in clinical trials following TLR agonist treatment. A potential issue of LRAs as part of a HIV-1 cure strategy is that the focus is on latently infected CD4+ T cells as the main target of the latency reversal. While infected memory CD4+ T cells constitutes a long-lived HIV-1 reservoir, other cell types have been shown to harbor replication competent virus such as monocytes, macrophages, and dendritic cells (77, 78). Additionally, infected cells reside in other compartments than the blood including the lymph nodes and gut associated lymphoid tissue, and potentially also reside in the brain, the genital tract, and the lungs (79–84). However, the latter compartments are notoriously difficult to sample in clinical trials.

Collectively, based on the current knowledge we believe there is evidence for latency reversal following TLR (particularly TLR9) agonist treatment in HIV-1-infected individuals. However, TLR agonists' potency as LRAs appear to be relatively modest but as we outline below, certain TLR agonists are potent immune stimulators and it is in this capacity that they may have the biggest role to play in HIV-1 cure strategies.

IMMUNOMODULATORY PROPERTIES OF TLR AGONISTS

Upon TLR activation of DCs, proinflammatory cytokines such as IL-12 and IFNs are secreted, leading to auto- and/or paracrine activation of immune cells including other DCs, macrophages, NK cells, and T cells (85, 86). Activation of the DCs additionally leads to a downregulation of the inflammatory chemokine receptor CCR6 on the DC surface and upregulated expression of the lymphoid-homing receptor CCR7. This triggers DC migration from tissues to lymph nodes where they can present antigen to T and B cells and thus mediate an adaptive immune response (22, 87, 88). IFNα-α, produced mainly by pDCs activates both CD4+ and CD8+ T cells via their interferon alpha receptor (IFNAR) (51, 89, 90). Krieg et al. demonstrated a significantly increased frequency of antigen specific CD8+ T cells (0.07–3.00%) in 8 of 8 melanoma patients receiving a melanoma antigen vaccine adjuvanted with CpG ODNs compared to eight control patients receiving the vaccine alone (91). Accordingly, several clinical studies from our group have demonstrated HIV-1 (re)activation through an IFNα-α induced CD4+ T-cell activation and increased HIV-1-specific polyfunctionality of

CD8+ T cells following TLR9 stimulation (74, 75, 92). Similar effects have been demonstrated *ex vivo* and *in vivo* in TL7TLR7 agonist studies (51, 93, 94).

NK cells can mediate direct killing upon interaction with foreign pathogens or cells exhibiting signs of stress, but they are also the primary effector cells in mediating antibody-dependent cellular cytotoxicity (ADCC) via their Fcγ receptor (CD16) (26, 95). The cytotoxic effect is executed through the release of perforins which allows secreted cytotoxic granzymes to enter the targeted cell (96). The analogous anti-viral effector function of activated macrophages is that of phagocytosis, where the macrophage will devour entire infected cells (96). This effect can, like ADCC, be enhanced by antibodies and is thus called antibody-dependent cellular phagocytosis (ADCP). Both macrophages and NK cells are important in clearing HIV-1 infected cells (97, 98), and TLR agonists can thus work to increase their effector functions both directly through TLRs expressed on macrophages and NK-cells (**Table 1**) and indirectly via activation of B-cells and DCs (**Figure 1**).

Our group demonstrated enhanced NK cell function following *ex vivo* MGN1703-stimulation of PBMCs from HIV-1-infected individuals on long-term ART (53). The cytotoxic ($CD56^{dim}$ CD16+) and cytokine-producing ($CD56^{bright}$ CD16±) NK cells showed a significant 7.5- and 2.2-fold increase in CD69-expression, respectively, after 48 h of stimulation. Compared to unstimulated NK cells, MGN1703-stimulated

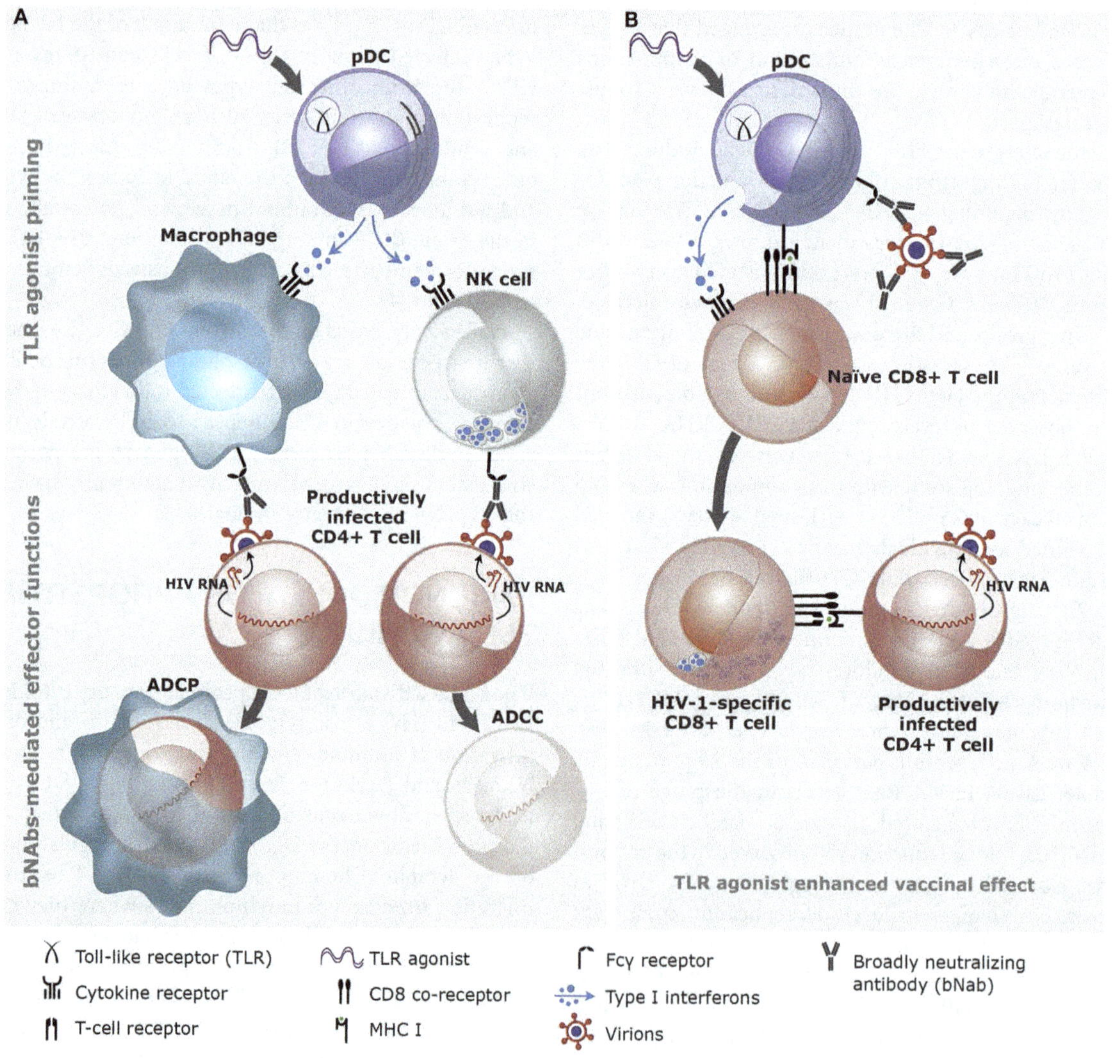

FIGURE 1 | A conceptual illustration of the effects of Toll-like receptor (TLR) agonists and broadly neutralizing antibodies (bNAbs) in combination. **(A)** TLR agonist priming of innate immune cells through plasmacytoid dendritic cells (pDC). The primed innate immune cells (here depicted macrophage and natural killer (NK) cell) bind the broadly neutralizing antibodies via the Fcγ receptors and mediate antibody-dependent cellular phagocytosis (ADCP) or cytotoxicity (ADCC) of the productively infected CD4+ T cells. **(B)** TLR agonists and bNAbs-antigen complexes cross-prime CD8+ T cells. TLR agonists and bNAbs-antigen complexes bind to pDCs which cross-presents viral antigens on the MHC class I molecule to the naïve CD8+ T cells leading to development of HIV-1-specific CD8+ T cells (graphics: Gitte Skovgaard Jensen, AUH).

NK cells additionally showed enhanced inhibition of HIV-1 production from autologous infected CD4+ T cells. Tsai et al. similarly demonstrated increased levels of activated NK cells (both CD56^{dim} CD16+ and CD56+ CD16-) upon GS-9620 stimulation of PBMCs from HIV-1-infected donors on long-term ART (51). Thus, both TLR7 and TLR9 agonists have demonstrated NK cell-activating properties *ex vivo* which have subsequently been confirmed *in vivo* (69, 70, 73–75, 99). Broad activation of antiviral immunity evidenced by enhanced transcription of interferon-stimulated genes (ISGs) have been observed with TLR3, TLR7, and TLR9 agonists *in vivo* (69–71, 74).

Thus, both TLR7 and TLR9 agonists are very potent enhancers of innate immune effector functions and broad stimulators of adaptive immunity. The activation of antigen presenting immune cells in the presence of relevant antigens helps focusing the adaptive immune response to effectively target HIV-1. The parallel activation of immune effector cells could boost the clearance of infected cells and hence the ability to control the infection. These features of TLR agonists could be valuable assets in the development of a functional cure for HIV-1, based on the induction of immune control of the infection.

Tissue Effects

As most TLRs are also expressed on epithelial cells throughout the body, TLR agonists may also affect resident cells in tissue (21). Our group investigated the effect of MGN1703 on gut mucosa epithelial cells, which express TLR9, using biopsies of the sigmoid colon from study participants of the short course MGN1703 treatment trial (74, 92). A global transcriptomic analysis showed that MGN1703 upregulated an ISG signature consistent with potent IFN-α induction. Furthermore, high levels of ISG proteins MX1 and ISG15 were detected by *in-situ* hybridization during MGN1703 stimulation in the epithelial cells. This induction was however not accompanied by excessive inflammation, evident by the lack of IFN-γ mRNA and absence of infiltrating neutrophils in the gut mucosa. These findings indicate that subcutaneously administered MGN1703 may have beneficial effects in the gut of infected individuals, but further investigations are needed to account for the exact mechanisms.

A sub-study to the 24-weeks MGN1703 treatment study (75) investigated the tissue-specific effects on lymph nodes (76). In LNMCs, augmented activation of pDCs, (CD86+ CD40+), NK cells (CD69+), and CD8+ effector memory T cells (HLA-DR+ CD38+) was detected and correlated with increased IFN levels and ISG15 expression. Interestingly, lymph node B cells displayed enhanced expression of activation-induced cytidine deaminase (AID) which is an essential enzyme in regulating B cell differentiation and somatic hypermutation. Consistently, a LNMC gene expression analysis showed markedly increased numbers of plasma cells post-MGN1703-treatment as well as increased levels of total IgG and subtypes IgG1, IgG2, and IgG3 antibodies. The induced antibodies showed specific neutralizing properties toward HIV-1 clade B and C, suggesting a possible autologous vaccinal effect of MGN1703. Finally, when assessing the architecture of the lymph nodes, it was demonstrated that the frequency of secondary follicles increased over the 24-weeks treatment period, suggestive of a restorative effect of the intervention.

In conclusion, these two studies from our group demonstrated broad immune enhancement and tissue restoration in the gut mucosa and lymph nodes following TLR9 agonist treatment. These results are encouraging for further clinical development as induction of potent immune responses in tissue compartments may be essential for the therapeutic success of HIV-1 cure strategies.

TLR-AGONISTS IN COMBINATION WITH OTHER THERAPEUTICS

TLR Agonists as Vaccine Adjuvants

Developing a therapeutic HIV-1 vaccine has long been an approach to boost immune control of HIV-1. Moody et al. tested the adjuvant properties of three different TLR agonists, both alone and in combination, to HIV-1 envelope protein immunogens in rhesus macaques (100). They found that the combination of TLR9 agonist CpG ODN and TLR7/8 agonist R848 mixed with base adjuvant Span85-Tween 80-squalene (STS+oCpG+R848) elicited the most potent antibody response against HIV-1 envelope gp140 and V1V2-gp70 as measured by antibody titers. The elicited antibodies were superior in terms of neutralizing HIV-1 when comparing animals treated with STS+oCpG+R848 to those treated with STS alone. Additionally, STS+oCpG+R848-elicited antibodies had greater capacity for inducing ADCC against HIV-antigen-covered cells compared to antibodies from control animals. However, the elicited antibodies were short-lived with an estimated half-life of 8.5 weeks.

Kasturi et al. attempted to assess the issue of short-lived antibodies by altering the formulation of the adjuvant in a NHP preventive vaccine study (101). The adjuvants R848 and TLR4 agonist monophosphoryl lipid A were packed in nanoparticles (NP) and administered with soluble recombinant SIVmac239-derived envelope gp140 and Gag protein 55, together referred to as the protein-NP vaccine. This protein-NP vaccine elicited a durable antibody response present in both serum and mucosa of the rhesus macaques. Ten NHPs in each group received 1 of 4 combinations of immunogens and adjuvants (virus-like particles or soluble envelope combined with either gag + NP or alum). The vaccines were administered 4 times: at week 0, 8, 16, and 25. The protein-NP group had a significantly greater peak in antibody responses at week 27 with an envelope-specific IgG level of 680.77 μg/mL compared to 104.47, 78.71, and 19.81 μg/mL, in the three other groups. The protein-NP group also showed significantly higher levels of envelope-specific plasma cells in bone marrow and draining lymph nodes. In addition, the protein-NP group exhibited the most potent protection when all study animals were challenged 12 times intravaginally with low-dose SIV once weekly starting at week 41 after the first vaccination. Although the protection against infection was stronger in the protein-NP vaccination group, 5 of 10 NHPs still became infected after 10 challenges, stressing that although the NP administration improved the adjuvating effect of the TLR agonists, this was not sufficient to elicit complete protection.

Borducchi et al. conducted a study on SIV-infected Indian origin rhesus macaques, testing a novel therapeutic vaccine compound named Ad26/MVA. The vaccine comprised an adenovirus vector (Ad26) expressing SIV gag-pol-env, which was boosted by modified vaccinia Ankara (MVA), also expressing gag-pol-env and adjuvanted by TLR7 agonist GS-986 (93). Levels of IFN-γ were increased and CD4+ and CD8+ T cell activation was evident by increased CD69-expression in the vaccine group, indicating effective immune stimulation. Upon ART discontinuation, the 9 NHPs receiving the Ad26/MVA vaccine adjuvanted with GS-986 showed a 2.5-fold delay in time to viral rebound compared to sham controls. Additionally, three of the nine animals that initially appeared to have rebounded after ART cessation regained durable virologic control throughout 160 days. None of the three components administered alone were able to induce similar levels of control suggesting a synergistic effect of the TLR7 agonist and the Ad26/MVA vaccine.

In 2008, our group investigated the immunostimulatory effect of TLR9 agonist CpG 7909 as adjuvant to pneumococcal vaccines in a randomized double-blinded, placebo-controlled trial among 97 HIV-1 infected individuals (102). All study participants received a 7-valent pneumococcal conjugate vaccine (7vPnC) at 0 and 3 months and a 23 valent pneumococcal polysaccharide vaccine (PPV-23) at 9 months. The experimental group received 1 mg of CPG 7909 as adjuvant with each vaccine dose, while the control group received a placebo adjuvant. At 9 months, the proportion of high vaccine responders, defined as a 2-fold increase in IgG levels for at least 5 of 7 of the 7vPnC serotypes, was 48% in the experimental group ($n = 48$) compared to 25% in the control group ($n = 49$). CpG 7909 significantly enhanced the immunogenicity of the pneumococcal vaccine. Interestingly, 10 individuals in each study group were treatment-naïve. In the experimental group, the treatment-naïve individuals had a slight increase in plasma-HIV-1 RNA compared to the control treatment-naïve individuals which may reflect broad immune activation (102). A *post-hoc* analysis by Winckelmann et al. showed a significant reduction of 12.6% in the level of total HIV-1 DNA in PBMCs among individuals receiving CPG 7909 as adjuvant, compared to those receiving placebo (saline) (103). These findings triggered the further investigation into the TLR9 agonist MGN1703 as immunomodulator and latency reversing agent described in the sections above.

TLR Agonists in Combination With bNAbs

Based on the immunological findings outlined above it has been proposed that administration of a TLR agonist in combination with bNAbs may enhance killing of infected cells by enhancing antibody-dependent effector mechanisms such as ADCC and ADCP (**Figure 1**). bNAbs function through three mechanisms: by direct viral neutralization, by opsonizing infected cells for immune mediated killing, and by activating the adaptive immune system via HIV-1-epitope-antibody-complexes (104–106).

Borducchi et al. investigated the effect of combining a bNAb (PGT121) with a TLR7 agonist (GS-9620) in a study with simian-human immunodeficiency virus (SHIV) infected rhesus macaques (99). The 44 NHPs were infected intrarectally with SHIV and ART was initiated at day 7 post-infection and continued for 96–104 weeks before bNAb and TLR7 agonist administration. ART was continued for another 16 weeks after the last administration of PGT121 before an ATI was initiated at week 130. By day 196 following ART cessation, only 6 of 11 NHPs in the PGT121+GS-9620 group had rebounded compared to 9 of 11 in the PGT121 group, 10 of 11 in the GS-9620 group, and 11 of 11 in the sham group. Of note, the viral reservoir measured as SHIV DNA in PBMCs was undetectable across all groups indicating that all animals hadvery small SHIV reservoirs, presumable due to the early initiation of ART. However, viral DNA was detectable in LNMCs and here, the PGT121+GS-9620 group had lower levels compared to the other groups. Subsequent anti-CD8α mediated CD8+ T-cell depletion in the non-rebounding NHPs failed to induce plasma viremia. Finally, adoptive transfer experiments where performed. PBMCs and LNMCs were first collected from the 2 PGT121+GS-9620 treated NHPs, who showed transcient rebound followed by durable virologic control. Cells were collected during the control phase of the ATI, but when transferred to SHIV-naïve NHPs, the cells induced infection. In contrast, adoptive transfer of cells from the 5 PGT121+GS-9620 treated NHPs who did not rebound upon ATI, did not cause infection in SHIV-naïve NHPs. These findings indicated that the viral SHIV reservoir was significantly reduced, maybe even completely eradicated in some animals by the combination of PGT121 and GS-9620 and have engouraged further investigations of this combination.

Along these lines, our group is performing an ongoing double-blinded randomized placebo controlled phase IIa clinical trial testing the TLR9 agonist MGN1703 and a combination of two bNAbs (3BNC117 and 101074) in HIV-1-infected donors on long-term ART, aiming to reduce the viral reservoir and induce immunological HIV-1 control (NCT03837756).

TLR Agonists and Programmed Death-1 (PD-1) Inhibition

The PD-1 receptor is a marker of T cell exhaustion, which is upregulated following prolonged antigen-stimulation during infection (107) and in cancer (108). By alleviating this T cell exhaustion, immunotherapy with antibodies blocking the PD-1 receptor has dramatically improved the prognosis of many different types of cancers such as malignant melanoma and renal cell carcinoma (109–111). In HIV-1 cure research the hope is that treatment with anti-PD-1 antibodies might lead to a more efficient targeting of the latently infected cells by HIV-specific T cells.

Bekerman et al. tested the immunomodulatory effect of a chimeric anti-PD-1 antibody and the TLR7 agonist GS-9620 in chronically SIV infected rhesus macaques (94). In a four-arm controlled design, NHPs received 0.15 mg/kg GS-9620 by oral gavage every other week for a total of 10 administrations, alone or in combination with 10 mg/kg anti-PD-1 antibody. Upon ART cessation all of the 20 NHPs rebounded within 14 days with no delay compared to the placebo group. Assessment of the viral reservoir measured by total SIV DNA levels in PBMCs similarly showed no reduction. Proportions of IFN-γ- and IL-2-producing SIV-specific T cells also did not differ between the groups. Previous studies have found beneficial effects of PD-1 receptor inhibition during SIV infection in rhesus macaques, when intervening in viremic animals or shortly after ART initiation (112, 113). Importantly, Bekerman et al. administered the PD-1 receptor antibody and TLR7 agonist after 2 years of suppressive ART. This suggests that the possible therapeutic benefits of PD-1 receptor blockade may depend on timing of administration in relation to ART initiation.

CONCLUDING REMARKS

Emerging preclinical and clinical studies strongly indicate that TLR agonists have great potential as immune boosting and priming agents in HIV-1 cure research. However, not all TLR agonist are created equally and so far, the most promising results have been observed following TLR7 and TLR9 administration. Expression patterns of TLRs in humans and the diverse response of the TLR subtypes are important factors to consider when assessing the potential clinical effect of TLR agonist treatment in HIV-1. Further investigation is needed into the physiological function of TLRs on immune cell subsets, differences in TLR expression in blood and tissue, as well as gender determined differences. TLR agonists should probably only be considered as moderately potent LRAs but while much interest in TLR agonists have evolved around their potential use as LRAs, we believe that pre-clinical and clinical findings demonstrate that the most important aspect of TLR agonists is their ability to enhance innate and adaptive immunity. This is underscored by the durable virologic control in the absence of ART achieved in NHPs by combining TLR agonists with AD26/MVA-vector SIV vaccines or bNAbs. Cross-priming of the CD8+ T cell response could be an important element of the antigen-dependent mechanisms seen with TLR agonist. Novel clinical trials testing these very concepts are now underway and their highly anticipated results will further inform the research field of the potential of TLR agonists as components in HIV-1 cure strategies.

AUTHOR CONTRIBUTIONS

JM, JG, and OS conceived and wrote the manuscript. All authors (+ JH and MT) contributed to manuscript revision and approved the submitted version.

REFERENCES

1. Richman DD, Margolis DM, Delaney M, Greene WC, Hazuda D, Pomerantz RJ. The challenge of finding a cure for HIV infection. *Science.* (2009) 323:1304–7. doi: 10.1126/science.1165706
2. Eisele E, Siliciano RF. Redefining the viral reservoirs that prevent HIV-1 eradication. *Immunity.* (2012) 37:377–88. doi: 10.1016/j.immuni.2012.08.010
3. Chun TW, Carruth L, Finzi D, Shen X, DiGiuseppe JA, Taylor H, et al. Quantification of latent tissue reservoirs and total body viral load in HIV-1 infection. *Nature.* (1997) 387:183–8. doi: 10.1038/387183a0
4. Finzi D, Hermankova M, Pierson T, Carruth LM, Buck C, Chaisson RE, et al. Identification of a reservoir for HIV-1 in patients on highly active antiretroviral therapy. *Science.* (1997) 278:1295–300. doi: 10.1126/science.278.5341.1295
5. Pierson T, McArthur J, Siliciano RF. Reservoirs for HIV-1: mechanisms for viral persistence in the presence of antiviral immune responses and antiretroviral therapy. *Annu Rev Immunol.* (2000) 18:665–708. doi: 10.1146/annurev.immunol.18.1.665
6. Chomont N, El-Far M, Ancuta P, Trautmann L, Procopio FA, Yassine-Diab B, et al. HIV reservoir size and persistence are driven by T cell survival and homeostatic proliferation. *Nat Med.* (2009) 15:893–900. doi: 10.1038/nm.1972
7. Medzhitov R. Recognition of microorganisms and activation of the immune response. *Nature.* (2007) 449:819–26. doi: 10.1038/nature06246
8. Kumar H, Kawai T, Akira S. Pathogen recognition by the innate immune system. *Int Rev Immunol.* (2011) 30:16–34. doi: 10.3109/08830185.2010.529976
9. Zicari S, Sessa L, Cotugno N, Ruggiero A, Morrocchi E, Concato C, et al. Immune activation, inflammation, and Non-AIDS co-morbidities in HIV-infected patients under long-term ART. *Viruses.* (2019) 11:200. doi: 10.3390/v11030200
10. Hemmi H, Akira S. TLR signalling and the function of dendritic cells. *Chem Immunol Allergy.* (2005) 86:120–35. doi: 10.1159/000086657
11. Hornung V, Rothenfusser S, Britsch S, Krug A, Jahrsdorfer B, Giese T, et al. Quantitative expression of toll-like receptor 1-10 mRNA in cellular subsets of human peripheral blood mononuclear cells and sensitivity to CpG oligodeoxynucleotides. *J Immunol.* (2002) 168:4531–7. doi: 10.4049/jimmunol.168.9.4531
12. Kapsenberg ML. Dendritic-cell control of pathogen-driven T-cell polarization. *Nat Rev Immunol.* (2003) 3:984–93. doi: 10.1038/nri1246
13. Ochoa MT, Legaspi AJ, Hatziris Z, Godowski PJ, Modlin RL, Sieling PA. Distribution of toll-like receptor 1 and toll-like receptor 2 in human lymphoid tissue. *Immunology.* (2003) 108:10–5. doi: 10.1046/j.1365-2567.2003.01563.x
14. Akira S, Uematsu S, Takeuchi O. Pathogen recognition and innate immunity. *Cell.* (2006) 124:783–801. doi: 10.1016/j.cell.2006.02.015
15. Kanzler H, Barrat FJ, Hessel EM, Coffman RL. Therapeutic targeting of innate immunity with Toll-like receptor agonists and antagonists. *Nat Med.* (2007) 13:552–9. doi: 10.1038/nm1589
16. Matsumoto M, Seya T. TLR3: interferon induction by double-stranded RNA including poly(I:C). *Adv Drug Deliv Rev.* (2008) 60:805–12. doi: 10.1016/j.addr.2007.11.005
17. Akira SB, Hartmann G. *Toll Like Receptors (TLRs) and Innate Immunity.* Berlin; Heidelberg: Springer-Verlag (2008).
18. Kawai T, Akira S. The role of pattern-recognition receptors in innate immunity: update on Toll-like receptors. *Nat Immunol.* (2010) 11:373–84. doi: 10.1038/ni.1863
19. Petes C, Odoardi N, Gee K. The toll for trafficking: toll-like receptor 7 delivery to the endosome. *Front Immunol.* (2017) 8:1075. doi: 10.3389/fimmu.2017.01075
20. Tartey S, Takeuchi O. Pathogen recognition and Toll-like receptor targeted therapeutics in innate immune cells. *Int Rev Immunol.* (2017) 36:57–73. doi: 10.1080/08830185.2016.1261318
21. McClure R, Massari P. TLR-dependent human mucosal epithelial cell responses to microbial pathogens. *Front Immunol.* (2014) 5:386. doi: 10.3389/fimmu.2014.00386
22. Iwasaki A, Medzhitov R. Toll-like receptor control of the adaptive immune responses. *Nat Immunol.* (2004) 5:987–95. doi: 10.1038/ni1112
23. Kawasaki T, Kawai T. Toll-like receptor signaling pathways. *Front Immunol.* (2014) 5:461. doi: 10.3389/fimmu.2014.00461
24. Verstak B, Nagpal K, Bottomley SP, Golenbock DT, Hertzog PJ, Mansell A. MyD88 adapter-like (Mal)/TIRAP interaction with TRAF6 is critical for TLR2- and TLR4-mediated NF-kappaB proinflammatory

responses. *J Biol Chem.* (2009) 284:24192–203. doi: 10.1074/jbc.M109.023044
25. Macedo AB, Novis CL, Bosque A. Targeting cellular and tissue HIV reservoirs with toll-like receptor agonists. *Front Immunol.* (2019) 10:2450. doi: 10.3389/fimmu.2019.02450
26. Altfeld M, Gale M Jr. Innate immunity against HIV-1 infection. *Nat Immunol.* (2015) 16:554–62. doi: 10.1038/ni.3157
27. Deeks SG, Lewin SR, Ross AL, Ananworanich J, Benkirane M, Cannon P, et al. International AIDS Society global scientific strategy: towards an HIV cure 2016. *Nat Med.* (2016) 22:839–50. doi: 10.1038/nm.4108
28. Sadowski I, Hashemi FB. Strategies to eradicate HIV from infected patients: elimination of latent provirus reservoirs. *Cell Mol Life Sci.* (2019) 76:3583–600. doi: 10.1007/s00018-019-03156-8
29. Deeks SG. HIV: Shock and kill. *Nature.* (2012) 487:439–40. doi: 10.1038/487439a
30. Sengupta S, Siliciano RF. Targeting the latent reservoir for HIV-1. *Immunity.* (2018) 48:872–95. doi: 10.1016/j.immuni.2018.04.030
31. Elliott JH, Wightman F, Solomon A, Ghneim K, Ahlers J, Cameron MJ, et al. Activation of HIV transcription with short-course vorinostat in HIV-infected patients on suppressive antiretroviral therapy. *PLoS Pathog.* (2014) 10:e1004473. doi: 10.1371/journal.ppat.1004473
32. Rasmussen TA, Tolstrup M, Brinkmann CR, Olesen R, Erikstrup C, Solomon A, et al. Panobinostat, a histone deacetylase inhibitor, for latent-virus reactivation in HIV-infected patients on suppressive antiretroviral therapy: a phase 1/2, single group, clinical trial. *Lancet HIV.* (2014) 1:e13–21. doi: 10.1016/S2352-3018(14)70014-1
33. Sogaard OS, Graversen ME, Leth S, Olesen R, Brinkmann CR, Nissen SK, et al. The depsipeptide romidepsin reverses HIV-1 latency *in vivo. PLoS Pathog.* (2015) 11:e1005142. doi: 10.1371/journal.ppat.1005142
34. Karn J, Stoltzfus CM. Transcriptional and posttranscriptional regulation of HIV-1 gene expression. *Cold Spring Harb Perspect Med.* (2012) 2:a006916. doi: 10.1101/cshperspect.a006916
35. Eckschlager T, Plch J, Stiborova M, Hrabeta J. Histone deacetylase inhibitors as anticancer drugs. *Int J Mol Sci.* (2017) 18:1414. doi: 10.3390/ijms18071414
36. Leth S, Schleimann MH, Nissen SK, Hojen JF, Olesen R, Graversen ME, et al. Combined effect of Vacc-4x, recombinant human granulocyte macrophage colony-stimulating factor vaccination, and romidepsin on the HIV-1 reservoir (REDUC): a single-arm, phase 1B/2A trial. *Lancet HIV.* (2016) 3:e463–472. doi: 10.1016/S2352-3018(16)30055-8
37. Bashiri K, Rezaei N, Nasi M, Cossarizza A. The role of latency reversal agents in the cure of HIV: a review of current data. *Immunol Lett.* (2018) 196:135–9. doi: 10.1016/j.imlet.2018.02.004
38. Kulkosky J, Sullivan J, Xu Y, Souder E, Hamer DH, Pomerantz RJ. Expression of latent HAART-persistent HIV type 1 induced by novel cellular activating agents. *AIDS Res Hum Retroviruses.* (2004) 20:497–505. doi: 10.1089/088922204323087741
39. Gutierrez C, Serrano-Villar S, Madrid-Elena N, Perez-Elias MJ, Martin ME, Barbas C, et al. Bryostatin-1 for latent virus reactivation in HIV-infected patients on antiretroviral therapy. *AIDS.* (2016) 30:1385–92. doi: 10.1097/QAD.0000000000001064
40. Elliott JH, McMahon JH, Chang CC, Lee SA, Hartogensis W, Bumpus N, et al. Short-term administration of disulfiram for reversal of latent HIV infection: a phase 2 dose-escalation study. *Lancet HIV.* (2015) 2:e520–9. doi: 10.1016/S2352-3018(15)00226-X
41. Saleh S, Wightman F, Ramanayake S, Alexander M, Kumar N, Khoury G, et al. Expression and reactivation of HIV in a chemokine induced model of HIV latency in primary resting CD4+ T cells. *Retrovirology.* (2011) 8:80. doi: 10.1186/1742-4690-8-80
42. Jiang G, Nguyen D, Archin NM, Yukl SA, Mendez-Lagares G, Tang Y, et al. HIV latency is reversed by ACSS2-driven histone crotonylation. *J Clin Invest.* (2018) 128:1190–8. doi: 10.1172/JCI98071
43. Lisziewicz J, Sun D, Weichold FF, Thierry AR, Lusso P, Tang J, et al. Antisense oligodeoxynucleotide phosphorothioate complementary to Gag mRNA blocks replication of human immunodeficiency virus type 1 in human peripheral blood cells. *Proc Natl Acad Sci USA.* (1994) 91:7942–6. doi: 10.1073/pnas.91.17.7942
44. Sereni D, Tubiana R, Lascoux C, Katlama C, Taulera O, Bourque A, et al. Pharmacokinetics and tolerability of intravenous trecovirsen (GEM 91), an antisense phosphorothioate oligonucleotide, in HIV-positive subjects. *J Clin Pharmacol.* (1999) 39:47–54. doi: 10.1177/00912709922007552
45. Krieg AM. CpG motifs in bacterial DNA and their immune effects. *Annu Rev Immunol.* (2002) 20:709–60. doi: 10.1146/annurev.immunol.20.100301.064842
46. Agrawal S, Martin RR. Was induction of HIV-1 through TLR9? *J Immunol.* (2003) 171:1621; author reply 1621-1622. doi: 10.4049/jimmunol.171.4.1621
47. Equils O, Schito ML, Karahashi H, Madak Z, Yarali A, Michelsen KS, et al. Toll-like receptor 2 (TLR2) and TLR9 signaling results in HIV-long terminal repeat trans-activation and HIV replication in HIV-1 transgenic mouse spleen cells: implications of simultaneous activation of TLRs on HIV replication. *J Immunol.* (2003) 170:5159–64. doi: 10.4049/jimmunol.170.10.5159
48. Novis CL, Archin NM, Buzon MJ, Verdin E, Round JL, Lichterfeld M, et al. Reactivation of latent HIV-1 in central memory CD4(+) T cells through TLR-1/2 stimulation. *Retrovirology.* (2013) 10:119. doi: 10.1186/1742-4690-10-119
49. Kaur J, Tsai A, Kukolj G, Cihlar T, Murry J. Pattern recognition receptor agonists induce HIV in ART suppressed HIV+ donor cells. *CROI 2018* abstract #321. Boston, MA (2018).
50. Thibault S, Imbeault M, Tardif MR, Tremblay MJ. TLR5 stimulation is sufficient to trigger reactivation of latent HIV-1 provirus in T lymphoid cells and activate virus gene expression in central memory CD4+ T cells. *Virology.* (2009) 389:20–5. doi: 10.1016/j.virol.2009.04.019
51. Tsai A, Irrinki A, Kaur J, Cihlar T, Kukolj G, Sloan DD, et al. Toll-Like Receptor 7 Agonist GS-9620 Induces HIV Expression and HIV-Specific Immunity in Cells from HIV-Infected Individuals on Suppressive Antiretroviral Therapy. *J Virol.* (2017) 91. doi: 10.1128/JVI.02166-16
52. Bam RA, Hansen D, Irrinki A, Mulato A, Jones GS, Hesselgesser J, et al. TLR7 Agonist GS-9620 Is a Potent Inhibitor of Acute HIV-1 Infection in Human Peripheral Blood Mononuclear Cells. *Antimicrob Agents Chemother.* (2016) 61:e01369–16. doi: 10.1128/AAC.01369-16
53. Offersen R, Nissen SK, Rasmussen TA, Ostergaard L, Denton PW, Sogaard OS, et al. A novel toll-like receptor 9 agonist, MGN1703, enhances HIV-1 transcription and NK cell-mediated inhibition of HIV-1-infected autologous CD4+ T cells. *J Virol.* (2016) 90:4441–53. doi: 10.1128/JVI.00222-16
54. Chaturvedi A, Pierce SK. How location governs toll-like receptor signaling. *Traffic.* (2009) 10:621–8. doi: 10.1111/j.1600-0854.2009.00899.x
55. Caron G, Duluc D, Fremaux I, Jeannin P, David C, Gascan H, et al. Direct stimulation of human T cells via TLR5 and TLR7/8: flagellin and R-848 up-regulate proliferation and IFN-gamma production by memory CD4+ T cells. *J Immunol.* (2005) 175:1551–7. doi: 10.4049/jimmunol.175.3.1551
56. Krieg AM. Development of TLR9 agonists for cancer therapy. *J Clin Invest.* (2007) 117:1184–94. doi: 10.1172/JCI31414
57. Schmidt M, Hagner N, Marco A, Konig-Merediz SA, Schroff M, Wittig B. Design and structural requirements of the potent and safe TLR-9 agonistic immunomodulator MGN1703. *Nucleic Acid Ther.* (2015) 25:130–40. doi: 10.1089/nat.2015.0533
58. Schlaepfer E, Speck RF. TLR8 activates HIV from latently infected cells of myeloid-monocytic origin directly via the MAPK pathway and from latently infected CD4+ T cells indirectly via TNF-alpha. *J Immunol.* (2011) 186:4314–24. doi: 10.4049/jimmunol.1003174
59. Macedo AB, Novis CL, De Assis CM, Sorensen ES, Moszczynski P, Huang SH, et al. Dual TLR2 and TLR7 agonists as HIV latency-reversing agents. *JCI Insight.* (2018) 3:e122673. doi: 10.1172/jci.insight.122673
60. Stoszko M, Ne E, Abner E, Mahmoudi T. A broad drug arsenal to attack a strenuous latent HIV reservoir. *Curr Opin Virol.* (2019) 38:37–53. doi: 10.1016/j.coviro.2019.06.001
61. Telwatte S, Moron-Lopez S, Aran D, Kim P, Hsieh C, Joshi S, et al. Heterogeneity in HIV and cellular transcription profiles in cell line models of latent and productive infection: implications for HIV latency. *Retrovirology.* (2019) 16:32. doi: 10.1186/s12977-019-0494-x
62. Ketloy C, Engering A, Srichairatanakul U, Limsalakpetch A, Yongvanitchit K, Pichyangkul S, et al. Expression and function of Toll-like receptors on dendritic cells and other antigen presenting cells from non-human primates. *Vet Immunol Immunopathol.* (2008) 125:18–30. doi: 10.1016/j.vetimm.2008.05.001

63. Gujer C, Sundling C, Seder RA, Karlsson Hedestam GB, Lore K. Human and rhesus plasmacytoid dendritic cell and B-cell responses to Toll-like receptor stimulation. *Immunology.* (2011) 134:257–69. doi: 10.1111/j.1365-2567.2011.03484.x
64. Caskey M, Lefebvre F, Filali-Mouhim A, Cameron MJ, Goulet JP, Haddad EK, et al. Synthetic double-stranded RNA induces innate immune responses similar to a live viral vaccine in humans. *J Exp Med.* (2011) 208:2357–66. doi: 10.1084/jem.20111171
65. Cheng L, Zhang Z, Li G, Li F, Wang L, Zhang L, et al. Human innate responses and adjuvant activity of TLR ligands *in vivo* in mice reconstituted with a human immune system. *Vaccine.* (2017) 35:6143–53. doi: 10.1016/j.vaccine.2017.09.052
66. Cheng L, Wang Q, Li G, Banga R, Ma J, Yu H, et al. TLR3 agonist and CD40-targeting vaccination induces immune responses and reduces HIV-1 reservoirs. *J Clin Invest.* (2018) 128:4387–96. doi: 10.1172/JCI99005
67. Kyi C, Roudko V, Sabado R, Saenger Y, Loging W, Mandeli J, et al. Therapeutic Immune Modulation against Solid Cancers with Intratumoral Poly-ICLC: A Pilot Trial. *Clin Cancer Res.* (2018) 24:4937–48. doi: 10.1158/1078-0432.CCR-17-1866
68. Wittig B, Schmidt M, Scheithauer W, Schmoll HJ. MGN1703, an immunomodulator and toll-like receptor 9 (TLR-9) agonist: from bench to bedside. *Crit Rev Oncol Hematol.* (2015) 94:31–44. doi: 10.1016/j.critrevonc.2014.12.002
69. Lim SY, Osuna CE, Hraber PT, Hesselgesser J, Gerold JM, Barnes TL, et al. TLR7 agonists induce transient viremia and reduce the viral reservoir in SIV-infected rhesus macaques on antiretroviral therapy. *Sci Transl Med.* (2018) 10:eaao4521. doi: 10.1126/scitranslmed.aao4521
70. Del Prete GQ, Alvord WG, Li Y, Deleage C, Nag M, Oswald K, et al. TLR7 agonist administration to SIV-infected macaques receiving early initiated cART does not induce plasma viremia. *JCI Insight.* (2019) 4:e127717. doi: 10.1172/jci.insight.127717
71. Saxena M, Sabado RL, La Mar M, Mohri H, Salazar AM, Dong H, et al. Poly-ICLC, a TLR3 agonist, induces transient innate immune responses in patients with treated hiv-infection: a randomized double-blinded placebo controlled trial. *Front Immunol.* (2019) 10:725. doi: 10.3389/fimmu.2019.00725
72. Salazar AM, Erlich RB, Mark A, Bhardwaj N, Herberman RB. Therapeutic in situ autovaccination against solid cancers with intratumoral poly-ICLC: case report, hypothesis, and clinical trial. *Cancer Immunol Res.* (2014) 2:720–4. doi: 10.1158/2326-6066.CIR-14-0024
73. Riddler S. *Vesatolimod (GS-9620) is Safe and Pharmacodynamically Active in HIV-Infected Individuals.* Mexico City: IAS 2019 oral #WEAA0304. (2019).
74. Vibholm L, Schleimann MH, Hojen JF, Benfield T, Offersen R, Rasmussen K, et al. Short-course toll-like receptor 9 agonist treatment impacts innate immunity and plasma viremia in individuals with human immunodeficiency virus infection. *Clin Infect Dis.* (2017) 64:1686–95. doi: 10.1093/cid/cix201
75. Vibholm LK, Konrad CV, Schleimann MH, Frattari G, Winckelmann A, Klastrup V, et al. Effects of 24-week toll-like receptor 9 agonist treatment in HIV type 1+ individuals. *AIDS.* (2019) 33:1315–25. doi: 10.1097/QAD.0000000000002213
76. Schleimann MH, Kobbero ML, Vibholm LK, Kjaer K, Giron LB, Busman-Sahay K, et al. TLR9 agonist MGN1703 enhances B cell differentiation and function in lymph nodes. *EBioMedicine.* (2019) 45:328–40. doi: 10.1016/j.ebiom.2019.07.005
77. Kumar A, Abbas W, Herbein G. HIV-1 latency in monocytes/macrophages. *Viruses.* (2014) 6:1837–60. doi: 10.3390/v6041837
78. Kandathil AJ, Sugawara S, Balagopal A. Are T cells the only HIV-1 reservoir? *Retrovirology.* (2016) 13:86. doi: 10.1186/s12977-016-0323-4
79. Sheth PM, Kovacs C, Kemal KS, Jones RB, Raboud JM, Pilon R, et al. Persistent HIV RNA shedding in semen despite effective antiretroviral therapy. *AIDS.* (2009) 23:2050–4. doi: 10.1097/QAD.0b013e3283303e04
80. Yukl SA, Shergill AK, Ho T, Killian M, Girling V, Epling L, et al. The distribution of HIV DNA and RNA in cell subsets differs in gut and blood of HIV-positive patients on ART: implications for viral persistence. *J Infect Dis.* (2013) 208:1212–20. doi: 10.1093/infdis/jit308
81. Costiniuk CT, Jenabian MA. The lungs as anatomical reservoirs of HIV infection. *Rev Med Virol.* (2014) 24:35–54. doi: 10.1002/rmv.1772
82. Sewald X, Ladinsky MS, Uchil PD, Beloor J, Pi R, Herrmann C, et al. Retroviruses use CD169-mediated trans-infection of permissive lymphocytes to establish infection. *Science.* (2015) 350:563–7. doi: 10.1126/science.aab2749
83. Ganor Y, Real F, Sennepin A, Dutertre CA, Prevedel L, Xu L, et al. HIV-1 reservoirs in urethral macrophages of patients under suppressive antiretroviral therapy. *Nat Microbiol.* (2019) 4:633–44. doi: 10.1038/s41564-018-0335-z
84. Wallet C, De Rovere M, Van Assche J, Daouad F, De Wit S, Gautier V, et al. Microglial cells: the main HIV-1 reservoir in the brain. *Front Cell Infect Microbiol.* (2019) 9:362. doi: 10.3389/fcimb.2019.00362
85. Rajasekaran N, Chester C, Yonezawa A, Zhao X, Kohrt HE. Enhancement of antibody-dependent cell mediated cytotoxicity: a new era in cancer treatment. *Immunotargets Ther.* (2015) 4:91–100. doi: 10.2147/ITT.S61292
86. Satoh T, and Akira S. Toll-Like Receptor Signaling and Its Inducible Proteins. *Microbiol Spectr.* (2016) 4. doi: 10.1128/microbiolspec.MCHD-0040-2016
87. Longhi MP, Trumpfheller C, Idoyaga J, Caskey M, Matos I, Kluger C, et al. Dendritic cells require a systemic type I interferon response to mature and induce CD4+ Th1 immunity with poly IC as adjuvant. *J Exp Med.* (2009) 206:1589–602. doi: 10.1084/jem.20090247
88. Tai Y, Wang Q, Korner H, Zhang L, Wei W. Molecular mechanisms of t cells activation by dendritic cells in autoimmune diseases. *Front Pharmacol.* (2018) 9:642. doi: 10.3389/fphar.2018.00642
89. Hervas-Stubbs S, Perez-Gracia JL, Rouzaut A, Sanmamed MF, Le Bon A, Melero I. Direct effects of type I interferons on cells of the immune system. *Clin Cancer Res.* (2011) 17:2619–27. doi: 10.1158/1078-0432.CCR-10-1114
90. Tolstrup M. *TLR Agonists and Latency Reversal: Can They Both Shock and Kill?* Amsterdam: AIDS 2018 oral #WESY0905. (2018).
91. Speiser DE, Lienard D, Rufer N, Rubio-Godoy V, Rimoldi D, Lejeune F, et al. Rapid and strong human CD8+ T cell responses to vaccination with peptide, IFA, and CpG oligodeoxynucleotide 7909. *J Clin Invest.* (2005) 115:739–46. doi: 10.1172/JCI23373
92. Krarup AR, Abdel-Mohsen M, Schleimann MH, Vibholm L, Engen PA, Dige A, et al. The TLR9 agonist MGN1703 triggers a potent type I interferon response in the sigmoid colon. *Mucosal Immunol.* (2018) 11:449–61. doi: 10.1038/mi.2017.59
93. Borducchi EN, Cabral C, Stephenson KE, Liu J, Abbink P, Ng'ang'a D, et al. Ad26/MVA therapeutic vaccination with TLR7 stimulation in SIV-infected rhesus monkeys. *Nature.* (2016) 540:284–7. doi: 10.1038/nature20583
94. Bekerman E, Hesselgesser J, Carr B, Nagel M, Hung M, Wang A, et al. PD-1 Blockade and TLR7 activation lack therapeutic benefit in chronic simian immunodeficiency virus-infected macaques on antiretroviral therapy. *Antimicrob Agents Chemother.* (2019) 63:e01163–19. doi: 10.1128/AAC.01163-19
95. Cassatella MA, Anegon I, Cuturi MC, Griskey P, Trinchieri G, Perussia B. Fc gamma R(CD16) interaction with ligand induces Ca2+ mobilization and phosphoinositide turnover in human natural killer cells. Role of Ca2+ in Fc gamma R(CD16)-induced transcription and expression of lymphokine genes. *J Exp Med.* (1989) 169:549–67. doi: 10.1084/jem.169.2.549
96. Molgora M, Supino D, Mavilio D, Santoni A, Moretta L, Mantovani A, et al. The yin-yang of the interaction between myelomonocytic cells and NK cells. *Scand J Immunol.* (2018) 88:e12705. doi: 10.1111/sji.12705
97. Mikulak J, Oriolo F, Zaghi E, Di Vito C, Mavilio D. Natural killer cells in HIV-1 infection and therapy. *AIDS.* (2017) 31:2317–30. doi: 10.1097/QAD.0000000000001645
98. Tay MZ, Wiehe K, Pollara J. Antibody-dependent cellular phagocytosis in antiviral immune responses. *Front Immunol.* (2019) 10:332. doi: 10.3389/fimmu.2019.00332
99. Borducchi EN, Liu J, Nkolola JP, Cadena AM, Yu WH, Fischinger S, et al. Antibody and TLR7 agonist delay viral rebound in SHIV-infected monkeys. *Nature.* (2018) 563:360–4. doi: 10.1038/s41586-018-0600-6
100. Moody MA, Santra S, Vandergrift NA, Sutherland LL, Gurley TC, Drinker MS, et al. Toll-like receptor 7/8 (TLR7/8) and TLR9 agonists cooperate to enhance HIV-1 envelope antibody responses in rhesus macaques. *J Virol.* (2014) 88:3329–39. doi: 10.1128/JVI.03309-13
101. Kasturi SP, Kozlowski PA, Nakaya HI, Burger MC, Russo P, Pham M, et al. Adjuvanting a Simian Immunodeficiency Virus Vaccine with Toll-Like Receptor Ligands Encapsulated in Nanoparticles Induces Persistent Antibody Responses and Enhanced Protection in TRIM5α Restrictive Macaques. *J Virol.* (2017) 91:e01844-16. doi: 10.1128/JVI.01844-16

102. Sogaard OS, Lohse N, Harboe ZB, Offersen R, Bukh AR, Davis HL, et al. Improving the immunogenicity of pneumococcal conjugate vaccine in HIV-infected adults with a toll-like receptor 9 agonist adjuvant: a randomized, controlled trial. *Clinical Infectious Diseases.* (2010) 51:42–50. doi: 10.1086/653112
103. Winckelmann AA, Munk-Petersen LV, Rasmussen TA, Melchjorsen J, Hjelholt TJ, Montefiori D, et al. Administration of a toll-like receptor 9 agonist decreases the proviral reservoir in virologically suppressed HIV-infected patients. *PLoS ONE.* (2013) 8:e62074. doi: 10.1371/journal.pone.0062074
104. Bournazos S, Klein F, Pietzsch J, Seaman MS, Nussenzweig MC, Ravetch JV. Broadly neutralizing anti-HIV-1 antibodies require Fc effector functions for *in vivo* activity. *Cell.* (2014) 158:1243–53. doi: 10.1016/j.cell.2014.08.023
105. Schoofs T, Klein F, Braunschweig M, Kreider EF, Feldmann A, Nogueira L, et al. HIV-1 therapy with monoclonal antibody 3BNC117 elicits host immune responses against HIV-1. *Science.* (2016) 352:997–1001. doi: 10.1126/science.aaf0972
106. Caskey M, Klein F, Nussenzweig MC. Broadly neutralizing anti-HIV-1 monoclonal antibodies in the clinic. *Nat Med.* (2019) 25:547–53. doi: 10.1038/s41591-019-0412-8
107. Barber DL, Wherry EJ, Masopust D, Zhu B, Allison JP, Sharpe AH, et al. Restoring function in exhausted CD8 T cells during chronic viral infection. *Nature.* (2006) 439:682–7. doi: 10.1038/nature04444
108. Ahmadzadeh M, Johnson LA, Heemskerk B, Wunderlich JR, Dudley ME, White DE, et al. Tumor antigen-specific CD8 T cells infiltrating the tumor express high levels of PD-1 and are functionally impaired. *Blood.* (2009) 114:1537–44. doi: 10.1182/blood-2008-12-195792
109. Weinstock M, McDermott D. Targeting PD-1/PD-L1 in the treatment of metastatic renal cell carcinoma. *Ther Adv Urol.* (2015) 7:365–77. doi: 10.1177/1756287215597647
110. Munhoz RR, Postow MA. Clinical Development of PD-1 in Advanced Melanoma. *Cancer J.* (2018) 24:7–14. doi: 10.1097/PPO.0000000000000299
111. Wu X, Gu Z, Chen Y, Chen B, Chen W, Weng L, et al. Application of PD-1 Blockade in Cancer Immunotherapy. *Comput Struct Biotechnol J.* (2019) 17:661–74. doi: 10.1016/j.csbj.2019.03.006
112. Velu V, Titanji K, Zhu B, Husain S, Pladevega A, Lai L, et al. Enhancing SIV-specific immunity *in vivo* by PD-1 blockade. *Nature.* (2009) 458:206–10. doi: 10.1038/nature07662
113. Mylvaganam GH, Chea LS, Tharp GK, Hicks S, Velu V, Iyer SS, et al. Combination anti-PD-1 antiretroviral therapy provides therapeutic benefit against SIV. *JCI Insight.* (2018) 3:e122940. doi: 10.1172/jci.insight.122940

14

Altered Immunity and Microbial Dysbiosis in Aged Individuals With Long-Term Controlled HIV Infection

*Nicholas Rhoades[1], Norma Mendoza[1], Allen Jankeel[1], Suhas Sureshchandra[1], Alexander D. Alvarez[1], Brianna Doratt[1], Omeid Heidari[2], Rod Hagan[3], Brandon Brown[4], Steven Scheibel[3], Theodore Marbley[3], Jeff Taylor[5] and Ilhem Messaoudi[1]**

[1] Molecular Biology and Biochemistry, University of California Irvine, Irvine, CA, United States, [2] School of Nursing, John Hopkins University, Baltimore, MD, United States, [3] Stonewall Medical Center, Borrego Health, Cathedral City, CA, United States, [4] School of Medicine, University of California, Riverside, Riverside, CA, United States, [5] HIV+ Aging-Palm Springs, Palm Springs, CA, United States

***Correspondence:**
Ilhem Messaoudi
imessaou@uci.edu

The introduction of highly active antiretroviral therapy (HAART) resulted in a significant increase in life expectancy for HIV patients. Indeed, in 2015, 45% of the HIV+ individuals in the United States were ≥55 years of age. Despite improvements in diagnosis and treatment of HIV infection, geriatric HIV+ patients suffer from higher incidence of comorbidities compared to age-matched HIV- individuals. Both chronic inflammation and dysbiosis of the gut microbiome are believed to be major contributors to this phenomenon, however carefully controlled studies investigating the impact of long-term (>10 years) controlled HIV (LTC-HIV) infection are lacking. To address this question, we profiled circulating immune cells, immune mediators, and the gut microbiome from elderly (≥55 years old) LTC-HIV+ and HIV- gay men living in the Palm Springs area. LTC-HIV+ individuals had lower frequency of circulating monocytes and CD4+ T-cells, and increased frequency CD8+ T-cells. Moreover, levels of systemic INFγ and several growth factors were increased while levels of IL-2 and several chemokines were reduced. Upon stimulation, immune cells from LTC-HIV+ individuals produced higher levels of pro-inflammatory cytokines. Last but not least, the gut microbiome of LTC-HIV+ individuals was enriched in bacterial taxa typically found in the oral cavity suggestive of loss of compartmentalization, while levels of beneficial butyrate producing taxa were reduced. Additionally, prevalence of *Prevotella* negatively correlated with CD4+ T-cells numbers in LTC-HIV+ individuals. These results indicate that despite long-term adherence and undetectable viral loads, LTC-HIV infection results in significant shifts in immune cell frequencies and gut microbial communities.

Keywords: HIV, HAART, aging, dysbiosis, inflammation

INTRODUCTION

Advances in the diagnosis and treatment of HIV infection has transformed what used to be a fatal diagnosis into a long-term chronic disease with individuals living up to 50 years after diagnosis (1, 2). In the United States, 450,000 of those living with HIV are ≥50 years of age, and this number is expected to grow over the coming decade (3). Highly active anti-retroviral therapy (HAART) must be taken continuously to maintain viral loads below detection (4, 5). However, low levels of viral replication can be detected in virtually all patients receiving HAART (6). Moreover, mortality rates among individuals living with long-term controlled HIV infection (LTC-HIV) remains higher than those seen in age-matched HIV- individuals due to HIV-associated non-AIDS (HANA) co-morbidities (7–9). HANA co-morbidities include neurocognitive disorders, cardiovascular disease, cancer, liver cirrhosis, kidney, and lung disease (10–16). The average number of comorbid conditions is higher in older HIV+ patients compared to age-matched HIV- subjects, indicative of accelerated aging (10, 17). The mechanisms underlying this increase in comorbidities and resulting mortality remain unclear. Consequently, very few interventions are available to counteract these adverse outcomes.

Some of these comorbidities could be explained by the high rates of co-infection among LTC-HIV patients, notably with Hepatitis C (18, 19). Moreover, HAART toxicity itself increases the risk of cardiovascular disease and metabolic dysfunction via mitochondrial dysfunction, but this does not fully explain the increase in neurocognitive disorders (20–23). Another potential factor is the increased systemic inflammation reported in LTC-HIV infection (24–27). While the initiation of HAART has been shown to reduce immune activation, the levels remain higher than those observed in HIV- individuals even after 2 years of treatment (28–31). The sources of this systemic inflammation are poorly understood. Some studies have suggested an association between shifts in the gut microbiome and systemic inflammation (32, 33). HIV-induced loss of Th17 CD4+ T cells in the gut is thought to disrupt the microbial community and impair the gut barrier resulting in the translocation of microbial products (34, 35). Indeed, increased levels of sCD14, LPS, IgM, iFABP, and endotoxin-bound IgM have been reported in HIV+ individuals at various stages of infection (36, 37). Some studies have reported an increase in the abundance of *Prevotella* in untreated, and HAART treated HIV+ individuals while others reported no changes (33, 38). Furthermore, disruption in tryptophan metabolism, reduction in short chain fatty acid (SCFA) production, and an increase in trimethylamine-n-oxide (TMAO) production have all been linked to increased HANA co-morbidities (39–41).

Our understanding of the role of circulating immune cells in the development and exacerbation of systemic inflammation also remains incomplete. While many have reported some recovery of CD4+ T cells upon initiation of HAART, this finding has only has been explored through the first 5 years of treatment (42–44). An increase in terminally differentiated T cells has also been listed as a potential source of aberrant immune activation (45). CD4+ T cells are not the only immune cells affected by HIV infection. Monocytes in particular are activated directly during initial infection by circulating viral proteins such as gp120 and Nef (45) and indirectly at later stages due to an increase in bacterial products such as LPS in circulation (46–48). Activated monocytes can release multiple immune mediators such as TNFα, IL-1β, IL-6 that can contribute to systemic inflammation (49). Natural Killer (NK) cells also play an important role in controlling HIV through the production of INFγ which suppresses infection, but can also contribute to excessive inflammation (50). HAART has been shown to restore NK populations over the first couple of years of treatment, but the durability of this recovery is not well-understood (51).

The lack of clear understanding of the impact of LTC-HIV infection on immune status, systemic inflammation, and microbiome communities is likely due to the paucity of well-controlled studies. Researchers often compare HIV+ and HIV- groups of differing socioeconomic status, sexual orientation, and geographic location. These factors can affect immunological status and the gut microbiome. To address this limitation, we obtained blood and rectal swabs from older ($\geq$55 years of age) LTC-HIV+ gay men (>10 years post-infection) and HIV- participants residing in the Palm Springs area. Our analysis shows that despite adherence to HAART treatment, HIV status is associated with a reduction in circulating CD4+ T-cells and monocytes, an increase in CD8+ T-cells, and greater activation/differentiation of NK cells. We also detected signs of heightened systemic inflammation and induced inflammatory response to polyclonal stimulation. Surprisingly, we detected a limited number of shifts in the gut microbial community with an increase in Fusobacteria, Bifidobacteriales, and Lactobacillales in LTC-HIV+ men. *Prevotella* was negatively correlated with CD4+ T-cell count in LTC-HIV+ but not HIV- individuals. Together these data suggest that significant differences in immunological and microbial communities persist in LTC-HIV infection.

METHODS

Study Population and Sample Collection

The Institutional Review Board of the University of California, Riverside reviewed and approved this study, and the University of California, Irvine obtained a reliance registry.

A total of 105 men $\geq$55 years of age (HIV- n = 47, LTC-HIV+ n = 58) were recruited from Palm Springs, CA. All LTC-HIV+ individuals have been on HAART therapy for >10 years with undetectable viral loads. Median CD4+ cell counts in the LTC-HIV cohort were 689 cells/mm^3 with only two individuals having CD4+ T cell count <200 cells/mm^3 while CD4+ cell counts in the HIV- cohort were 1198 cells/mm^3. Each participant submitted a blood sample, a rectal swab, and completed a paper demographics/co-morbidities survey (**Table 1**). Complete blood cell counts (CBC) were determined using a hematology analyzer (Beckman Coulter). Peripheral blood mononuclear cells (PBMC) and plasma were obtained by standard density gradient centrifugation over the blood separation polymer Ficoll (GE Healthcare Life Sciences, Pittsburg, PA, United States). PBMC were frozen in 10% DMSO/FBS and stored in liquid nitrogen while plasma was stored at 80°C until analysis.

Flow Cytometry

1–2 × 10^6 PBMC were stained using antibodies against: CD4, CD8b, CD95, CD28, CCR7, CD20, CD27, IgD, PD-1, KLRG1, and Ki-67 to delineate naïve and memory T and B cell populations, as well as measure activation and proliferation (**Supplementary Figure 1**). A second tube of 1–2 × 10^6 PBMC was stained using antibodies against: CD3, CD20,

TABLE 1 | Demographics and co-morbidities.

	Total *n* [S.D.](%)	LTC-HIV + *n* [S.D.](%)	HIV – *n* [S.D.](%)	*p*
DEMOGRAPHICS				
Age	64 [6.8]	65.7 [7.3]	62.7 [6.03]	0.02*
Race				0.82
Non-hispanic white	90 (84.6)	49 (84.5)	41 (87.2)	
Other	15 (15.5)	9 (15.5)	6 (12.8)	
Education				0.299
High school	8 (8.3)	7 (12.5)	1 (2.4)	
Some college	32 (33.3)	21 (37.5)	11 (26.8)	
Four-year university	25 (24.0)	13 (23.2)	12 (29.3)	
Graduate school	32 (33.3)	15 (26.8)	17 (41.4)	
Relationship status				0.10
Single	43 (41.7)	29 (49.2)	14 (31.8)	
In a relationship	18 (17.5)	10 (16.9)	8 (18.2)	
Engaged	2 (1.9)	1 (1.7)	1 (2.3)	
Married	34 (33.0)	14 (23.7)	20 (45.5)	
Widowed	6 (5.8)	5 (8.5)	1 (2.3)	
On disability	28 (28.28)	25 (43.86)	3 (7.14)	0.001***
COMORBIDITIES				
Depression	27 (25.96)	21 (35.59)	6 (13.33)	0.013*
Arthritis	30 (28.85)	17 (28.81)	13 (28.89)	1.000
Hepatitis	8 (7.69)	8 (13.56)	0 (0)	0.009***
Neuropathy	33 (31.73)	24 (40.68)	9 (20)	0.033*
Hypertension	38 (36.54)	18 (30.51)	20 (44.44)	0.156
Dermatitis	12 (11.54)	10 (16.95)	2 (4.44)	0.064
Herpes	13 (12.50)	8 (13.56)	5 (11.11)	0.773
Vision loss	17 (16.35)	9 (15.25)	8 (17.78)	0.792
Diabetes	13 (12.5)	8 (13.56)	5 (11.11)	0.773
Hearing loss	25 (24.04)	11 (18.64)	14 (31.11)	0.168
Respiratory problems	6 (5.78)	3 (5.08)	3 (6.67)	1.000
Heart condition	11 (10.58)	4 (6.78)	7 (15.56)	0.201
Broken bones	1 (0.96)	0 (0)	1 (2.22)	0.433

*Chi-squared or Fisher's exact tests were conducted to determine significant differences between the two *p < 0.05, ***p < 0.001.*

HLA-DR, CD14, CD11c, CD123, CD56, CD16, granzymeB, and CD57 to delineate monocytes, myeloid dendritic cells (mDC), plasmacytoid dendritic cells (pDC), and natural killer (NK) cell subsets, respectively (**Supplementary Figure 2**). All flow cytometry samples were acquired with Attune NxT (Life Technologies, Carlsbad, CA, United States) and analyzed using FlowJo (TreeStar, Ashland, OR, United States).

PBMC Stimulation

5×10^5 PBMC were incubated for 16 h in the absence (unstimulated) or presence (stimulated) of 5 ng/ml PMA and 1 μg/ml Ionomycin at 37°C in a humidified incubator (5% CO_2). At the end of the incubation, cells were spun down for 5 min at 2,000 rpm. Supernatants were collected to measure production of immune mediators and cell pellets were used for RNA extraction.

Analysis of Immune Mediator Production

Plasma levels of immune mediators were assessed using a human 45-plex assay (Thermo Fisher Scientific, Waltham, MA, United States). Immune mediators produced by PBMC in response to PMA/ionomycin stimulation were measured using Magnetic 33-plex assay (R&D Systems, Minneapolis, MN, United States). All samples were analyzed using a MAGPIX instrument (Luminex, Austin, TX, United States).

RNAseq Library Prep

Total RNA was isolated from PBMC pellets obtained from control and stimulated wells using the Qiagen mRNAeasy kit (Qiagen, Valencia, CA, United States). RNA concentration and integrity was verified using Agilent 2,100 Bioanalyzer. Total RNA was depleted of ribosomal fraction using Ribo-Gone rRNA removal kit. Libraries were then constructed using SMARTer Stranded RNA-Seq Kit (Clontech, Mountain View, CA, United States). Following assessment of size, quality, and concentrations, libraries were multiplexed and subject to sequencing (75 bp single end) on the NextSeq platform (Illumina, San Diego, CA, United States).

RNAseq Data Analysis

Quality control of raw reads was performed retaining bases with quality scores of 20 and reads at least 50 base pair long. Reads were aligned to human genome (hg38) using splice aware aligner TopHat as previously described (52) using annotations available from Ensembl (GRCh38.85) database. Quantification and statistical validation of differentially expressed genes (DEGs) was performed using edgeR (https://bioconductor.org/packages/release/bioc/html/edgeR.html), with candidate genes defined by at least two-fold change in expression with multiple hypothesis corrected (Benjamini-Hochberg procedure) FDR <0.05. Functional enrichment of DEGs was performed using open source functional enrichment tool Metascape (53) and disease associations analyzed using MetaCore™. Heatmaps were generated in R. Gene expression data have been deposited in NCBI's Sequence Read Archive BioProject (PRJNA518909).

16S rRNA Gene Library Construction and Sequencing

Total DNA was extracted from rectal swabs using the PowerSoil DNA Isolation Kit (MO BIO Laboratories, Carlsbad, CA, USA), and a 30-s bead-beating step using a Mini-Beadbeater-16 (BioSpec Products, Bartlesville, OK, USA). This genomic DNA was used as the template to amplify the hypervariable V4 region of the 16S rRNA gene using PCR primers (515F/806R with the reverse primers including a 12-bp barcode) and reactions containing: 50 mM Tris (pH 8.3), 500 μg/ml bovine serum albumin (BSA), 2.5 mM MgCl2, 250 μM of each deoxynucleotide triphosphate (dNTP), 400 nM of each primer, 5 μl of DNA template, and 0.25 units of JumpStart Taq DNA polymerase (Sigma-Aldrich, St Louis, MO, USA). Thermal cycling parameters were 94°C for 5 min; 35 cycles of 94°C for 20 s, 50°C for 20 s, 72°C for 30 s, followed by 72°C for 5 min. PCR products were purified using a MinElute 96 UF PCR Purification

Kit (Qiagen, Valencia, CA, USA). Libraries were sequenced (1 × 300 bases) using an Illumina MiSeq.

16S rRNA Gene Sequence Processing

Raw FASTQ sequence files of 16S rRNA genes were processed with the UPARSE pipeline (54). We used a custom Python script to demultiplex and prepare sequence files for clustering. Sequences were then filtered at a maxee value of 1.0 (allowing only one nucleotide per sequence to be incorrect) to remove low-quality sequences. The remaining sequences were dereplicated and singletons were removed. Operational taxonomic units (OTUs) were assigned with UPARSE at a 97% sequence identity threshold. Taxonomy was assigned to sequences for each OTU using the Ribosomal Database Project (RDP) classifier with a confidence threshold of 0.5 against the Greengenes 13_8 database using Quantitative Insights Into Microbial Ecology (QIIME) version 1.9.1 (55). To eliminate any bias due to sequencing depth, all samples were rarefied to 13,000 sequences per sample before calculating diversity metrics. 16S amplicon sequencing data have been deposited in NCBI's Sequence Read Archive BioProject (PRJNA518910).

RESULTS

Long-Term HIV Infection Is Associated With Significant Shifts in Circulating Immune Cell Populations.

It has been well-established that HIV infection is associated with alterations of lymphocyte subsets both in circulation and lymphoid tissues (56). This can be partially remediated using HAART (57), but the long-term outcomes of HAART (>10 years) on immune cell frequencies has not been addressed. To this end, we compared frequencies of circulating lymphocyte and myeloid populations within peripheral blood mononuclear cells (PBMC) between HIV- and LTC-HIV+ older men (≥55 years of age). As previously reported, our CBC data showed a reduced number of total lymphocytes in the blood with LTC-HIV infection (**Supplementary Figure 3C**) with no additional changes in total leukocytes, granulocytes or monocyte numbers (**Supplementary Figures 3A,B,D**). Since CBC data is based on cell size and granularity rather than specific cell markers, we next investigated the impact of LTC-HIV infection on circulating immune population via flow cytometry.

Total T and B cell numbers (CD3+ and CD19+, respectively) did not differ significantly between the two groups (**Figures 1A,B**). However, a significant reduction in the number of CD4+ helper T cells was detected in LTC-HIV+ individuals (**Figure 1C**). Conversely, the number of circulating CD8+ cytotoxic T cells was increased in the LTC-HIV+ group (**Figure 1D**). We next determined the effect of LTC-HIV infection on the relative frequencies of naïve, transitional effector memory (TEMRA), central memory (TCM), and effector memory (TEM) (**Supplementary Figure 1**). This analysis showed that the frequency of CD4+TCM cells was significantly reduced, while the frequency of CD4+TEM cells was significantly increased (**Figure 1E**). No changes in frequency of naïve and memory CD8+ T cell subsets were detected (**Figure 1F**). Moreover, no changes in the frequency of naïve and memory B cell subsets were noted (**Supplementary Figures 3E–G**). In terms of homeostatic proliferation, we detected an increase in the TEM CD8+ cells subset but none of the other subsets (**Supplementary Figures 4A–D**). No differences in homeostatic proliferation of CD4+ subsets were detected (**Supplementary Figures 4E–H**). Interestingly, we found no differences in T cell activation measured via KLRG1 expression levels, or exhaustion measured via PD-1 expression levels, in either CD4+ (**Supplementary Figures 5A,B**) or CD8+ (**Supplementary Figures 5C,D**) T cell subsets.

We next characterized the frequency of circulating innate immune cells. No significant differences were seen in the abundance of total dendritic cells (DC) or in the relative frequencies of myeloid DC (mDC) and plasmacytoid DC (pDC) with LTC-HIV infection (**Figures 2A–C**). In contrast, the number of circulating monocytes was reduced in LTC-HIV+ individuals (**Figure 2D**), with no differences observed within monocyte subsets (**Figures 2E,F**). Lastly, no differences were detected in natural killer (NK) cell frequencies (**Figure 2G**). However, the relative abundances of activated CD57+ and cytotoxic CD16+GrzmB+ NK cells were higher in LTC-HIV+ group (**Figures 2H,I**).

Long-Term HIV Infection Leads to a Heightened Pro-Inflammatory Response at Baseline and After Stimulation

To explore the impact of LTC-HIV on systemic inflammatory markers, we measured plasma levels of cytokines, chemokines, and growth factors using Luminex technology. This analysis revealed significantly higher levels of the pro-inflammatory cytokine INFγ as well as growth factors BDNF, SCF, and VEGF (**Figure 3A**). On the other hand, levels of anti-inflammatory cytokines IL-1RA, T cell cytokine IL-2, eosinophil maturation factor IL-5, inhibitory cytokine LIF, growth factor SDF1a, as well as chemo-attractants MCP-1, MIP-1b, and IL-8 were reduced in LTC-HIV+ individuals (**Figure 3A**).

To further explore the effect of LTC-HIV infection on immune mediator production, we stimulated a subset of PBMC samples (HIV- $n = 9$, LTC-HIV $n = 11$) with PMA/ionomycin for 16 h and measured the production of cytokines, chemokines, and growth factors via Luminex technology. Samples from LTC-HIV patients generated a more pronounced and variable response to stimulation (**Figure 3B**). After correcting for baseline spontaneous production, 21 of 33 measured analytes were produced in higher amounts in response to stimulation by samples from the LTC-HIV+ group compared to the HIV- group. These included the pro-inflammatory cytokines IL-6, TNFα, INFγ as well as anti-inflammatory cytokine IL-10 (**Figure 3C**).

We next interrogated whether the increased response of LTC-HIV PBMCs to PMA/ionomycin was mirrored by an increased transcriptional response using RNA sequencing (RNA-Seq). Principal component analysis (PCA) shows that the samples clustered based on group and treatment (**Figure 4A**). At baseline,

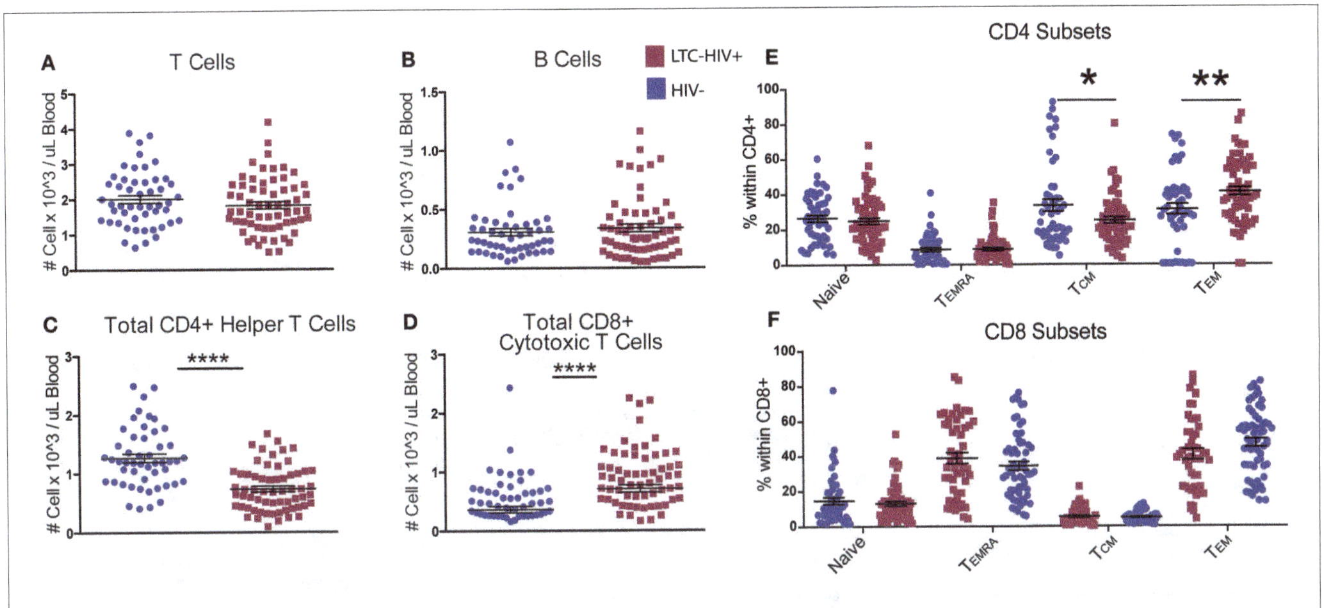

FIGURE 1 | LTC-HIV results in alterations in T but not B cell subsets. **(A)** Numbers of circulating CD3+ T cells **(B)** CD20+ B cells **(C)** CD3+CD4+ helper T cells, and **(D)** CD3+CD8+ cytotoxic T cells. **(E,F)** Relative frequencies of CD4+ **(E)** and CD8+ **(F)** T cell subsets **(E)**. Each point represents a study subject. Horizontal bars and whiskers indicate the mean ± SEM. Significance was determined using an unpaired *t*-test. $^{*}p < 0.05$, $^{**}p < 0.01$, $^{****}p < 0.0001$.

we identified only 11 protein coding differentially expressed genes (DEGs) all of which were down-regulated in LTC-HIV samples (*TNFRSF1B, IL7R, ARHGDIB, RPS27, PPBP, CTSL, HIST1H2BJ, TNKS2, TTC37, SEC24B,* and *EEF1A1).* Following PMA/ionomycin stimulation, a larger number of DEGs were detected in the HIV- group (334) compared to the LTC-HIV+ group (183), with 85 DEGs detected in both groups (**Figure 4A**). To better understand the biological significance of these changes, we carried out an initial functional enrichment using Metascape (53). DEGs detected in the samples from the HIV- group enriched to gene ontology (GO) terms associated with host defense including "cell chemotaxis," "response to TNF," and "leukocyte degranulation" (**Figure 4B**). On the other hand, DEGs detected in the LTC-HIV+ group enriched to GO terms associated with metabolic processes (**Figure 4B**). DEGs detected in both groups enriched to GO terms associated with signaling (**Figure 4B**).

Additional functional enrichment using Metacore™ showed that the 85 common DEGs enriched to GO terms such as "response to LPS" and "response to molecule of bacterial origin" characteristic of a response to antigenic stimulation (**Table 2**). Several of 32 genes that were downregulated upon stimulation in both groups were important for cell adhesion, and proliferation such as: *IL-24, ZNF740, MAP3K3, THBS1,* and *THBS4* (**Figure 4C**). Some of the 53 genes that were upregulated in both groups include genes important for myeloid activation and interferon regulation such as: *CD300LB, TNFAIP8L1, MMP1, SLC35F5,* and *IRF4* (**Figure 4C**).

In line with the output of Metascape, functional enrichment using Metacore™ showed that DEGs that were only detected in PBMCs from HIV- individuals enriched to GO terms such as "inflammatory response," and "response to cytokines" (**Table 2**). Some of the notable DEGs that were only significantly up-regulated in PBMCs from HIV- individuals included: *CXCL9, TNFSF8, NFKBIE, CXCR3,* and *STAT4* (**Figure 4D**). Downregulated DEGs that enriched to the same GO terms included: *LYZ, CCL2,* and *CD14* (**Figure 4D**). Similar to the Metascape output, DEGs that were only detected in PBMC from the LTC-HIV+ group enriched to GO terms associated with signaling (**Table 2**). Genes that were uniquely up-regulated in PBMCs from LTC-HIV+ individuals included: *HIF1A, DHE3,* and solute carrier gene *SLC3A2* which are unique to CD8+ T cells as well as *CXCR5, IL17C,* and *TRPA1* (**Figure 4E**).

To elucidate the source of the DEGs detected, we used the Immunological Genome Project Consortium database (ImmGen), which delineates gene expression patterns across different leukocyte subsets (58). This analysis revealed that DEGs detected only in LTC-HIV+ samples are predicted to be expressed by DCs, monocytes, macrophages, and to a lesser extent T cells and B cells (**Supplementary Figure 6A**). DEGs detected only in the HIV- samples were mostly expressed by monocytes/macrophages and DCs (**Supplementary Figure 6B**), while common DEGs exhibited broad distribution (**Supplementary Figure 6C**). To gain a better understanding of alterations in immune cells frequencies following stimulation, we employed Immquant, which uses the digital cell quantification algorithm (59) to predict changes in immune cell subsets based on total transcriptional profiles using the IRIS database (60). This analysis predicted that the transcriptional changes observed were associated with a significant increase of stimulated Th1 CD4+ T cells in both LTC-HIV+ and HIV- individuals upon PMA stimulation (**Supplementary Figure 6D**). Additionally, transcriptional changes in LTC-HIV+ individuals were associated with an

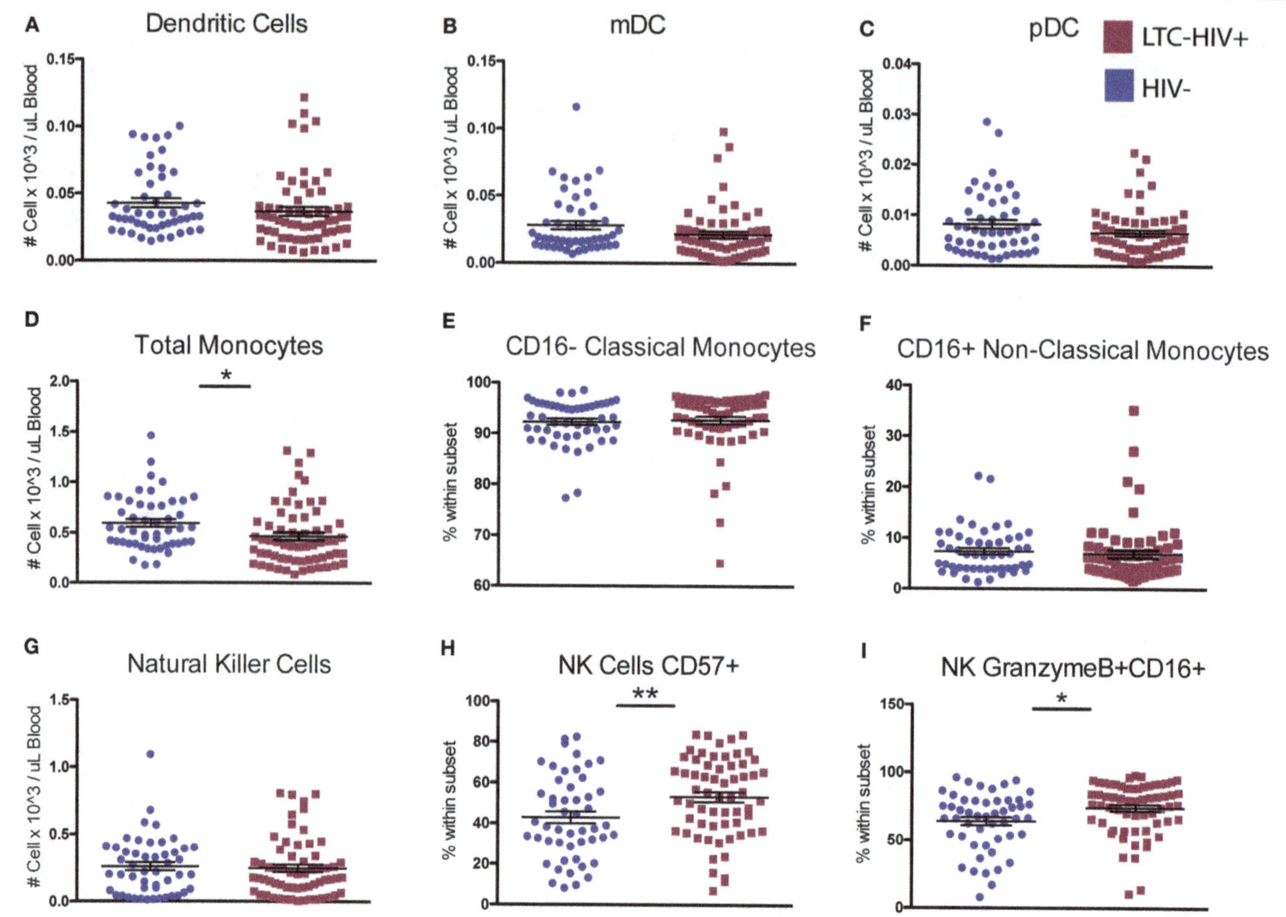

FIGURE 2 | A reduction in circulating monocytes and increase in NK cell activation seen with LTC-HIV infection. **(A)** Number of total circulating dendritic cells (DC) **(B)** myeloid DCs, and **(C)** plasmacytoid (DC). **(D)** Number of total circulating CD14+ monocytes and **(E)** relative abundance of CD16- Classical monocytes, and **(F)** CD16+ non-classical monocytes. **(G)** Number of total circulating CD56+ natural killer (NK) cells and **(H)** relative frequency of CD57+ NK cells and **(I)** granzymeB+CD16+ cytotoxic NK cells. Horizontal bar and whisker indicate the mean ± SEM. Significance was determined using an unpaired *t*-test. $^{*}p < 0.05$, $^{**}p < 0.01$.

increase in stimulated Th2 CD4+ T cells and LPS stimulated DCs upon PMA stimulation (**Supplementary Figure 6D**).

Long-Term HIV Infection Leads to Dysbiosis

Several studies have suggested that HIV infection results in increased gut permeability and translocation of microbial products into circulation (46, 47, 61, 62). To determine if those changes were evident in an older population with LTC-HIV infection, we evaluated several markers of barrier function. Analysis of circulating levels of sCD14, fatty acid binding protein (iFABP), IgM-bound endotoxin and Limulus amebocyte lysate (LAL) did not reveal significant differences between the two group (**Supplementary Figures 7A–D**).

Next, we investigated whether LTC-HIV infection is associated with alterations in the gut microbiome using 16S amplicon sequencing. The overall taxonomic landscape of the gut microbiome was not significantly different as measured by alpha- and beta-diversity (**Figure 5A**, **Supplementary Figures 7E–G**). Specifically, principal coordinate analysis (PCoA) of unweighted UniFrac distance showed significant overlap in the overall gut microbiome communities of HIV- and LTC-HIV+ individuals (**Supplementary Figure 7E**). Both groups also had similar numbers of observed species and Pielou evenness (**Supplementary Figures 7F,G**).

At the phyla level, microbiomes from both groups were dominated by Firmicutes and Bacteroidetes with smaller contributions from Actinobacteria and Proteobacteria (**Figure 5A**). Fusobacteria was the fourth most abundant phyla across all samples and significantly enriched in LTC-HIV+ individuals (**Figure 5B**). Clostridiales and Bacteroidales were the most abundant bacterial orders and *Prevotella* was the most abundant genus across both groups (**Figure 5A**). Ten genera were differentially abundant between LTC-HIV+ and HIV- individuals. The gut microbiomes of LTC-HIV+ individuals were enriched in; *Garnerella*, *Snethia*, *Fusobacterium*, *Lactobacillus*, and *Helicobater* (**Figure 5B**). While the gut microbiomes of HIV- individuals had a significantly higher relative abundance of; *Oxalobacter*, *Streptococcus*, *Enhydrobacter*, *Eggerthella*, and *Clostridiaceae* 02d06 (**Figure 5B**).

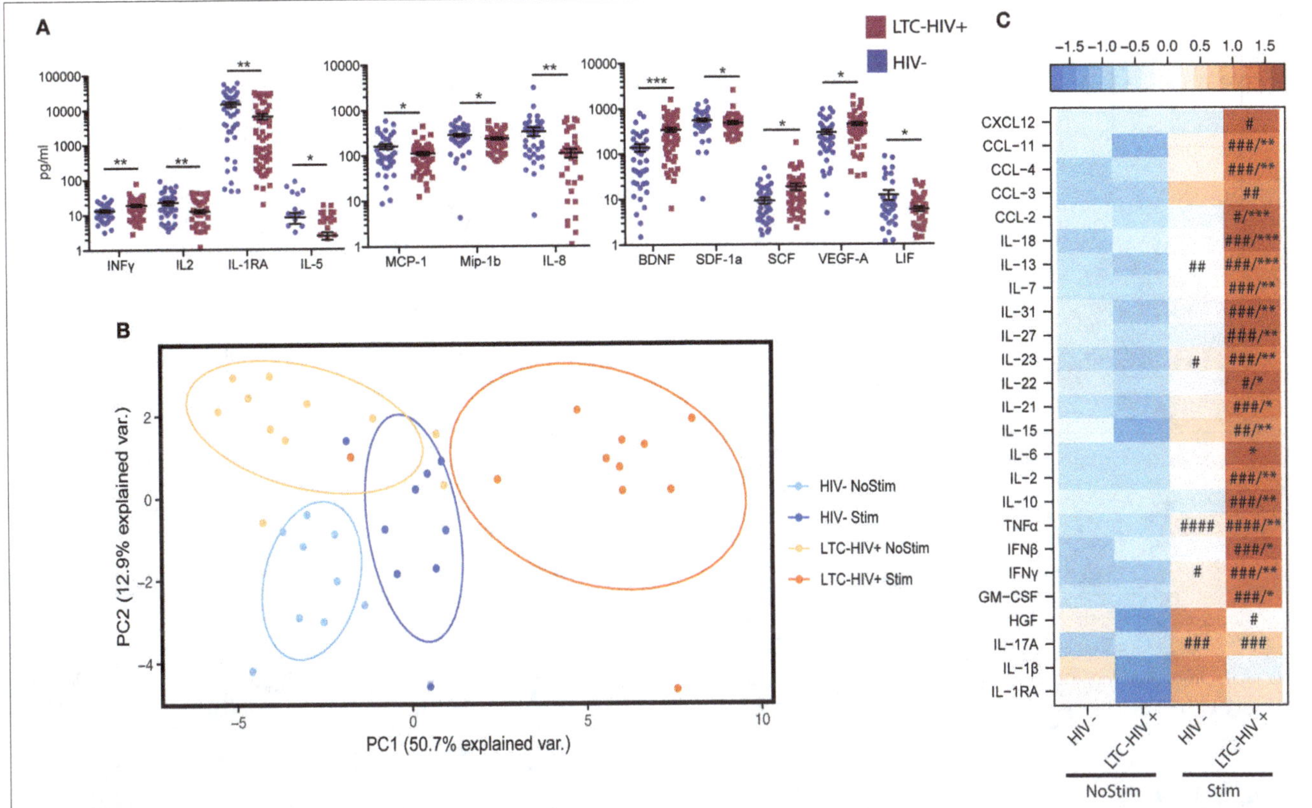

FIGURE 3 | Change in circulating and production of immune mediators following stimulation. **(A)** Serum level of immune mediators measured using a multiplexed ELISA assay. Horizontal bar and whiskers indicate the mean ± SEM. Significance was determined using an unpaired *t*-test. *$p < 0.05$, **$p < 0.01$, ***$p < 0.001$ **(B)** Principal component analysis of immune mediators released by PBMC's from HIV- and LTC-HIV+ individuals in the absence and presence of PMA/ionomycin. **(C)** Heat map of differentially abundant immune mediators produced by PBMCs upon stimulation (all immune mediators statistically significant via 1-way ANOVA, Significant Tukeys *post-hoc* comparison of stimulated samples vs. corresponding baseline samples) #$p < 0.05$, ##$p < 0.01$, ###$p < 0.001$, ####$p < 0.0001$. Unpaired *T*-tests of absolute change followed by Welch's correction [Stimulation—baseline] in immune mediator production *$p < 0.05$, **$p < 0.01$, ***$p < 0.001$.

To further explore the relationship between the microbial communities of the gut microbiome and LTC-HIV, we stratified our LTC-HIV+ individuals into quartiles based on the CD4+ T cell numbers and compared the microbial communities of individuals in the highest and lowest quartile. This analysis revealed seven differentially abundant genera between the highest and lowest CD4+ T cell quartiles (**Figure 5C**). Of note, *Prevotella* was significantly more abundant in individuals with a low CD4+ individuals (**Figure 5C**) and negatively correlated with CD4+ T cell count across all LTC-HIV+ individuals (**Figure 5D**), a pattern not seen in HIV- individuals (**Figure 5E**).

DISCUSSION

The advent and rapid adoption of HAART treatment in the U.S. has turned HIV infection into a chronic disease. Indeed, the average life expectancy of individuals diagnosed with HIV at age 20 has risen from 32 in the late 1980's to 71 in 2018 (63). Consequently, the majority of HIV+ individuals in the U.S. are expected to be older than 50 years of age by 2020 (64). However, HAART treatment is associated with significant adverse outcomes, and individuals who have received long-term HAART are experiencing a higher incidence of several morbidities compared to age-matched HIV- individuals (17). These HANA co-morbidities include cardiovascular disease, neurocognitive disorders, osteoporosis, cancer, liver cirrhosis, kidney, and lung disease (10–16). The mechanisms underlying this increased susceptibility are poorly understood due to the lack of carefully controlled studies on older HIV+ individuals who have been on HAART for >5 years. In this study, we addressed this question using samples collected from a large cohort of LTC-HIV+ gay men who have received HAART treatment for at least 10 years. Importantly, the control population was matched with the LTC-HIV+ cohort for age, sexual preference, location, and socioeconomic status. This experimental set up allowed us to determine the effects of LTC-HIV infection on immunological and microbial shifts that can be subsequently targeted for intervention to reduce HANA co-morbidities.

HAART treatment within the first 3 years results in a rebound in CD4 T cell count that is strongly linked to the CD4 count at the time of treatment initiation (42–44, 57). However, our data showed a significant reduction in total circulating CD4+ T cells. Thirty-six of the fifty-seven participants in this study were initially infected with HIV in the 1980's well before the introduction of HAART. Consequently, 28 of these individuals did not have access to therapy for ~10 years prior to starting

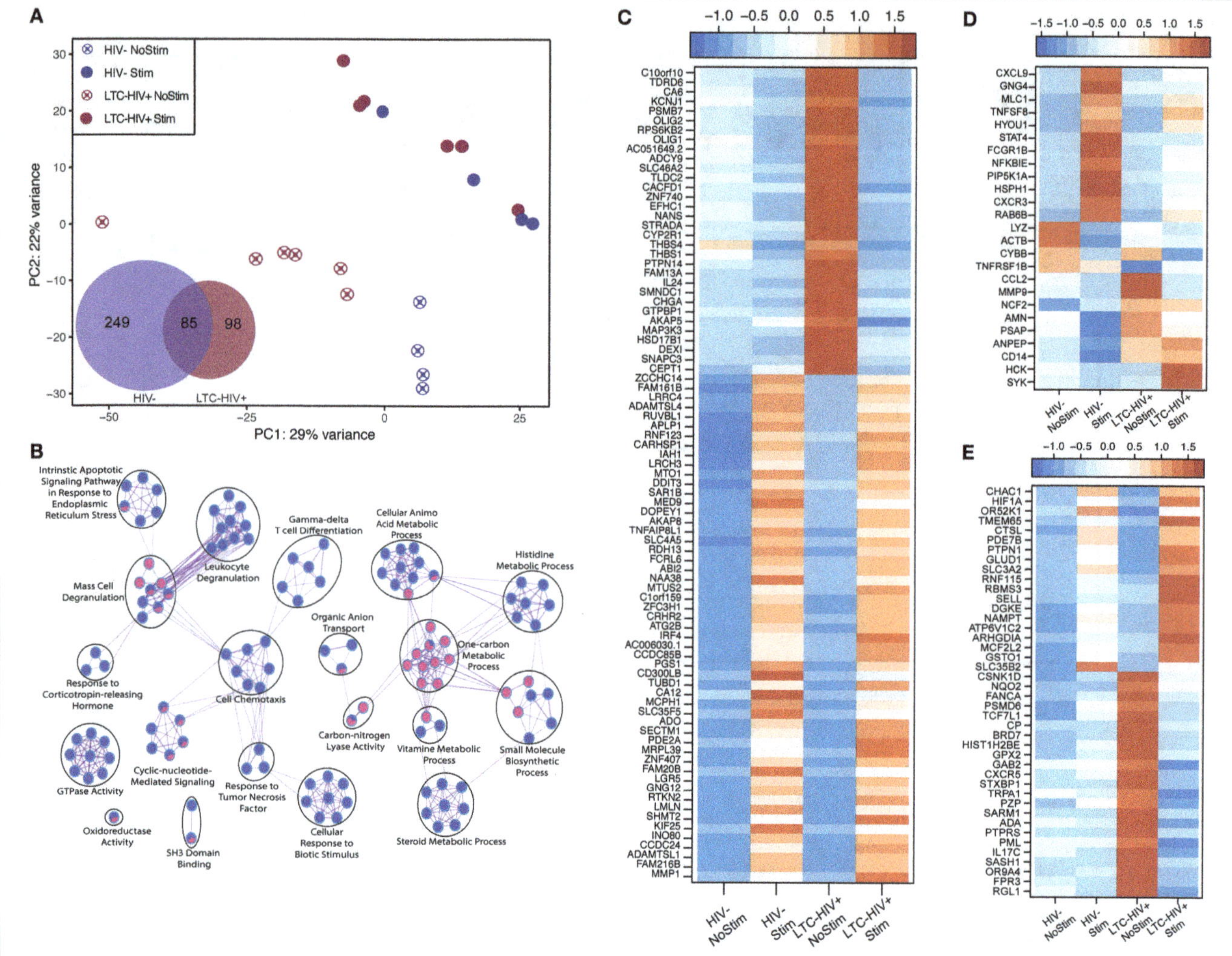

FIGURE 4 | LTC-HIV infection alters PBMC transcriptional response to PMA/Ionomycin. **(A)** Principal component analysis of unstimulated and PMA/ionomycin stimulated PBMCs from HIV- and LTC-HIV and Venn diagram of stimulation DEGs showing unique and common protein coding genes. **(B)** Network visualization using Cytoscape of functional enrichment output of DEGs detected in PBMC from LTC-HIV+ and HIV- subjects following PMA stimulation obtained using Metascape. The size of node represents the number of DEGs associated with each gene ontology (GO) term and the pie chart filling represents relative proportion of each group's DEGs that enriched to that GO term. Heat maps of select DEGs for Common **(C)**, HIV- **(D)**, and LTC-HIV+ **(E)**.

this treatment and likely began with very low CD4+ counts. Unfortunately we did not have access to the nadir CD4+ counts for our study population, which were shown to be predictive of CD4+ levels during HAART treatment (42, 65, 66). Levels of IL-2, a cytokine critical for T cell survival were also reduced and could partially explain the reduced CD4+ T cell numbers we observed in LTC-HIV+ individuals (67). Both aging and long-term HIV infection have been associated with an accumulation of terminally differentiated T cells (68, 69). In line with these earlier studies, we found a greater shift toward terminally differentially CD4+ T cells in this group indicative of accelerated differentiation of memory T cells.

CD8+ T cells play an important role in the control of HIV infection and their numbers become elevated rapidly upon HIV infection and persist after initiation of HAART (70, 71). Although the numbers of CD8+ T cells were significantly higher in LTC-HIV+ individuals, no differences were observed in the relative abundance of naïve and memory subsets. We did however detect a significant increase in homeostatic proliferation within the CD8+ T cell EM subset, suggestive of accelerated conversion to memory T cells. Additionally, a large percentage of circulating NK cells showed higher activation with LTC-HIV infection. Collectively, this increased differentiation/proliferation of circulating lymphocytes could contribute to heightened systemic inflammation in LTC-HIV infection. Analysis of circulating immune mediators showed increased serum levels of the antiviral cytokine INFγ. This is in line with previous studies that reported increased levels of INFγ, but not IL-6 and TNFα in HAART treated HIV patients (49). The source of INFγ could be the activated NK cells, CD8+ T cells, or TEM CD4+ T cells, but testing this hypothesis will require additional studies such as single cell RNA sequencing.

The effect of LTC-HIV infection on the innate arm of the immune system is not well-understood. Acute HIV infection is associated with a dramatic increase in inflammatory (non-classical CD16+) monocytes (28). This population has been shown to remain elevated throughout the first year of HAART treatment (72). In contrast, we observed a reduction in total circulating monocytes, and no differences in the relative proportions of CD16+ and CD16- monocytes. Monocytes are susceptible to HIV infection and can serve as a reservoir for latent HIV (48). The reduction in circulating monocyte numbers could potentially be due to low levels of viral reactivation (73), or alternatively mediated by lower levels circulating chemokines MCP-1, MIP-1b, and IL-8. Further analysis of the functional capacity (e.g., phagocytosis and wound healing) of monocytes is needed to assess their contribution to the development of HANA co-morbidities.

TABLE 2 | Functional enrichment of DEGs detected in response to PMA stimulation.

	No of genes	FDR *p*-value
COMMON DEGs		
Regulation of purine nucleotide metabolic process	12	1.517E-05
Response to lipopolysaccharide	10	1.565E-02
Response to molecule of bacterial origin	10	1.888E-02
Regulation of phosphorus metabolic process	21	2.026E-02
DEGs DETECTED IN LTC-HIV SAMPLES ONLY		
Regulation of signaling	46	1.711E-03
Neutrophil homeostasis	23	2.506E-03
Regulation of communication	44	2.506E-03
Regulation of blood circulation	11	2.574E-03
DEGs DETECTED IN HIV- SAMPLES ONLY		
Intracellular signal transduction	63	1.190E-08
Cell chemotaxis	19	1.335E-06
Response to cytokine	52	1.740E-06
Inflammatory response	32	2.492E-06

We also observed a substantial increase in circulating BDNF, and VEGF-A in the serum of LTC-HIV. Both of these factors have been previously linked to HIV associated neurological disorders including depression (74, 75). HIV protein gp120 has been shown to both increase the production and negatively alter neuronal processing of BDNF (76, 77). It is possible that the buildup of circulating BDNF is a compensatory mechanism due to decreased bioavailability of BDNF in the brain. The continuation of this process despite low viral load seen in LTC-HIV could explain the higher incidence of depression and neuropathy that we and others have observed (78–80). We also detected a reduction in the anti inflammatory cytokine IL-1RA, which could indicate a higher level of systemic inflammation. These changes are consistent with, but are not as pronounced as what has been reported in HIV+ patients on HAART for a shorter duration

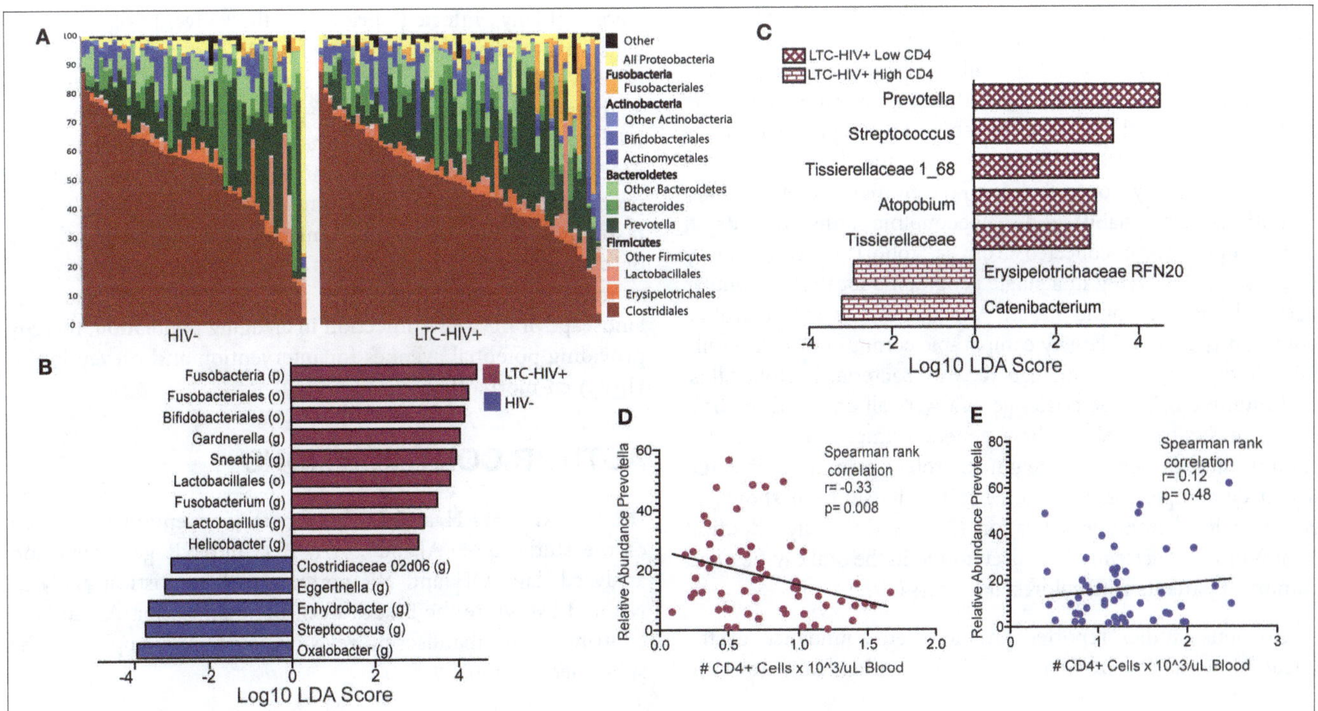

FIGURE 5 | Taxonomic differences in the gut microbiome of LTC-HIV **(A)** Stack bar plot illustrating the abundance of bacterial orders and phyla in HIV- and LTC-HIV+ individuals. **(B)** Differentially abundant bacterial taxa between LTC-HIV+/HIV- determined using LEfSE (Log_{10} LDA score >2) at the Phyla, Order and Genus level. **(C)** Differentially abundant genera between LTC-HIV+ High CD4+ and LTC-HIV+ Low CD4+ individuals (Log_{10} LDA score > 2). **(D)** Spearman rank correlation between CD4+ T cell abundance and relative abundance of *Prevotella* in LTC-HIV+ individuals. **(E)** Spearman rank correlation between CD4+ T cell abundance and relative abundance of *Prevotella* in HIV- individuals.

(81) or during acute infection prior to the initiation of HAART treatment (82).

Upon polyclonal activation of PBMC we observed a significantly heightened inflammatory response by PBMCs from LTC-HIV individuals. While our study design does not allow us to decisively identify the source of these immune mediators, these data clearly indicate functional abnormalities in circulating immune populations. HIV infection has been shown to alter the epigenetic landscape of both T-cells and monocytes during acute and HAART controlled infections (83–85). Future studies should investigate the link between these epigenetic changes and aberrant inflammatory and anti-microbial responses. Interestingly, our transcriptional analysis showed a smaller number of DEGs in PBMC from LTC-HIV+ subjects despite a greater production of immune mediators. Moreover, while DEGs detected in PBMC from HIV- subjects enriched to GO terms associated with leukocyte activation, those detected in LTC-HIV+ samples enriched to GO terms associated with signaling. One possible explanation is that the response to stimulation peaked earlier in the LTC-HIV+ samples. While the luminex data captures accumulation of immune mediators, RNA-Seq only provides a snap shot of the specific time point selected. Future studies can address this question through a kinetic analysis.

Dysbiosis in the gut microbiome during HIV infection has been implicated as a source of aberrant immune activation and inflammation in acute infection and chronic HIV (32, 33, 86). The host immune system tightly regulates the large reservoir of microbes in the human gut; and loss of key immune cells due to HIV infection (87) can result in changes in composition of microbial communities and their compartmentalization. However, data on HIV-associated shifts in the gut microbiome have been inconsistent likely due to the lack of studies that appropriately controlled for race/ethnicity, diet, sanitary conditions, sexual habits, and socioeconomic status. In contrast, our samples were collected from a cohort of gay, mostly Caucasian, men living in a single geographic location of similar age and socioeconomic status. Analysis of the gut microbial community revealed largely comparable communities with only 10 differentially abundant genera. Fusobacteria, Lactobacillus, and multiple Bifidobacteriales genera were all enriched in LTC-HIV+ individuals. Since these genera primarily colonize the mouth, their presence in the gut microbial communities could signal de-compartmentalization has previously been shown to result in local immune activation (88). Additionally, identical strains of *Fusobacterium* have been found in the oral cavities, and tumors of patients with colorectal cancers (89).

Previous studies reported an increased abundance of the bacterial genus *Prevotella* in LTC-HIV+ individuals; however, many of these studies did not control for sexual orientation, and geographic location, which can influence abundance of *Prevotella* (90, 91). Although we did not find a difference in the abundance of *Prevotella* based on HIV status, we observed a negative correlation between CD4+ T cell counts and *Prevotella* abundance. *Prevotella* has previously been linked to high circulating levels of trimethylamine-N-oxide (TMAO) a compound strongly associated with cardiovascular disease (92). Future metabolomics, and transcriptomic studies will be needed to determine if this higher abundance of *Prevotella* leads to more inflammatory microbial products and if this activity varies in LTC-HIV vs. age matched controls. Abundance of other bacterial genera such as *Streptococcus* and *Atopbium* was also negatively correlated with CD4+ T cell counts and are both commonly found in the oral cavity (93). On the other hand, abundance of the short chain fatty acid (SCFA)-producing Clostridia *Catenibacterium* was higher in LTC-HIV+ individuals in the highest CD4+ T cell quartile. SCFAs produced by gut microbes play an important role in maintaining gut homeostasis and local immune function (94–96). While the abundances of these taxa were too sparse to obtain meaningful correlations with CD4+ T cell counts, this could indicate a greater capacity for beneficial SCFA production in LTC-HIV+ patients with a higher CD4+ count.

In summary, this study provides novel insight into the impact of LTC-HIV infection on systemic immunity and microbial gut communities in older patient populations (≥55 years). A little over half of the subjects in our study were initially infected prior to the advent of HAART. This delay may have interfered with the restorative effect of HAART as shown by a lower abundance of CD4+ T cells and monocytes when compared to age-matched HIV- individuals; immune dysregulation, as evidenced by differences in circulating immune mediators and a more pronounced response to stimulation in LTC-HIV; and taxonomic shifts in the gut microbiome indicative of loss of compartmentalization. Taken together these data provide a more complete picture of the immune and microbial landscape of LTC-HIV infection in an aging population, thereby providing potential avenues for intervention and prevention of HANA co-morbidities.

AUTHOR CONTRIBUTIONS

IM, JT, TM, StS, RH, and BB contributed conception and design of the study. NM, AJ, SuS, AA, BD, and NR generated and analyzed data. OH and NR performed the statistical analysis. NR and IM wrote the first draft of the manuscript. All authors contributed to manuscript revision, read, and approved the submitted version.

REFERENCES

1. Siddiqi AE, Hall HI, Hu X, Song R. Population-based estimates of life expectancy after HIV diagnosis: United States 2008-2011. *J Acquir Immune Defic Syndr.* (2016) 72:230–6. doi: 10.1097/QAI.0000000000000960
2. Harrison KM, Song R, Zhang X. Life expectancy after HIV diagnosis based on national HIV surveillance data from 25 states, United States. *J Acquir Immune Defic Syndr.* (2010) 53:124–30. doi: 10.1097/QAI.0b013e3181b563e7
3. Center for Disease Control and Prevention. Estimated HIV Incidence and Prevalence in the United States, 2010–2015. (2018). Available online at: http://www.cdc.gov/hiv/library/reports/hiv-surveillance.html

4. Le T, Farrar J, Shikuma C. Rebound of plasma viremia following cessation of antiretroviral therapy despite profoundly low levels of HIV reservoir: implications for eradication. *AIDS.* (2011) 25:871–2; author reply 872–3. doi: 10.1097/QAD.0b013e32834490b1
5. Maldarelli F, Palmer S, King MS, Wiegand A, Polis MA, Mican J, et al. ART suppresses plasma HIV-1 RNA to a stable set point predicted by pretherapy viremia. *PLoS Pathog.* (2007) 3:e46. doi: 10.1371/journal.ppat.0030046
6. Martinez-Picado J, Deeks SG. Persistent HIV-1 replication during antiretroviral therapy. *Curr Opin HIV AIDS.* (2016) 11:417–23. doi: 10.1097/COH.0000000000000287
7. de Coninck Z, Hussain-Alkhateeb L, Bratt G, Ekström AM, Gisslén M, Petzold M, et al. Non-AIDS mortality is higher among successfully treated people living with HIV compared with matched HIV-negative control persons: a 15-year follow-up cohort study in Sweden. *AIDS Patient Care STDS.* (2018) 32:297–305. doi: 10.1089/apc.2018.0015
8. Engsig FN, Zangerle R, Katsarou O, Dabis F, Reiss P, Gill J, et al. Long-term mortality in HIV-positive individuals virally suppressed for >3 years with incomplete CD4 recovery. *Clin Infect Dis.* (2014) 58:1312–21. doi: 10.1093/cid/ciu038
9. Marin B, Thiébaut R, Bucher HC, Rondeau V, Costagliola D, Dorrucci M, et al. Non-AIDS-defining deaths and immunodeficiency in the era of combination antiretroviral therapy. *AIDS.* (2009) 23:1743–53. doi: 10.1097/QAD.0b013e32832e9b78
10. Knobel H, Domingo P, Suarez-Lozano I, Gutierrez F, Estrada V, Palacios R, et al. Rate of cardiovascular, renal and bone disease and their major risks factors in HIV-infected individuals on antiretroviral therapy in Spain. (2018) *Enferm Infecc Microbiol Clin.* doi: 10.1016/j.eimc.2018.09.015
11. Rogalska-Płonska M, Rogalski P, Leszczyszyn-Pynka M, Stempkowska J, Kocbach P, Kowalczuk-Kot A, et al. Hypertension, dyslipidaemia, and cardiovascular risk in HIV-infected adults in Poland. *Kardiol Pol.* (2017) 75:1324–31. doi: 10.5603/KP.a2017.0148
12. Friis-Møller N, Weber R, Reiss P, Thiébaut R, Kirk O, d'Arminio Monforte A, et al. Cardiovascular disease risk factors in HIV patients–association with antiretroviral therapy. Results from the DAD study. *AIDS.* (2003) 17:1179–93. doi: 10.1097/00002030-200305230-00010
13. Clifford GM, Polesel J, Rickenbach M, Dal Maso L, Keiser O, Kofler A, et al. Cancer risk in the Swiss HIV Cohort Study: associations with immunodeficiency, smoking, and highly active antiretroviral therapy. *J Natl Cancer Inst.* (2005) 97:425–32. doi: 10.1093/jnci/dji072
14. Cohen RA, Gullett JM, Porges EC, Woods AJ, Lamb DG, Bryant VE, et al. Age effects on HIV-associated neurocognitive function. (2018) *Alcohol Clin Exp Res.* 32:519–28. doi: 10.1111/acer.13915
15. Chan P, Brew BJ. HIV associated neurocognitive disorders in the modern antiviral treatment era: prevalence, characteristics, biomarkers, and effects of treatment. *Curr HIV/AIDS Rep.* (2014) 11:317–24. doi: 10.1007/s11904-014-0221-0
16. Thio CL, Seaberg EC, Skolasky R, Phair J, Visscher B, Muñoz A, et al. HIV-1, hepatitis B virus, and risk of liver-related mortality in the Multicenter Cohort Study (MACS). *Lancet.* (2002) 360:1921–6. doi: 10.1016/S0140-6736(02)11913-1
17. Guaraldi G, Orlando G, Zona S, Menozzi M, Carli F, Garlassi E, et al. Premature age-related comorbidities among HIV-infected persons compared with the general population. *Clin Infect Dis.* (2011) 53:1120–6. doi: 10.1093/cid/cir627
18. Sterling RK, Lissen E, Clumeck N, Sola R, Correa MC, Montaner J, et al. Development of a simple noninvasive index to predict significant fibrosis in patients with HIV/HCV coinfection. *Hepatology.* (2006) 43:1317–25. doi: 10.1002/hep.21178
19. Matthews GV, Dore GJ. HIV and hepatitis C coinfection. *J Gastroenterol Hepatol.* (2008) 23:1000–8. doi: 10.1111/j.1440-1746.2008.05489.x
20. Parsons TD, Tucker KA, Hall CD, Robertson WT, Eron JJ, Fried MW, et al. Neurocognitive functioning and HAART in HIV and hepatitis C virus co-infection. *AIDS.* (2006) 20:1591–5. doi: 10.1097/01.aids.0000238404.16121.47
21. Ganta KK, Mandal A, Chaubey B. Depolarization of mitochondrial membrane potential is the initial event in non-nucleoside reverse transcriptase inhibitor efavirenz induced cytotoxicity. *Cell Biol Toxicol.* (2017) 33:69–82. doi: 10.1007/s10565-016-9362-9
22. Nomura R, Sato T, Sato Y, Medin JA, Kushimoto S, Yanagisawa T. Azidothymidine-triphosphate impairs mitochondrial dynamics by disrupting the quality control system. *Redox Biol.* (2017) 13:407–17. doi: 10.1016/j.redox.2017.06.011
23. Foli Y, Ghebremichael M, Li M, Paintsil E. Upregulation of apoptosis pathway genes in peripheral blood mononuclear cells of HIV-infected individuals with antiretroviral therapy-associated mitochondrial toxicity. *Antimicrob Agents Chemother.* (2017) 61:e00522-17. doi: 10.1128/AAC.00522-17
24. Heron SE, Elahi S. HIV Infection and compromised mucosal immunity: oral manifestations and systemic inflammation. *Front Immunol.* (2017) 8:241. doi: 10.3389/fimmu.2017.00241
25. Erlandson KM, Ng DK, Jacobson LP, Margolick JB, Dobs AS, Palella FJ Jr, et al. Inflammation, immune activation, immunosenescence, and hormonal biomarkers in the frailty-related phenotype of men with or at risk for HIV infection. *J Infect Dis.* (2017) 215:228–37. doi: 10.1093/infdis/jiw523
26. Fukui SM, Piggott DA, Erlandson KM. Inflammation strikes again: frailty and HIV. *Curr HIV/AIDS Rep.* (2018) 15:20–9. doi: 10.1007/s11904-018-0372-5
27. Montoya JL, Campbell LM, Paolillo EW, Ellis RJ, Letendre SL, Jeste DV, et al. Inflammation relates to poorer complex motor performance among adults living with HIV on suppressive antiretroviral therapy. *J Acquir Immune Defic Syndr.* (2018) 80:15–23. doi: 10.1097/QAI.0000000000001881
28. Han J, Wang B, Han N, Zhao Y, Song C, Feng X, et al. CD14(high)CD16(+) rather than CD14(low)CD16(+) monocytes correlate with disease progression in chronic HIV-infected patients. *J Acquir Immune Defic Syndr.* (2009) 52:553–9. doi: 10.1097/QAI.0b013e3181c1d4fe
29. Sereti I, Krebs SJ, Phanuphak N, Fletcher JL, Slike B, Pinyakorn S, et al. Persistent, albeit reduced, chronic inflammation in persons starting antiretroviral therapy in acute HIV infection. *Clin Infect Dis.* (2017) 64:124–31. doi: 10.1093/cid/ciw683
30. Lichtfuss GF, Cheng WJ, Farsakoglu Y, Paukovics G, Rajasuriar R, Velayudham P, et al. Virologically suppressed HIV patients show activation of NK cells and persistent innate immune activation. *J Immunol.* (2012) 189:1491–9. doi: 10.4049/jimmunol.1200458
31. Rajasuriar R, Wright E, Lewin SR. Impact of antiretroviral therapy (ART) timing on chronic immune activation/inflammation and end-organ damage. *Curr Opin HIV AIDS.* (2015) 10:35–42. doi: 10.1097/COH.0000000000000118
32. Gootenberg DB, Paer JM, Luevano JM, Kwon DS. HIV-associated changes in the enteric microbial community: potential role in loss of homeostasis and development of systemic inflammation. *Curr Opin Infect Dis.* (2017) 30:31–43. doi: 10.1097/QCO.0000000000000341
33. Monaco CL, Gootenberg DB, Zhao G, Handley SA, Ghebremichael MS, Lim ES, et al. Altered virome and bacterial microbiome in human immunodeficiency virus-associated acquired immunodeficiency syndrome. *Cell Host Microbe.* (2016) 19:311–322. doi: 10.1016/j.chom.2016.02.011
34. Prendergast A, Prado JG, Kang YH, Chen F, Riddell LA, Luzzi G, et al. HIV-1 infection is characterized by profound depletion of CD161+ Th17 cells and gradual decline in regulatory T cells. *AIDS.* (2010) 24:491–502. doi: 10.1097/QAD.0b013e3283344895
35. Mudd JC, Brenchley JM. Gut mucosal barrier dysfunction, microbial dysbiosis, and their role in HIV-1 disease progression. *J Infect Dis.* (2016) 214 (Suppl. 2):S58–66. doi: 10.1093/infdis/jiw258
36. Sandler NG, Wand H, Roque A, Law M, Nason MC, Nixon DE, et al. Plasma levels of soluble CD14 independently predict mortality in HIV infection. *J Infect Dis.* (2011) 203:780–90. doi: 10.1093/infdis/jiq118
37. Hunt PW, Sinclair E, Rodriguez B, Shive C, Clagett B, Funderburg N, et al. Gut epithelial barrier dysfunction and innate immune activation predict mortality in treated HIV infection. *J Infect Dis.* (2014) 210:1228–38. doi: 10.1093/infdis/jiu238
38. Dubourg G, Lagier JC, Hüe S, Surenaud M, Bachar D, Robert C, et al. Gut microbiota associated with HIV infection is significantly enriched in bacteria tolerant to oxygen. *BMJ Open Gastroenterol.* (2016) 3:e000080. doi: 10.1136/bmjgast-2016-000080
39. Missailidis C, Neogi U, Stenvinkel P, Trøseid M, Nowak P, Bergman P. The microbial metabolite trimethylamine-N-oxide in association with inflammation and microbial dysregulation in three HIV cohorts at various disease stages. *AIDS.* (2018) 32:1589–98. doi: 10.1097/QAD.0000000000001813

40. Keegan MR, Chittiprol S, Letendre SL, Winston A, Fuchs D, Boasso A, et al. Tryptophan metabolism and its relationship with depression and cognitive impairment among HIV-infected individuals. *Int J Tryptophan Res.* (2016) 9:79–88. doi: 10.4137/IJTR.S36464
41. Das B, Dobrowolski C, Shahir AM, Feng Z, Yu X, Sha J, et al. Short chain fatty acids potently induce latent HIV-1 in T-cells by activating P-TEFb and multiple histone modifications. *Virology.* (2015) 474:65–81. doi: 10.1016/j.virol.2014.10.033
42. Clouse K, Pettifor A, Maskew M, Bassett J, Van Rie A, Gay C, et al. Initiating antiretroviral therapy when presenting with higher CD4 cell counts results in reduced loss to follow-up in a resource-limited setting. *AIDS.* (2013) 27:645–50. doi: 10.1097/QAD.0b013e32835c12f9
43. Collazos J, Knobel H, Casado JL, Grupo Español para el Estudio Multifactorial de la Adherencia. CD4 count and viral load time-courses in patients treated with highly active antiretroviral therapy and association with the CDC staging system. *HIV Med.* (2006) 7:504–13. doi: 10.1111/j.1468-1293.2006.00405.x
44. Chaisson RE, Keruly JC, Moore RD. Association of initial CD4 cell count and viral load with response to highly active antiretroviral therapy. *JAMA.* (2000) 284:3128–9. doi: 10.1001/jama.284.24.3123
45. Appay V, Sauce D. Immune activation and inflammation in HIV-1 infection: causes and consequences. *J Pathol.* (2008) 214:231–41. doi: 10.1002/path.2276
46. Ancuta P, Kamat A, Kunstman KJ, Kim EY, Autissier P, Wurcel A, et al. Microbial translocation is associated with increased monocyte activation and dementia in AIDS patients. *PLoS ONE.* (2008) 3:e2516. doi: 10.1371/journal.pone.0002516
47. Brenchley JM, Price DA, Schacker TW, Asher TE, Silvestri G, Rao S, et al. Microbial translocation is a cause of systemic immune activation in chronic HIV infection. *Nat Med.* (2006) 12:1365–71. doi: 10.1038/nm1511
48. Campbell JH, Hearps AC, Martin GE, Williams KC, Crowe SM. The importance of monocytes and macrophages in HIV pathogenesis, treatment, and cure. *AIDS.* (2014) 28:2175–87. doi: 10.1097/QAD.0000000000000408
49. Amirayan-Chevillard N, Tissot-Dupont H, Capo C, Brunet C, Dignat-George F, Obadia Y, et al. Impact of highly active anti-retroviral therapy (HAART) on cytokine production and monocyte subsets in HIV-infected patients. *Clin Exp Immunol.* (2000) 120:107–112. doi: 10.1046/j.1365-2249.2000.01201.x
50. Terunuma H, Deng X, Dewan Z, Fujimoto S, Yamamoto N. Potential role of NK cells in the induction of immune responses: implications for NK cell-based immunotherapy for cancers and viral infections. *Int Rev Immunol.* (2008) 27:93–110. doi: 10.1080/08830180801911743
51. Luo Z, Li Z, Martin L, Hu Z, Wu H, Wan Z, et al. Increased natural killer cell activation in HIV-infected immunologic non-responders correlates with CD4+ T cell recovery after antiretroviral therapy and viral suppression. *PLoS ONE.* (2017) 12:e0167640. doi: 10.1371/journal.pone.0167640
52. Trapnell C, Pachter L, Salzberg SL. TopHat: discovering splice junctions with RNA-Seq. *Bioinformatics.* (2009) 25:1105–11. doi: 10.1093/bioinformatics/btp120
53. Tripathi S, Pohl MO, Zhou Y, Rodriguez-Frandsen A, Wang G, Stein DA, et al. Meta- and orthogonal integration of influenza "OMICs" data defines a role for UBR4 in virus budding. *Cell Host Microbe.* (2015) 18:723–35. doi: 10.1016/j.chom.2015.11.002
54. Edgar RC. UPARSE: highly accurate OTU sequences from microbial amplicon reads. *Nat Methods.* (2013) 10:996–8. doi: 10.1038/nmeth.2604
55. Caporaso JG, Kuczynski J, Stombaugh J, Bittinger K, Bushman FD, Costello EK, et al. QIIME allows analysis of high-throughput community sequencing data. *Nat Methods.* (2010) 7:335–6. doi: 10.1038/nmeth.f.303
56. Wei X, Ghosh SK, Taylor ME, Johnson VA, Emini EA, Deutsch P, et al. Viral dynamics in human immunodeficiency virus type 1 infection. *Nature.* (1995) 373:117–22. doi: 10.1038/373117a0
57. Li TS, Tubiana R, Katlama C, Calvez V, Ait Mohand H, Autran B. Long-lasting recovery in CD4 T-cell function and viral-load reduction after highly active antiretroviral therapy in advanced HIV-1 disease. *Lancet.* (1998) 351:1682–6. doi: 10.1016/S0140-6736(97)10291-4
58. Heng TS, Painter MW, Immunological Genome Project Consortium. Immunological genome project, the immunological genome project: networks of gene expression in immune cells. *Nat Immunol.* (2008) 9:1091–4. doi: 10.1038/ni1008-1091
59. Frishberg A, Brodt A, Steuerman Y, Gat-Viks I. ImmQuant: a user-friendly tool for inferring immune cell-type composition from gene-expression data. *Bioinformatics.* (2016) 32:3842–3. doi: 10.1093/bioinformatics/btw535
60. Abbas AR, Baldwin D, Ma Y, Ouyang W, Gurney A, Martin F, et al. Immune response *in silico* (IRIS): immune-specific genes identified from a compendium of microarray expression data. *Genes Immun.* (2005) 6:319–31. doi: 10.1038/sj.gene.6364173
61. Dinh DM, Volpe GE, Duffalo C, Bhalchandra S, Tai AK, Kane AV, et al. Intestinal microbiota, microbial translocation, and systemic inflammation in chronic HIV infection. *J Infect Dis.* (2015) 211:19–27. doi: 10.1093/infdis/jiu409
62. Li SK, Leung RK, Guo HX, Wei JF, Wang JH, Kwong KT, et al. Detection and identification of plasma bacterial and viral elements in HIV/AIDS patients in comparison to healthy adults. *Clin Microbiol Infect.* (2012) 18:1126–33. doi: 10.1111/j.1469-0691.2011.03690.x
63. Center for Disease Control and Prevention. Today's HIV/AIDS Epidemic. (2018). Available online at: https://www.cdc.gov/nchhstp/newsroom/docs/factsheets/todaysepidemic-508.pdf
64. Center for Disease Control and Prevention. HIV Among People Aged 50 and Older. (2016). Available online at: https://www.cdc.gov/hiv/group/age/olderamericans/index.html
65. Grimsrud A, Cornell M, Schomaker M, Fox MP, Orrell C, Prozesky H, et al. CD4 count at antiretroviral therapy initiation and the risk of loss to follow-up: results from a multicentre cohort study. *J Epidemiol Commun Health.* (2016) 70:549–55. doi: 10.1136/jech-2015-206629
66. Mberi MN, Kuonza LR, Dube NM, Nattey C, Manda S, Summers R. Determinants of loss to follow-up in patients on antiretroviral treatment, South Africa, 2004-2012: a cohort study. *BMC Health Serv Res.* (2015) 15:259. doi: 10.1186/s12913-015-0912-2
67. Onwumeh J, Okwundu CI, Kredo T. Interleukin-2 as an adjunct to antiretroviral therapy for HIV-positive adults. *Cochrane Database Syst Rev.* (2017) 5:CD009818. doi: 10.1002/14651858.CD009818.pub2
68. Appay V, Zaunders JJ, Papagno L, Sutton J, Jaramillo A, Waters A, et al. Characterization of CD4(+) CTLs *ex vivo*. *J Immunol.* (2002) 168:5954–8. doi: 10.4049/jimmunol.168.11.5954
69. Salam N, Rane S, Das R, Faulkner M, Gund R, Kandpal U, et al. T cell ageing: effects of age on development, survival & function. *Indian J Med Res.* (2013) 138:595–608.
70. Cao W, Mehraj V, Kaufmann DE, Li T, Routy JP. Elevation and persistence of CD8 T-cells in HIV infection: the Achilles heel in the ART era. *J Int AIDS Soc.* (2016) 19:20697. doi: 10.7448/IAS.19.1.20697
71. Mudd JC, Lederman MM. CD8 T cell persistence in treated HIV infection. *Curr Opin HIV AIDS.* (2014) 9:500–5. doi: 10.1097/COH.0000000000000086
72. Tippett E, Cheng WJ, Westhorpe C, Cameron PU, Brew BJ, Lewin SR, et al. Differential expression of CD163 on monocyte subsets in healthy and HIV-1 infected individuals. *PLoS ONE.* (2011) 6:e19968. doi: 10.1371/journal.pone.0019968
73. Palmer S, Maldarelli F, Wiegand A, Bernstein B, Hanna GJ, Brun SC, et al. Low-level viremia persists for at least 7 years in patients on suppressive antiretroviral therapy. *Proc Natl Acad Sci USA.* (2008) 105:3879–84. doi: 10.1073/pnas.0800050105
74. Sporer B, Koedel U, Paul R, Eberle J, Arendt G, Pfister HW. Vascular endothelial growth factor (VEGF) is increased in serum, but not in cerebrospinal fluid in HIV associated CNS diseases. *J Neurol Neurosurg Psychiatry.* (2004) 75:298–300. doi: 10.1136/jnnp.2003.016287
75. Del Guerra FB, Fonseca JL, Figueiredo VM, Ziff EB. Konkiewitz EC. Human immunodeficiency virus-associated depression: contributions of immuno-inflammatory, monoaminergic, neurodegenerative, and neurotrophic pathways. *J Neurovirol.* (2013) 19:314–27. doi: 10.1007/s13365-013-0177-7
76. Bachis A, Avdoshina V, Zecca L, Parsadanian M, Mocchetti I. Human immunodeficiency virus type 1 alters brain-derived neurotrophic factor processing in neurons. *J Neurosci.* (2012) 32:9477–84. doi: 10.1523/JNEUROSCI.0865-12.2012
77. Wang Y, Liao J, Tang SJ, Shu J, Zhang W. HIV-1 gp120 upregulates brain-derived neurotrophic factor (BDNF) expression in BV2 cells via the Wnt/beta-catenin signaling pathway. *J Mol Neurosci.* (2017) 62:199–208. doi: 10.1007/s12031-017-0931-z
78. Schütz SG, Robinson-Papp J. HIV-related neuropathy: current perspectives. *HIV AIDS.* (2013) 5:243–51. doi: 10.2147/HIV.S36674
79. Simioni S, Cavassini M, Annoni JM, Rimbault Abraham A, Bourquin I, Schiffer V, et al. Cognitive dysfunction in HIV patients despite

long-standing suppression of viremia. *AIDS.* (2010) 24:1243–50. doi: 10.1097/QAD.0b013e3283354a7b

80. Abas M, Ali GC, Nakimuli-Mpungu E, Chibanda D. Depression in people living with HIV in sub-Saharan Africa: time to act. *Trop Med Int Health.* (2014) 19:1392–6. doi: 10.1111/tmi.12382
81. Keating SM, Golub ET, Nowicki M, Young M, Anastos K, Crystal H, et al. The effect of HIV infection and HAART on inflammatory biomarkers in a population-based cohort of women. *AIDS.* (2011) 25:1823–32. doi: 10.1097/QAD.0b013e3283489d1f
82. Haissman JM, Vestergaard LS, Sembuche S, Erikstrup C, Mmbando B, Mtullu S, et al. Plasma cytokine levels in Tanzanian HIV-1-infected adults and the effect of antiretroviral treatment. *J Acquir Immune Defic Syndr.* (2009) 52:493–7. doi: 10.1097/QAI.0b013e3181b627dc
83. Espíndola MS, Soares LS, Galvão-Lima LJ, Zambuzi FA, Cacemiro MC, Brauer VS, et al. Epigenetic alterations are associated with monocyte immune dysfunctions in HIV-1 infection. *Sci Rep.* (2018) 8:5505. doi: 10.1038/s41598-018-23841-1
84. Horvath S, Stein DJ, Phillips N, Heany SJ, Kobor MS, Lin DTS, et al. Perinatally acquired HIV infection accelerates epigenetic aging in South African adolescents. *AIDS.* (2018) 32:1465–74. doi: 10.1097/QAD.0000000000001854
85. Horvath S, Levine AJ. HIV-1 Infection accelerates age according to the epigenetic clock. *J Infect Dis.* (2015) 212:1563–73. doi: 10.1093/infdis/jiv277
86. Vujkovic-Cvijin I, Dunham RM, Iwai S, Maher MC, Albright RG, Broadhurst MJ, et al. Dysbiosis of the gut microbiota is associated with HIV disease progression and tryptophan catabolism. *Sci Transl Med.* (2013) 5:193ra191. doi: 10.1126/scitranslmed.3006438
87. Brenchley JM, Schacker TW, Ruff LE, Price DA, Taylor JH, Beilman GJ, et al. CD4+ T cell depletion during all stages of HIV disease occurs predominantly in the gastrointestinal tract. *J Exp Med.* (2004) 200:749–59. doi: 10.1084/jem.20040874
88. Atarashi K, Suda W, Luo C, Kawaguchi T, Motoo I, Narushima S, et al. Ectopic colonization of oral bacteria in the intestine drives TH1 cell induction and inflammation. *Science.* (2017) 358:359–65. doi: 10.1126/science.aan4526
89. Komiya Y, Shimomura Y, Higurashi T, Sugi Y, Arimoto J, Umezawa S, et al. Patients with colorectal cancer have identical strains of Fusobacterium nucleatum in their colorectal cancer and oral cavity. *Gut.* (2018) doi: 10.1136/gutjnl-2018-316661 [Epub ahead of print]
90. Noguera-Julian M, Rocafort M, Guillén Y, Rivera J, Casadellà M, Nowak P, et al. Gut microbiota linked to sexual preference and HIV infection. *EBioMedicine.* (2016) 5:135–46. doi: 10.1016/j.ebiom.2016.01.032
91. De Filippo C, Di Paola M, Ramazzotti M, Albanese D, Pieraccini G, Banci E, et al. Diet, environments, and gut microbiota. a preliminary investigation in children living in rural and urban burkina faso and Italy. *Front Microbiol.* (2017) 8:1979. doi: 10.3389/fmicb.2017.01979
92. Koeth RA, Wang Z, Levison BS, Buffa JA, Org E, Sheehy BT, et al. Intestinal microbiota metabolism of L-carnitine, a nutrient in red meat, promotes atherosclerosis. *Nat Med.* (2013) 19:576–85. doi: 10.1038/nm.3145
93. Paster BJ, Olsen I, Aas JA, Dewhirst FE. The breadth of bacterial diversity in the human periodontal pocket and other oral sites. *Periodontol 2000.* (2006) 42:80–7. doi: 10.1111/j.1600-0757.2006.00174.x
94. Kau AL, Ahern PP, Griffin NW, Goodman AL, Gordon JI. Human nutrition, the gut microbiome and the immune system. *Nature.* (2011) 474:327–36. doi: 10.1038/nature10213
95. Liu J, Kandasamy S, Zhang J, Kirby CW, Karakach T, Hafting J, et al. Prebiotic effects of diet supplemented with the cultivated red seaweed Chondrus crispus or with fructo-oligo-saccharide on host immunity, colonic microbiota and gut microbial metabolites. *BMC Complement Altern Med.* (2015) 15:279. doi: 10.1186/s12906-015-0802-5
96. Rooks MG, Garrett WS. Gut microbiota, metabolites and host immunity. *Nat Rev Immunol.* (2016) 16:341–52. doi: 10.1038/nri.2016.42

15

Safety and Immunological Evaluation of Interleukin-21 Plus Anti-α4β7 mAb Combination Therapy in Rhesus Macaques

Maria Pino[1], Srijayaprakash Babu Uppada[2], Kabita Pandey[2], Colin King[1], Kevin Nguyen[1], Inbo Shim[1], Kenneth Rogers[3], Francois Villinger[3], Mirko Paiardini[1,4†] and Siddappa N. Byrareddy[2,5,6*†]*

[1] Division of Microbiology and Immunology, Yerkes National Primate Research Center, Emory University, Atlanta, GA, United States, [2] Department of Pharmacology and Experimental Neuroscience, University of Nebraska Medical Center, Omaha, NE, United States, [3] New Iberia Research Center, University of Louisiana at Lafayette, New Iberia, LA, United States, [4] Department of Pathology and Laboratory Medicine, Emory University School of Medicine, Atlanta, GA, United States, [5] Department of Genetics, Cell Biology and Anatomy, University of Nebraska Medical Center, Omaha, NE, United States, [6] Department of Biochemistry and Molecular Biology, University of Nebraska Medical Center, Omaha, NE, United States

***Correspondence:**
Mirko Paiardini
mirko.paiardini@emory.edu
Siddappa N. Byrareddy
sid.byrareddy@unmc.edu

† These authors have contributed equally to this work

Human immunodeficiency virus (HIV) and simian immunodeficiency virus (SIV) infections compromise gut immunological barriers, inducing high levels of inflammation and a severe depletion of intestinal $CD4^+$ T cells. Expression of α4β7 integrin promotes homing of activated T cells to intestinal sites where they become preferentially infected; blockade of α4β7 with an anti-α4β7 monoclonal antibody (mAb) prior to infection has been reported to reduce gut SIV viremia in rhesus macaques (RMs). Interleukin-21 (IL-21) administration in antiretroviral therapy-treated, SIV-infected RMs reduces gut inflammation and improves gut integrity. We therefore hypothesized that the combination of IL-21 and anti-α4β7 mAb therapies could synergize to reduce inflammation and HIV persistence. We co-administered two intravenous doses of rhesus anti-α4β7 mAb (50 mg/kg) combined with seven weekly subcutaneous infusions of IL-21–IgFc (100 μg/kg) in four healthy, SIV-uninfected RMs to evaluate the safety and immunological profiles of this intervention in blood and gut. Co-administration of IL-21 and anti-α4β7 mAb showed no toxicity at the given dosages as assessed by multiple hematological and chemical parameters and did not alter the bioavailability of the therapeutics or result in the generation of antibodies against the anti-α4β7 mAb or IL-21–IgFc. Upon treatment, the frequency of CD4 memory T cells expressing β7 increased in blood and decreased in gut, consistent with an inhibition of activated CD4 T-cell homing to the gut. Furthermore, the frequency of T cells expressing proliferation and immune activation markers decreased in blood and, more profoundly, in gut. The combined IL-21 plus anti-α4β7 mAb therapy is well-tolerated in SIV-uninfected RMs and reduces the gut homing of $\alpha4\beta7^+$ CD4 T cells as well as the levels of gut immune activation.

Keywords: anti-α4β7, IL-21, immune activation, T- cell homing, macaques, rhesus macaques, combined immune intervention

INTRODUCTION

Human immunodeficiency virus (HIV) infection induces high and persistent levels of immune activation and inflammation, which are associated with the loss of $CD4^+$ T cells and accelerated disease progression (1, 2). With the advances in antiretroviral therapy (ART), the incidence of HIV infection and transmission has been reduced significantly. However, despite effective viral suppression in plasma, ART does not cure HIV infection, with virus persisting in long-lived $CD4^+$ T cells or macrophages in different tissues and organs (3). Furthermore, ART-treated HIV-infected individuals can still present persistent chronic inflammation, limited $CD4^+$ T-cell reconstitution, and mucosal immune dysfunction (1, 4–6), which have all been linked to increased HIV- and non–HIV-associated comorbidities and mortality. Therefore, new therapeutic strategies aimed at reducing both viral reservoir and chronic immune activation in combination with ART could be beneficial for a potential cure strategy.

Interleukin-21 (IL-21) is a pleiotropic cytokine, member of the common ɣ-chain-signaling family, which includes IL-2, IL-4, IL-7, IL-9, and IL-15, and it is mainly produced by CD4 T helper (T_H) cells (including T_H17 and Tfh), ɣδ T cells, CD8 T, and natural killer (NK) T cells. Interleukin-21 affects multiple pathways of both humoral and cell-mediated immune responses (7). Previously, we showed that in simian immunodeficiency virus (SIV)-infected rhesus macaques (RMs) loss of IL-21–producing $CD4^+$ T cells in the gut is associated with T_H17 cell depletion, loss of gut mucosa integrity, and mucosal immune dysfunction (8). Moreover, we have shown that administration of a rhesus IL-21–IgFc fusion protein in acute (9) or chronic ART-treated SIV-infected RMs (10) resulted in the preservation of intestinal T_H17 cells, improved mucosal immune function, and reduced microbial translocation. Finally, we also showed that IL-21 treatment resulted in a reduction of the replication competent viral reservoir in lymph nodes (10). Importantly, a cross-sectional human study showed that IL-21 production is decreased at the very early stage of HIV infection and that serum IL-21 concentrations correlate with $CD4^+$ T-cell counts (11). In contrast, normal levels of IL-21–producing $CD4^+$ T cells were observed in HIV elite controllers, individuals able to naturally (without ART) control HIV replication to very low levels (11). Furthermore, it has been shown that IL-21 promotes degranulation and effector functions of $CD8^+$ T cells (12, 13) and that IL-21–producing HIV-1–specific $CD8^+$ T cells are more abundant in elite controllers (14).

α4β7 integrin is a key molecule for mucosal homing of lymphocytes (15), and $\alpha4\beta7^+$ CD4 T cells, including T_H17 cells, are the primary targets and thus rapidly depleted during the initial phase of HIV and SIV infection (2, 16, 17). Previous studies in RMs suggest that α4β7 blockade could limit the number of activated and preferentially infected cells to gastrointestinal-associated lymphoid tissues (GALTs), with the potential to reduce both viral loads and chronic inflammation within the gut. Treatment with a primatized anti-α4β7 monoclonal antibody (mAb) initiated prior to SIV infection in RMs has been shown to reduce mucosal transmission and reduce the viral loads within the gut (18).

Collectively, data generated with these single interventions showed that α4β7 blockade limited viremia in mucosal sites of HIV persistence, and IL-21 promoted the reconstitution of mucosal T_H17 cells, critical to maintain mucosal integrity and limit microbial translocation, one key cause of chronic immune activation in HIV and SIV infection. Therefore, we propose that a combined strategy based on administration of IL-21 and anti-α4β7 mAb could have the potential to limit inflammation and, as a consequence, improve antiviral immune responses and reduce viral persistence in ART-suppressed HIV-infected individuals. Although IL-21 and anti-α4β7 mAb administration has been tested individually and found to be safe, co-administration of the two compounds has never been tested or reported. Here, we conducted a pilot study aimed at determining the safety, tolerability, and biological activity of the combined IL-21 and anti-α4β7 mAb treatment in healthy, SIV-uninfected RMs. The data generated from this pilot study will guide future combined interventions in ART-treated SIV-infected non-human primates, aimed at limiting residual inflammation and viral persistence.

MATERIALS AND METHODS

Animal Ethical Consideration and Treatment

All animal experiments were conducted following guidelines established by the Animal Welfare Act and the National Institutes of Health (NIH) for Housing and Care of Laboratory Animals and performed in accordance with institutional regulations after review and approval by the Institutional Animal Care and Usage Committees at the Yerkes National Primate Research Center (YNPRC). Anesthesia was administered prior to performing any procedure, and proper steps were taken to minimize the suffering of the animals in this study. A total of four Indian origin RMs (*Macaca mulatta*) were enrolled in this pilot study (**Supplementary Table 1**). All macaques were housed and maintained at the YNPRC (Atlanta, GA, USA). All animals received two doses of rhesus anti-α4β7 mAb (50 mg/kg, intravenous route) obtained from NIH Non-human Primate Reagent Resource, University of Massachusetts Medical School, Worcester, MA, USA, at 3-week interval (days 0 and 21) and seven weekly doses (days 0, 7, 14, 21, 28, 35, and 42) of recombinant rhesus IL-21–IgFc (IL-21-Fc, 100 μg/kg, subcutaneous route) obtained from Resource for Nonhuman Primate Immune Reagents of the New Iberia Research Center.

Sample Collection and Processing

Blood and rectal biopsies (RBs) were collected at multiple time points before, during, and after the interventions. Blood samples were used for complete blood counts and comprehensive serum chemistry panels. Plasma was separated from EDTA-anticoagulated blood by centrifugation within 1 h of phlebotomy. Density centrifugation was used to isolate peripheral blood mononuclear cells (PBMCs). Up to 20 RBs were collected with biopsy forceps under visual control via an anoscope. Rectal biopsy-derived lymphocytes were isolated by digestion with 1 mg/mL collagenase for 2 h at 37°C and then passed through a 70-μm cell strainer to remove residual tissue fragments. All samples were processed, stained, fixed (1% paraformaldehyde), and analyzed by flow cytometry within 24 h of collection as described previously (10).

Flow Cytometric Analysis

Flow cytometric analysis was performed on PBMCs and RB-derived cells according to standard procedures using a panel of mAbs that others and we have shown to be cross-reactive with RM immune cells (10, 19) (**Supplementary Table 2**). The following Abs were used: anti-CD4-APCCy7 (clone OKT4), anti-HLA-DR-BV711 (clone L243), and anti-CD20 PerCpCy5.5 (clone 2H7) all from Biolegend, San Diego, CA, USA; anti-CD95-CF594 (clone DX2), anti-beta7-PECy5 (clone FIB504), anti-CCR7-PECy7 (clone 3D12), anti-Ki67-Alexa700 (clone B56), anti-CD3-BUV395 (clone SP34-2), anti-CD8-BUV496 (clone RPA-T8), anti-CD56-BV605 (clone B159), and anti-CD16-BV650 (clone 3G8) all from Becton-Dickinson, BD Biosciences, San Jose, CA, USA; anti-NKG2A-APC (clone Z199), from Beckman Coulter, Brea, CA, USA; Aqua Live/Dead amine dye-AmCyan from ThermoFisher Scientific, Invitrogen, Waltham, MA, USA; anti-CD38-FITC (clone AT-1) from STEMCELL Technologies, Vancouver, British Columbia, Canada; and anti-α4β7-PE (clone Act-1) obtained from the NIH Non-human Primate Reagent Resource, University of Massachusetts Medical School. Flow cytometric acquisition was performed on at least 100,000 $CD3^+$ T cells on a BD LSRII Flow Cytometer driven by BD FACSDiva software. Analyses of the acquired data were performed by FlowJo software, Tree Star, Inc., Ashland, OR, USA.

Measurement of Rhesus Anti-α4β7 mAb in Plasma

Levels of rhesus anti-α4β7 mAb in plasma samples from the four macaques were quantified as previously described (20). Briefly, HuT78 cells were first incubated at 37°C for 3 days in RPMI 1640 media containing 1 μM retinoic acid to increase surface expression of α4β7; 1×10^5 cells/well were dispensed into 96-well plates and incubated with plasma (1:10, diluted in phosphate-buffered saline (PBS)/2% fetal bovine serum) for 30 min at 4°C. Cells in the wells were washed and incubated with biotinylated antirhesus IgG1 kappa (clone 7H11; NIH Non-human Primate Reagent Resource, University of Massachusetts Medical School) for 30 min at 4°C and then washed again and resuspended in neutravidin-PE (A-2660; ThermoFisher Scientific) for 20 min at 4°C. Cells were washed, fixed in 2% paraformaldehyde, and analyzed on a flow cytometer (Attune NxT; ThermoFisher Scientific). Rhesus anti-α4β7 antibody was quantified using a standard curve method by comparing the mean channel fluorescence intensity mean channel fluorescent intensity (MFI) of cells treated with macaque plasma to the mean channel fluorescence intensity MFI of cells treated with serially diluted rhesus anti-α4β7 mAb (clone Act-1, obtained from NIH Non-human Primate Reagent Resource, University of Massachusetts Medical School).

Measurement of Rhesus Anti-rhesus (Anti-drug) Antibodies

To determine whether the rhesus may potentially generate antibodies against the infused recombinant rhesus anti-a4b7 mAb, an enzyme-linked immunosorbent assay (ELISA)-based assay was developed to monitor the detection of such rhesus anti-rhesus Ig antibodies (RARA), also named anti-drug antibodies (ADAs). Detection of antibodies generated against rhesus IgG1 kappa chain in RM plasma was measured by detecting monoclonal anti-lambda light chain bound to immobilized rhesus recombinant anti-α4β7 antibody by ELISA assays. In brief, ELISA plates (ThermoFisher Scientific) were coated with anti-α4β7 antibody (NIH NHP RR-Rhesus Recombinant IgG1 kappa, CDR-g, lot no. 092012G) in coating buffer (1× PBS) at 10 μg/mL. 100 μl were added to individual wells of the 96-well microtiter plate and left overnight at 4°C. Plates were then washed six times with wash buffer (PBS/0.05% Tween 20) and blocked with 300 μL per well of Superblock solution (ThermoFisher Scientific) for 15 min at room temperature (RT) followed by washing six additional times with wash buffer. The test sera from the monkeys to be screened for ADAs were 4-fold diluted (starting at 1:10) in dilution buffer (PBS/2% bovine serum albumin) and dispensed into duplicate wells at 100 μL per well. After 1-h incubation at RT, plates were washed six times with wash buffer followed by the addition of 100 μL of a 1:100 dilution of a monoclonal anti-lambda light chain-biotin (clone IS7-24C7; Miltenyi Biotech, Cologne, Germany) per well. After 1-h incubation at RT, plates were washed six times with wash buffer followed by the addition of 100 μL of a 1:10,000 dilution of streptavidin-horseradish peroxidase (HRP) (Invitrogen) per well. After 1-h incubation at RT, wells were washed six times with wash buffer followed by the addition of TMB substrate (SeraCare, Gaithersburg, MD, USA) at 100 μL per well to develop color and finally halted with stop solution containing H_2SO_4 (KPL). The optical density (OD) was recorded at 450 nm on Spectramax i3x plate reader (Molecular Devices, San Jose, CA, USA). Controls consisted of wells with baseline monkey sera and PBS alone (negative control); sera from a previously titered ADAs containing positive sera served as a positive control. Briefly, the positive control RNo13 was a RM infected intravenously with SIV_{mac239}, which initiated ART at week 5 of infection for a 90-day course. At week 9 of infection, and similarly to our study, this animal received 50 mg/kg of mAb against α4β7 intravenously every 3 weeks (21). The end point was noted as the highest dilution of the test sera with OD >2× pretreatment sample, and this dilution was considered positive for the assay.

Measurement of Rhesus IL-21–Fc in Plasma

Maxisorp 96-well plates were precoated overnight at 4°C with 2 μg/mL purified anti-human IL-21 capture mAb (clone J148-1134; BD Biosciences) in 100 μL bicarbonate buffer pH 9.6 per well. The next morning, the unbound antibody was removed, and the coated plates were blocked for 2 h with 300 μL per well of PBS with 2% bovine serum albumin at 37°C. The plates were then washed four times with PBS supplemented with 0.05%

Tween 20, added serial 2-fold dilutions of test plasma samples in duplicates and a dilution series of a IL-21–Fc standard, and incubated for 2 h at RT. Plates were washed and added 100 μL of anti-IL-21-biotin detection mAb (clone I76-539; BD Biosciences) at a 1:2,000 dilution and incubated for 2 h at RT. After washing, the plates were added HRP-conjugated Avidin D (Vector Laboratories, Burlingame, CA, USA) at a 1:2,000 dilution followed by TMB substrate (KPL) in sequential steps. The reaction was stopped by the addition of 20 μL of 1 M H_2SO_4, and the absorbance read at 450 nm using a Bio-Tek Synergy HT multimode microplate reader. Baseline plasma samples for each test subject collected prior to IL-21 administration were included to determine background values. The lower detection limit of IL-21–Fc was 15.6 pg/mL.

Measurement of Rhesus Anti–IL-21–Fc Antibodies

To determine whether the rhesus may potentially generate antibodies against the infused recombinant rhesus IL-21–Fc, an ELISA-based assay was performed. Maxisorp 96-well plates were precoated overnight at 4°C with 4 μg/mL recombinant rhesus IL-21–Fc in 100 μL of 1× coating solution (KPL) per well. The next morning, plates were washed with PBS 0.05% Tween-20 and blocked by adding 200 μL/well of PBS with 1% bovine serum albumin (blocking buffer) at 4°C overnight. After washing the plates, 100 μL plasma samples diluted (1:100, 1:1,000, and 1:10,000) in blocking buffer were added in duplicate to wells, or blocking buffer was added to wells for negative and positive control wells. Following an incubation at 4°C overnight, the plates were washed, and 100 μL of monkey cross-reactive goat anti–human kappa-Biot (Southern Biotech, Birmingham, AL, USA) diluted 1:1,000 in blocking buffer was added to sample and negative control wells. To positive control wells, 100 μL of goat anti–monkey IgG biotin (Rockland, Limerick, PA, USA) diluted 1:1,000 in blocking buffer was added. The plate was incubated for 2 h at RT. After washing, HRP-conjugated avidin D at a 1:1,000 dilution was added to wells and incubated for 1 h. Plates were washed and developed with TMB substrate and read on a microplate reader as described above for the IL-21–Fc capture ELISA. Baseline plasma samples for each test subject collected prior to IL-21 administration were included to determine background values. The positive control confirmed the correct coating of the wells and consisted of a mouse anti–human IL-21 mAb (clone I76-539, BD #558502) that cross-reacts with the rhesus IL-21–Fc, and it specifically binds to this cytokine. Of note, with this assay, we do not detect the lambda chain antibodies, but across multiple isotypes (IgA, IgG, IgM).

Statistical Analysis

Data analyses were performed using GraphPad Prism (GraphPad Software, Inc., La Jolla, CA, USA). The results are expressed as the mean ± SD. Statistical significance (*P*-value) of immunophenotyping data between time points was not reported because of the limited number of animals included in the pilot study.

RESULTS

The Combined Administration of IL-21 and Anti-α4β7 mAb Is Safe and Tolerated in RMs

IL-21 and anti-α4β7 mAbs have been previously administered as single interventions in naive or SIV-infected RMs with an acceptable safety profile (10, 18, 21–25). However, combined administration of the two reagents has not yet been tested. To determine the safety and tolerability of the combined IL-21 and anti-α4β7 mAb administration in non-human primates, four healthy, SIV-uninfected RMs were treated with two doses of anti-α4β7 mAb (50 mg/kg, intravenous) at a 3-week interval (days 0 and 21) and seven weekly doses (from days 0 to 42) of recombinant rhesus IL-21–IgFc (IL-21-Fc, 100 μg/kg, subcutaneous) (see section Materials and Methods and **Figure 1A**). First, we measured variations in weight and multiple hematological parameters. All four RMs included in the study showed stable or increased weights up to day 78 post-infusion of the combined treatment, the latest assessed experimental point, when compared with pre-treatment baseline (**Figure 1B**). Multiple hematological parameters were analyzed to determine possible anemias [red blood cell (RBC) count and hemoglobin (HGB)] or kidney dysfunction [blood urea nitrogen (BUN)]. We did not find any significant changes in RBC, HGB, and BUN levels, which remained stable over the entire follow-up period (**Figures 1C–E**). Then, we monitored serum chemistry parameters such as creatinine (kidney function), alanine aminotransferase (ALT; liver function), total protein (T-Prot; kidney and liver functions), and aspartate aminotransferase (AST; kidney, liver, and heart function) and found no significant variation from baseline with all measured values for the entire follow-up period (**Figures 1F–I**). Thus, at the doses administered, combined administration of IL-21 and anti-α4β7 mAb is well-tolerated and has no detectable toxic effects.

Co-administration of IL-21 and Anti-α4β7 mAb Does Not Induce ADAs Or Alter the Bioavailability of the Two Compounds

Previous studies have shown that the administration of anti-α4β7 mAb can lead to the development of ADA in a subset of RMs, which resulted in loss of anti-α4β7 mAb biological activity (21, 23, 24). In one of those studies, in which 11 RMs received eight intravenously doses of the anti-α4β7 mAb (50 mg/kg each; at weeks 9, 12, 16, 18, 20, 24, 28, and 32 post-SIV infection), three animals developed ADA responses starting either after two, three, or six doses (21). In order to test whether repeated and combined infusions of IL-21 and anti-α4β7 mAb induced ADA responses, we measured the levels of rhesus ADA against the anti-α4β7 mAb in the plasma of the four treated RMs. The plasma end point titers for all RMs before infusion as well as after infusion and until day 78 remained unchanged (**Figure 2A**). A positive control serum from monkey RNo13 was used as a positive control, which was collected during the aforementioned *in vivo* study (21), with a titer of 1:10,000 (**Figure 2A**). Similarly, we did not find any measurable levels of anti–IL-21–Fc in the plasma of the four RMs

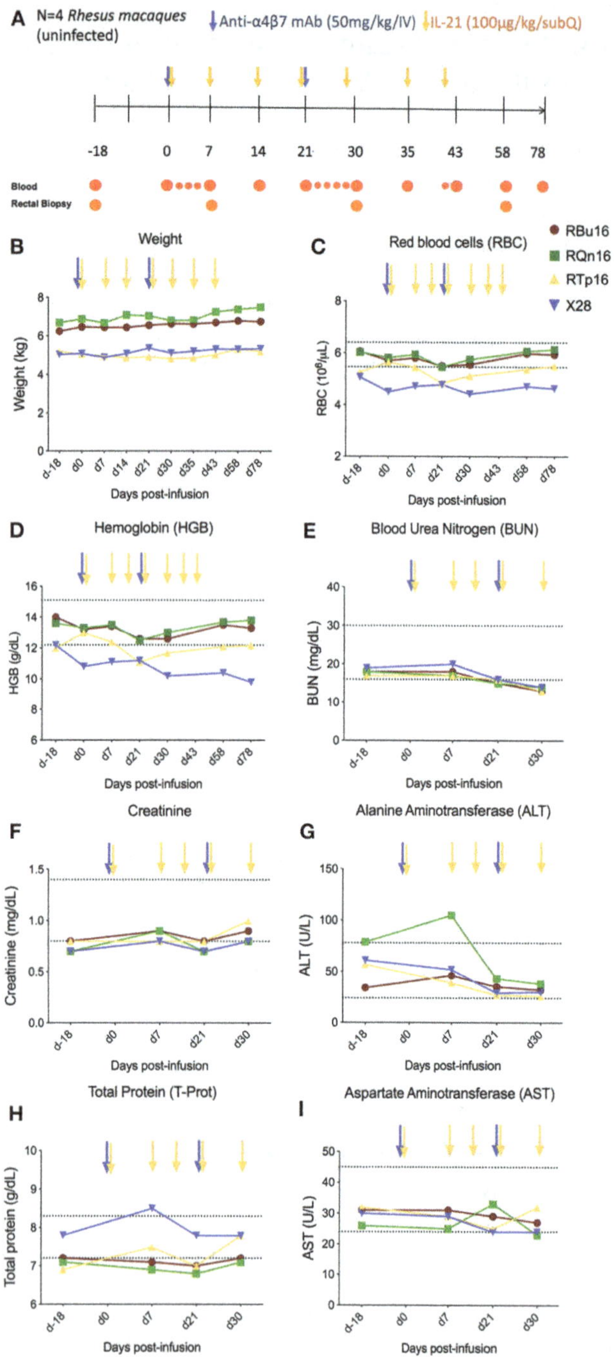

FIGURE 1 | Co-administration of anti-α4β7 mAb and IL-21. **(A)** Schematic study design of co-administration of anti-α4β7 mAb and IL-21 in uninfected RMs ($n = 4$). Prior to treatment, baseline blood and RBs were collected. On day 0, 50 mg/kg of anti-α4β7 mAb was administered intravenously along with 100 µg/kg of IL-21 subcutaneously. IL-21 was given weekly up to 6 weeks (day 42 post-infusion). 50 mg/kg of anti-α4β7 mAb was infused in two doses on day 0, week 3 (day 21 post-infusion). Blood samples were collected at regular intervals as shown in the schema. **(B)** Weight changes were recorded regularly until the end of treatment. **(C)** Red blood cells, **(D)** hemoglobin, **(E)** BUN, **(F)** creatinine, **(G)** ALT, **(H)** total protein, and **(I)** AST were analyzed from the blood collected at regular intervals until the end of the study. Individual *(Continued)*

FIGURE 1 | animals are represented with different colors and symbols. Baseline days are indicated as d-18 and d0. Normal range levels of each parameter analyzed are indicated in dashed lines. Blue arrows indicate the anti-α4β7 mAb intravenous infusions, and yellow arrows indicate IL-21 subcutaneous infusions.

neither at any tested time points or at any tested dilutions (1:100, 1:1,000, and 1:10,000) (**Figure 2B**), whereas positive control showed measurable anti–IL-21–Fc levels, confirming the correct coating of the plate (data not shown). These results indicate that, at least under the conditions used in this study, the co-administration of IL-21 and anti-α4β7 mAb did not promote the induction of ADA against either therapeutic agent. Next, we quantified the levels of anti-α4β7 mAb in plasma using flow cytometry as described in section Materials and Methods and as previously published (20). Mean baseline levels of anti-α4β7 mAb in all RMs before anti-α4β7 mAb administration were less than 40 µg/mL (**Figure 2C**); this is likely due to pre-existing antibodies against anti-α4β7 or assay background. The mean plasma levels of anti-α4β7 mAb increased to 95.6 µg/mL and to 213 µg/mL by day 7 after the first and second dose of 50 mg/kg infusion of anti-α4β7 mAb, respectively; the mean plasma levels were maintained at 92 µg/mL until day 42 post-infusion (**Figure 2C**). The stable levels of anti-α4β7 mAb during weekly administration of IL-21 suggest that IL-21 did not markedly influence levels of the anti-α4β7 mAb and that there were no drug–drug interactions. Finally, we quantified IL-21–Fc levels in plasma by ELISA. IL-21–Fc plasma levels increased after IL-21 infusion for all four animals compared with their baseline levels (<15.625 pg/mL in all animals). Its maximum concentration was achieved at day 1 post-infusion for RTp16 (323.24 pg/mL), and day 3 post-infusion for the remaining animals (RBu16: 696.54 pg/mL, RQn16: 228.3 pg/mL, and X28: 116.6 pg/mL) (**Figure 2D**). Increased plasma levels of IL-21 were still evident on day 22, 1 day after the fourth IL-21 infusion (performed on day 21), but attenuated afterward.

The Combined IL-21 and Anti-α4β7 mAb Treatment Reduces Gut Homing of Memory CD4 T Cells Expressing α4β7

To investigate the impact of combined IL-21 and anti-α4β7 mAb therapy impact on T-cell gut homing, we quantified the frequency of memory CD4 ($CD3^+CD4^+CD95^+$) and CD8 ($CD3^+CD8^+CD95^+$) T cells expressing $\alpha4\beta7^{hi}$ or β7 in blood (**Figures 3A–C**, and **Supplementary Figures 1A–C**) and RBs (**Figures 3D–F** and **Supplementary Figures 1D–F**) collected longitudinally during the study. The frequencies of $\alpha4\beta7^{hi}$ CD4 memory T cells decreased by greater than 99% in blood (**Figure 3B**) and 92.5% in RBs (**Figure 3E**) already at 1 week after the first anti-α4β7 mAb infusion; these measured levels remained constant up to day 58 post-infusion, ~5 weeks after the second dose of anti-α4β7 mAb and gradually increased thereafter, although they remained still below baseline on day 78 post-infusion, the latest time point of the study (**Figures 3B,E**). Similar results were found for CD8 T cells, with the frequencies

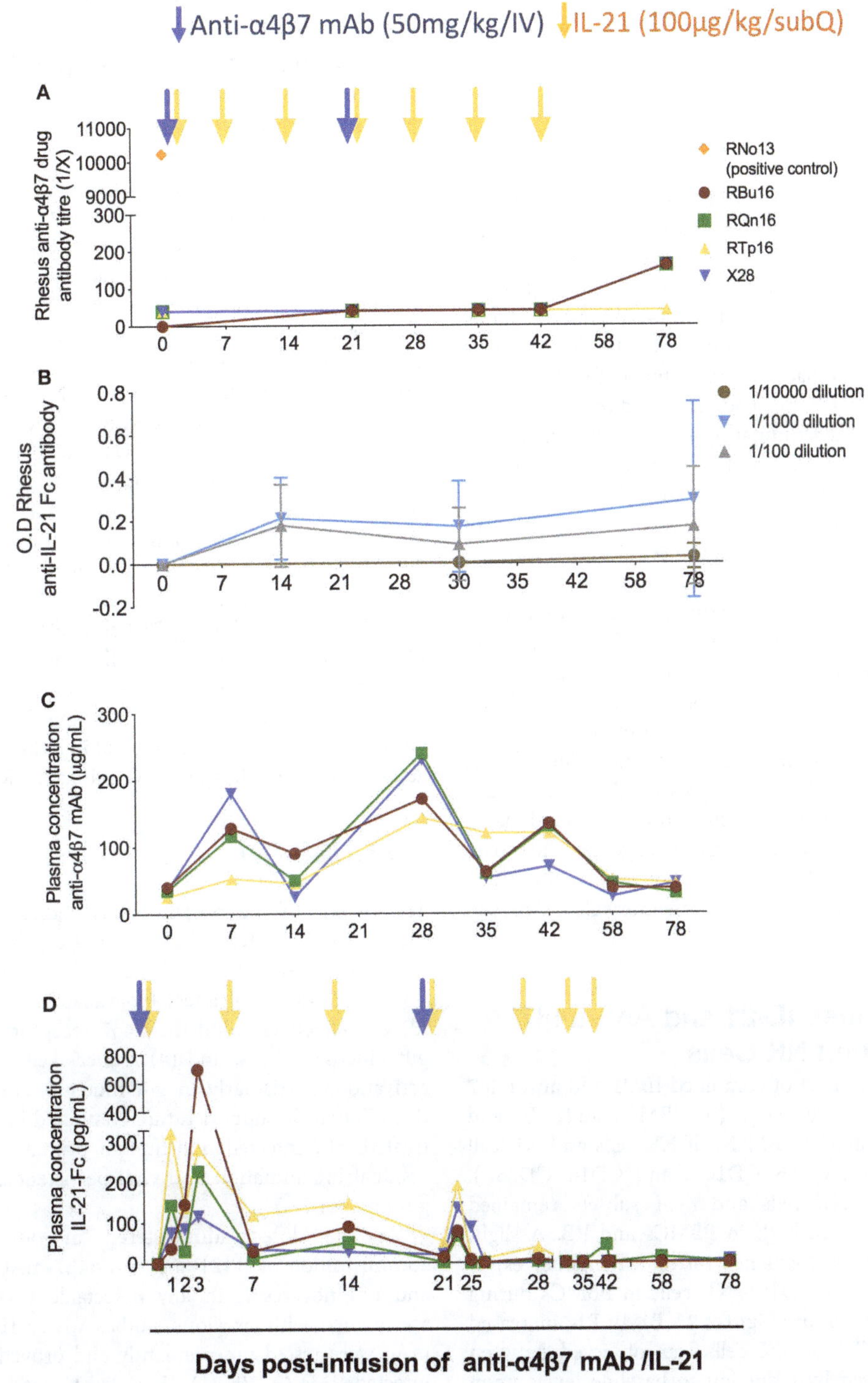

FIGURE 2 | Co-administration of anti-α4β7 mAb and IL-21 does not elicit reactive antibodies. **(A)** Analysis of rhesus antibodies anti-α4β7 mAb in plasma at different time points. The anti-drug antibodies levels were measured by ELISA end point titer method as described in the Materials and Methods section. RNo13, indicated in orange, corresponds to the plasma of an animal from a previous study that developed ADAs (21), and it was used as a positive control. **(B)** Measurement of anti–IL-21–Fc antibodies in plasma at different time points. Anti–IL-21–Fc antibodies were measured by ELISA longitudinally until the end of the study with three different dilutions (1:100, 1:1,000, and 1:10,000). **(C)** Measurement of anti-α4β7 mAb plasma levels (μg/mL) in RMs (*n* = 4). The assay was performed using flow cytometry with HuT 78 cells. The levels of anti-α4β7 mAb were measured employing standard curve method. Mean fluorescence intensity (MFI) of known concentration of anti-α4β7 mAb was obtained, and then the MFI of plasma levels of anti-α4β7 mAb was plotted. **(D)** Measurement of IL-21–Fc plasma levels (pg/mL) in RMs (*n* = 4). ELISA background and plasma baseline values were subtracted from the values analyzed at each time point. Individual animals are represented with different colors and symbols. Blue arrows indicate the anti-α4β7 mAb intravenous infusions, and yellow arrows indicate IL-21 subcutaneous infusions.

of $\alpha4\beta7^{hi}$ CD8 memory T cells decreased by greater than 99% in blood (**Supplementary Figure 1B**) and 97% in RB (**Supplementary Figure 1E**). Because the mAb used for flow cytometry staining recognizes the same epitope as the anti-α4β7 mAb used *in vivo*, these data indicate the biological activity of the anti-α4β7 mAb in targeting α4β7 expressed on CD4 and CD8 T cells in blood and gut. Of note, the very low frequencies of $\alpha4\beta7^{hi}$ CD4 and CD8 memory T cells were maintained during the IL-21 only administrations (days 30, 35, and 43 post-infusion) that followed the last dose of anti-α4β7 mAb (day 21 post-infusion), showing that the administration of IL-21 did not influence the expression of α4β7 or the ability of the anti-α4β7 mAb to target it. Furthermore, PBMCs were monitored for the expression of β7 using an anti-β7 mAb that does not compete for the epitope recognized by the anti-α4β7 mAb administered *in vivo*; as such, this analysis allows for discriminating whether the inability to stain for α4β7 results from *in vivo* depletion of α4β7 expressing cells or masking of the α4β7 molecule on cells, as well as to determine the impact of the treatment on the trafficking of $\beta7^{+}$ cells to the gut. As shown in **Figure 3C**, β7 expression on blood memory CD4 T cells was increased up to 2-fold at day 30 post-infusion as compared to pre-treatment levels (**Figure 3C**; from 30.25 to 61.88%). In RBs, frequencies of $\beta7^{+}$ cells were significantly lower up to day 58 post-infusion as compared to pre-treatment (**Figure 3F**, from 49.7 to 4.74%). Interestingly, β7 expression on memory CD8 T cells differed from that of memory CD4 T cells after anti-α4β7 mAb administration. Specifically, frequencies of memory CD8 T cells expressing β7 were reduced from 38.7 to 10.77% in blood, whereas they remained stable in the gut (**Supplementary Figures 1C, F**). Together, these data indicate that anti-α4β7 mAb treatment combined with IL-21 effectively reduces the homing of $\alpha4\beta7^{hi}$ memory CD4 T cells to the gut mucosa.

Effect of Combined IL-21 and Anti-α4β7 mAb Treatment on NK Cells

We then measured the effect of combined IL-21 and anti-α4β7 mAb treatment on the frequency (in PBMCs and RB) and absolute number (limited to PBMCs) of NK cells and NK cell subsets ($CD56^{-}CD16^{+}$, $CD56^{+}CD16^{-}$, and $CD16^{-}CD56^{-}$). Overall, the levels of NK cells and their subsets remained stable during the treatment both in PBMCs and RB. A slight increase was noted in the frequency (of total lymphocytes) of $CD56^{+}CD16^{-}$ and $CD56^{-}CD16^{-}$ NK cells in PBMCs during the treatment (**Supplementary Figures 2A,B**). In RB, increased frequency (of live cells) of NK cells was observed between days 7 and 30, followed by reduction to baseline levels upon interruption of IL-21 therapy (d58; **Supplementary Figure 2C**). This slight increase of bulk NK cells resulted in an increased frequency of $CD56^{-}CD16^{+}$ from baseline (d-18) to day 30 (**Supplementary Figure 2D**) and of $CD56^{+}CD16^{-}$ from baseline to day 7 (**Supplementary Figure 2E**), which return to baseline levels at day 58. In RB, $CD56^{-}CD16^{-}$ NK cells remained constant across the course of the study and were not affected by withdrawal of IL-21 therapy (not shown).

Combined IL-21 and Anti-α4β7 mAb Treatment Limits Immune Activation and Cell Cycling of Gut Memory CD4 T Cells

We assessed the effects of the combined IL-21 and anti-α4β7 mAb therapy on systemic and gut immune activation. For this aim, we measured the frequency of memory T cells expressing markers of activation (HLA-DR and CD38) and cell cycling (Ki67). The frequency of blood memory CD4 and CD8 T cells with an $HLA\text{-}DR^{+}CD38^{+}$ (**Figures 4A,C**) or $Ki67^{+}$ (**Figures 4B,D**) phenotype remained similar overall, with a slight decrease at specific time points. Specifically, the frequency of $HLA\text{-}DR^{+}CD38^{+}$ T cells was lower as compared to baseline on days 30, 58, and 78 after IL-21 plus anti-α4β7 mAb treatments for memory CD4 and at day 58 post-treatment for memory CD8 T cells. The frequency of $Ki67^{+}$ T cells was lower as compared to baseline only at day 14 post-treatment both for memory CD4 and CD8 T cells. Importantly, differences were more pronounced in gut, with a progressive reduction in the frequency of memory CD4 and CD8 T cells that are $HLA\text{-}DR^{+}CD38^{+}$ (**Figures 4E,G**) or $Ki67^{+}$ (**Figures 4F,H**) from baseline to day 30 post-treatment. The reduction in both immune activation and cell cycling in the gut is consistent with CD4 T cells expressing $\alpha4\beta7^{hi}$ being retained in blood as a result of the combined treatment. Collectively, our data show that a strategy based on the combined administration of IL-21 and anti-α4β7 mAb is effective in blocking the homing of memory $CD4^{+}$ $\alpha4\beta7^{hi}$ T cells to the gut and in reducing mucosal immune activation, even in healthy, SIV-uninfected RMs.

DISCUSSION

The results of the present study indicate that treatment of healthy, SIV-uninfected RMs with a combined IL-21 and anti-α4β7 mAb intervention (1) is safe and well-tolerated (at the tested doses), (2) does not affect bioavailability of both compounds, (3) can effectively bind the α4β7 receptor on both blood and gut mucosa T cells, and (4) reduces cell cycling and immune activation, particularly in gut mucosa. The data generated in this pilot study support future combined interventions in ART-treated, SIV-infected non-human primates, aimed at limiting residual inflammation and viral persistence, particularly in the gut mucosa.

At the doses administered in our study, combined administration of IL-21 and anti-α4β7 mAb was well-tolerated and did not result in any detectable toxicity. These results are aligned with previous studies where IL-21 and anti-α4β7 mAb were tested independently and proved to be safe in SIV-infected RMs (9, 10, 21). IL-21 treatment in RMs can increase the JAK/STAT signaling pathway, implicated to have roles in inflammation processes (10), whereas gene expression studies in vedolizumab-treated patients revealed dysregulated expression of genes related to cell cycle, cell growth, and inflammation (26). In our study, the combined treatment was not associated with any increase in parameters related to inflammation or immune activation.

The production of antibodies against drugs administered *in vivo* not only can reduce the bioavailability and biological

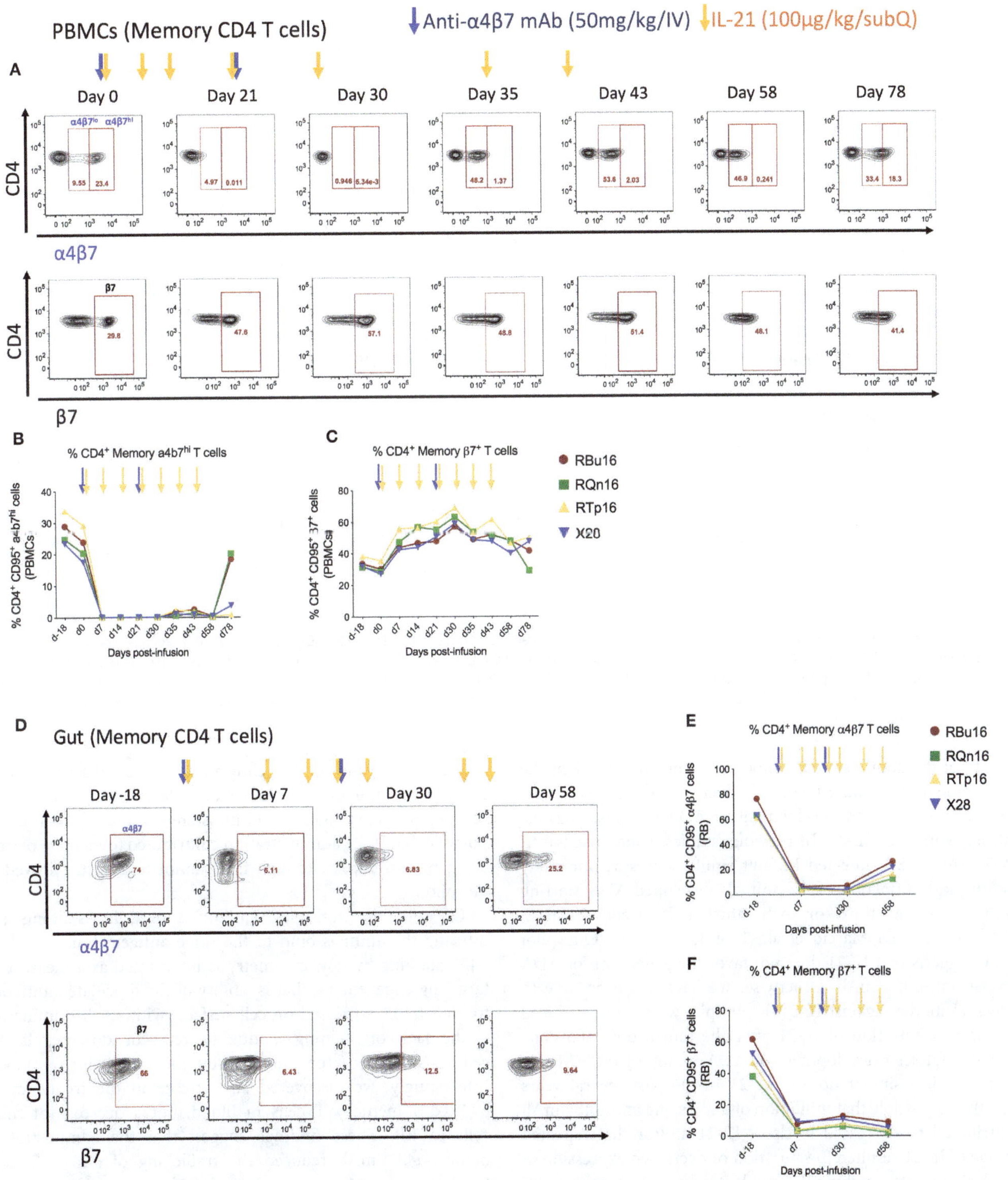

FIGURE 3 | Co-administration of anti-α4β7 mAb and IL-21 decreases gut homing of CD4 $\alpha 4\beta 7^{hi}$ to gut. **(A)** Representative flow cytometry staining of memory CD4 T cells expressing $\alpha 4\beta 7^{hi}$ (top panel) and $\beta 7^{+}$ (bottom panels) in PBMCs. **(B)** Frequency of $\alpha 4\beta 7^{hi}$ and **(C)** $\beta 7^{+}$ memory CD4 T cells in PBMCs. **(D)** Representative flow cytometry staining of memory CD4 T cells expressing $\alpha 4\beta 7^{+}$ (top panel) and $\beta 7^{+}$ (bottom panels) in gut. **(E)** Frequency of $\alpha 4\beta 7^{+}$ and **(F)** $\beta 7^{+}$ memory CD4 T cells in gut. Individual animals are represented with different colors and symbols. Baseline days are indicated as d-18 and d0. Blue arrows indicate the anti-α4β7 mAb intravenous infusions, and yellow arrows indicate IL-21 subcutaneous infusions.

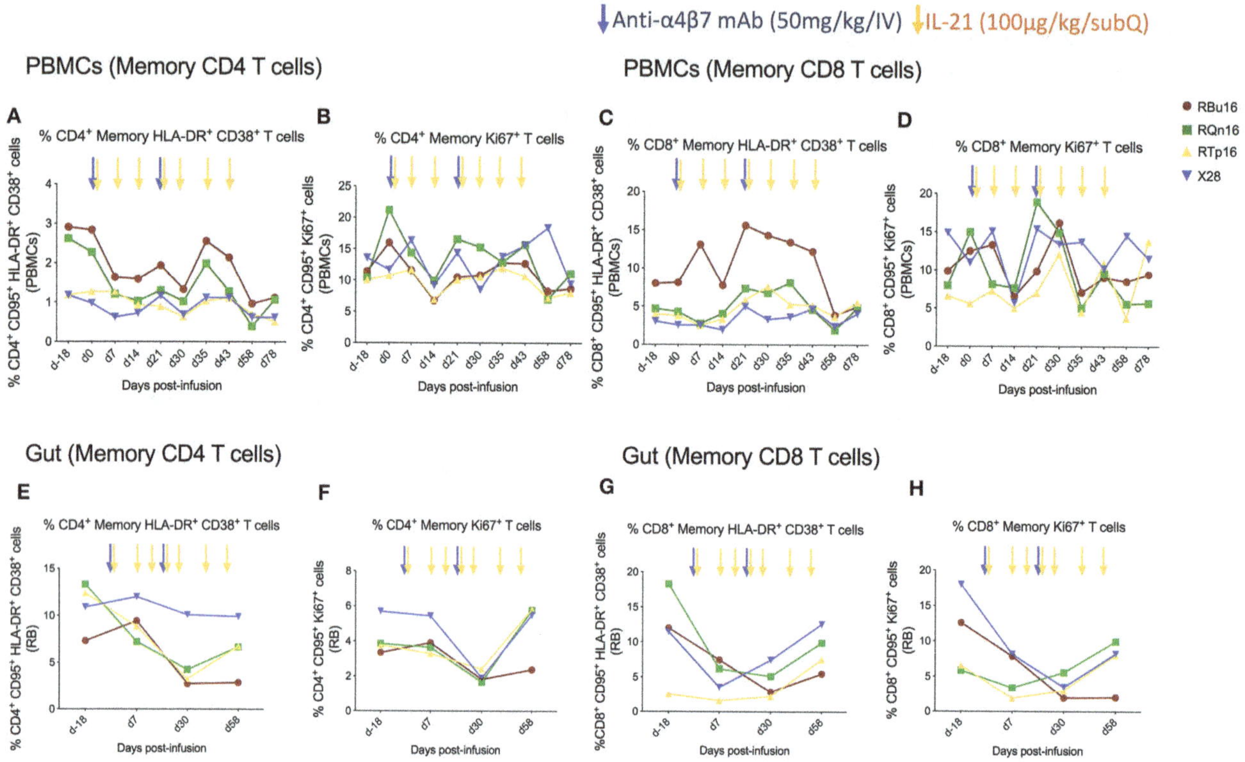

FIGURE 4 | Co-administration of anti-α4β7 mAb and IL-21 limits immune activation and cell cycling of memory CD4 T cells in gut. **(A)** Percentage of memory CD4 T cells expressing HLA-DR$^+$CD38$^+$, **(B)** Ki67$^+$, **(C)** memory CD8 T cells expressing HLA-DR$^+$CD38$^+$, and **(D)** Ki67$^+$ in PBMCs. **(E)** Percentage of memory CD4 T cells expressing HLA-DR$^+$CD38$^+$, **(F)** Ki67$^+$, **(G)** memory CD8 T cells expressing HLA-DR$^+$CD38$^+$, and **(H)** Ki67$^+$ in gut mucosa. Individual animals are represented with different colors and symbols. Baseline days are indicated as d-18 and d0. Blue arrows indicate the anti-α4β7 mAb intravenous infusions, and yellow arrows indicate IL-21 subcutaneous infusions.

activity of the administered compounds, but can also elicit the development of immune-mediated adverse events. In our study, we have not observed development of ADA responses against anti-α4β7 mAb or IL-21. In previous studies, which used anti-α4β7 mAb in SIV-infected RMs at similar doses as our study (500 μg/kg), a fraction of the animals developed ADA starting from the second, third, or sixth infusion (Byrareddy et al., 3 of 11 animals; Di Mascio et al., 1 of 12 animals). Our pilot study suggests that IL-21 does not favor the generation of ADA against anti-α4β7 mAb. Otherwise, we have not been able to detect antibodies against IL-21–Fc, despite we found a reduced plasma concentration of IL-21 after the fourth dose. To date, we have not seen development of ADA in any of the RMs we treated with a similar dose of IL-21 in the past several years (9, 10). It is possible that inhibition of α4β7 using anti-α4β7 mAb contributed to decreased levels of IL-21 and/or that repeated dosage of IL-21 resulted in saturation or decreased expression of the IL-21 receptor, making IL-21 to be freely available for a faster clearance as compared to bound IL-21. The consistent increase of plasma concentration of anti-α4β7 mAb during IL-21 infusions indicates that IL-21 does not negatively affect anti-α4β7 mAb bioavailability. Interestingly, there is an unexpected increase of anti-α4β7 plasma levels at day 42, present in three of the four treated RMs, without any new anti-α4β7 mAb administration. One possibility is that this results from differences in receptor activation (27) and or recycling processes, as observed for β1 integrin receptor in a previous study (28), altering the number of receptors able to bind the administered anti-α4β7 Ab. It is also possible that IL-21 administration contributed to increase plasma levels of anti-α4β7, although this cannot be directly proved in our pilot.

Of note, the anti-α4β7 antibodies used for staining and infusing the animals bind to the same antigen; thus, a lack of α4β7 staining by flow cytometry is interpreted as a measure of targeting engagement, that is, ability of the inoculated antibody to bind α4β7 expressed on cell surface, without discriminating if the lack of staining is due to receptor downregulation, cell lysis, or receptor blockage by the competing antibody. Interestingly, we discovered an increase in the frequency of β7$^+$ CD4 memory T cells in blood, but a decrease of these cells in RB. These findings suggest that the administration of anti-α4β7 mAb reduced the trafficking of α4β7^{hi} T cells to the gut, confirming the mode of action, prevention of trafficking of activated T cells to the gut, of vedoluzimab as adjunctive therapy in inflammatory bowel disease and Crohn disease (IBD/CD) (29–34). As such, a similar strategy is of interest in the context of HIV infection, where CD4 T cells that express CCR5 and α4β7 are the preferred target for HIV infection in the gut, a major site for early HIV infection and replication (2, 35–37).

Combined administration of IL-21 and anti-α4β7 antibody decreased the frequency of T cells expressing immune activation and proliferation markers in the gut of healthy RMs, despite the low baseline level. This result supports the use of this combined treatment in the context of SIV infection in RMs. Our previous studies showed that, by favoring maintenance of T_H17 and T_H22 cells, IL-21 improves mucosal integrity and reduces inflammation when administered in acute (9) or chronic, ART-treated (10) SIV-infected RMs. Similarly, anti-α4β7 antibody reduced SIV infection in the GALT when animals were challenged either intravenously, intrarectally, and intravaginally (18, 38, 39). In another recent study, the combination of primatized anti-α4β7 and VRC01 significantly delayed vaginal SHIV exposure and reduced viral loads in rectal tissues compared to control (40). The effect of anti-α4β7 mAb administered in SIV-infected RMs during ART continues to be a highly debatable issue. While an earlier study showed that this treatment can limit viral rebound after ART interruption (21), more recent pre-clinical (23–25) and clinical (41) studies did not show any significant benefit from anti-α4β7 mAb treatment in ART-suppressed, HIV-infected individuals or SIV-infected RMs in inducing viral remission in the absence of ART (42). Recently, using samples obtained from various gastrointestinal sites from IBD/CD patients, it was found that anti-α4β7 therapy led to a significant reduction of lymphoid aggregates, mostly in the terminal ileum (43). Because lymphoid aggregates serve as important sanctuary sites for maintaining viral reservoirs, the authors proposed that their ablation by anti-α4β7 mAb should be considered in developing novel therapies for HIV remission. These findings highlight that much has yet to be learned about the mechanisms of action and biologic effects of anti-α4β7 therapy, as well as on the combination of anti-α4β7 mAb with additional immunotherapies to provide immunologic and virologic benefits.

This is the first study in non-human primates showing that anti-α4β7 mAb and IL-21 treatment can be administered safely and can reduce cell cycling and immune activation, particularly in gut mucosa. As such, our study provides rationale to explore this combined treatment as a strategy aimed at limiting immune activation and viral persistence in ART-suppressed, SIV-infected RMs.

ETHICS STATEMENT

The animal study was reviewed and approved by Institutional Animal Care and Usage Committees at the Yerkes National Primate Research Center, Emory University.

AUTHOR CONTRIBUTIONS

MPi, MPa, and SB contributed to study design. MPi, SU, KP, CK, KN, IS, and KR contributed to data collection. MPi, SU, KP, KR, and SB contributed to data quality and analysis. MPi, SU, FV, MPa, and SB wrote the manuscript. All authors contributed to manuscript development and have critically reviewed and approved the final version.

ACKNOWLEDGMENTS

We thank Lepakshe S. Madduri for help in ADA assays and Robin Taylor for editorial help. Anti-α4β7 mAb was obtained from Non-human Primate Reagents Resources (University of Massachusetts Medical School); IL-21 was obtained from Resource for Non-human Primate Immune Reagents of New Iberia Research Center.

REFERENCES

1. Hileman CO, Funderburg NT. Inflammation, immune activation, and antiretroviral therapy in HIV. *Curr HIV AIDS Rep.* (2017) 14:93–100. doi: 10.1007/s11904-017-0356-x
2. Sivro A, Schuetz A, Sheward D, Joag V, Yegorov S, Liebenberg LJ, et al. Integrin α4β7 expression on peripheral blood CD4(+) T cells predicts HIV acquisition and disease progression outcomes. *Sci Transl Med.* (2018) 10:eaam6354. doi: 10.1126/scitranslmed.aam6354
3. Sengupta S, Siliciano RF. Targeting the latent reservoir for HIV-1. *Immunity.* (2018) 48:872–95. doi: 10.1016/j.immuni.2018.04.030
4. Hunt PW, Lee SA, Siedner MJ. Immunologic biomarkers, morbidity, and mortality in treated HIV infection. *J Infect Dis.* (2016) 214(Suppl. 2):S44–50. doi: 10.1093/infdis/jiw275
5. Martinez-Picado J, Deeks SG. Persistent HIV-1 replication during antiretroviral therapy. *Curr Opin HIV AIDS.* (2016) 11:417–23. doi: 10.1097/COH.0000000000000287
6. Rasmussen TA, Mcmahon JH, Chang JJ, Audsley J, Rhodes A, Tennakoon S, et al. The effect of antiretroviral intensification with dolutegravir on residual virus replication in HIV-infected individuals: a randomised, placebo-controlled, double-blind trial. *Lancet HIV.* (2018) 5:e221–30. doi: 10.1016/S2352-3018(18)30040-7
7. Spolski R, Leonard WJ. Interleukin-21: a double-edged sword with therapeutic potential. *Nat Rev Drug Discov.* (2014) 13:379–95. doi: 10.1038/nrd4296
8. Micci L, Cervasi B, Ende ZS, Iriele RI, Reyes-Aviles E, Vinton C, et al. Paucity of IL-21-producing CD4(+) T cells is associated with Th17 cell depletion in SIV infection of rhesus macaques. *Blood.* (2012) 120:3925–35. doi: 10.1182/blood-2012-04-420240
9. Pallikkuth S, Micci L, Ende ZS, Iriele RI, Cervasi B, Lawson B, et al. Maintenance of intestinal Th17 cells and reduced microbial translocation in SIV-infected rhesus macaques treated with interleukin (IL)-21. *PLoS Pathog.* (2013) 9:e1003471. doi: 10.1371/journal.ppat.1003471
10. Micci L, Ryan ES, Fromentin R, Bosinger SE, Harper JL, He T, et al. Interleukin-21 combined with ART reduces inflammation and viral reservoir in SIV-infected macaques. *J Clin Invest.* (2015) 125:4497–513. doi: 10.1172/JCI81400
11. Iannello A, Boulassel MR, Samarani S, Debbeche O, Tremblay C, Toma E, et al. Dynamics and consequences of IL-21 production in HIV-infected individuals: a longitudinal and cross-sectional study. *J Immunol.* (2010) 184:114–26. doi: 10.4049/jimmunol.0901967
12. Casey KA, Mescher MF. IL-21 promotes differentiation of naive CD8 T cells to a unique effector phenotype. *J Immunol.* (2007) 178:7640–8. doi: 10.4049/jimmunol.178.12.7640
13. White L, Krishnan S, Strbo N, Liu H, Kolber MA, Lichtenheld MG, et al. Differential effects of IL-21 and IL-15 on perforin expression, lysosomal degranulation, and proliferation in CD8 T cells of patients with human immunodeficiency virus-1 (HIV). *Blood.* (2007) 109:3873–80. doi: 10.1182/blood-2006-09-045278

14. Williams LD, Bansal A, Sabbaj S, Heath SL, Song W, Tang J, et al. Interleukin-21-producing HIV-1-specific CD8 T cells are preferentially seen in elite controllers. *J Virol.* (2011) 85:2316–24. doi: 10.1128/JVI.01476-10
15. Berlin C, Berg EL, Briskin MJ, Andrew DP, Kilshaw PJ, Holzmann B, et al. Alpha 4 beta 7 integrin mediates lymphocyte binding to the mucosal vascular addressin MAdCAM-1. *Cell.* (1993) 74:185–95. doi: 10.1016/0092-8674(93)90305-A
16. Cicala C, Arthos J, Fauci AS. HIV-1 envelope, integrins and co-receptor use in mucosal transmission of HIV. *J Transl Med.* (2011) 9(Suppl. 1):S2. doi: 10.1186/1479-5876-9-S1-S2
17. Stieh DJ, Matias E, Xu H, Fought AJ, Blanchard JL, Marx PA, et al. Th17 cells are preferentially infected very early after vaginal transmission of SIV in macaques. *Cell Host Microbe.* (2016) 19:529–40. doi: 10.1016/j.chom.2016.03.005
18. Byrareddy SN, Kallam B, Arthos J, Cicala C, Nawaz F, Hiatt J, et al. Targeting α4β7 integrin reduces mucosal transmission of simian immunodeficiency virus and protects gut-associated lymphoid tissue from infection. *Nat Med.* (2014) 20:1397–400. doi: 10.1038/nm.3715
19. Mcgary CS, Deleage C, Harper J, Micci L, Ribeiro SP, Paganini S, et al. CTLA-4(+)PD-1(-) memory CD4(+) T cells critically contribute to viral persistence in antiretroviral therapy-suppressed, SIV-infected rhesus macaques. *Immunity.* (2017) 47:776–88 e775. doi: 10.1016/j.immuni.2017.09.018
20. Calenda G, Keawvichit R, Arrode-Bruses G, Pattanapanyasat K, Frank I, Byrareddy SN, et al. Integrin α4β7 blockade preferentially impacts CCR6(+) lymphocyte subsets in blood and mucosal tissues of naive rhesus macaques. *J Immunol.* (2018) 200:810–20. doi: 10.4049/jimmunol.1701150
21. Byrareddy SN, Arthos J, Cicala C, Villinger F, Ortiz KT, Little D, et al. Sustained virologic control in SIV+ macaques after antiretroviral and alpha4beta7 antibody therapy. *Science.* (2016) 354:197–202. doi: 10.1126/science.aag1276
22. Pallikkuth S, Rogers K, Villinger F, Dosterii M, Vaccari M, Franchini G, et al. Interleukin-21 administration to rhesus macaques chronically infected with simian immunodeficiency virus increases cytotoxic effector molecules in T cells and NK cells and enhances B cell function without increasing immune activation or viral replication. *Vaccine.* (2011) 29:9229–38. doi: 10.1016/j.vaccine.2011.09.118
23. Abbink P, Mercado NB, Nkolola JP, Peterson RL, Tuyishime H, Mcmahan K, et al. Lack of therapeutic efficacy of an antibody to α4β7 in SIVmac251-infected rhesus macaques. *Science.* (2019) 365:1029–33. doi: 10.1126/science.aaw8562
24. Di Mascio M, Lifson JD, Srinivasula S, Kim I, Degrange P, Keele BF, et al. Evaluation of an antibody to α4β7 in the control of SIVmac239-nef-stop infection. *Science.* (2019) 365:1025–9. doi: 10.1126/science.aav6695
25. Iwamoto N, Mason RD, Song K, Gorman J, Welles HC, Arthos J, et al. Blocking α4β7 integrin binding to SIV does not improve virologic control. *Science.* (2019) 365:1033–6. doi: 10.1126/science.aaw7765
26. Arijs I, De Hertogh G, Lemmens B, Van Lommel L, De Bruyn M, Vanhove W, et al. Effect of vedolizumab (anti-α4β7-integrin) therapy on histological healing and mucosal gene expression in patients with UC. *Gut.* (2018) 67:43–52. doi: 10.1136/gutjnl-2016-312293
27. Askari JA, Buckley PA, Mould AP, Humphries MJ. Linking integrin conformation to function. *J Cell Sci.* (2009) 122:165–70. doi: 10.1242/jcs.018556
28. Arjonen A, Alanko J, Veltel S, Ivaska J. Distinct recycling of active and inactive beta1 integrins. *Traffic.* (2012) 13:610–25. doi: 10.1111/j.1600-0854.2012.01327.x
29. Amiot A, Serrero M, Peyrin-Biroulet L, Filippi J, Pariente B, Roblin X, et al. Three-year effectiveness and safety of vedolizumab therapy for inflammatory bowel disease: a prospective multi-centre cohort study. *Aliment Pharmacol Ther.* (2019) 50:40–53. doi: 10.1111/apt.15294
30. Battat R, Dulai PS, Jairath V, Vande Casteele N. A product review of vedolizumab in inflammatory bowel disease. *Hum Vaccin Immunother.* (2019) 15:2482–90. doi: 10.1080/21645515.2019.1591139
31. Battat R, Ma C, Jairath V, Khanna R, Feagan BG. Benefit-risk assessment of vedolizumab in the treatment of crohn's disease and ulcerative colitis. *Drug Saf.* (2019) 42:617–32. doi: 10.1007/s40264-018-00783-1
32. Brandes A, Groth A, Gottschalk F, Wilke T, Ratsch BA, Orzechowski HD, et al. Real-world biologic treatment and associated cost in patients with inflammatory bowel disease. *Z Gastroenterol.* (2019) 57:843–51. doi: 10.1055/a-0903-2938
33. Loftus EV. A SPECIAL MEETING REVIEW EDITION: Highlights in inflammatory bowel disease from the 14th Congress of ECCO. *Gastroenterol Hepatol.* (2019) 15:1–24.
34. Tamilarasan AG, Cunningham G, Irving PM, Samaan MA. Recent advances in monoclonal antibody therapy in IBD: practical issues. *Frontline Gastroenterol.* (2019) 10:409–16. doi: 10.1136/flgastro-2018-101054
35. Arthos J, Cicala C, Martinelli E, Macleod K, Van Ryk D, Wei D, et al. HIV-1 envelope protein binds to and signals through integrin α4β7, the gut mucosal homing receptor for peripheral T cells. *Nat Immunol.* (2008) 9:301–9. doi: 10.1038/ni1566
36. Cicala C, Martinelli E, Mcnally JP, Goode DJ, Gopaul R, Hiatt J, et al. The integrin α4β7 forms a complex with cell-surface CD4 and defines a T-cell subset that is highly susceptible to infection by HIV-1. *Proc Natl Acad Sci USA.* (2009) 106:20877–82. doi: 10.1073/pnas.0911796106
37. Kader M, Wang X, Piatak M, Lifson J, Roederer M, Veazey R, et al. Alpha4(+)beta7(hi)CD4(+) memory T cells harbor most Th-17 cells and are preferentially infected during acute SIV infection. *Mucosal Immunol.* (2009) 2:439–49. doi: 10.1038/mi.2009.90
38. Ansari AA, Reimann KA, Mayne AE, Takahashi Y, Stephenson ST, Wang R, et al. Blocking of α4β7 gut-homing integrin during acute infection leads to decreased plasma and gastrointestinal tissue viral loads in simian immunodeficiency virus-infected rhesus macaques. *J Immunol.* (2011) 186:1044–59. doi: 10.4049/jimmunol.1003052
39. Kwa S, Kannanganat S, Nigam P, Siddiqui M, Shetty RD, Armstrong W, et al. Plasmacytoid dendritic cells are recruited to the colorectum and contribute to immune activation during pathogenic SIV infection in rhesus macaques. *Blood.* (2011) 118:2763–73. doi: 10.1182/blood-2011-02-339515
40. Calenda G, Frank I, Arrode-Bruses G, Pegu A, Wang K, Arthos J, et al. Delayed vaginal SHIV infection in VRC01 and anti-α4β7 treated rhesus macaques. *PLoS Pathog.* (2019) 15:e1007776. doi: 10.1371/journal.ppat.1007776
41. Sneller MC, Clarridge KE, Seamon C, Shi V, Zorawski MD, Justement JS, et al. An open-label phase 1 clinical trial of the anti-α4β7 monoclonal antibody vedolizumab in HIV-infected individuals. *Sci Transl Med.* (2019) 11:eaax344. doi: 10.1126/scitranslmed.aax3447
42. Berg J. Editorial expression of concern. *Science.* (2019) 365:991. doi: 10.1126/science.aaz2722
43. Uzzan M, Tokuyama M, Rosenstein AK, Tomescu C, Sahbandar IN, Ko HM, et al. Anti-α4β7 therapy targets lymphoid aggregates in the gastrointestinal tract of HIV-1-infected individuals. *Sci Transl Med.* (2018) 10:eaau4711. doi: 10.1126/scitranslmed.aau4711

16

TLR10 Senses HIV-1 Proteins and Significantly Enhances HIV-1 Infection

Bethany M. Henrick[1,2], Xiao-Dan Yao[3], Muhammad Atif Zahoor[3], Alash'le Abimiku[4], Sophia Osawe[4] and Kenneth L. Rosenthal[3] for the InFANT Study Team*

[1] Evolve Biosystems, Davis, CA, United States, [2] Department of Food Science and Technology, University of Nebraska, Lincoln, NE, United States, [3] Department of Pathology and Molecular Medicine, McMaster University, Hamilton, ON, Canada, [4] Institue of Human Virology-Nigeria, Abuja, Nigeria

***Correspondence:**
Kenneth L. Rosenthal
rosenthl@mcmaster.ca

Toll-like receptors (TLRs) play a crucial role in innate immunity and provide a first line of host defense against invading pathogens. Of the identified human TLRs, TLR10 remains an orphan receptor whose ligands and functions are poorly understood. In the present study, we sought to evaluate the level of TLR10 expression in breast milk (BM) and explore its potential function in the context of HIV-1 infection. We evaluated HIV-1-infected (Nigerian: $n = 40$) and uninfected (Nigerian: $n = 27$; Canadian: $n = 15$) BM samples for TLR expression (i.e., TLR10, TLR2, and TLR1) and report here that HIV-1-infected BM from Nigerian women showed significantly higher levels of TLR10, TLR1, and TLR2 expression. Moreover, the level of TLR10 expression in HIV-1-infected BM was upregulated by over 100-fold compared to that from uninfected control women. *In vitro* studies using TZMbl cells demonstrated that TLR10 overexpression contributes to higher HIV-1 infection and proviral DNA integration. Conversely, TLR10 inhibition significantly decreased HIV-1 infection. Notably, HIV-1 gp41 was recognized as a TLR10 ligand, leading to the induction of IL-8 and NF-κBα activation. The identification of a TLR10 ligand and its involvement in HIV-1 infection enhances our current understanding of HIV-1 replication and may assist in the development of improved future therapeutic strategies.

Keywords: human breast milk, HIV-1, gp41, p17, p24, TLR10, IL-8, NF-κBα

INTRODUCTION

Toll-like receptors (TLRs) are the most well-known and researched family of pattern recognition receptors (PRRs) that recognize conserved regions of pathogen-associated molecular patterns (PAMPs) and endogenous danger-associated molecular patterns (DAMPs) responsible for driving cellular activation central to innate immunity. To date, 10 TLRs have been identified in humans, with TLR10 being the only remaining family member without a clearly defined ligand (1, 2); however, a number of ligands, including synthesized TLR2 ligands (i.e., Pam3CSK4 and PamCysPamSK$_4$), have been identified as potential TLR10 PAMPs through computational protein modeling (3).

Once believed to be only preferentially expressed on various types of immune cells (4), TLR10 has now been identified in multiple mucosal sites, including the small intestine, fallopian tubes, eye, and stomach (5–8). Interestingly, many of these sites are also highly affected during acute viral infections, including HIV-1; therefore, identifying ligands for TLR10 and defining the mechanisms of host defense following viral infection is of particular interest for the development of novel vaccines and drug therapies.

Immune activation is critical to HIV-1 infection and pathogenesis, leading to increased proinflammatory cytokine production, T cell exhaustion, and the eventual development of opportunistic infections (9); however, our understanding of immunopathogenesis remains incomplete. Historically, research has focused on HIV-1-specific adaptive immune responses, whereas the role of innate immunity has been largely overlooked, despite the fact that it provides the first line of defense and shapes subsequent adaptive responses. Although the identification of HIV-1 PAMPs recognized by PRRs remain poorly elucidated, data indicate that peripheral blood mononuclear cells (PBMCs) and plasmacytoid dendritic cells (pDCs) derived from HIV-1 infected individuals have increased levels of TLR2, TLR3, TLR4, TLR6, TLR7, and TLR8 mRNA at various stages of disease progression (10, 11). In addition, our laboratory has previously investigated the genital epithelium of Kenyan commercial sex workers and found significant modification in TLR expression, which correlates with resistance to HIV-1 (12). Furthermore, we were the first to demonstrate that soluble TLR2 (sTLR2), which is highly prevalent in human breast milk (BM) (13) serves as an innate antiviral factor in BM and significantly inhibits HIV-1 infection and integration *in vitro* (14, 15). We further reported a significant increase in TLR2 expression in BM cells, and that the overexpression of TLR2 in reporter cells greatly enhanced HIV-1 infection *in vitro* (15). We further identified HIV-1-specific structural proteins, p17, p24, and gp41, which serve as PAMPs, leading to significantly increased immunopathogenesis and infection *in vitro* (16).

Given that TLR10 is a homolog of both TLR2 and TLR1, we hypothesized that TLR10 is involved in sensing specific HIV-1 structural proteins, which leads to increased cellular activation and HIV-1 infection. In this study, we report highly significantly increased TLR10 and TLR1 expression in HIV-1-infected human primary BM cells. Additionally, for the first time, TLR10 was found to be involved in innate immune sensing and cellular activation induced by HIV-1, leading to increased infection *in vitro*. Taken together, we provide clear evidence that specific HIV-1 structural proteins trigger TLR10-dependent cellular activation. These findings indicate that TLR10 and its heterodimers, TLR1 and TLR2, play a central role in the innate immune response to HIV-1 infection by sensing viral proteins, leading to increased immunopathogenesis.

RESULTS

Healthy Human BM Derived Macrophages and Mammary Epithelial Cells Express TLR10, TLR2, and TLR1

Depending on the stage of lactation, the predominant cell types in BM consist of a variety of leukocytes in colostrum (4×10^6 cells/mL) and mature BM (10^5-10^6 cells/mL), as well as mammary epithelial cells (MECs) (16–18). The majority of leukocytes present in BM display an activated phenotype (19) and are comprised primarily of macrophages (55–60%) and neutrophils (30–40%), with the remaining 5–10% composed of lymphocytes (~65% CD8+ T cells, 15% CD4+ T cells, and 20% B cells) (18). Macrophages and MECs are thought to facilitate mother-to-child transmission (MTCT) of HIV-1, and both cell types express several canonical HIV-1 receptors, (e.g., CD4 and CCR5), readily endocytose cell-free HIV-1, and can function as a viral reservoir (20). To explore how TLR expression is linked to HIV-1 infection, we first analyzed the phenotype of the macrophages and MECs present in HIV-1 uninfected human BM using flow cytometry. We found that the majority of cells that were CD14+ and CD45+ (>10%) expressed TLR1 (3.03%), TLR2 (58.6%), and TLR10 (99.3%). Similarly, MUC1+ (75.4%) MECs also expressed TLR1, TLR2, and TLR10 exhibiting 3.67, 69.1, and 0.39%, respectively (**Figure 1**). Based on our flow cytometry data our findings suggest that BM derived macrophages predominantly express TLR10 which implies that these cells may play an important role in innate immunity against invading pathogens in suckling infants.

TLR10 and TLR1 Are Highly Expressed in HIV-1 Infected Human Primary BM Cells

The biological relevance of primary BM cells in HIV MTCT remains unclear. BM derived TLRs such as TLR2, TLR3, and TLR5 along with other bioactive molecules are known to play an important role in intestinal protection, inflammatory responses and even microbial recognition (21). Indeed, it has been suggested that certain cytokines such as interferon gamma secreted by primary BM cells reduce the rate of BM transmission of HIV-1 in breastfeeding infants (22, 23); therefore, we next sought to determine the level of TLR10 and TLR1 expression in BM collected from HIV-1 infected women from Nigeria and compared to HIV-1 uninfected women. Both HIV-1 infected as well as uninfected control women were recruited from Plateau State, Nigeria and a series of BM samples from first week to 52 weeks postpartum were collected and shipped to Canada. All HIV-1 positive women were on antiretroviral therapy (ART) and receiving antiretroviral drugs according to the regimen set by Nigerian Government and world Health Organization (WHO) as described (24) We evaluated HIV-1-infected (Nigerian: $n = 40$) and uninfected (Nigerian: $n = 27$; Canadian: $n = 15$) BM samples for the expression of TLR10 and TLR1. Our results clearly demonstrated a highly significant increase in the expression of both TLR1 and TLR10 cDNA in HIV-1-infected compared to uninfected primary BM cells from the same geographical location (**Figure 2**; $P = 0.0006$ and $P < 0.0001$, respectively). Specifically, TLR10 expression was ~100-fold higher in HIV-1 infected vs. HIV-1 uninfected primary BM cells. In addition to HIV-1 infected and uninfected women from Nigeria, we also collected BM samples from uninfected healthy women from Hamilton region, Ontario, Canada and compared their TLR1 and TLR10 expression levels with uninfected healthy control women from Nigeria. Interestingly, it was found that TLR1 and TLR10 expression on Nigerian HIV-1 uninfected primary BM cells was significantly lower compared to that on Canadian HIV-1

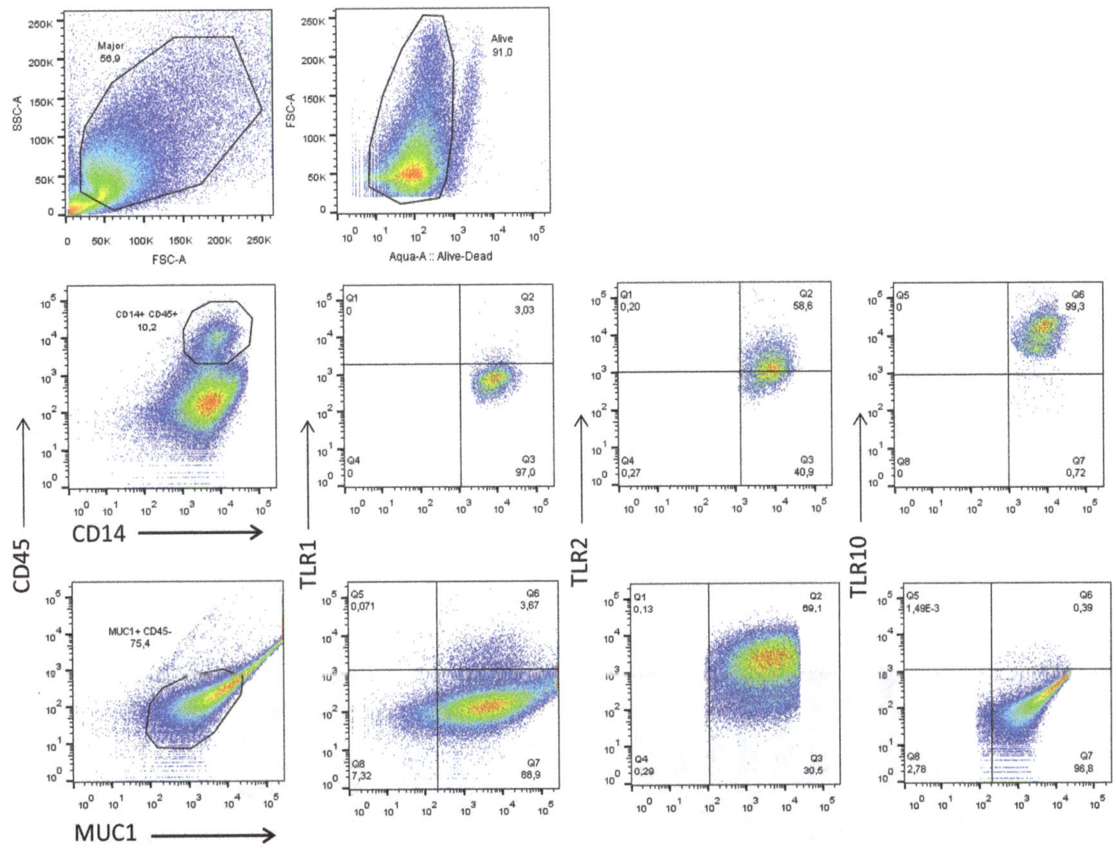

FIGURE 1 | Flow cytometry analyses of TLR1, TLR2, and TLR10 expression in the two major types of primary BM cells obtained from HIV-1 uninfected women at 3 months post-partum. Leucocytes were gated with CD45-PerCP-Cy5.5 and CD14-V450 whereas the epithelial cells were gated with MUC1-PE-Cy7 and CD45-. The antibodies TLR1-APC TLR2-APC and TLR10-PE were separately used to detect TLR1, TLR2, and TLR10 in CD14$^+$-CD45$^+$-MUC1$^-$ and MUC1$^+$-CD45$^-$ cell types to differentiate the two major constituents of BM. Representative images are shown with TLR1, TLR2, and TLR10 expression depicted as percentages on right corner of each image.

uninfected primary BM cells thus highlighting the demographic differences. Taken together, these results show that TLRs are highly expressed on primary BM cells, and this expression may be closely associated with an individual's HIV-1 infection and innate immune status.

The Level of TLR10 Expression Significantly Alters HIV-1 Infection and Integration

Since the extracellular expression of TLR10, TLR1, and TLR2 are innate immune molecules involved in pathogen signaling and are highly expressed on cells in BM (**Figures 1, 2**) and PBMCs (1, 25) we decided to utilize human mammary epithelial (Michigan Cancer Foundation-10A; MCF-10A) cells and macrophage cell lines (human acute monocytic leukemia; THP-1) for further downstream experiments. MCF-10A is a human non-tumorigenic epithelial cell line with no signs of terminal differentiation and has been used in our previous studies (15). THP-1 is an immortalized monocyte-like cell line derived from the peripheral blood of a childhood case of acute monocytic leukemia (26, 27) and has been utilized previously (28). First we determined whether the expression levels could influence HIV-1 infection *in vitro*. For this purpose, HIV-1 reporter TZMbl cells (29) were transiently transfected alone or in combination with plasmids overexpressing TLR10 and the heterodimers, TLR2 and TLR1 (**Figure 3A**), followed by HIV-1 infection and measurement of luciferase activity. The results showed a significantly increased rate of HIV-1 infection in TZMbl cells overexpressing TLR10 and heterodimers TLR1 or TLR2 compared to the empty vector alone, uninfected control or a T20 control (Enfuvirtide; HIV-1 fusion inhibitor) (30, 31) (**Figure 3A**; $P < 0.05$). In addition, HIV-1 infection was significantly elevated in TZMbl cells, which were either co-transfected with TLR1/10 or TLR2/10 compared to the control (**Figure 3A**; $P < 0.05$).

Next, we determined the extent of HIV-1 infection in TLR10 and TLR2 stable reporter cell lines. TZMbl-T2 and TZMbl-T10 displayed significantly higher levels of proviral DNA compared to TZMbl cells, which served as a control (**Figure 3B**; $P < 0.05$). Furthermore, stable TZMbl-T2 transiently over-expressing

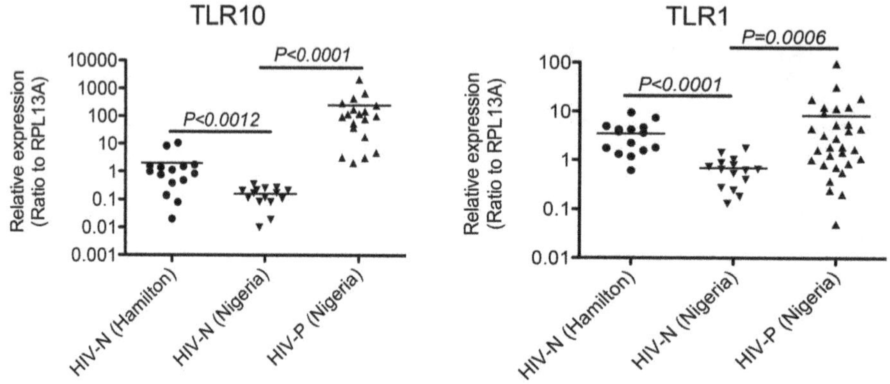

FIGURE 2 | Significantly elevated expression level of TLR1 and TLR10 in HIV-1 infected human primary BM cells. Expression of TLR1 and TLR10 as measured by qRT-PCR with the mRNA extracted from primary BM cells collected from HIV-1 negative Hamilton, Canada women (HIV-N Hamilton) and Nigerian HIV-1 negative (HIV-N) and HIV-1 positive (HIV-P) women. TLR1 expression is shown on right ($p = 0.0006$) whereas TLR10 expression is shown on left ($p < 0.0001$).

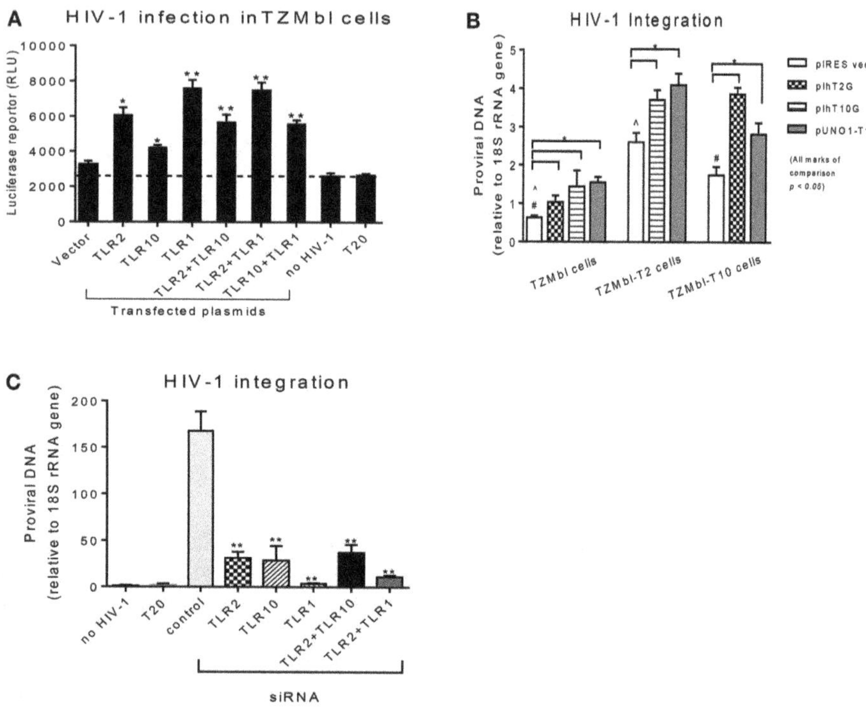

FIGURE 3 | Overexpression or siRNA mediated knockdown of TLR10 significantly alters HIV-1 infection and integration **(A)** HIV-1 infection was significantly enhanced in HIV-1 reporter TZMbl cells transiently overexpressing TLR10 alone and co-transfected with TLR2 or TLR1 expression plasmids by measuring luciferase activity in relative light units (RLU). **(B)** HIV-1 integration was significantly increased in stable TZMbl reporter cells overexpressing TLR10, TLR2, and TLR1. TZMbl, TLR2- stable, and TLR10-stable cells were used for co-transfection with plasmids: empty vector, TLR2, TLR10, and TLR1 vector, TLR10 and TLR1 vector, and TLR2 and TLR1 vector. Proviral DNA (DNA pol) was detected by PCR and normalized to the 18S rRNA gene. **(C)** Proviral DNA was obviously decreased in macrophages with TLR10 knocked down prior to HIV-1 infection. T20: Enfuvirtide, an HIV-1 fusion inhibitor used as a negative control. Data set is representative of three different experiments completed in triplicate (Statistic marks in the plots: $^{*}p < 0.05$, $^{**}p < 0.01$ for Mann Whitney *t*-tests, each group compared to the vector group in A and B, or to the control group in C; pair comparison ∧, # in B, respectively).

TLR10 or TLR1 also enhanced HIV-1 pol gene expression. Similarly, stable TZMbl-T10 cells transiently over-expressing TLR2 or TLR1 also enhanced proviral pol DNA at 8 h post-infection compared with the empty vector-transient stable cells (**Figure 3B**; $P < 0.05$).

In order to observe the HIV-1 infection in susceptible cells, macrophages were differentiated from THP-1 cells to determine whether siRNA-mediated knockdown of TLR1, 2 and/or 10 for 2 days prior to CCR5-tropic HIV-1 (BAL strain) exposure for 7 days would affect the HIV-1 infection rate. THP-1 cells were first transfected with siRNAs targeting TRL1, TLR2, or TLR10, and their knockdown was confirmed by Western blot. TLR1 and TLR2 knockdown was complete compared to TLR10 where it was partial (**Supplementary Figure 1**). After the confirmation of the siRNA-mediated knockdown, HIV-1 integration was determined by PCR, which showed significantly decreased proviral DNA production in the cells that received siRNAs against TLR1, TLR2, TLR10, or combinations of TLR2 with TRL10 or TLR1 compared to the control siRNA (**Figure 3C**). In addition, since we observed incomplete TLR10 knockdown in THP-1 cells, it is likely that upon complete knockdown of TLR10, HIV-1 integration and proviral DNA production will be impacted. Together, these data indicate that the expression of TLR1, 2 and TLR10 alone or in combination significantly enhances HIV-1 infection and integration *in vitro*. Moreover, based on TLR10 and TLR2 co-transfection or co-depletion through siRNA and effect on HIV-1 infection or integration, TLR10 appears to play a role in HIV-1 infection and integration independent of TLR2 since no additive effect of TLR10 and TLR2 was observed (**Figures 3B,C**). Therefore, it is highly likely that TLR2 and TLR10 are independently involved in the regulation of HIV-1 infection in a non-heterodimeric form.

Expression of TLR10, TLR1, and TLR2 Is Up-Regulated by PAMPs and HIV-1

We next determined whether the expression of TLR1, 2, or 10 changes in response to various TLR ligands. MCF-10A, THP-1, and primary BM cells were stimulated with TLR ligands of interest at the following doses: 100 ng/mL Pam3Cys-Ser-(Lys)4 (Pam3CSK4); 10 ng/mL lipopolysaccharide (LPS), ssRNA40 1 μg/mL, and cell-free HIV-1 overnight. Total RNA was isolated from the cells and qRT-PCR was performed. Data showed that compared to medium control, MCF-10A cells exposed to the TLR2/1 ligand, Pam3CSK4, significantly increased the level of TLR1, 2, and 10 expression (**Figure 4A**). Similarly, exposure to TLR4 ligand, LPS, significantly increased TLR1 and 2 expression (**Figure 4A**). In contrast, although ssRNA40 showed a significant increase in TLR1 and TLR10, but had no significant effect on TLR2 expression (**Figure 4A**). Conversely, HIV-1 exposure significantly increased the level of TLR10 expression on MCF-10A cells (**Figure 4A**) despite the fact that HIV-1 does not productively infect this cell type (20). In THP-1 cells, Pam3CSK4 exposure significantly increased the level of TLR2 and 10 expression, whereas LPS exposure resulted in an increase in TLR1 and 2 expression (**Figure 4B**). Following exposure to ssRNA40, the expression of TLR1, 2, and 10 was significantly increased. Similarly, HIV-1 exposure significantly increased the level of TLR1, 2, and 10 expression in THP-1 cells (**Figure 4B**). Primary BM cells exposed to specific PAMPs also exhibited significantly increased levels of TLR1 and TLR2 expression following exposure to Pam3CSK4 and LPS (**Figure 4C**). Elevated TLR2 expression was also observed after exposure to ssRNA40 and cell-free HIV-1 (**Figure 4C**). Most importantly, the data indicated that TLR10 was significantly elevated after exposure to ssRNA40 and HIV-1 (**Figure 4C**). Taken together, these data indicate that specific HIV-1 PAMPs, as well as cell-free HIV-1, significantly increase TLR10, TLR1, and TLR2 expression in primary BM cells.

HIV-1 Proteins Regulate TLR Expression Levels and Induce IL-8 Secretion

HIV-1 structural proteins and glycoproteins have been detected in BM (15) and have been shown to exert immunological effects typical of a proinflammatory response (32–37). Based on our recent findings that HIV-1 structural proteins bind to TLR2 (16), we hypothesized that HIV-1 components may contact the cell surface and trigger TLR10 signaling. Therefore, we next investigated whether specific HIV-1 structural proteins increased cellular activation in primary BM cells. To characterize which HIV-1 structural proteins were involved in this process, we used purified p17 (200 ng/mL), p24 (200 ng/mL), gp41 (1 μg/mL), and gp120 (1 μg/mL) to treat MCF-10A and THP-1 cells and detected the cellular responses. The results demonstrated that the expression of TLR10 and TLR2 mRNA was significantly altered following exposure to gp41 alone compared to untreated medium, as well as Pam3CSK4, which served as a positive control in MCF-10A cells (**Figure 5A**). IL-8 production increased in a dose-dependent manner in the supernatants of MCF-10A cell cultures containing gp41 and Pam3CSK4 (**Figure 5B**). However, TLR10 was significantly highly expressed in THP-1 cells in the presence of gp41 as well as p17 (**Figure 5C**). TLR2 and TLR1 were obviously increased in the presence of gp41, p17, and p24. In the THP-1 cell culture, IL-8 was also correspondingly produced with increases in the amount of Pam3CSK4 and structural proteins, except gp120 (**Figure 5D**). Together, this data indicates that HIV-1 gp41 is able to induce the innate immune response and alters the level of TLR10 expression, similar to TLR2 (16) and is not cell-type-sensitive.

Furthermore, we confirmed our observations by transfecting THP-1 cells with siRNA specific to target genes (**Figure 6A**). Compared to the cells treated with the control siRNA, TLR10 siRNA suppressed more than 3-fold of IL-8 production in the cells treated with HIV-1 PAMPs. Treatment with TLR2 siRNA decreased IL-8 production by ~2-fold. The combination of TLR10 and TLR2 siRNAs decreased IL-8 production more than 2-fold. In addition, we used antibodies to neutralize TLR10, TLR2, and TLR1 in gp41 and p17-treated THP-1 cells. As shown in **Figure 6B**, treatment with anti-TLR10 and TLR1 antibodies significantly reduced IL-8 production in gp41- and p17-treated cells, respectively. Anti-TLR2 antibodies exhibited a similar trend but without a statistical difference. Since the primary focus of this study was TLR10-related events, we only used anti-TLR10 antibodies to treat MCF-10A cells in the neutralization experiments. The results revealed that gp41-induced IL-8 production was also significantly decreased in the presence of the anti-TLR10 antibody (**Figure 6C**). Similarly, primary BM cells were incubated with the anti-TLR10 antibody before treatment with HIV-1 proteins. The data revealed that gp41-induced IL-8 production was also significantly decreased in the presence of TLR10 antibodies in primary BM cells

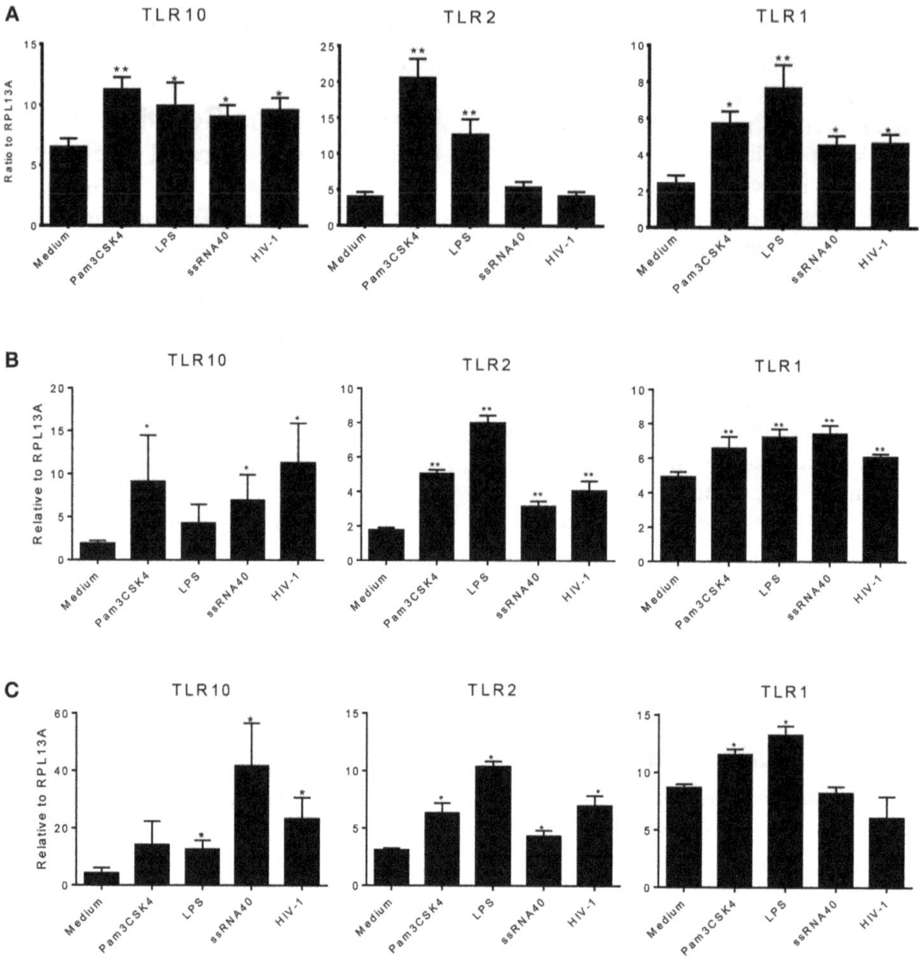

FIGURE 4 | Effects of PAMPs and HIV-1 on the level of TLR expression in cell cultures. **(A)** qRT-PCR of TLR10, TLR2, and TLR1 mRNA from MCF-10A cells treated with TLR2 PAMP Pam3CSK4, TLR4 PAMP LPS, TLR7/TLR8 PAMP ssRNA40, and cell-free HIV-1 BAL. **(B)** q-RT-PCR in THP-1 cells. **(C)** qRT-PCR in primary BM cells. Data set is representative of three different experiments completed in triplicate. Statistic marks: $^{*}p < 0.05$, $^{**}p < 0.01$ for the Mann-Whitney *t*-tests, each group compared to medium-treated group (Medium).

(**Figure 6D**). These results suggest that HIV-1 gp41 is capable of upregulating both TLR2 (15) and TLR10 in all cells under our experimental conditions.

HIV-1 Proteins Induce TLR10, TLR2, and TLR1 Signaling Through the Activation of NF-κBα

TLR2 and TLR1-mediated signaling pathways have been well-studied. We have recently discovered that the HIV-1 structural proteins p17, p24, and gp41 directly interact with TLR2, inducing NF-κBα activation. We then asked whether these structural proteins also induce NF-κBα activation via their PAMP effects on TLR10. Cells were treated with Pam3CSK4, p17, p24, and gp41, followed by a Western blot of the lysates with anti-phospho-IκBα, a subunit of NF-κBα that is representative of active NF-κBα. The results in **Figure 7A** demonstrate that activated NF-κBα was substantially expressed in MCF-10A cells treated with gp41, compared to the positive control (Pam3CSK4) and negative control (medium)-treated cells. In contrast, moderate expression of P-IκBα was observed in the MCF-10A cells treated with p17. However, in both the macrophages derived from THP-1 and BM cells, the three HIV-1 proteins greatly stimulated the production of active NF-κBα. In addition, translocation of the NF-κBα p65 subunit into the nuclei occurred in MCF-10A cells treated with Pam3CSK4 and gp41 (**Figure 7B**). p65 translocation was observed in a number of MCF-10A cells in the presence of p17 and p24. Compared to the medium control, treatment with Pam3CSK4 and each of the three HIV-1 proteins led to p65 translocation to the nuclei of THP-1 cells.

When TLR10 expression was knocked down using siRNA, NF-κBα activation in response to HIV-1 proteins was significantly reduced in THP-1 cells (**Figure 8**). The signaling activity induced by the ligation of TLR2 and TLR1 by the positive siRNA control was similar to the response induced by TLR10 activation by the three HIV-1 proteins (p17, p24, and gp41), suggesting that these proteins are involved in the activation of NF-κBα. Considering the possibility that endotoxin

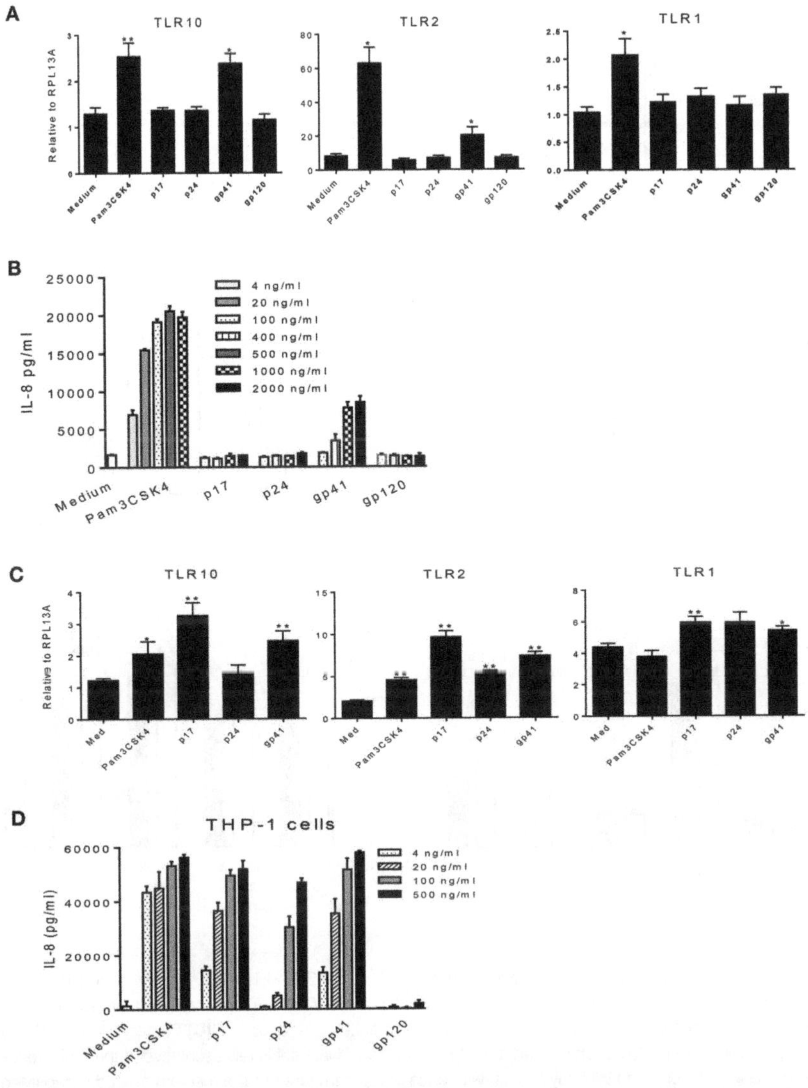

FIGURE 5 | Effects of HIV-1 proteins on TLR expression and cellular responses. **(A)** MCF-10A cells were treated with Pam3CSK4 and the HIV-1 structural proteins: p17, p24, gp41, and gp120. Cellular TLR10, TLR2, and TLR1 mRNAs were analyzed by qRT-PCR. **(B)** IL-8 production in cell culture supernatants in the presence of different concentrations of Pam3CSK4 and HIV-1 proteins were analyzed by ELISA. **(C)** The expression of TLR mRNAs analyzed by qRT-PCR in THP-1 cells treated with Pam3CSK4 and the HIV-1 structural proteins: p17, p24, and gp41. **(D)** IL-8 production in THP-1 cell culture supernatants in the presence of different concentrations of Pam3CSK4 and HIV-1 proteins was analyzed by ELISA. Data set is representative of three different experiments completed in triplicate. Statistic marks: $^*p < 0.05$, $^{**}p < 0.01$ for the Mann-Whitney *t*-tests, each group was compared to the medium-treated group (Medium).

was present in the HIV-1 products, we used TLR4 siRNA in the same experiment. The Western blot results clearly showed that knocking down TLR4 did not change the cellular response to p17 and gp41 in activating NF-κBα, which excluded endotoxin or LPS contamination in the two proteins. A 50% reduction in NF-κBα activation was observed in TLR4 siRNA transfected cells treated with Pam3CSK4 and p24, thus indicating cross-talk and a convergence between the different TLR signaling pathways.

DISCUSSION

To date, a total of 10 (1–10) human TLRs have been identified, which are known to play an important role in the innate immune sensing of invading pathogens (38, 39). Although the ligands for TLRs 1 through 9 are well-known, TLR10 has remained the only orphan receptor with no known ligand, despite being identified >17 years ago (4). To our knowledge, we are the first to report that TLR10 is involved in HIV-1 infection and most importantly, that gp41 acts as a ligand for TLR10 in human macrophages and MECs.

We initially attempted to identify and screen TLRs present in human BM and previously reported that soluble TLR2 (sTLR2) is present in human BM and significantly inhibits HIV-1 infection (15). Furthermore, we also showed that the HIV-1 structural proteins, p17, p24, and gp41, serve as PAMPs for TLR2, leading to the activation of the NF-κBα signaling pathway (16).

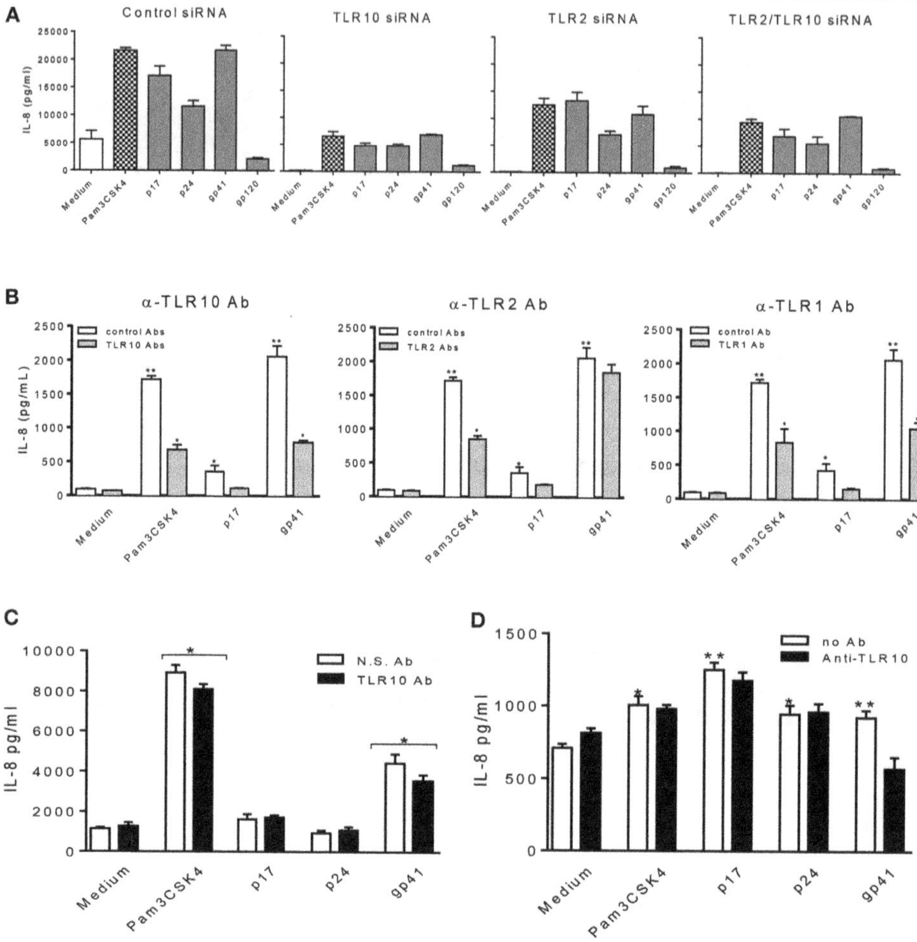

FIGURE 6 | HIV-1 proteins, p17 and gp41 elicit cellular responses through sensing TLR10, TLR2, and TLR1. IL-8 production stimulated by Pam3CSK4, p17, p24, and gp41 was greatly suppressed in THP-1 cells knocked-down of TLR10 with specific siRNA **(A)** and THP-1 cells neutralized with anti-TLR10 antibody **(B)**. **(C)** IL-8 stimulated by Pam3CSK4 and gp41 was reduced in MCF-10A cells neutralized with an anti-TLR10 antibody. **(D)** Primary BM cells displayed a significant decrease in IL-8 production induced by HIV-1 gp41 following neutralization with an anti-TLR10 antibody. Data set is representative of three different experiments completed in triplicate. Statistic marks: $^{*}p < 0.05$; $^{**}p < 0.01$ for Mann Whitney *t*-tests, with each group compared to the medium treated group (Medium).

Surprisingly, with the exception of TLR1 and TLR2, we found significantly higher levels of TLR10 (>100-fold) expression in BM samples collected from HIV-1 infected Nigerian women (**Figure 2**), thus indicating that TLR10 might play an important role in HIV-1 infection and pathogenesis. In addition, uninfected BM samples from Canadian women exhibited higher basal levels of TLR10 and TLR1 expression compared to uninfected Nigerian women. Although whether there is a significant difference in the level of these two TLRs in healthy populations remains unknown, it is tempting to speculate that the genetic differences present in these two populations might affect the outcome of HIV-1 infection.

TLR1, TLR6, and TLR10 share a common locus on chromosome 4p14 and are structurally similar to each another (40) and are thought to have arisen from several gene duplication events (41). Furthermore, it has been established that TLR10, TLR1, and TLR6 form a single cluster and provide an important first line of defense against infectious agents. Previous work related to TLR1, TLR2, TLR6, and TLR10 has failed to provide the agonist for TLR10 but suggests that the TLR10 ligand might be of a viral origin, leading to the activation of NF-κBα (40, 42). Our current study confirms that one ligand for TLR10 is indeed of viral origin, notably HIV-1 gp41.

TLR10 is known to possess point mutations in its TIR domain that play a critical role in its proper functioning (43). Furthermore, it has been shown that genetic variations in TLR10 can lead to various ailments, such as Crohn's disease (44) and asthma (45). Moreover, TLR10 has been shown to be involved in osteoarthritis (46), Crimean Congo hemorrhagic fever (47), *Listeria monocytogenes*, *Salmonella* Typhimurium (28), *Helicobacter pylori* (7), and influenza (2). Nevertheless, the involvement of TLR10 in various diseases paves the way for future exploratory studies.

Interestingly, recent data concerning early hominins, Neandertals, and Denisovans, who lived in Europe and Western Asia for over 200,000 years, likely interbred and

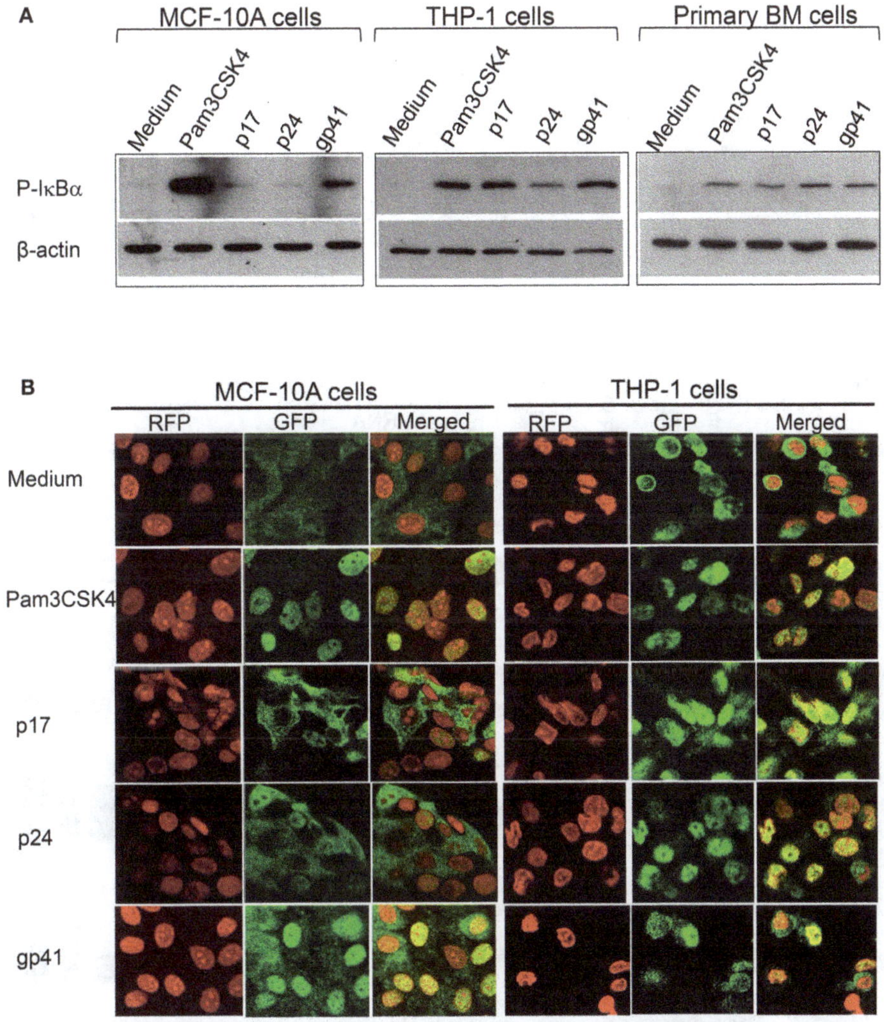

FIGURE 7 | HIV-1 proteins lead to NF-κBα activation **(A)** Western blot analysis of the cell lysates extracted from MCF-10A, THP-1, and primary BM cells treated with HIV-1 proteins and detected with an antibody against the active NF-κBα subunit, phospho(P)-IκBα, with anti β-actin used as the loading control on the same membranes **(B)** Confocal microscopy of HIV-treated MCF-10A and THP-1 cells fixed and stained with an anti- NF-κBα subunit p65 antibody and visualized with a second antibody, anti-rabbit-IgG-alexa488 (GFP; green), p65 was translocated upon activation into the nuclei (RFP; red with propidium iodide staining) displayed in yellow (Merged).

contributed advantageous genetic alleles to the immune systems of modern humans (48–50). Indeed, TLR genes, which are critical components of innate immunity, have also gained advantageous alleles through this mixing of the gene pool. Notably, adaptive introgression and local positive selection led to the significantly increased expression of the TLR6, TLR1, and TLR10 genes, which facilitated resistance to infectious diseases but may also be associated with increased hypersensitivity to non-pathogenic allergens.

Primary BM cells, MCF-10A MECs, and macrophages display significantly higher levels of TLR10 expression in response to HIV-1. In particular, gp41, not p17, and p24, was able to act as a ligand for TLR10. Since primary BM cells express TLR2, TLR1, and TLR10 (**Figures 1, 2**); thus, it is plausible that these TLRs could form heterodimers.

Our data have shown that macrophages and MECs are human BM constituents that express TLR1, TLR2, and TLR10. Although gp41 was found to act as a ligand for both TLR2 (16) and TLR10 in the current study. Whether TLR2 and TLR10 interact and associate with each other in the context of an HIV-1 infection remains unclear and will be intriguing to investigate in future studies. However, since macrophages derived from THP-1 cells sensed gp41 in addition to p17 and p24, it is suggested that BM derived macrophages actively participates in HIV-1-induced innate immunity.

Although the induction of TLR10 by immune cells (e.g., B-cells, plasmacytoid dendritic cells, and macrophages) is well-reported (28, 40); the induction of TLR10 by non-immune cells (e.g., intestinal epithelial cells or MECs) raises the possibility of a

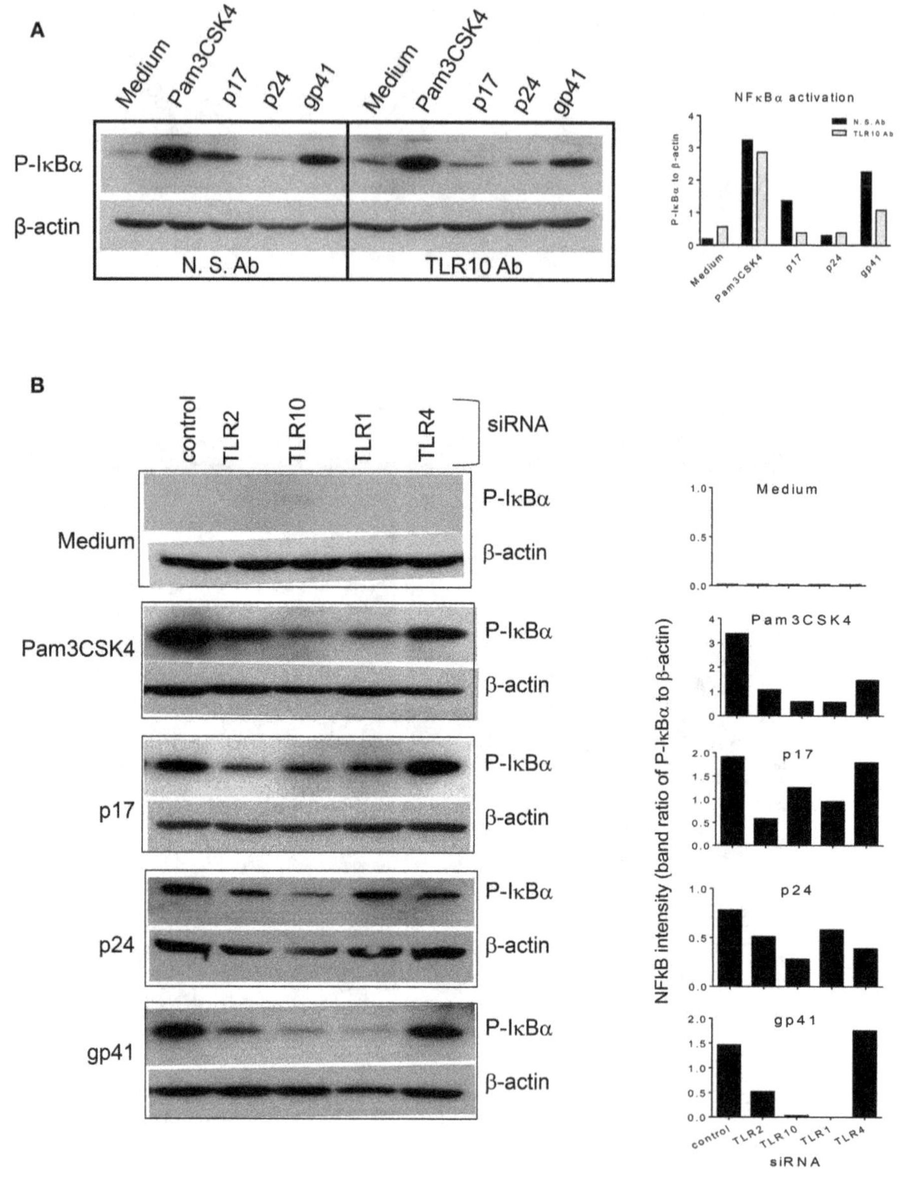

FIGURE 8 | siRNA mediated knockdown or antibody mediated blocking of TLR10 inhibits NF-κBα activation induced by HIV-1 proteins **(A)** anti-TLR10 antibody decreased gp41 induced P-IκBα by half in MCF-10A cells. **(B)** TLR10 siRNA ablated the induction of P-IκBα by gp41 in THP-1 cells.

conserved mechanism regarding TLR10 expression by epithelial cells (28).

We suggest that TLR10 and TLR1 both work cooperatively as the transfection of TRL10 and TLR1 alone or in combination significantly enhanced HIV-1 infection, indicating that TLR10 and TLR1 likely form heterodimers. This is evidenced by the observation that a depletion of TLR10 by a siRNA-mediated knockdown negatively impacted the proviral integration of HIV-1. Moreover, TLR10 knockdown led to significantly lower levels of IL-8 production in cells treated with gp41, p17, and p24. Furthermore, gp41, p17, and p24 were able to activate NF-κBα, which was readily blocked using an anti-TLR10 antibody or TLR10-specific siRNA-treated cells, suggesting that TLR10 signaling led to the activation of NF-κBα and ultimately the production of IL-8.

Importantly, the present study provides the first evidence that HIV-1 gp41 functions as a ligand for TLR10 in MCF-10A and THP-1 cells. Recently, double-stranded RNA (dsRNA) has been shown to act as a ligand for TLR10 (51). In addition, the same study demonstrated that TLR10 competes with TLR3 for binding to ligands in various endocytic pathways, ultimately leading to the induction of interferons. Similarly, synergy between TLR3 and TLR10 has been suggested in the context of an influenza virus infection. Although our current data demonstrates the involvement of TLR10 in HIV-1 infection, the existence of such synergy between TLR10 and TLR3 in an HIV-1 infection cannot be dismissed and requires further future investigation.

Our data demonstrated that HIV-1 gp41 acts as a ligand for TLR10 and leads to the induction of IL-8 and NF-κBα activation. However, our observation is contradictory to some previous reports where TLR10 expression has been shown to suppress the cytokine responses (1, 52). These contradictions could be due to differences in cell-type use, ligand specificity or geographical location. Further, divergent roles of TLR10 have been suggested to be due to the mechanism of cross-talking between TLR10 and TLR3 (51) or perhaps the interaction of TLR10 with TLR2, TLR1 and TLR6 (1). Although, the exact mechanism is not known; we cannot exclude the possibility of spontaneous heterodimerization of TLR2 and TLR10 (1) due to HIV-1 gp41 which acts as a ligand for both TLR2 (16) and TLR10.

The present investigation demonstrated that TLR10 acts as an innate immune sensor for HIV-1 infection and leads to the induction of IL-8. Furthermore, we showed that blocking TLR10 with either an anti-TLR10 antibody or siRNA attenuates gp41-mediated NF-κBα activation (**Figure 8**). Interestingly, TLR1 depletion through siRNA knockdown also inhibited gp41-mediated NF-κB activation, suggesting that TLR1 and TLR10 might form a heterodimer. Recent evidence shows that TLR10 plays a key role in the innate immune response following an influenza infection (2). Specifically, it was found that silencing of the TLR10 gene impacted IL-8 production in human influenza virus-infected macrophages. Similarly, we observed that when TRL10 is silenced in HIV-1 infected macrophages, IL-8 production is severely impaired, thus raising the possibility that there is a conserved mechanism during HIV-1 and influenza virus infections in human macrophages.

Our studies have shown that human primary BM cells express significantly higher levels of TLR1, TLR2, and TLR10. Currently, the precise role of these TLRs in infants following BM ingestion remains unknown. However, in our other ongoing studies, we have identified some novel exosomal miRNAs in BM samples exclusive to HIV-1 infection present in mother's milk (data not shown) that could potentially play a protective role during MTCT of HIV-1 in conjunction with these TLRs.

Taken together, our data reveal for the first time that TLR10 is involved in HIV-1 infection. Furthermore, gp41 was found to act as a novel ligand for TLR10. We believe that the data shown in the present study describing an HIV-1 ligand for TLR10 will advance our current knowledge, as well as further our understanding of the role of TLR10 in innate immunity during HIV-1 infection.

MATERIALS AND METHODS

Human Subjects

HIV-1-uninfected (Hamilton, Ontario, Canada and Nigeria) and HIV-infected (Nigeria) women were recruited to participate in the present study. All HIV-infected women were in the chronic phase of infection as determined by at least two positive HIV-1 serological tests separated by at least 1 year. All women were sampled during voluntary "healthy" research visits as per the cohort protocol, and therefore, were not acutely ill at the time of assessment. Written as well as informed consent for the collection of demographics, behavioral data and biological samples were obtained from all study participants. Inclusion criteria included breastfeeding women who were HIV-uninfected and did not report complications *in utero* during their full-term pregnancies or intrapartum. Women were excluded if they had cesarean sections, their pregnancies were not full-term, or they were diagnosed with mastitis post-partum. Samples included in these analyses were obtained from women who were not taking medications other than vitamin supplements intra- or post-partum and did not receive an epidural intra-partum. Three mothers reported minor colic and one reported silent reflux in their infants. The study was approved by the institutional review boards of the University of Manitoba Hospital ethical review committee. All clinical investigations were conducted according to the principles of the Helsinki Declaration. The study was approved by the McMaster Research Ethics Board (REB Approval #08-176) and the CCI of Children's Hospital, Los Angeles.

Sample Acquisition and Preparation

Milk samples were self-collected into sterile tubes within the first week and at 1, 3, and 6 months post-partum, and immediately shipped on ice for processing in our laboratory. The samples were separated into lipid, supernatant, and cellular fractions and stored at −80°C and liquid nitrogen, respectively. BM supernatant fractions were used for Western blotting or were filter-sterilized (0.45 μm) for functional assays to avoid cellular contamination.

Cells and Reagents

THP-1 and primary BM cells were cultured in RMPI-1640 supplemented with 10% FBS, 2 mM L-glutamine, 10 mM HEPES, 1 mM Sodium Pyruvate, and 1% penicillin/streptomycin (Invitrogen). MCF-10A cells (American Type Culture Collection, Manassas, VA) were maintained in Dulbecco's modified Eagle's medium-F12 (DMEM/F12, Invitrogen) supplemented with 5% horse serum (Invitrogen), 100 ng/mL cholera toxin (Sigma), 10 μg/mL insulin (Sigma), 20 ng/mL recombinant human EGF (Peprotech), 0.5 μg/mL hydrocortisone (Sigma), and 1% penicillin/streptomycin (Invitrogen). The TZMbl cells were cultured in DMEM supplemented with 10% FBS and 1% (vol/vol) each of L-glutamine, penicillin, and streptomycin with and without 0.8 mg/mL geneticin (G418; Invitrogen, Burlington, ON, Canada), respectively, as described previously (16, 29). HIV-1 proteins included p17 (Virogen, Mississauga, ON, Canada), p24, and gp41 (Genway Biotech, Inc., San Diego, CA, USA). TLR ligands, ssRNA40 (Mobix, McMaster University), LPS, Pam3CSK4 (InvivoGen), and poly I:C (Sigma-Aldrich, Burlington, ON, Canada) were diluted in phosphate-buffered saline (PBS).

Quantitative Reverse-Transcriptase Real-Time Polymerase Chain Reaction

Total RNA was extracted from the cells using Trizol as per the manufacturer (Invitrogen, Carlsbad, California, USA) and treated with DNase I, DNA-free (Ambion, Austin, Texas, USA).

Reverse transcription (RT) reactions and quantitative real-time PCR (qRT-PCR) was performed as previously described (11).

Small Interfering RNA Knockdown

siRNA molecules targeting human TLR1 (Sigma-Aldrich, SASI_Hs01_00162170/AS), TLR2 (Sigma-Aldrich, SASI_Hs01_ 00081589/AS), TLR4 (Sigma-Aldrich, SASI_Hs01_00122250/AS), TLR10 (Sigma-Aldrich, SASI_Hs01_00099892), or non-targeting siRNA (Invitrogen, 129201 H07/129296 H05) were purchased and used as previously described (16). The cells were exposed to specific HIV-1 proteins, and the supernatants were collected to quantify the level of pro-inflammatory cytokine production as previously described (16).

Flow Cytometry

Flow cytometry analysis was performed as previously described (53). Briefly, 10 mL of fresh healthy human BM containing ~5 × 10^6 cells collected within 3 months of lactation, was centrifuged at 2,000 × g at room temperature for 10 min, washed with PBS, and centrifuged two more times. The cells were first incubated with Live/Dead Fixable Aqua (ThermoFisher) at room temperature for 30 min and subsequently washed twice with PBS. Besides compensation and FMO controls, two sets of cells were immune-stained at room temperature for 30 min in 0.5% BSA-PBS containing a combination of conjugated antibodies (CD45-PerCP-Cy5.5 BD, CD14-V450 BD, MUC1-PE-Cy7 BioLegend, TLR2-APC R&D Systems, TLR10-PE BioLegend) and (CD45-PerCP-Cy5.5, CD14-V450, MUC1-PE-Cy7, TLR1-APC R&D Systems, TLR10-PE), respectively. The cells were washed twice with PBS and fixed with 1% PFA-PBS. The samples were run on a BD LSRFortessa and analyzed using FlowJo software.

Establishment of a Stable TLR10 Reporter Cell Line

The TLR10 expression plasmid, pIhT10G, was subcloned from pUNO1-hTLR10 (InvivoGen) into pIRES2-Green1 vector (Clontech), with a *SacI-BamHI* fragment via PCR using Phusion DNA polymerase (New England Biolabs, USA). Transfection with 2.5 μg pIhT10G and 5 μL Lipofectamine 2,000 into TZMbl cells was performed in a six-well plate for 2 days. The cells were trypsinized and re-suspended in 0.2–1.4 mg/mL series of G418 geneticin (Thermo Fisher Scientific, MA, USA) containing growth medium in a 96-well plate, and cultured for at least 7 days, followed by repeating the selection for a total of three times in the same manner. The established cells were named TZMbl-10 and cultured in 0.2–0.4 mg/mL geneticin growth medium.

HIV-1 Infection and Integration

TZMbl and the derived TZMbl-2 and TZMbl-10 cells were transfected with plasmids, phT2G (16), phT10G, and pUNO1-hT1 (InvivoGen) expressing TLR10, TLR2, and TLR1, with PolyJet (SignaGen Rockville, MD, USA) in a 96-well plate for 24 h. The cells were infected with HIV-1 BAL 30-50 $TCID_{50}$/96-well plus 12 μg/mL DEAE-dextran for 45 h for HIV-1 infection. The proviral DNA analysis was performed by measuring the relative light units of luciferase activity for 8 h.

THP-1 cells grown in a 96-well plate were expanded in 8 mM PMA-growth medium for 3 days and PMA-free medium for another 2 days. The cells were then transfected with specific siRNAs using Lipofectamine RNAiMAX reagent (Thermo Fisher Scientific, MA, USA) for 2 days. The cells were infected with HIV-1 BAL 100 $TCID_{50}$/well plus 4 μg/mL polybrene overnight and washed with growth medium and cultured for a total of 7 days. HIV-1 integration was detected by the isolation of total cellular DNA using proteinase K digestion and phenol extraction, followed by PCR of the viral pol gene. The proviral DNA was normalized to the cellular 18S rRNA gene in a same sample.

IL-8 ELISA

IL-8 production from the cell culture was assessed via an EB ELISA in 20–100-fold dilution as per the manufacturer's instruction as described previously (16).

Stimulation of Primary BM Cells *in vitro* and Neutralization

Healthy BM was diluted 2-fold in PBS and the cells were isolated by centrifugation at 800 × g for 20 min. The lipid layer and fluid were removed, and the cell pellet was washed twice with PBS. The cells were resuspended in a 96-well plate at a density of 1.5 × 10^5 per well with RPMI-1640 medium and cultured overnight.

Since none of the available anti-TLR10 antibodies were able to efficiently neutralize TLR10 alone under our experimental conditions (data not shown), we used a cocktail of TLR10 antibodies from different sources comprising rabbit polyclonal sc-30198 (Santa Cruz Biotechnology, Santa Cruz, CA, USA), mouse monoclonal sc-293300 (Santa Cruz Biotechnology, Santa Cruz, CA, USA), mouse anti-human TLR10 H00081793-M01 (Novus Biologicals), and mouse monoclonal MA6619 (R&D Systems) compared to a cocktail control which consisted of rabbit and mouse isotype IgG controls (Santa Cruz Biotechnology, Santa Cruz, CA, USA).

Western Blot

The cells were washed with PBS and the lysates were prepared as previously described (16). Protein quantification was performed using a DC™ protein assay kit (Bio-Rad) and run on SDS-PAGE gels. The primary antibodies consisted of anti-TLR1, anti-TLR2 (R&D Systems), anti-TLR4 (Novus Biologicals), anti-TLR10 (Santa Cruz Biotechnology, Santa Cruz, CA, USA), phospho-IκBα #9246 (Cell Signaling), NF-κBα p65 sc-372 (Santa Cruz Biotechnology, Santa Cruz, CA, USA), and anti-β-actin antibodies. HRP-labeled goat anti-mouse IgG 1706516 (Bio-Rad) and HRP-labeled goat anti-rabbit IgG 1706515 (Bio-Rad) were used as secondary antibodies.

Confocal Microscopy

Immunofluorescence staining was performed as previously described (54). MCF-10A and THP1 cells grown on an eight-well BD Falcon culture slides (BD Biosciences) were either left untreated or treated with Pam3CSK4, or the HIV-1 proteins p17, p24, and gp41. The cells were fixed and immune-stained with NF-κBα p65 (1:500) to detect the nuclear translocation of NF-κBα p65. Corresponding Alexa Fluor 488 conjugated IgG (Molecular Probes, Eugene, OR, USA) was used as a secondary antibody. The images were acquired using an inverted laser-scanning confocal microscope (LSM 510, Zeiss, Oberkochen, Germany).

Statistical Analysis

The data were plotted and analyzed using Microsoft Excel, SPSS, and Prism 4.0 software and shown as Mean ± SEM (GraphPad Software, San Diego, California, USA). Non-parametric tests were used, including Mann-Whitney U-tests for unmatched comparisons, Wilcoxon paired *t*-tests for matched samples, and a Spearman's rank test for matched correlations.

AUTHOR CONTRIBUTIONS

BH, X-YD and MZ performed the experiments and wrote the manuscript. AA and SO performed clinical studies and collected the human samples. BH and KR conceived the idea. KR supervised the work, obtained the grant and wrote the manuscript.

ACKNOWLEDGMENTS

This work was supported by a grant from the Canadian Institute of Health Research (CIHR) as a part of the Canadian HIV-1 Vaccine Initiative (CHVI). We would like to thank the Canadian and Nigerian women who participated in our study.

REFERENCES

1. Oosting M, Cheng S-C, Bolscher JM, Vestering-Stenger R, Plantinga TS, Verschueren IC, et al. Human TLR10 is an anti-inflammatory pattern-recognition receptor. *Proc Natl Acad Sci USA.* (2014) 111:E4478–84. doi: 10.1073/pnas.1410293111
2. Lee SMY, Kok K-H, Jaume M, Cheung TKW, Yip T-F, Lai JCC, et al. Toll-like receptor 10 is involved in induction of innate immune responses to influenza virus infection. *Proc Natl Acad Sci USA.* (2014) 111:3793–98. doi: 10.1073/pnas.1324266111
3. Guan Y, Ranoa DRE, Jiang S, Mutha SK, Li X, Baudry J, Tapping RI. Human TLRs 10 and 1 Share Common Mechanisms of Innate Immune Sensing but Not Signaling. *J Immunol.* (2010) 184:5094–103. doi: 10.4049/jimmunol.0901888
4. Chuang TH, Ulevitch RJ. Identification of hTLR10: a novel human toll-like receptor preferentially expressed in immune cells. *Biochim Biophys Acta.* (2001) 1518:157–61. doi: 10.1016/S0167-4781(00)00289-X
5. Hart KM, Murphy AJ, Barrett KT, Wira CR, Guyre PM, Pioli PA. Functional expression of pattern recognition receptors in tissues of the human female reproductive tract. *J Reprod Immunol.* (2009) 80:33–40. doi: 10.1016/j.jri.2008.12.004
6. Mohammed I, Abedin A, Tsintzas K, Abedin SA, Otri AM, Hopkinson A, et al. Increased expression of hepcidin and toll-like receptors 8 and 10 in viral keratitis. *Cornea.* (2011) 30:899–904. doi: 10.1097/ICO.0b013e31820126e5
7. Nagashima H, Iwatani S, Cruz M, Abreu JAJ, Uchida T, Mahachai V, et al. Toll-like receptor 10 in helicobacter pylori infection. *J Infect Dis.* (2015) 212:1666–76. doi: 10.1093/infdis/jiv270
8. Chougule P, Herlenius G, Hernandez NM, Patil PB, Xu B, Sumitran-Holgersson S. Isolation and characterization of human primary enterocytes from small intestine using a novel method. *Scand J Gastroenterol.* (2012) 47:1334–43. doi: 10.3109/00365521.2012.708940
9. Deeks SG. Immune dysfunction, inflammation, and accelerated aging in patients on antiretroviral therapy. *Top HIV Med.* (2008) 17:118–23. doi: 10.1109/ICASSP.2005.1416298
10. Lester RT, Yao XD, Ball TB, McKinnon LR, Omange WR, Kaul R, et al. HIV-1 RNA dysregulates the natural TLR response to subclinical endotoxemia in Kenyan female sex-workers. *PLoS ONE.* (2009) 4:e5644. doi: 10.1371/journal.pone.0005644
11. Lester RT, Yao XD, Ball TB, McKinnon LR, Kaul R, Wachihi C, ET AL. Toll-like receptor expression and responsiveness are increased in viraemic HIV-1 infection. *AIDS.* (2008) 22:685–94. doi: 10.1097/QAD.0b013e3282f4de35
12. Yao XD, Omange RW, Henrick BM, Lester RT, Kimani J, Ball TB, et al. Acting locally: innate mucosal immunity in resistance to HIV-1 infection in kenyan commercial sex workers. *Mucos Immun.* (2014) 7:268–79. doi: 10.1038/mi.2013.44
13. LeBouder E, Rey-Nores JE, Rushmere NK, Grigorov M, Lawn SD, Affolter M, et al. Soluble forms of Toll-Like Receptor (TLR)2 capable of modulating TLR2 signaling are present in human plasma and breast milk. *J Immunol.* (2003) 171:6680–9. doi: 10.4049/jimmunol.171.12.6680
14. Henrick BM, Nag K, Yao X-D, Drannik AG, Aldrovandi GM, Rosenthal KL. Milk matters: soluble Toll-Like Receptor 2 (sTLR2) in breast milk significantly inhibits HIV-1 infection and inflammation. *PLoS ONE.* (2012) 7:e40138. doi: 10.1371/journal.pone.0040138
15. Henrick BM, Yao XD, Drannik AG, Abimiku A, Rosenthal KL, INFANT Study Team. Soluble Toll-like receptor 2 is significantly elevated in HIV-1 infected breast milk and inhibits HIV-1 induced cellular activation, inflammation and infection. *AIDS.* (2014) 28:2023–32. doi: 10.1097/QAD.00000000000000381
16. Henrick BM, Yao XD, Rosenthal KL. HIV-1 structural proteins serve as PAMPs for TLR2 heterodimers significantly increasing infection and innate immune activation. *Front Immunol.* (2015) 6:426. doi: 10.3389/fimmu.2015.00426
17. Goldman AS. Human milk, leukocytes, and immunity. *J Pediatr.* (1977) 90:167–8. doi: 10.1016/S0022-3476(77)80805-6
18. Jain N, Mathur NB, Sharma VK, Dwarkadas AM. Cellular composition including lymphocyte subsets in preterm and full term human colostrum and milk. *Acta Paediatr Scand.* (1991) 80:395–9.
19. Michie CA, Tantscher E, Schall T, Rot A. Physiological secretion of chemokines in human breast milk. *Eur Cytokine Netw.* (1998) 9:123–9.
20. Dorosko SM, Connor RI. Primary human mammary epithelial cells endocytose HIV-1 and facilitate viral infection of CD4 $^{+}$ T lymphocytes. *J Virol.* (2010) 84:10533–42. doi: 10.1128/JVI.01263-10
21. Cacho NT, Lawrence RM. Innate immunity and breast milk. *Front Immunol.* (2017) 8:584. doi: 10.3389/fimmu.2017.00584
22. Satomi M, Shimizu M, Shinya E, Watari E, Owaki A, Hidaka C, et al. Transmission of macrophage-tropic HIV-1 by breast-milk macrophages via DC-SIGN. *J Infect Dis.* (2005) 191:174–81. doi: 10.1086/426829
23. Lohman-Payne B, Slyker JA, Moore S, Maleche-Obimbo E, Wamalwa DC, Richardson BA, et al. Breast milk cellular HIV-specific interferon gamma responses are associated with protection from peripartum HIV transmission. *AIDS.* (2012) 26:2007–16. doi: 10.1109/ICFHR.2014.121
24. Dalhatu I, Onotu D, Odafe S, Abiri O, Debem H, Agolory S, et al. Outcomes of Nigeria's HIV/AIDS treatment program for patients initiated on

antiretroviral treatment between 2004-2012. *PLoS ONE.* (2016) 11:e0165528. doi: 10.1371/journal.pone.0165528
25. Sindhu S, Akhter N, Kochumon S, Thomas R, Wilson A, Shenouda S, et al. Increased expression of the innate immune receptor TLR10 in obesity and type-2 diabetes: association with ROS-mediated oxidative stress. *Cell Physiol Biochem.* (2018) 45:572–590. doi: 10.1159/000487034
26. Tsuchiya S, Yamabe M, Yamaguchi Y, Kobayashi Y, Konno T, Tada K. Establishment and characterization of a human acute monocytic leukemia cell line (THP-1). *Int J Cancer.* (1980) 26:171–6. doi: 10.1002/ijc.29102 60208
27. Bosshart H, Heinzelmann M. THP-1 cells as a model for human monocytes. *Ann Transl Med.* (2016) 4: 438. doi: 10.21037/atm.2016.08.53
28. Regan T, Nally K, Carmody R, Houston A, Shanahan F, MacSharry J, et al. Identification of TLR10 as a key mediator of the inflammatory response to listeria monocytogenes in intestinal epithelial cells and macrophages. *J Immunol.* (2013) 191:6084–92. doi: 10.4049/jimmunol.1203245
29. Nazli A, Dizzell S, Zahoor MA, Ferreira VH, Kafka J, Woods MW, et al. Interferon- β induced in female genital epithelium by HIV-1 glycoprotein 120 via toll-like-receptor 2 pathway acts to protect the mucosal barrier. *Cell Mol Immunol.* (2018) 16:178–94. doi: 10.1038/cmi.2017.168
30. Lalezari JP, Henry K, O'Hearn M, Montaner JSG, Piliero PJ, Trottier B, et al. Enfuvirtide, an HIV-1 fusion inhibitor, for drug-resistant HIV infection in North and South America. *N Engl J Med.* (2003) 348:2175–85. doi: 10.1056/NEJMoa035026
31. Ding X, Zhang X, Chong H, Zhu Y, Wei H, Wu X, et al. Enfuvirtide (T20)-based lipopeptide is a potent HIV-1 cell fusion inhibitor: implications for viral entry and inhibition. *J Virol.* (2017) 91:e00831-17. doi: 10.1128/JVI. 00831-17
32. De Francesco MA, Baronio M, Fiorentini S, Signorini C, Bonfanti C, Poiesi C, et al. HIV-1 matrix protein p17 increases the production of proinflammatory cytokines and counteracts IL-4 activity by binding to a cellular receptor. *Proc Natl Acad Sci USA.* (2002) 99:9972–7. doi: 10.1073/pnas.142274699
33. De Francesco MA, Baronio M, Poiesi C. HIV-1 p17 matrix protein interacts with heparan sulfate side chain of CD44v3, syndecan-2, and syndecan-4 proteoglycans expressed on human activated CD4+ T cells affecting tumor necrosis factor α and interleukin 2 production. *J Biol Chem.* (2011) 286:19541–8. doi: 10.1074/jbc.M110.191270
34. De Francesco MA, Caruso A, Fallacara F, Canaris AD, Dima F, Poiesi C, et al. HIV p17 enhances lymphocyte proliferation and HIV-1 replication after binding to a human serum factor. *AIDS.* (1998) 12:245–52. doi: 10.1097/00002030-199803000-00001
35. Chirmule N, Pahwa S. Envelope glycoproteins of human immunodeficiency virus type 1: profound influences on immune functions. *Microbiol Rev.* (1996) 60:386–406.
36. Nazli A, Chan O, Dobson-Belaire WN, Ouellet M, Tremblay MJ, Gray-Owen SD, et al. Exposure to HIV-1 directly impairs mucosal epithelial barrier integrity allowing microbial translocation. *PLoS Pathog.* (2010) 6:e1000852. doi: 10.1371/journal.ppat.1000852
37. Caccuri F, Giagulli C, Bugatti A, Benetti A, Alessandri G, Ribatti D, et al. HIV-1 matrix protein p17 promotes angiogenesis via chemokine receptors CXCR1 and CXCR2. *Proc Natl Acad Sci USA.* (2012) 109:14580–5. doi: 10.1073/pnas.1206605109
38. Kawai T, Akira S. Antiviral signaling through pattern recognition receptors. *J Biochem.* (2007) 141:137–45. doi: 10.1093/jb/mvm032
39. Kawai T, Akira S. The role of pattern-recognition receptors in innate immunity: update on toll-like receptors. *Nat Immunol.* (2010) 11:373–84. doi: 10.1038/ni.1863
40. Hasan U, Chaffois C, Gaillard C, Saulnier V, Merck E, Tancredi S, et al. Human TLR10 is a functional receptor, expressed by B cellsand plasmacytoid dendritic cells, which activates gene transcription through MyD88. *J Immunol.* (2005) 174:2942–50. doi: 10.4049/jimmunol.174.5.2942
41. Mikacenic C, Reiner AP, Holden TD, Nickerson DA, Wurfel MM. Variation in the TLR10/TLR1/TLR6 locus is the major genetic determinant of interindividual difference in TLR1/2-mediated responses. *Genes Immun.* (2013) 14:52–7. doi: 10.1038/gene.2012.53
42. Loré K, Betts MR, Brenchley JM, Kuruppu J, Khojasteh S, Perfetto S, et al. Toll-like receptor ligands modulate dendritic cells to augment cytomegalovirus- and HIV-1-specific T cell responses 1. *J Immunol.* (2003) 171:4320–8. doi: 10.4049/jimmunol.171.8.4320
43. Hess NJ, Jiang S, Li X, Guan Y, Tapping RI. TLR10 is a B cell intrinsic suppressor of adaptive immune responses. *J Immunol.* (2017) 198:699–707. doi: 10.4049/jimmunol.1601335
44. Morgan AR, Lam WJ, Han DY, Fraser AG, Ferguson LR. Genetic variation within TLR10 is associated with Crohn's disease in a New Zealand population. *Hum Immunol.* (2012) 73:416–20. doi: 10.1016/j.humimm.2012. 01.015
45. Lazarus R, Raby BA, Lange C, Silverman EK, Kwiatkowski DJ, Vercelli D, et al. TOLL-like receptor 10 genetic variation is associated with asthma in two independent samples. *Am J Respir Crit Care Med.* (2004) 170:594–600. doi: 10.1164/rccm.200404-491OC
46. Vrgoc G, Vrbanec J, Eftedal RK, Dembic PL, Balen S, Dembic Z, et al. Interleukin-17 and toll-like receptor 10 genetic polymorphisms and susceptibility to large joint osteoarthritis. *J Orthop Res.* (2018) 36:1684–93. doi: 10.1002/jor.23823
47. Kizildag S, Arslan S, Özbilüm N, Engin A, Bakir M. Effect of TLR10 (2322A/G, 720A/C, and 992T/A) polymorphisms on the pathogenesis of crimean congo hemorrhagic fever disease. *J Med Virol.* (2018) 90:19–25. doi: 10.1002/jmv.24924
48. Dannemann M, Andrés AM, Kelso J. Introgression of neandertal- and denisovan-like haplotypes contributes to adaptive variation in human toll-like receptors. *Am J Hum Genet.* (2016) 98:22–33. doi: 10.1016/j.ajhg.2015. 11.015
49. Deschamps M, Laval G, Fagny M, Itan Y, Abel L, Casanova JL, et al. Genomic signatures of selective pressures and introgression from archaic hominins at human innate immunity genes. *Am J Hum Genet.* (2016) 98:5–21. doi: 10.1016/j.ajhg.2015.11.014
50. Laayouni H, Oosting M, Luisi P, Ioana M, Alonso S, Ricano-Ponce I, et al. Convergent evolution in european and rroma populations reveals pressure exerted by plague on toll-like receptors. *Proc Natl Acad Sci USA.* (2014) 111:2668–73. doi: 10.1073/pnas.1317723111
51. Lee SMY, Yip TF, Yan S, Jin DY, Wei HL, Guo RT, et al. Recognition of double-stranded RNA and regulation of interferon pathway by toll-like receptor 10. *Front Immunol.* (2018) 9:516. doi: 10.3389/fimmu.2018.00516
52. Jiang S, Li X, Hess NJ, Guan Y, Tapping RI. TLR10 is a negative regulator of both MyD88-dependent and-independent TLR signaling. *J Immunol.* (2016) 4:211. doi: 10.4049/jimmunol.1502599
53. Jiang JQ, Patrick A, Moss RB, Rosenthal KL. CD8+ T-cell-mediated cross-clade protection in the genital tract following intranasal immunization with inactivated human immunodeficiency virus antigen plus cpg oligodeoxynucleotides. *J Virol.* (2005) 79:393–400. doi: 10.1128/JVI.79.1.393-400.2005
54. Drannik AG, Nag K, Yao XD, Henrick BM, Ball TB, Plummer FA, et al. Anti-HIV-1 activity of elafin depends on its nuclear localization and altered innate immune activation in female genital epithelial cells. *PLoS ONE.* (2012) 7:e52738. doi: 10.1371/journal.pone.0052738

17

Poly-ICLC, a TLR3 Agonist, Induces Transient Innate Immune Responses in Patients With Treated HIV-Infection: A Randomized Double-Blinded Placebo Controlled Trial

Mansi Saxena[1], Rachel L. Sabado[1†], Melissa La Mar[2], Hiroshi Mohri[2], Andres M. Salazar[3], Hanqing Dong[1], Joel Correa Da Rosa[4], Martin Markowitz[2], Nina Bhardwaj[1‡] and Elizabeth Miller[1,4†‡]*

[1] Icahn School of Medicine at Mount Sinai, New York, NY, United States, [2] Aaron Diamond AIDS Research Center, Rockefeller University, New York, NY, United States, [3] Oncovir, Inc., Washington, DC, United States, [4] Laboratory of Investigative Dermatology, The Rockefeller University, New York, NY, United States

***Correspondence:**
Nina Bhardwaj
nina.bhardwaj@mssm.edu

†Present Address:
Rachel L. Sabado, Genentech, South San Francisco, CA, United States
Elizabeth Miller, Regeneron Pharmaceuticals, Tarrytown, NY, United States

‡These authors share co-senior authorship

Objective: Toll-like receptor-3 agonist Poly-ICLC has been known to activate immune cells and induce HIV replication in pre-clinical experiments. In this study we investigated if Poly-ICLC could be used for disrupting HIV latency while simultaneously enhancing innate immune responses.

Design: This was a randomized, placebo-controlled, double-blinded trial in aviremic, cART-treated HIV-infected subjects. Participants ($n = 15$) were randomized 3:1 to receive two consecutive daily doses of Poly-ICLC (1.4 mg subcutaneously) vs. placebo. Subjects were observed for adverse events, immune activation, and viral replication.

Methods: Besides primary outcomes of safety and tolerability, several longitudinal immune parameters were evaluated including immune cell phenotype and function via flowcytometry, ELISA, and transcriptional profiling. PCR assays for plasma HIV-1 RNA, $CD4^+$ T cell-associated HIV-1 RNA, and proviral DNA were performed to measure HIV reservoirs and latency.

Results: Poly-ICLC was overall safe and well-tolerated. Poly-ICLC-related adverse events were Grade 1/2, with the exception of one Grade 3 neutropenia which was short-lived. Mild Injection site reactions were observed in nearly all participants in the Poly-ICLC arm. Transcriptional analyses revealed upregulation of innate immune pathways in PBMCs following Poly-ICLC treatment, including strong interferon signaling accompanied by transient increases in circulating IP-10 (CXCL10) levels. These responses generally peaked by 24–48 h after the first injection and returned to baseline by day 8. $CD4^+$ T cell number and phenotype were unchanged, plasma viral control was maintained and no significant effect on HIV reservoirs was observed.

Conclusions: These finding suggest that Poly-ICLC could be safely used for inducing transient innate immune responses in treated HIV$^+$ subjects indicating promise as an adjuvant for HIV therapeutic vaccines.

Trial Registration: www.ClinicalTrials.gov, identifier: NCT02071095.

Keywords: HIV-1, vaccine, adjuvant, poly-ICLC, toll-like receptor ligand

INTRODUCTION

Innate immune dysregulation during HIV infection hinders the formation of anti-HIV adaptive immunity (1–6) resulting in rampant viral dissemination and progression to AIDS. Adherence to combination anti-retroviral therapy (cART) regimens controls viremia, restores CD4$^+$T cell counts and reverses immune dysfunction to a larg extent. However, cART fails to eradicate latent viral reservoirs, posing a major barrier to achieving sterilizing cure (7). Thus, safe and effective adjuvants that stimulate innate immune responses (8) and reactivate latent HIV, allowing for killing of infected cells, are likely to be a vital element of successful therapeutic immunization strategies in aviremic patients (9).

Pattern recognition receptors, such as Toll-like receptors (TLRs), are key activators of innate immunity. These germ line encoded receptors induce rapid inflammation in response to a wide range pathogen associated molecular patterns (PAMPs) (10). Of the 10 TLRs expressed in humans, TLRs 1,2,4,5,6, and 10 are expressed on the cell surface and recognize pathogenic cell membrane components such as lipoproteins, peptidoglycans, flagellin, etc. TLR 3, TLR 7/8, and TLR9 are intracellular receptors that respond to double stranded RNA, single stranded RNA and unmethylated DNA, respectively. TLR3 is expressed multiple cell types including myeloid dendritic cells (DCs), macrophages, Natural killer cells (NK cells), neuronal cells, fibroblasts, endothelial cells, mast cells, and epithelial cells (11). While TLR7 is also expressed on myeloid DCs, NK cells, macrophages, and mast cells, its expression is enriched in plasmacytoid DCs (pDCs), B cells and T cells (12). TLR9 expression pattern is similar to that of TLR7 as it is also primarily expressed in human memory B cells, NK cells, and pDCs (13). Once activated by their cognate ligands, the TLRs signal through the downstream receptors MyD88 (TLR1, 2, 4, 5, 6, 7, 8, 9) or TRIF (TLRs4 and 3) to initiate a complex signaling cascade that culminates in transcriptional induction of inflammatory genes (14).

TLR agonists are potent immune adjuvants. In general their primary adjuvant effects are orchestrated through activation of immune cells like Natural Killer (NK) cells and antigen presenting cells such as DCs (15). DC maturation, induced by TLR agonists, is marked by up regulation of MHC-I and MHC-II and induction of co-stimulatory markers such CD40, CD80, and CD86. TLR activation also leads to secretion of cytokines in immune cells, such as interleukin (IL) 12 secretion by DCs and interferon-gamma (IFNγ) secretion by NK cells. The cumulative net effect is the induction of T cell activation and other specific or general adaptive immune responses (16). Interestingly, TLR agonists have also been shown to reactivate latent HIV both *ex vivo* (17–19) and in patients (20, 21).

Polyinosinic-polycytidylic acid, and poly-L-lysine (Poly-ICLC) is a double stranded RNA complex that serves as a viral mimic recognized by endosomal receptor TLR3 and cytoplasmic sensors MDA-5 and DHX/DDX RNA helicases (22–24). Its adjuvant effects are multi-faceted, including activation of classical DCs to express high levels of IL-12 and type I IFN (16) to promote Th1 polarization (25). Studies in humanized mice models have validated the significance of Poly-IC as a potent adjuvant for driving DC-induced inflammation and activation of antigen specific cytotoxic T cells (26). Furthermore, Poly-IC has been reported to reverse viral latency in human microglial cells *in vitro* (27).

In clinical trials with healthy volunteers and cancer patients, Poly-ICLC has been found to be overall safe and immunogenic (28–33). Interestingly, Poly-IC has been reported to be more efficient than other TLR ligands at improving immunogenicity and inducing viral control when it is either administered alone (34) or in combination with other components (35–38).

A major challenge in using TLR ligands as therapy during HIV infection is the profound host immune dysfunction induced by the virus, including dampening of TLR responsiveness (6, 39, 40). While viremia suppression by cART has been reported to rescue DC activation (39); whether Poly-ICLC can be safely used as an adjuvant and a latency reversing agent in this setting remains to be determined.

Here we report the results of a randomized, placebo-controlled, double-blinded trial investigating the use of Poly-ICLC in HIV setting (NCT02071095). The primary end point of the study was to establish if Poly-ICLC is safe and well-tolerated in HIV-1-infected subjects on cART. The secondary end points were; (a) to determine whether Poly-ICLC disrupts viral latency in HIV-1-infected individuals on cART and (b) to confirm that Poly-ICLC enhances innate immune responses in HIV-infected subjects on cART, and that its immunostimulatory properties are transient in nature. The secondary endpoints include measuring innate immune activation (DC, NK Cells, soluble factors, and transcriptional responses), and measures of viral RNA and DNA. A special consideration for the use of an immunostimulant during HIV infection is the risk of inducing inappropriate immune activation resulting in increased number of cellular targets of infection. Therefore, multiple parameters of generalized immune activation and exhaustion were monitored as additional safety measures. While we did not observe any clear effects of Poly-ICLC in reversing HIV latency or on the size of viral reservoirs; we did determine that Poly-ICLC was safe and well-tolerated in the HIV-infected population studied.

Furthermore, Poly-ICLC lead to transient innate immune stimulation without undue generalized immune activation. These findings suggest that Poly-ICLC may enhance the formation of HIV-specific immune responses when administered with HIV therapeutic vaccines.

METHODS

Study Design and Eligibility

This was a randomized, placebo-controlled, double-blinded, trial in cART-suppressed subjects with HIV infection (NCT02071095). Participants ($N = 15$) were randomized 3:1 to receive 2 consecutive daily doses of Poly-ICLC (Hiltonol®, Oncovir) [1.4 mg subcutaneously (SQ)] vs. placebo (normal saline) (**Figure 1**) and followed for 48 weeks. Subjects were randomized into blocks of 4 4 8 4. In total 12 participants received Poly-ICLC and 3 participants received the placebo (**Figure 2**).

Eligible participants included non-pregnant, non-lactating men, and women aged 18–55 years with HIV-infection on cART. Further eligibility was determined based on documented plasma HIV-1 RNA suppression below 50 copies/ml for at least 48 weeks and CD4$^+$ T cells >500 cells/mm^3. Persons with co-morbidities including vascular disease, poorly controlled hypertension, diabetes, hyperlipidemia, renal disease, active hepatitis B/C co-infection, autoimmunity, or multi-drug resistant HIV were excluded. Subjects were recruited from the New York City area from Mount Sinai Hospital Clinics, Rockefeller University Recruitment Office and IRB-approved advertising.

Plasma HIV-1 RNA Levels

HIV-1 RNA levels in plasma were determined using the Roche COBAS AmpliPrep/COBAS TaqMan HIV-1 Assay, Version 2.0, which detects 10 to 20 × 10^6 copies per ml.

DC Enumeration and Activation

To enumerate and assess maturation of CD11c$^+$ DCs and pDCs, fresh peripheral blood mononuclear cells (PBMCs) were stained with Live/Dead Violet, HLA-DR PerCP-Cy5.5, CD123 PE-Cy7, Lin1 FITC, CD11c PE-CF594, CD40 APC, CD86 Alexa700, and CD83 PE. Fresh PBMCs, plated for 1 h, were treated with Golgi Plug (1:1,000) for 5 h and stained for surface expression of HLA-DR PerCP-Cy5.5, CD123 PE-Cy7, Lin1 FITC, CD11c PE-CF594, and Live/Dead Violet followed by intracellular cytokine staining with IFNα APC, IL-12 p40/70 PE, and TNFα Alexa700. For the control fluorescence minus one (FMO) wells, the corresponding antibody was omitted from the cocktail. Stained and fixed cells were acquired using BD Fortessa Cytometer.

NK Cell Enumeration and Activation

Fresh PBMCs were stained with Live/Dead Violet, CD3 PE-CF594, CD16 PerCP-Cy5.5, CD56 BV605, CD69 Alexa700, NKp44 APC, NKG2D PE-Cy7, TIM3 Alexa488, and KIR3DS1/DL1 PE. Stained and fixed cells were acquired using BD Fortessa Cytometer.

T Cell Phenotype

Thawed PBMCs were stained with CD4 FITC, CD8 Alexa700, HLA-DR PerCP-Cy5.5, CD38 APC, PD-1 BV605, CTLA-4 PE, CD3 PE-CF594, and Live/Dead Violet and acquired using BD Fortessa Cytometer.

ELISA

Presence of plasma IFNα (PBL Assay Science), IP-10 (R&D systems), sCD14 (R&D systems), TNFα (R&D systems), D-Dimer (Abcam), and C-Reactive Protein (CRP) (Abcam) was evaluated by ELISA per manufacturers protocol.

Transcriptional Responses

Transcriptional responses profiling 249 inflammation-related genes were evaluated in PBMCs at baseline and days 2, 4, and 8 in a subset of participants ($N = 12$) via NanoString Technologies including statistical analysis (nCounter® gene expression panel, human inflammation kit).

Quantification of Cell-Associated HIV-1 RNA and DNA in Peripheral CD4$^+$T Cells

Cell-associated HIV-1 proviral DNA was measured at baseline and week 4, and cell-associated HIV-1 RNA was measured at each visit through week 16 (baseline, days 2, 4, 8, week 4 and 16). CD4$^+$T cells were isolated from PBMCs using Dynabeads FlowComp Human CD4 Kit (Invitrogen). DNA and RNA isolation was performed with AllPrep DNA/RNA Mini Kit (Qiagen). Isolated RNA was treated with DNase I, Amplification Grade (Invitrogen) and purified with RNeasy Mini Kit (Qiagen). Real time PCR was performed with AmpliTaq Gold with Buffer A or AmpliTaq Gold DNA Polymerase with Buffer II and MgCl2 with ROX Reference Dye (Applied Biosystems) using the Stratagene Mx3000P QPCR System (Agilent Technologies). PCR reactions were performed in quadruplicate. Note that for each case an optimal primers/probe set was determined, which gave the highest amplification efficiency among three primer/probe sets tested. Accordingly two primer/probe sets were used, RF/RR/PB (41) for 9 participants and 6F/84R/HIV gag probe (42) for 6 participants.

Cell-associated RNA was primed with random hexamers and reverse transcribed with Superscript II (Invitrogen). PCR reagent mix containing primers, probe, and AmpliTaq Gold was added to each of RT product, and quantitative rtPCR was performed as described above in quadruplicate. No reverse transcriptase control was also included.

Statistical Methods

Comparisons among the treatment Arms on the proportions of related adverse events was made using Fisher's exact test. Immunologic and virologic parameters between and within treatment Arms were compared at each time points from baseline to post-administration of Poly-ICLC vs. placebo using a linear mixed effect model. Parameters between treatment arms were compared using analysis of covariance, with baseline values as a covariate, after a Box-Cox family variance stabilizing transformation.

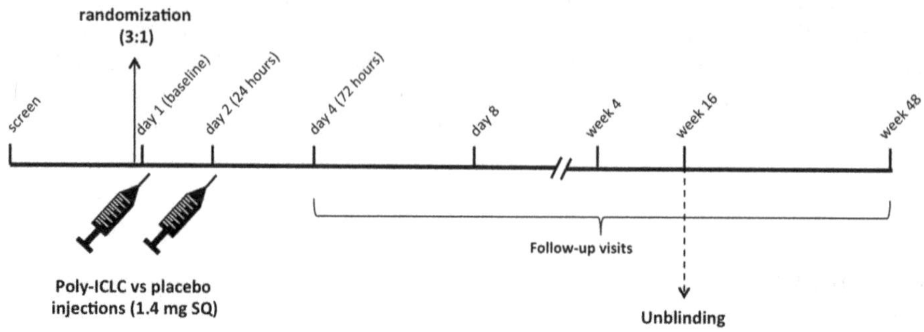

FIGURE 1 | Study Schema. Following screening, eligible subjects are randomized 3:1 to receive Poly-ICLC (1.4 mg SQ) vs. Placebo on days 1 and 2. Participants returned for follow up visits on days 4 and 8, weeks 4, 16, and 48. Unblinding of the study occurred after all subjects completed the week 16 follow up visit as specified by the protocol.

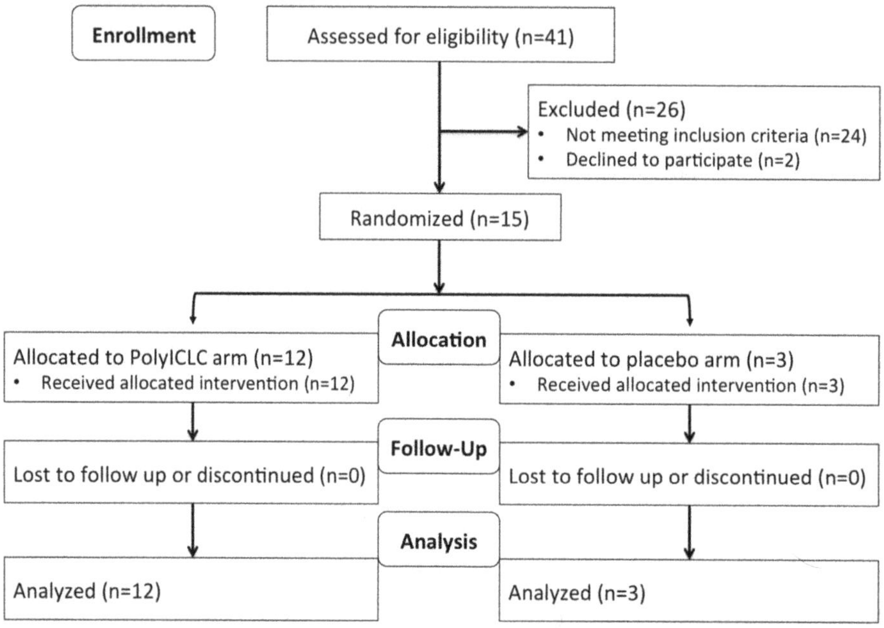

FIGURE 2 | Study flow diagram.

For primary end-point of safety, power of Fisher's Exact Test for difference between two proportions when sample sizes are $n1 = 12$ and $n2 = 3$ was determined (data not shown) and deemed appropriate. For the secondary endpoint, assuming a modest correlation between baseline and follow-up, maximum cellular associated HIV-1 RNA ($r = 0.32$), a sample size of 12 patients in the active arm and 3 patients in the control arm can detect a difference of $|2.23|$ standard deviations in cellular associated HIV-1 RNA maximum fold change between Poly-ICLC SQ and placebo with 2-sided $\alpha = 0.05$ and power = 92% (calculations from PASS version 12) (43). The assumptions used in this power calculation are consistent with the effect sizes, variability, and correlation over time for the primary outcome in work by Archin et al. (44). Considering the endpoints for cellular phenotype: the sample size provides 80% power at 5% of significance for detecting a minimum difference of $|1.95|$ standard deviations between the two study arms when using a two-sided unpaired *t*-test.

RESULTS

Participants and Demographic Details

Participants included 14 males and 1 transgender female with HIV infection. Participants hailed from diverse racial and ethnic backgrounds (40% white, 26.6% black or AA, 6.7% Native American, 6.7% Asian, and 20% multiple or unspecified race, with 46.6% Hispanic or Latino ethnicity). The median age was 39.73 years old (range 26–54), and median baseline $CD4^+$ T cell count was 619 cells/mm^3. A detailed description of baseline patient demographics across the two arms of the study can be found in **Table 1**.

TABLE 1 | Tabulated view of baseline patient demographics in each arm.

		Arm A: Poly:ICLC	Arm B: Placebo	Total
Number of participants		12	3	15
Age (years)	Continuous Mean (Standard Deviation)	41.1 (9.32)	34.33 (4.03)	39.73 (8.61)
Sex (Number)	Female	0	0	0
	Male	12	3	15
Ethnic Category (Number)	Hispanic or Latino	6	1	7
	Not Hispanic or Latino	6	2	8
Racial Categories (Number)	American Indian/Alaska Native	1	0	1
	Asian	1	0	1
	Native Hawaiian or Other Pacific Islander	0	0	0
	Black or African American	4 (1 Hispanic)	0	4
	White	4 (3 Hispanic)	2	6
	More than one race	1 (Hispanic)	0	1
	Unknown/ Unreported	1 (Hispanic)	1 (Hispanic)	2

TABLE 2 | Tabulated view of treatment related Adverse Events (AEs).

	Placebo (n = 3)			Poly:ICLC (n = 12)		
	Grade 1-2	Grade 3	Grade 4	Grade 1-2	Grade 3	Grade 4
GENERAL DISORDERS AND ADMINISTRATION SITE CONDITIONS						
Chills	0	0	0	3	0	0
Injection site reaction–erythema	0	0	0	5	0	0
Injection site reaction–pain	0	0	0	10	0	0
Fatigue	3	0	0	7	0	0
Fever	0	0	0	4	0	0
Malaise	1	0	0	2	0	0
NERVOUS SYSTEM DISORDERS						
Headache	2	0	0	1	0	0
MUSCULOSKELETAL AND CONNECTIVE TISSUE DISORDERS						
Myalgias	0	0	0	2	0	0
HEMATOLOGICAL						
Low neutrophils count	0	0	0	0	1	0

Safety and Tolerability

All study participants received both doses of Poly-ICLC or placebo as planned, and all subjects completed visits through week 48 (**Figure 2**). Overall, Poly-ICLC was safe and well-tolerated with only Grade 1/2 adverse events (AEs) attributed to the study agent, with the exception of one Grade 3 transient neutropenia without clinical sequelae. Injection site reactions (ISR) were the most frequent AE, all of which were Grade 1. Pain was the most common ISR, occurring at 66% of injection sites. Erythema was present at 33% of injection sites. Fever, generally low-grade, was also common (26.6%), lasting 24–48 h. Other frequently reported AEs include chills, myalgias, fatigue, malaise, and headache (**Table 2**). AEs deemed treatment-related were more common in the Poly-ICLC arm compared with the placebo arm (P = 0.012), as was injection site pain (P = 0.022). All subjects completed the protocol's dosing regimen, and there were no cases of discontinuation. Two serious adverse events (SAEs) occurred during the study which were deemed unrelated to Poly-ICLC, and both of these occurred in the placebo group.

There was no impact on subjects' CD4$^+$ T cell counts following Poly-ICLC injections. The median CD4$^+$ T cell count in the Poly-ICLC group increased from 604.5 cells/mm^3 at baseline to 698 cells/mm^3 and 656 cells/mm^3 at day 8 and week 16, respectively, but was not a statistically significant change (**Figure 3**).

All subjects maintained virologic control with plasma HIV-1 RNA remaining below the limit of detection (<20 copies/ml) throughout the study, with the exception of two discrete

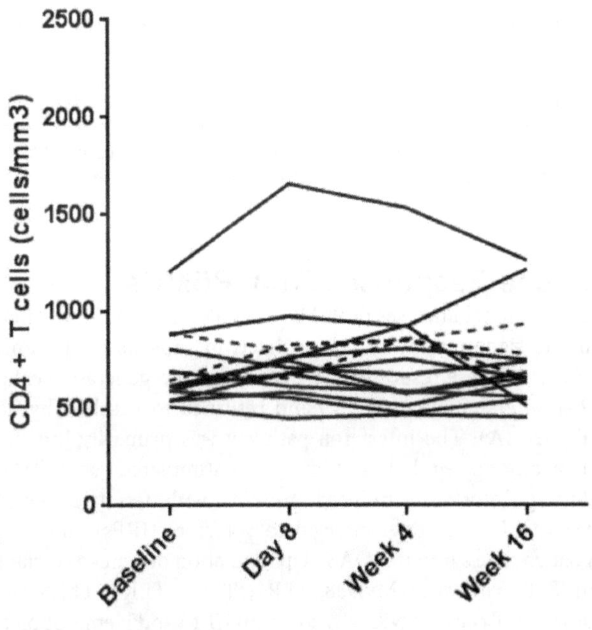

FIGURE 3 | No overall change in CD4$^+$ T cells counts in the treatment arm. CD4$^+$ T cell counts (cells/mm^3) for each subject are shown over the course of the study. Values for subjects in Arm A (Poly-ICLC) and Arm B (Placebo) are depicted by solid and dashed lines, respectively.

measurements of detectable HIV RNA, both in Poly-ICLC arm, with <200 copies/ml. One participant experienced a transient elevation in plasma HIV RNA to 110 copies/ml in the setting of a genital herpes simplex virus outbreak that occurred at their week 4 visit, and another participant was found to have a level of 190 copies/ml that occurred at their week 48 visit (data not shown).

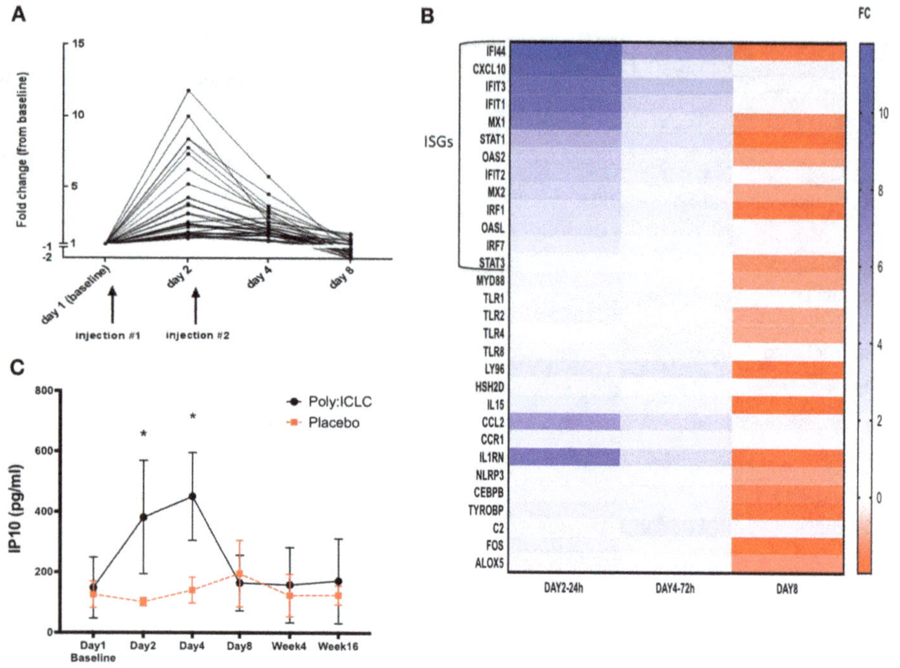

FIGURE 4 | Transient upregulation of pro-inflammatory genes in subjects who received Poly-ICLC, with strong induction of interferon pathway. Transcriptional responses were evaluated longitudinally in subjects' PBMCs using NanoString Technologies (nCounter® gene expression panel, human inflammation kit). **(A)** Fold change (FC) from baseline of significantly upregulated genes from subjects in Arm A (Poly-ICLC) are depicted graphically over time through day 8. Transient upregulation of several genes occurred ($N = 31$), generally peaking at 24 h and returning to baseline shortly thereafter. No significant changes were observed in subjects' PBMCs in Arm B (Placebo) (not shown). **(B)** Heat map of all significantly induced genes in Arm A (Poly-ICLC) represented as a FC over baseline. Most of the highly upregulated genes were found to be interferon-stimulated genes (ISGs) FDR < 1, FC $\geq \pm 1.5$. **(C)** In concordance with strong upregulation of ISGs, plasma levels of IP-10 were transiently upregulated in subjects in Arm A Poly-ICLC ($N = 12$) vs. those in Arm B Placebo ($N = 3$). $^{*}p < 0.001$.

Immune Responses From PBMCs

Transcriptional analyses of PBMCs revealed that multiple innate immune signatures were up regulated in subjects in the Poly-ICLC arm. These responses were transient and generally peaked at 24 h after injection (day 2) and returned to baseline by day 8 (**Figure 4A**). The interferon pathway was primarily induced, with strong up regulation of interferon-stimulated genes (ISGs) including Interferon Induced proteins with tetratricopeptide repeats (IFITs), interferon regulatory factors (IRFs), and 2′-5′ oligoadenylate synthase (OAS). Up regulation of genes associated with TLR pathways (MyD88, TLR1, TLR2, TLR4, TLR8, and Ly96) (45), T cell and NK cell activation [IL15 and Hematopoietic SH2 Domain Containing (HSH2D)] (46–48) inflammasome activation [NLR Family Pyrin Domain Containing 3 (NLRP3)] (49) and other inflammatory transcription factors, chemokines, and cytokines (FOS, CCL2, CCR1, etc.) was observed to a lesser extent (**Figure 4B** and **Supplemental Table 1**). In accordance with the strong up regulation of ISGs found on transcriptional analyses, transient increases in plasma IP-10 in the Poly-ICLC arm were observed on days 2 and 4 compared with baseline and subsequent time points ($p < 0.001$), while no changes were observed in the placebo arm (**Figure 4C**). Changes in levels of circulating IFNα and other inflammatory markers (IFNβ, TNFα, sCD14, D-dimer, and C reactive protein) were not detected following Poly-ICLC administration, though certain individuals did experience transient increases in D-dimer and CRP that quickly returned to baseline (**Supplemental Figure 1**).

T Cell Exhaustion

Immune activation on T cells was assessed by surface expression of HLA-DR and CD38. Programmed Cell Death 1 (PD-1) and Cytotoxic T-Lymphocyte Associated Protein 4 (CTLA-4) expression was used as an indicator of T cell exhaustion. Please note that PD1 and CTLA-4 maybe up regulated very early in activated T cells but in later stages are considered markers of exhaustion. Neither HLA-DR nor PD1 and CTLA-4 on $CD4^{+}$ and $CD8^{+}$ T cells was found to be overall changed from baseline following Poly-ICLC administration. However, CD38 was significantly upregulated on day 4 compared with baseline on $CD8^{+}$ T cells and normalized by day 8 ($P < 0.001$; **Figure 5**).

DC and NK Cell Activation

Many different subsets of DCs have been identified such as $CD141^{+}$ cDC1s, $CD1c^{+}$cDC2s, Langerhans cells, pDCs, and inflammatory DCs. We focused on analyzing the effect of Poly-ICLC on pDCs and mDCs (most similar to cDC2) as these two are the most abundant DC subsets in blood. DCs were identified by a lack of lineage marker expression (CD3, CD14, CD16, CD20, and CD56) and positive for HLA-DR (a heterodimeric MHC-II cell surface receptor). pDCs and mDCs were identified by

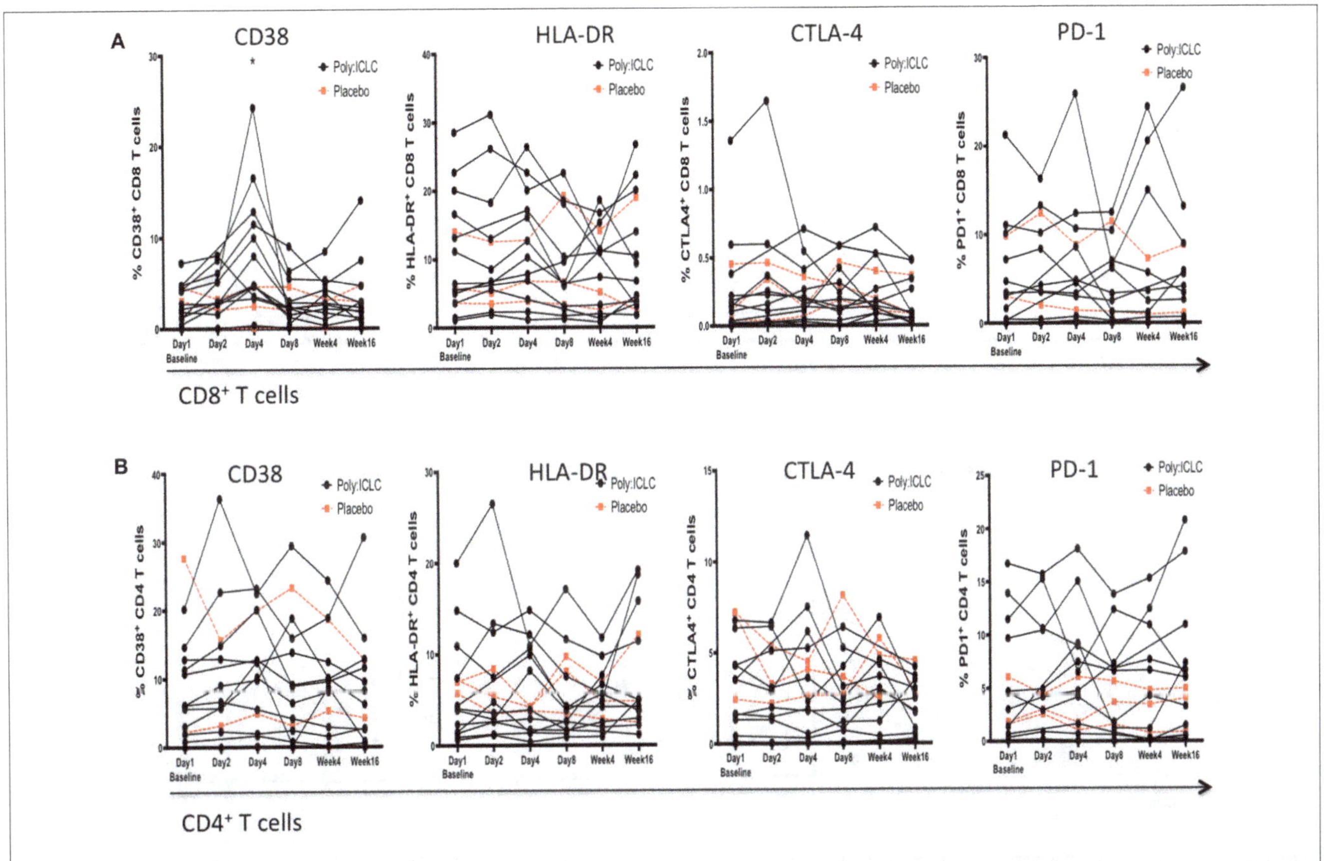

FIGURE 5 | Markers of immune activation and exhaustion on CD4+ and CD8+ T cells following Poly-ICLC administration. In order to monitor for the secondary induction of generalized immune activation following Poly-ICLC administration, surface expression of CD38, HLA-DR, PD-1, and CTLA-4 was evaluated at each time point via flowcytometry on subjects'; **(A)** CD8+ T cells and **(B)** CD4+ T cells. No longitudinal changes were found to be statistically significant following Poly-ICLC administration with the exception of transient upregulation of CD38 on CD8+ T cells at Day 4. $^{*}p < 0.001$.

mutually exclusive expression of CD123 and CD11c, respectively (16, 50). NK cells were identified as being negative for CD3 and by co-expression of CD16 and CD56. $CD16^{+}CD56^{dim}$ NK cells are considered mature NK cells that are highly cytolytic and inflammatory while $CD16^{+/-}CD56^{bright}$ NK cells are highly proliferative and known for producing high levels of IFNγ upon stimulation. $CD16^{+}CD56^{-}$ NK cells have been previously described in healthy cord blood samples and chronic HIV donors (51, 52), however it is unclear if these are immature, dysfunctional NK cells or an artifact due to contamination from the myeloid fraction. There was no significant difference in percentage of pDCs and mDCs in circulation post Poly-ICLC treatment. The $CD56^{dim}$ NK cell subsets appeared to transiently decrease on day 2 compared with baseline but subsequently returned to baseline by day 8 ($P < 0.05$; **Figure 6**).

To determine the phenotype of circulating DCs expression of co-stimulatory cell surface proteins CD40, CD83, CD86, all of which are required for optimally engaging and activating T cells, was examined (8, 16). A unique array of activating and inhibitory receptors control NK cell effector functions by either recognizing the presence or absence of their ligands on target cells. For our study we analyzed the expression of two activating receptors, NKp44 and NKG2D and two inhibitory receptors, TIM3, and KIR3DS1/DL1 on circulating NK cells (53, 54). The activation status of both, DCs and NK cells, remained overall unchanged from baseline. There were also no changes in intracellular cytokine secretion of TNFα, IFNα, or IL-12 observed in DCs from baseline (not shown).

HIV-1 Latency and Reservoirs

$CD4^{+}$ T cell-associated HIV-1 RNA was measured to determine changes in HIV latency from baseline. Though certain individuals experienced increases in cell-associated HIV RNA following administration of Poly-ICLC at various time points, these were low in magnitude and overall was not a statistically significant finding (**Figure 7A**). Cell-associated HIV-1 proviral DNA was measured as an estimate of reservoir size at baseline and week 4, and there was no observed difference in this measure (**Figure 7B**).

DISCUSSION

The innate immune environment during vaccination plays a crucial role in the induction of strong and durable immunity. Here, we report multiple outcomes of the first study of Poly-ICLC, a TLR3 agonist, during treated HIV infection. In a

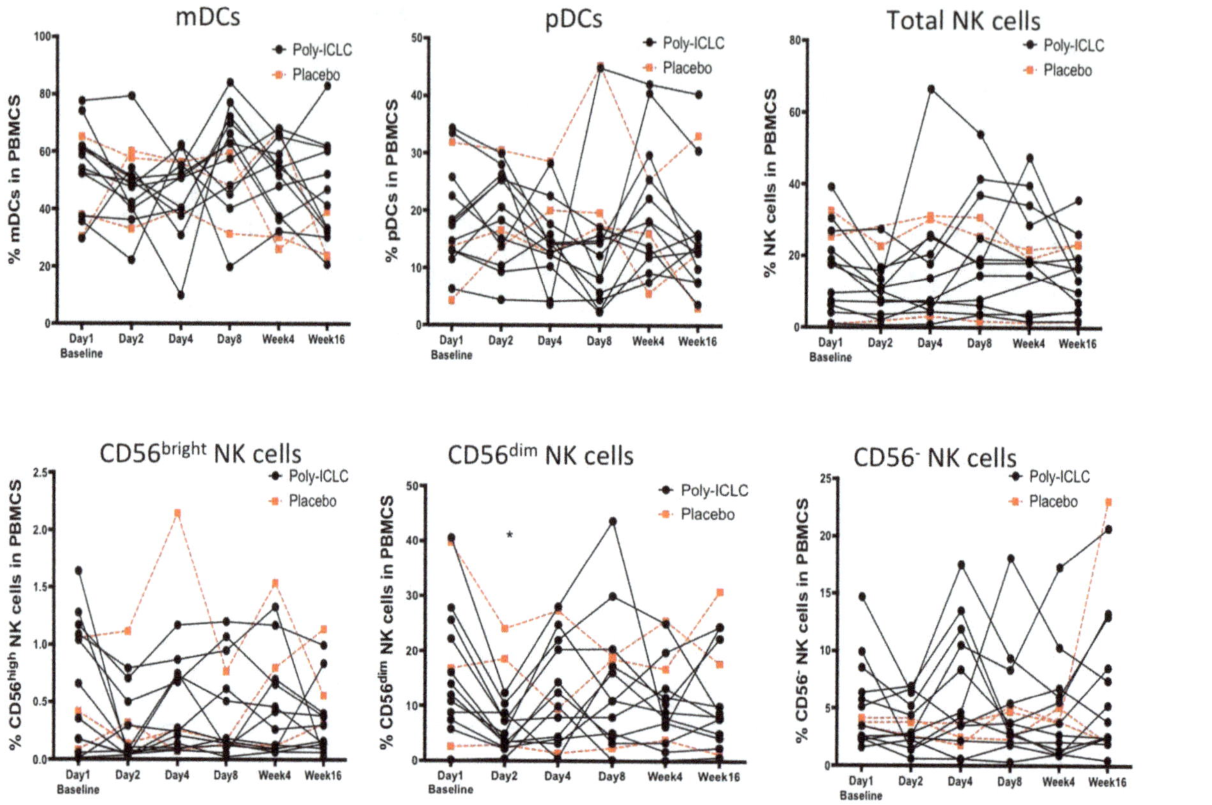

FIGURE 6 | No changes in DC and NK cell numbers and activation following Poly-ICLC treatment. DC and NK cell subsets were enumerated as described following Poly-ICLC vs. placebo. Percentage of mDCs, pDCs, total NK cells, CD56 bright, CD56 dim, and CD56 negative cells in PBMCs for each subject are shown over the course of the study as measured by flowcytometry. Values for subjects in Arm A (Poly-ICLC) and Arm B (Placebo) are depicted by solid and dashed lines, respectively. Though multiple NK cell subsets declined following Poly-ICLC, the only CD56 dim NK cells were found to be statistically significant. (*$p < 0.05$, FDR <1).

previous study of eight healthy volunteers who received a single dose of Poly-ICLC (1.6 mg SQ), majority of participants had reported moderate or severe ISRs, along with a high frequency of systemic AEs (31). However, in our study, Poly-ICLC was very well-tolerated in the HIV-infected population studied; with AEs primarily consisting of mild ISRs in nearly all subjects and less frequent fevers and other systemic symptoms. It is unclear as to why the AEs were relatively mild in our study. It has been suggested that there may be some Poly-ICLC lot variability in terms of reactogenicity on the other hand it is also possible that dampening of innate immune responses during HIV infection may be responsible for this outcome (6, 39, 40). Though favorable adjuvant tolerability during HIV infection is advantageous, it remains unclear what effect, if any, this may have on its potency when administered with a vaccine.

Nevertheless, we observed strong upregulation of numerous ISGs and increases in circulating levels of IP-10. These responses were transient, generally peaking by 24–48 h after injection and returning to baseline by day 8. In previous studies also, the transcriptional responses following Poly-ICLC, in healthy volunteers (31) and cancer patients (28), reported transient upregulation of ISGs with accompanying induction in other innate immune pathways but to a lesser extent. Similarly, in addition to ISGs, we detected transcriptional upregulation of other innate immune pathways but did not find associated significant increases in circulating pro-inflammatory cytokines beyond IP-10. It remains unclear if a lack of secreted inflammatory signature in our study was a result of a diminished effect of Poly-ICLC during HIV infection or due to low dosing over a short period of time.

Poly-ICLC administration also did not induce activation of circulating DCs and NK cells, as gleaned from flowcytometry analysis. However, local effects on tissue DCs and other innate immune cells were likely induced as evidenced by ISRs in the vast majority of individuals. Furthermore, we observed a transient decrease in circulating NK cells subsets ($CD56^{dim}$) following Poly-ICLC treatment, which may possibly reflect trafficking of this subset of NK cells to the tissues. In preclinical studies, Poly-ICLC has been shown to secondarily activate NK cells to enhance their cytotoxicity which may in turn augment the killing and elimination of latently infected cells alone (25, 55) or in combination with other TLR ligands (56).

Prior trials have primarily evaluated the formation of antigen-specific adaptive immune responses in patients administered with Poly-ICLC in combination with either tumor associated peptides or specific targeting antibodies (29, 30, 32, 57, 58), thus

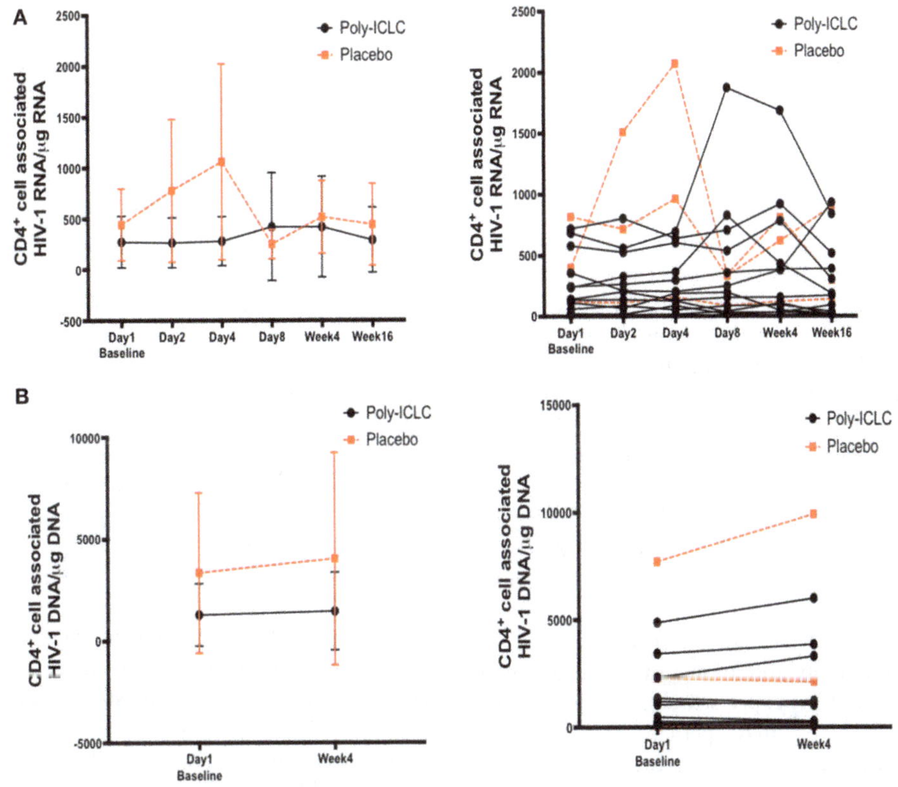

FIGURE 7 | Longitudinal assessment of cell associated HIV-1 RNA and DNA values show no significant changes overall following discrete dosing of Poly-ICLC. **(A)** Following RNA extraction from purified $CD4^+$ T cells at baseline and multiple time points following Poly-ICLC, rtPCR for HIV-1 RNA was performed in quadruplicate. Cell-associated HIV-1 RNA copy number is expressed as copy number per 1 µg of RNA in purified $CD4^+$ T cells. The left graph depicts pooled values from all participants in Arm A (Poly-ICLC) and Arm B (placebo), with the mean values and standard deviation. The right graph depicts this data as individual values over time for each participant in Arm A and Arm B. **(B)** Following DNA extraction from purified $CD4^+$ T cells at baseline and at week 4, rtPCR for HIV-1 DNA was performed in quadruplicate. Cell-associated HIV-1 DNA copy number is expressed as copy number per 1 µg of DNA in purified $CD4^+$ T cells. Left graph depicts pooled values from all participants in Arm A and Arm B. The right graph shows individual values for each participant in Arm A and Arm B. Values for subjects in Arm A (Poly-ICLC) and Arm B (Placebo) are depicted by solid and dashed lines, respectively.

making comparison to the current study of Poly-ICLC-alone difficult. Specially given our focus on induction of innate immune responses. In future trials, vaccination with Poly-ICLC combined with HIV related peptides will serve as the true test of its potential role as an adjuvant during HIV infection.

An ongoing safety concern associated with the use of novel adjuvants in HIV-infection is the potential for induction of generalized immune activation that could increase cellular targets of infection and contribute to immunopathogenesis. Therefore, in addition to monitoring viral parameters, we gauged levels of generalized immune activation and exhaustion on $CD4^+$ and $CD8^+$ T cells via flowcytometry and measured circulating markers of inflammation including D-dimer, CRP, sCD14. We did not find any upregulation in markers of immune activation on $CD4^+$ T cells that would lead to increased risk for infection. Similarly, markers of immune activation and exhaustion were not found to be significantly upregulated in plasma or on $CD8^+$ T cells except for a transient increase in CD38, a maker of T cell activation (59), expression on $CD8^+$ T cells on day 4 that returned to baseline by day 8. The elevated levels of CD38 on $CD8^+$ T cells in this study were likely a result of temporary increases in IFNs induced by Poly-ICLC (60). Given the fleeting nature of this upregulation, along with the stability of other surface markers including HLA-DR, PD-1, and CTLA-4, it is unlikely that deleterious effects on adaptive immune function are imparted overall.

TLR ligands may not only serve as vaccine adjuvants during HIV infection but may also impact viral latency (17–21). Indeed, TLR ligand driven activation of innate immune cells induces inflammatory cytokines, several of which are known to promote viral reactivation (61, 62). Here, we observed no overall effect within the Poly-ICLC-treated group on viral latency via measurement of $CD4^+$ T cell-associated HIV-1 RNA, despite increases detected in certain individuals following Poly-ICLC treatment that remains of unclear significance. Furthermore, there was no significant change in $CD4^+$ T cell-associated HIV-1 proviral DNA, suggesting that HIV reservoirs were largely unchanged following Poly-ICLC administration. Larger studies, possibly with more frequent dosing of poly-ICLC will be needed to assess whether this adjuvant will ultimately impact the HIV reservoir. These findings are in contrast to preclinical studies with TLR ligands during HIV/Simian immunodeficiency virus (SIV) infection *in vivo* and *in vitro* (18, 21, 63). TLR9 agonist (MGN1703) has been shown to enhance HIV-1 transcription *in vitro* in PBMCs from aviremic donors (18). Moreover, recent preclinical studies of TLR7 agonists (GS-9620 and GS-980, Gilead) in SIV-infected non-human primates receiving cART, revealed transient increases in plasma SIV RNA levels and decreased viral reservoirs in PBMCs and lymph nodes (21). Additionally, viral load in two of the treated animals remained undetectable for more than 90 days after ART interruption (21).

There remains scant clinical data regarding the use of TLR ligands alone during HIV infection with the exception of a clinical trial that administered TLR9 agonist MGN-1703, twice weekly for 4 weeks, in cART suppressed patients (20). The study demonstrated a significant increase in plasma viremia in 6 out 15 patients along with increase in pDC, NK cell, and $CD8^+$ T cell activation and induction of plasma IFNα, TNFα, IFNγ during the course of the study. The differential findings in these studies with other TLR ligands vs. the current trial may be related to distinct effects of the TLR ligands themselves and to the dissimilar dosing strategies utilized. Though each of these TLR ligands (3, 7, 9) are involved in anti-viral immunity and known to stimulate type I IFN responses, TLRs 7 and 9 are expressed on pDC, as opposed to TLR3 which is expressed on mDC, perhaps accounting for divergent effects of these ligands on innate immunity in a vaccine context (64). Moreover, latency reversal effects of TLR7 ligands in SIV infection setting was not observed following the first two doses, but became evident after 3 more doses of the 10–19 received in total, indicating a net cumulative effect (21). It is possible that additional and/or higher doses of Poly-ICLC would have resulted in similar effects on viral latency. Given the early phase of this clinical trial with a primary emphasis on safety, such dosing regimens were not suitable. Exploration of increased or expanded dosing strategies and routes of administration in future studies will help clarify Poly-ICLC's effect on HIV latency.

There are several limitations to this study that must be considered, including relatively small sample size. This prevented the evaluation of multiple sub-group analyses, including the influence of individual ART regimens on immunologic and virologic parameters, which have been shown to alter TLR responsiveness *in vitro* (65). Other limitations include the overall homogeneity of the study population in terms of gender, though racially and ethnically diverse. Furthermore, due to strict study entry criteria designed to maximize safety, the exclusion of older individuals (>55 years) and common comorbidities such as cardiovascular disease and diabetes further limit the generalizability of the safety findings in the HIV-infected population as a whole. Additional studies that increase the diversity of the HIV-infected individuals included will help to bolster these safety findings.

In summary, the TLR3 ligand, Poly-ICLC, was safe and tolerable in the HIV-infected population studied and transiently stimulated innate immune responses without resulting in undue immune activation. Given the promising safety profile of PolyICLC in our trial, future studies may now be designed; enlisting a larger cohort, with a wider inclusion criteria, longer duration, and more frequent dosing to further optimize the potential use for PolyICLC as a latency reversal agent. Moreover, this study paves the way for HIV therapeutic vaccines trials that combine Poly-ICLC with HIV antigen vaccines to enhance adaptive immunity to ultimately reduce viral reservoirs.

ETHICS STATEMENT

This study was carried out in accordance with the good clinical practice (GCP), with written informed consent from all participants in accordance with the Declaration of Helsinki. The protocol was approved by Ethics Committees and IRBs at Icahn School of Medicine at Mount Sinai and Rockefeller University Hospital.

AUTHOR CONTRIBUTIONS

MS: critical data analysis, manuscript writing, reviewing, and editing. RS and EM: protocol immunologists. RS and HD: specimen handling and processing at Vaccine and Cell Therapy Laboratory at Icahn School of Medicine at Mount Sinai. HM: protocol virologist and manuscript review. ML: data and regulatory management. JC: biostatistician. AS: study design and reagents. MM: co-principal investigator, manuscript revision, and study design. NB and EM: co-principal investigators, senior authors, study design, data interpretation and manuscript writing and reviewing.

ACKNOWLEDGMENTS

This study was supported by funding from NIH/NIAID (R37 AI044628 to NB, R21 AI110736 to EM) and the Campbell Foundation to NB and EM. This research was also supported in part by grant # UL1 TR000043 from the National Center for Advancing Translational Sciences (NCATS, National Institutes of Health (NIH) Clinical and Translational Science Award (CTSA) program. NB is a member of the Parker Institute for Cancer Immunotherapy, which supports the Icahn School of Medicine at Mount Sinai, NY, Cancer Immunotherapy Program.

SUPPLEMENTARY MATERIAL

Supplemental Figure 1 | No induction of soluble mediators of inflammation upon Poly-ICLC administration. Plasma levels of IFN alpha, IFN beta, TNF alpha, sCD14, D-dimer, and C-reactive protein (CRP) for each subject are shown as a mean with standard deviation over the course of the study as measured by ELISA. Values for subjects in Arm A (Poly-ICLC) and Arm B (Placebo) are depicted by solid (black) and dashed (red) lines, respectively. No longitudinal changes were found to be statistically significant following Poly-ICLC administration.

Supplemental Table 1 | Transient upregulation of pro-inflammatory genes in subjects whom received Poly-ICLC. Transcriptional responses were evaluated longitudinally in subjects' PBMCs using NanoString Technologies (nCounter® gene expression panel, human inflammation kit). Fold change (FC) from baseline of all significantly up regulated genes ($p < 0.05$, FDR < 1, FC ≥ +/−1.5) from subjects in Arm A (Poly-ICLC) are shown through day 8. No significant changes were observed in subjects' PBMCs in Arm B (Placebo) (not shown).

REFERENCES

1. Espindola MS, Soares LS, Galvao-Lima LJ, Zambuzi FA, Cacemiro MC, Brauer VS, et al. HIV infection: focus on the innate immune cells. *Immunol Res.* (2016) 64:1118–32. doi: 10.1007/s12026-016-8862-2
2. Miller E, Spadaccia M, Sabado R, Chertova E, Bess J, Trubey CM, et al. Autologous aldrithiol-2-inactivated HIV-1 combined with polyinosinic-polycytidylic acid-poly-L-lysine carboxymethylcellulose as a vaccine platform for therapeutic dendritic cell immunotherapy. *Vaccine.* (2015) 33:388–95. doi: 10.1016/j.vaccine.2014.10.054
3. Miller EA, Gopal R, Valdes V, Berger JS, Bhardwaj N, O'Brien MP. Soluble CD40 ligand contributes to dendritic cell-mediated T-cell dysfunction in HIV-1 infection. *AIDS.* (2015) 29:1287–96. doi: 10.1097/QAD.0000000000000698
4. Buisson S, Benlahrech A, Gazzard B, Gotch F, Kelleher P, Patterson S. Monocyte-derived dendritic cells from HIV type 1-infected individuals show reduced ability to stimulate T cells and have altered production of interleukin (IL)-12 and IL-10. *J Infect Dis.* (2009) 199:1862–71. doi: 10.1086/599122
5. Smed-Sorensen A, Lore K, Walther-Jallow L, Andersson J, Spetz AL. HIV-1-infected dendritic cells up-regulate cell surface markers but fail to produce IL-12 p70 in response to CD40 ligand stimulation. *Blood.* (2004) 104:2810–7. doi: 10.1182/blood-2003-07-2314
6. Frleta D, Ochoa CE, Kramer HB, Khan SA, Stacey AR, Borrow P, et al. HIV-1 infection-induced apoptotic microparticles inhibit human DCs via CD44. *J Clin Invest.* (2012) 122:4685–97. doi: 10.1172/JCI64439
7. Battistini A, Sgarbanti M. HIV-1 latency: an update of molecular mechanisms and therapeutic strategies. *Viruses.* (2014) 6:1715–58. doi: 10.3390/v6041715
8. Saxena M, Bhardwaj N. Turbocharging vaccines: emerging adjuvants for dendritic cell based therapeutic cancer vaccines. *Curr Opin Immunol.* (2017) 47:35–43. doi: 10.1016/j.coi.2017.06.003
9. Katlama C, Deeks SG, Autran B, Martinez-Picado J, van Lunzen J, Rouzioux C, et al. Barriers to a cure for HIV: new ways to target and eradicate HIV-1 reservoirs. *Lancet.* (2013) 381:2109–17. doi: 10.1016/S0140-6736(13)60104-X
10. Swaminathan G, Navas-Martin S, Martin-Garcia J. Interplay between microRNAs, Toll-like receptors, and HIV-1: potential implications in HIV-1 replication and chronic immune activation. *Discov Med.* (2014) 18:15–27.
11. Matsumoto M, Seya T. TLR3: interferon induction by double-stranded RNA including poly(I:C). *Adv Drug Deliv Rev.* (2008) 60:805–12. doi: 10.1016/j.addr.2007.11.005
12. Petes C, Odoardi N, Gee K. The toll for trafficking: toll-like receptor 7 delivery to the endosome. *Front Immunol.* (2017) 8:1075. doi: 10.3389/fimmu.2017.01075
13. Muller T, Hamm S, Bauer S. TLR9-mediated recognition of DNA. *Handb Exp Pharmacol* 2008:51–70. doi: 10.1007/978-3-540-72167-3_3
14. Satoh T, Akira S. Toll-like receptor signaling and its inducible proteins. *Microbiol Spectr.* (2016) 4. doi: 10.1128/microbiolspec.MCHD-0040-2016
15. Sivori S, Carlomagno S, Pesce S, Moretta A, Vitale M, Marcenaro E. TLR/NCR/KIR: which one to use and when? *Front Immunol.* (2014) 5:105. doi: 10.3389/fimmu.2014.00105
16. Saxena M, Bhardwaj N. Re-emergence of dendritic cell vaccines for cancer treatment. *Trends Cancer.* (2018) 4:119–37. doi: 10.1016/j.trecan.2017.12.007
17. Novis CL, Archin NM, Buzon MJ, Verdin E, Round JL, Lichterfeld M, et al. Reactivation of latent HIV-1 in central memory CD4(+) T cells through TLR-1/2 stimulation. *Retrovirology.* (2013) 10:119. doi: 10.1186/1742-4690-10-119
18. Offersen R, Nissen SK, Rasmussen TA, Ostergaard L, Denton PW, Sogaard OS, et al. A novel toll-like receptor 9 agonist, MGN1703, enhances hiv-1 transcription and nk cell-mediated inhibition of hiv-1-infected autologous CD4+ T cells. *J Virol.* (2016) 90:4441–53. doi: 10.1128/JVI.00222-16
19. Tsai A, Irrinki A, Kaur J, Cihlar T, Kukolj G, Sloan DD, et al. Toll-like receptor 7 agonist gs-9620 induces HIV expression and HIV-specific immunity in cells from HIV-infected individuals on suppressive antiretroviral therapy. *J Virol.* (2017) 91:e02166-16. doi: 10.1128/JVI.02166-16
20. Vibholm L, Schleimann MH, Hojen JF, Benfield T, Offersen R, Rasmussen K, et al. Short-course toll-like receptor 9 agonist treatment impacts innate immunity and plasma viremia in individuals with human immunodeficiency virus infection. *Clin Infect Dis.* (2017) 64:1686–95. doi: 10.1093/cid/cix201
21. Lim SY, Osuna CE, Hraber PT, Hesselgesser J, Gerold JM, Barnes TL, et al. TLR7 agonists induce transient viremia and reduce the viral reservoir in SIV-infected rhesus macaques on antiretroviral therapy. *Sci Transl Med.* (2018) 10:eaao4521. doi: 10.1126/scitranslmed.aao4521
22. Martins KA, Bavari S, Salazar AM. Vaccine adjuvant uses of poly-IC and derivatives. *Expert Rev Vaccines.* (2015) 14:447–59. doi: 10.1586/14760584.2015.966085
23. McCartney S, Vermi W, Gilfillan S, Cella M, Murphy TL, Schreiber RD, et al. Distinct and complementary functions of MDA5 and TLR3 in poly(I:C)-mediated activation of mouse NK cells. *J Exp Med.* (2009) 206:2967–76. doi: 10.1084/jem.20091181
24. Zhang Z, Kim T, Bao M, Facchinetti V, Jung SY, Ghaffari AA, et al. DDX1, DDX21, and DHX36 helicases form a complex with the adaptor molecule TRIF to sense dsRNA in dendritic cells. *Immunity.* (2011) 34:866–78. doi: 10.1016/j.immuni.2011.03.027
25. Longhi MP, Trumpfheller C, Idoyaga J, Caskey M, Matos I, Kluger C, et al. Dendritic cells require a systemic type I interferon response to mature and induce CD4+ Th1 immunity with poly IC as adjuvant. *J Exp Med.* (2009) 206:1589–602. doi: 10.1084/jem.20090247
26. Cheng L, Zhang Z, Li G, Li F, Wang L, Zhang L, et al. Human innate responses and adjuvant activity of TLR ligands in vivo in mice reconstituted with a human immune system. *Vaccine.* (2017) 35:6143–53. doi: 10.1016/j.vaccine.2017.09.052
27. Alvarez-Carbonell D, Garcia-Mesa Y, Milne S, Das B, Dobrowolski C, Rojas R, et al. Toll-like receptor 3 activation selectively reverses HIV latency in microglial cells. *Retrovirology.* (2017) 14:9. doi: 10.1186/s12977-017-0335-8
28. Kyi C, Roudko V, Sabado R, Saenger YM, Loging W, Mandeli J, et al. Therapeutic immune modulation against solid cancers with intratumoral poly-ICLC: a pilot trial. *Clin Cancer Res.* (2018) 24:4937–48. doi: 10.1158/1078-0432.CCR-17-1866
29. Liu H, Zha Y, Choudhury N, Malnassy G, Fulton N, Green M, et al. WT1 peptide vaccine in Montanide in contrast to poly ICLC, is able to induce WT1-specific immune response with TCR clonal enrichment in myeloid leukemia. *Exp Hematol Oncol.* (2018) 7:1. doi: 10.1186/s40164-018-0093-x
30. Griffiths EA, Srivastava P, Matsuzaki J, Brumberger Z, Wang ES, Kocent J, et al. NY-ESO-1 vaccination in combination with decitabine induces antigen-specific t-lymphocyte responses in patients with myelodysplastic syndrome. *Clin Cancer Res.* (2018) 24:1019–29. doi: 10.1158/1078-0432.CCR-17-1792
31. Caskey M, Lefebvre F, Filali-Mouhim A, Cameron MJ, Goulet JP, Haddad EK, et al. Synthetic double-stranded RNA induces innate immune responses similar to a live viral vaccine in humans. *J Exp Med.* (2011) 208:2357–66. doi: 10.1084/jem.20111171
32. Tsuji T, Sabbatini P, Jungbluth AA, Ritter E, Pan L, Ritter G, et al. Effect of Montanide and poly-ICLC adjuvant on human self/tumor antigen-specific CD4+ T cells in phase I overlapping long peptide vaccine trial. *Cancer Immunol Res.* (2013) 1:340–50. doi: 10.1158/2326-6066.CIR-13-0089
33. Salazar AM, Erlich RB, Mark A, Bhardwaj N, Herberman RB. Therapeutic in situ autovaccination against solid cancers with intratumoral poly-ICLC: case report, hypothesis, and clinical trial. *Cancer Immunol Res.* (2014) 2:720–4. doi: 10.1158/2326-6066.CIR-14-0024
34. Aravantinou M, Frank I, Hallor M, Singer R, Tharinger H, Kenney J, et al. PolyICLC exerts pro- and anti-HIV effects on the DC-T cell milieu *in vitro* and *in vivo*. *PLoS ONE.* (2016) 11:e0161730. doi: 10.1371/journal.pone.0161730
35. Vagenas P, Aravantinou M, Williams VG, Jasny E, Piatak M Jr, Lifson JD, et al. A tonsillar PolyICLC/AT-2 SIV therapeutic vaccine maintains low viremia following antiretroviral therapy cessation. *PLoS ONE.* (2010) 5:e12891. doi: 10.1371/journal.pone.0012891
36. Park H, Adamson L, Ha T, Mullen K, Hagen SI, Nogueron A, et al. Polyinosinic-polycytidylic acid is the most effective TLR adjuvant for SIV gag protein-induced T cell responses in nonhuman primates. *J Immunol.* (2013) 190:4103–15. doi: 10.4049/jimmunol.1202958
37. Zurawski G, Zurawski S, Flamar AL, Richert L, Wagner R, Tomaras GD, et al. Targeting HIV-1 Env gp140 to LOX-1 elicits immune responses in rhesus macaques. *PLoS ONE.* (2016) 11:e0153484. doi: 10.1371/journal.pone.0153484
38. Flynn BJ, Kastenmuller K, Wille-Reece U, Tomaras GD, Alam M, Lindsay RW, et al. Immunization with HIV Gag targeted to dendritic cells followed by recombinant New York vaccinia virus induces robust T-cell immunity

in nonhuman primates. *Proc Natl Acad Sci USA.* (2011) 108:7131–6. doi: 10.1073/pnas.1103869108
39. Miller EA, Spadaccia MR, O'Brien MP, Rolnitzky L, Sabado R, Manches O, et al. Plasma factors during chronic HIV-1 infection impair IL-12 secretion by myeloid dendritic cells via a virus-independent pathway. *J Acquir Immune Defic Syndr.* (2012) 61:535–44. doi: 10.1097/QAI.0b013e31826afbce
40. Miller EA, Spadaccia MR, Norton T, Demmler M, Gopal R, O'Brien M, et al. Attenuated Listeria monocytogenes vectors overcome suppressive plasma factors during HIV infection to stimulate myeloid dendritic cells to promote adaptive immunity and reactivation of latent virus. *AIDS Res Hum Retroviruses.* (2015) 31:127-36. doi: 10.1089/aid.2014.0138
41. Markowitz M, Evering TH, Garmon D, Caskey M, La Mar M, Rodriguez K, et al. A randomized open-label study of 3- versus 5-drug combination antiretroviral therapy in newly HIV-1-infected individuals. *J Acquir Immune Defic Syndr.* (2014) 66:140–7. doi: 10.1097/QAI.0000000000000111
42. Palmer S, Wiegand AP, Maldarelli F, Bazmi H, Mican JM, Polis M, et al. New real-time reverse transcriptase-initiated PCR assay with single-copy sensitivity for human immunodeficiency virus type 1 RNA in plasma. *J Clin Microbiol.* (2003) 41:4531-6. doi: 10.1128/JCM.41.10.4531-4536.2003
43. Hintze J. *P"ASS12. NCSS.* Kaysville, UT: LLC (2012). Available online at: www.ncss.com
44. Archin NM, Liberty AL, Kashuba AD, Choudhary SK, Kuruc JD, Crooks AM, et al. Administration of vorinostat disrupts HIV-1 latency in patients on antiretroviral therapy. *Nature.* (2012) 487:482–5. doi: 10.1038/nature11286
45. Chang JJ, Lacas A, Lindsay RJ, Doyle EH, Axten KL, Pereyra F, et al. Differential regulation of toll-like receptor pathways in acute and chronic HIV-1 infection. *AIDS.* (2012) 26:533–41. doi: 10.1097/QAD.0b013e32834f3167
46. Rautela J, Huntington ND. IL-15 signaling in NK cell cancer immunotherapy. *Curr Opin Immunol.* (2017) 44:1–6. doi: 10.1016/j.coi.2016.10.004
47. Shapiro MJ, Spruce L, Sundsbak R, Thapa P, Shapiro VS. Phosphorylation at serine 318 is not required for inhibition of T cell activation by ALX. *Biochem Biophys Res Commun.* (2010) 396:994–8. doi: 10.1016/j.bbrc.2010.05.043
48. Cornish GH, Sinclair LV, Cantrell DA. Differential regulation of T-cell growth by IL-2 and IL-15. *Blood.* (2006) 108:600–8. doi: 10.1182/blood-2005-12-4827
49. Saxena M, Yeretssian G. NOD-like receptors: master regulators of inflammation and cancer. *Front Immunol.* (2014) 5:327. doi: 10.3389/fimmu.2014.00327
50. Balan S, Arnold-Schrauf C, Abbas A, Couespel N, Savoret J, Imperatore F, et al. Large-scale human dendritic cell differentiation revealing notch-dependent lineage bifurcation and heterogeneity. *Cell Rep.* (2018) 24:1902–15.e1906. doi: 10.1016/j.celrep.2018.07.033
51. Milush JM, Lopez-Verges S, York VA, Deeks SG, Martin JN, Hecht FM, et al. CD56negCD16(+) NK cells are activated mature NK cells with impaired effector function during HIV-1 infection. *Retrovirology.* (2013) 10:158. doi: 10.1186/1742-4690-10-158
52. Jacobson A, Bell F, Lejarcegui N, Mitchell C, Frenkel L, Horton H. Healthy neonates possess a CD56-negative NK cell population with reduced anti-viral activity. *PLoS ONE.* (2013) 8:e67700. doi: 10.1371/journal.pone.0067700
53. da Silva IP, Gallois A, Jimenez-Baranda S, Khan S, Anderson AC, Kuchroo VK, et al. Reversal of NK-cell exhaustion in advanced melanoma by Tim-3 blockade. *Cancer Immunol Res.* (2014) 2:410–22. doi: 10.1158/2326-6066.CIR-13-0171
54. Gonzalez-Gugel E, Saxena M, Bhardwaj N. Modulation of innate immunity in the tumor microenvironment. *Cancer Immunol Immunother.* (2016) 65:1261–8. doi: 10.1007/s00262-016-1859-9
55. Akazawa T, Ebihara T, Okuno M, Okuda Y, Shingai M, Tsujimura K, et al. Antitumor NK activation induced by the Toll-like receptor 3-TICAM-1 (TRIF) pathway in myeloid dendritic cells. *Proc Natl Acad Sci USA.* (2007) 104:252–7. doi: 10.1073/pnas.0605978104
56. Nouri-Shirazi M, Tamjidi S, Nourishirazi E, Guinet E. TLR8 combined withTLR3 or TLR4 agonists enhances DC-NK driven effector Tc1 cells. *Immunol Lett.* (2018) 193:58–66. doi: 10.1016/j.imlet.2017.10.015
57. Dhodapkar MV, Sznol M, Zhao B, Wang D, Carvajal RD, Keohan ML, et al. Induction of antigen-specific immunity with a vaccine targeting NY-ESO-1 to the dendritic cell receptor DEC-205. *Sci Transl Med.* (2014) 6:232ra251. doi: 10.1126/scitranslmed.3008068
58. Okada H, Butterfield LH, Hamilton RL, Hoji A, Sakaki M, Ahn BJ, et al. Induction of robust type-I CD8+ T-cell responses in WHO grade 2 low-grade glioma patients receiving peptide-based vaccines in combination with poly-ICLC. *Clin Cancer Res.* (2015) 21:286–94. doi: 10.1158/1078-0432.CCR-14-1790
59. Quarona V, Zaccarello G, Chillemi A, Brunetti E, Singh VK, Ferrero E, et al. CD38 and CD157: a long journey from activation markers to multifunctional molecules. *Cytometry B Clin Cytom.* (2013) 84:207–17. doi: 10.1002/cyto.b.21092
60. Urban SL, Berg LJ, Welsh RM. Type 1 interferon licenses naive CD8 T cells to mediate anti-viral cytotoxicity. *Virology.* (2016) 493:52–9. doi: 10.1016/j.virol.2016.03.005
61. Castro-Gonzalez S, Colomer-Lluch M, Serra-Moreno R. Barriers for a HIV cure: the latent reservoir. *AIDS Res Hum Retroviruses.* (2018) 34:739–59. doi: 10.1089/aid.2018.0118
62. Kent SJ, Reece JC, Petravic J, Martyushev A, Kramski M, De Rose R, et al. The search for an HIV cure: tackling latent infection. *Lancet Infect Dis.* (2013) 13:614–21. doi: 10.1016/S1473-3099(13)70043-4
63. Jones RB, Mueller S, O'Connor R, Rimpel K, Sloan DD, Karel D, et al. A subset of latency-reversing agents expose HIV-infected resting CD4+ T-cells to recognition by cytotoxic T-lymphocytes. *PLoS Pathog.* (2016) 12:e1005545. doi: 10.1371/journal.ppat.1005545
64. Saxena M, Balan S, Roudko V, Bhardwaj N. Towards superior dendritic-cell vaccines for cancer therapy. *Nat Biomed Eng.* (2018) 2:341–6. doi: 10.1038/s41551-018-0250-x
65. Melchjorsen J, Risor MW, Sogaard OS, O'Loughlin KL, Chow S, Paludan SR, et al. Tenofovir selectively regulates production of inflammatory cytokines and shifts the IL-12/IL-10 balance in human primary cells. *J Acquir Immune Defic Syndr.* (2011) 57:265–75. doi: 10.1097/QAI.0b013e3182185276

18

Circulating LPS and (1→3)-β-D-Glucan: A Folie à Deux Contributing to HIV-Associated Immune Activation

*Rayoun Ramendra[1,2,3], Stéphane Isnard[1,2], Vikram Mehraj[4], Jun Chen[1,2], Yonglong Zhang[5], Malcolm Finkelman[5] and Jean-Pierre Routy[1,2,6]**

[1] Chronic Viral Illness Service, McGill University Health Centre, Montreal, QC, Canada, [2] Infectious Diseases and Immunity in Global Health Program, Research Institute, McGill University Health Centre, Montreal, QC, Canada, [3] Department of Microbiology and Immunology, McGill University, Montreal, QC, Canada, [4] Centre de Recherche du Centre Hospitalier de l'Université de Montréal, Montreal, QC, Canada, [5] Associates of Cape Cod Inc., Falmouth, MA, United States, [6] Division of Hematology, McGill University Health Centre, Montreal, QC, Canada

***Correspondence:**
Jean-Pierre Routy
jean-pierre.routy@mcgill.ca

Immune activation is the driving force behind the occurrence of AIDS and non-AIDS events, and is only partially reduced by antiretroviral therapy (ART). Soon after HIV infection, intestinal CD4+ T cells are depleted leading to epithelial gut damage and subsequent translocation of microbes and/or their products into systemic circulation. Bacteria and fungi are the two most abundant populations of the gut microbiome. Circulating lipopolysaccharide (LPS) and (1→3)-β-D-Glucan (βDG), major components of bacterial and fungal cell walls respectively, are measured as markers of microbial translocation in the context of compromised gut barriers. While LPS is a well-known inducer of innate immune activation, βDG is emerging as a significant source of monocyte and NK cell activation that contributes to immune dysfunction. Herein, we critically evaluated recent literature to untangle the respective roles of LPS and βDG in HIV-associated immune dysfunction. Furthermore, we appraised the relevance of LPS and βDG as biomarkers of disease progression and immune activation on ART. Understanding the consequences of elevated LPS and βDG on immune activation will provide insight into novel therapeutic strategies against the occurrence of AIDS and non-AIDS events.

Keywords: HIV, LPS, (1→3)-β-D-Glucan, immune activation, microbial translocation, antiretroviral therapy, non-AIDS events

INTRODUCTION

The gastrointestinal tract (GI) is a dynamic setting constantly in contact with nutrients, allergens, commensal microbes, and pathogens. As such, this milieu is equipped with a complex and well balanced system of physical and immunological barriers to allow the absorption of nutrients while preventing the translocation of microbes and their products (1). A physical barrier is formed by firmly linked intestinal epithelial cells (enterocytes) connected via tight junctions. These cells form villi to maximize the absorption of nutrients. The base of each villus forms crypts composed of intestinal stem cells and Paneth cells which secrete growth factors that promote intestinal stem cell proliferation, antimicrobial peptide secretion, and digestive enzyme production (2, 3). In the upper regions of the villus, goblet cells contribute to the physical and chemical barriers by secreting a mucous layer that protects the gut epithelium from the microbiota (4). Patrolling leukocytes in the lamina propria constitute an immunological barrier that ensures any pathogens in the lamina propria are phagocytosed, cleared, and sent to the draining mesenteric lymph nodes (5).

HIV-infection is characterized by the depletion of gut CD4+ T cells, epithelial gut damage, and translocation of microbes and their products into systemic circulation (6). People living with HIV (PLWH) have damage to the gut epithelium which has been shown to precede immune activation in models of SIV-infected rhesus macaques (7, 8). As systemic immune activation is considered the driving force of CD4+ T cell depletion and development of acquired immunodeficiency syndrome (AIDS), it is important to understand the link between epithelial gut damage and systemic immune activation in PLWH.

In 2006, Brenchley et al. were the first to report that increased plasma levels of gram-negative bacterial cell wall antigen lipopolysaccharide (LPS) induces systemic immune activation in both PLWH and SIV-infected rhesus macaques (9). Estes et al. in 2010, demonstrated that elevated plasma levels of LPS in PLWH is a result of HIV-induced epithelial gut damage allowing for the translocation of microbial products from the gut microbiota into systemic circulation (10). Despite the success of antiretroviral therapy (ART), epithelial gut damage, microbial translocation, and to a lesser extent systemic immune activation are not reversed. In parallel, Cani et al. coined the term "metabolic endotoxemia" to describe the phenomenon of obese individuals with high plasma levels of LPS linked to reduced insulin sensitivity and increased risk of metabolic diseases (11). Furthermore, conserved parts of the LPS molecule act as a pathogen-associated molecular patterns (PAMPs) that have been associated *in vitro*, in animal models, and epidemiologically with increased innate immune activation, inflammation, and risk of developing non-AIDS events in ART-treated PLWH (9, 12).

Increasing awareness about the human gut microbiota reveals that it is a complex community of bacteria, fungi, archaea, viruses, and parasites influencing health and disease (13). However, studies regarding microbial translocation in PLWH have primarily focused on bacterial translocation. (1→3)-β-D-Glucan (βDG), a major component of most fungal cell walls, is commonly used as a biomarker for the diagnosis and management of invasive fungal infections (IFI) and has been recently used as a marker of fungal translocation in people without IFI (14). In 2012, Morris et al. were the first to show elevated plasma levels of βDG in PLWH (15). We and others have found that plasma levels of βDG are associated with epithelial gut damage, immune activation, inflammation, and risk of developing non-AIDS events (16–20). Like epithelial gut damage, plasma levels of βDG do not normalize despite long-term ART (20). These findings show converging evidence that like LPS, βDG also plays a significant role in chronic immune activation and development of non-AIDS events in PLWH (**Figure 1**).

Currently, persistence of systemic immune activation and development of non-AIDS events despite long-term ART represents one of the hurdles in caring for PLWH (21). Herein, we look to comprehensively review the existing English literature regarding the contribution of circulating LPS and βDG in systemic immune activation in PLWH. Understanding the consequences of LPS and βDG antigenemia will help with the development of therapeutic strategies against this "folie à deux."

GUT DAMAGE

In homeostatic conditions, the microbiota is contained within the gut by the mucous layer, epithelial barrier, and residential leukocytes (22–25).

HIV infection leads to early disruption of the gut epithelial barrier characterized by villous atrophy, crypt hyperplasia, increased gastrointestinal inflammation, and increased intestinal permeability (7, 26–28). Such damage is not completely restored despite long-term ART. Deterioration of the gastrointestinal landscape in PLWH and SIV-infected rhesus macaques has been shown to cause microbial translocation and resultant immune activation (9, 10, 29). Interestingly, SIV-infected sooty mangabeys, which do not progress to AIDS, present without disruption of the GI epithelial layer nor increased microbial translocation, and limited immune activation (30, 31). Thus, understanding the cause(s) and implications of epithelial gut damage in PLWH may help to understand the source(s) of systemic immune activation.

The precise mechanisms responsible for HIV-associated epithelial gut damage remain poorly understood and are now known to precede mucosal immune dysfunction (7). HIV gp120 and Tat proteins have been shown to have detrimental effects on intestinal epithelial cells (32–36). HIV induces inflammasome to produce IL-18, resulting in intestinal epithelial cell death and reduced expression of tight junction proteins, contributing to intestinal permeability and resultant microbial translocation (37, 38). Globally, HIV contributes to epithelial gut damage which is partially improved on ART (39, 40). Markers of epithelial gut damage such as soluble suppressor of tumorigenicity 2 (sST2) and intestinal fatty acid binding protein (I-FABP) have been reported to be elevated in inflammatory bowel diseases, graft vs. host disease, and HIV (41, 42).

As reported by Hensley-McBain et al., alterations to the intestinal epithelial structure precede mucosal immune dysfunction (7). Early mucosal damage in PLWH is partially explained by a substantially high expression of CCR5, a HIV co-receptor, on CD4+ T cells in the gut as compared to peripheral blood (43, 44). This is in line with findings that HIV is 10 times more likely to infect CD4+ T cells in the gut compared to peripheral blood (45). IL-17 producing cells, such as Th17 and Th22 CD4+ T cells, are known to homeostatically maintain the epithelial barrier (7). We and others have reported alterations of the Th17/Treg ratio in PLWH, owing to increased frequency of Tregs and decreased frequency of Th17 CD4+ T cells (46, 47). This in turn impairs the homeostatic response to prevent and restore epithelial gut damage in PLWH. HIV-associated gastrointestinal abnormalities have also been associated with changes in the composition of the gut microbiome (dysbiosis) and translocation of microbial products in PLWH.

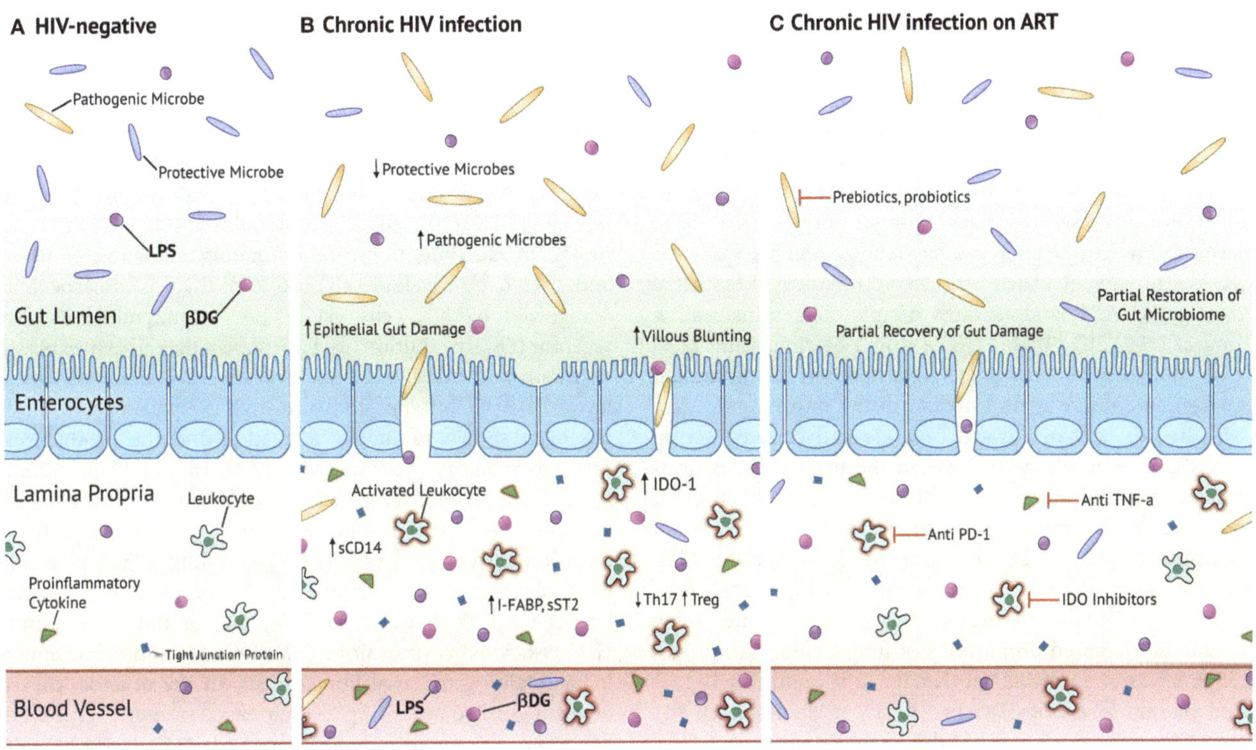

FIGURE 1 | Proposed mechanism of microbial translocation in chronic HIV-infection and chronic HIV-infection on ART compared to HIV- homeostasis. **(A)** Healthy, HIV-uninfected individuals have an abundance of protective microbes in the gut and tight junctions connecting enterocytes to prevent the translocation of gut microbes and their products. Patrolling leukocytes in the lamina propria are not activated and there is an almost negligible level of inflammation and epithelial damage. **(B)** PLWH in the chronic stage of infection have increased proportions of pathogenic microbes and decreased proportions of protective microbes in the gut. There is severe villous blunting, epithelial gut damage, and microbial translocation. Patrolling leukocytes are activated and secrete large quantities of pro-inflammatory cytokines. There is elevated circulation of markers of epithelial gut damage, microbial translocation, and inflammation. **(C)** PLWH on long-term ART have partially restored composition of the gut microbiota, epithelial gut damage, and reduced microbial translocation. Activated leukocytes and systemic inflammation persists. Prebiotics and probiotics are potential therapeutic strategies to fully recover the composition of the gut microbiota. Anti PD-1, anti TNF-α, and IDO inhibitors represent potential therapeutic strategies against persistent immune activation and inflammation. LPS, lipopolysaccharide; βDG, (1→3)-β-D-Glucan; sCD14, soluble cluster of differentiation 14; I-FABP, intestinal fatty acid binding protein; sST2, soluble suppressor of tumorigenicity 2; IDO-1, indoleamine-2,3-dioxygenase 1.

BACTERIAL AND FUNGAL TRANSLOCATION

In homeostatic conditions, microbial translocation is limited by physical and immunological barriers in the intestine (48). However, when the gut epithelium is damaged and the mucosal immune system is compromised, microbial products translocate out of the gut into systemic circulation via the lamina propria (49, 50). Microbial translocation has been implicated in several conditions including Crohn's disease, ulcerative colitis, graft-vs.-host disease, and HIV (40).

SIV-infected rhesus macaques were shown to have elevated plasma levels of LPS that could be partially reversed with antibiotics. Immunohistochemistry and immunofluorescence of gut biopsies demonstrated that such elevation was a result of bacterial translocation from the gut lumen into systemic circulation via the lamina propria (9, 10). Interestingly, SIV-infected African green monkeys, a natural host of SIV, receiving intravenous injection of LPS had increased viral replication, mucosal CD4+ T cell depletion, and systemic immune activation without inducing epithelial gut damage (51, 52). Altogether, this suggests that translocation of microbial products plays a major role in systemic immune activation and inflammation.

We and others have shown elevation of microbial products in the blood of PLWH (9, 15, 46). Most published studies measured microbial translocation using plasma levels of bacterial DNA fragments, LPS, LPS binding protein (LBP), soluble CD14 (sCD14), and EndoCab (50). Bacterial DNA fragments were quantified using 16S rDNA PCR. Most studies in PLWH use the Limulus Amebocyte Lysate (LAL) assay to measure plasma levels of LPS, a major component of the outer membrane of gram-negative bacteria. LPS binds to LBP, which transfers LPS onto monocytes/macrophages causing the release of soluble CD14 (sCD14) (53). EndoCab is a group of antibodies specific for the core of LPS that are produced by B cells in response to enteric gram-negative bacteria (54). LBP, sCD14, and EndoCab are commonly measured in plasma/serum using solid-phase enzyme-linked immunosorbent assay (ELISA) as circulating biomarkers of LPS-induced innate immune activation (9, 39).

Most research on microbial translocation in PLWH has been focused on bacterial translocation (13). Morris et al. were the first to show elevation of circulating levels of fungal cell wall antigen, βDG, in PLWH (15). Hoenigl et al. have shown that plasma βDG is inversely correlated with the abundance of *Lactobacilli* in the distal gut (19). *Lactobacillus* is a protective genus of bacteria that is inversely associated with gut integrity and distal gut permeability. Furthermore, we have shown that plasma levels of βDG is strongly correlated with classical marker of epithelial gut damage, I-FABP, and markers of microbial translocation LPS and sCD14 (20) (**Table 1**). The origin of circulating βDG was first studied in murine models. As opposed to the human gut microbiome, there is no *Candida* in the murine gut. Mice fed with live or heat-inactivated *Candida* had elevated serum levels of βDG. Such elevation induced the production of pro-inflammatory cytokines IL-6 and TNF-α. Administration of Fluconazole, an anti-fungal small molecule, partially inhibited the elevation of serum βDG and systemic inflammation (55). Similar results were found in a murine model of lupus and sepsis (56, 57). As PLWH without invasive fungal infections are highly susceptible to increased proportions of fungal colonization and have high levels of epithelial gut damage, it is highly likely that elevated plasma levels of βDG in PLWH originates from the gut (14). Thus, there is a need to definitely determine whether elevated plasma levels of βDG in PLWH is a result of microbial translocation and involved in systemic immune activation.

MICROBIAL TRANSLOCATION AND SYSTEMIC IMMUNE ACTIVATION

Microbial products such as LPS and βDG represent potent PAMPs that trigger a significant immune response. Several studies have provided convincing evidence that elevated plasma levels of LPS induces immune activation in sepsis, Crohn's disease, ulcerative colitis, obesity, and HIV (9, 11, 58, 59).

LPS is captured by LBP and complexed with CD14, myeloid differentiation 2 protein, and Toll like receptor 4 (TLR4). The formation of this complex is crucial for the immune system to mount a response to LPS. Classical antigen presenting cells (APCs) recognize this complex using TLR4 and subsequently phagocytose LPS while shedding sCD14. B cells also express TLR4 to recognize different parts of the LPS core lipids and secrete EndoCAb to facilitate the phagocytosis of the antigen (60). LPS has been shown to induce the secretion of several pro-inflammatory cytokines including IL-6, IL-8, and TNF-α by APCs (61). Plasma levels of LPS correlated with plasma levels of IFN-α and frequency of activated CD4+ and CD8+ T cells in PLWH (9). Similarly, plasma levels of sCD14 correlated with plasma levels of IL-6 and C reactive protein in PLWH (62).

Meanwhile, βDG is predominantly recognized by complement receptor 3 (CR3), Dectin-1, NKp30, Ephrin type-A receptor 2 (EphA2), and Langerin. CR3 is a ubiquitous heterodimer receptor composed of CD11b and CD18. Recent findings have shown reduced expression of CR3 on both myeloid and plasmacytoid dendritic cells (DC) in PLWH. βDG-specific interactions with CR3 on DC have been shown to increase IL-6 and TNF-α production by activating the Syk-JNK-AP-1 pathway (63). Dectin-1 represents the most prominent myeloid cell receptor for βDG and is expressed on monocytes, macrophages, DCs, and neutrophils (63–65). We have shown that Dectin-1 expression on monocytes is reduced in PLWH and that such expression is inversely correlated with plasma levels of βDG but not LPS (20). βDG-specific binding to Dectin-1 leads to the production of pro-inflammatory cytokines IL-6, IL-8, and TNF-α by myeloid cells (66, 67). βDG is also specifically recognized by NK cells via NKp30, a functional activation receptor (68). In addition, we have shown that NKp30 expression is diminished in PLWH and inversely correlated with plasma levels of βDG but not LPS (20, 69). NKp30-specific binding has been shown to induce activation and the production of pro-inflammatory cytokines such as IL-1β and TNF-α (70, 71). EphA2 is a βDG-specific receptor expressed on epithelial cells, predominantly in the colon and small intestine, that has yet to be measured in PLWH (72). Interestingly, EphA2 has also been identified as a receptor for Kaposi Sarcoma associated herpes virus (also called HHV8), one of the most common HIV-associated co-infections (73). DCs play an important role in maintaining mucosal homeostasis. In the mucosa, they can be distinguished according to their expression of C-type lectins: Langerin [expressed by Langerhans cells (LCs)] and DC-SIGN (expressed by classical DCs). LCs reside in the epithelium of most mucosal surfaces and are thus one of the first APCs to encounter HIV as well as products of microbial translocation. Langerin has been shown to be an important receptor for βDG during *Candida* and *Saccharomyces* infections that has yet to be assessed in PLWH without IFI (74). βDG induces the secretion of pro-inflammatory cytokines IL-1β, IL-6, IL-8, IL-23, TNF-α, and chemokine CCL22 that has been shown to increase monocyte recruitment to the colon (66, 75, 76). Indeed, we and others have shown that elevated plasma levels of βDG is correlated with plasma levels of IL-6 and IL-8 in PLWH (15, 20).

Microbial translocation in PLWH is associated with Indoleamine-2,3-deoxygenase-1 (IDO-1) activity and HIV disease progression (77). IDO-1 is expressed in all myeloid cells and activated after PAMPs recognition to metabolize Tryptophan into Kynurenines (78). As such, IDO-1 activity is considered a marker of inflammation and immune activation. We and others have shown that IDO-1 activity is increased in PLWH and does not normalize with early ART. In PLWH, IDO-1 activity is associated with plasma levels of LPS and βDG, increased frequency of Tregs, epithelial gut damage, microbial translocation, immune activation, and HIV reservoir size (20, 46, 79, 80).

Persistent epithelial gut damage and elevated plasma levels of LPS and βDG, despite long-term ART, likely contribute to inflammation and chronic immune activation leading to the development of non-AIDS events in PLWH. In the ART-era, the development of non-AIDS events represents one of the challenges to caring for PLWH. Therefore, both LPS and βDG represent important therapeutic targets to reduce the risk of developing non-AIDS events.

TABLE 1 | Overview of studies associating elevation of plasma levels of βDG with immune activation and immune dysfunction in PLWH.

References (country)	Sample size	Study populations	Major findings
Morris et al. (15) (USA)	132	Chronic ART-treated PLWH; cross-sectional analysis	βDG was elevated in the plasma of PLWH and associated with plasma levels of IL-8, TNF-α, and frequency of CD38+ and HLA-DR+ CD8+ T cells. Elevated βDG was associated with cardiopulmonary dysfunction.
Hoenigl et al. (17) (USA)	41	Chronic ART-treated PLWH; cross-sectional analysis	Plasma level of βDG was positively associated with plasma levels of neopterin and IL-6.
Hoenigl et al. (19) (USA)	11	PLWH in early stage of infection, before and after ART; cross-sectional analysis	Elevated plasma levels of βDG was inversely correlated with abundance of *Lactobacillales* in the distal gut.
Hoenigl et al. (16) (USA)	21	Chronic ART-treated PLWH; cross-sectional analysis	βDG was elevated in the plasma and CSF of PLWH and positively associated with neurocognitive dysfunction.
Hoenigl et al. (18) (USA)	451	PLWH before and after ART; cross-sectional analysis	Multivariate analysis showed that pre-event plasma levels of βDG and LBP was independently associated with increased risk of non-AIDS events.
Mehraj et al. (20) (Canada)	146	PLWH in early and chronic stages, ART-treated and untreated; longitudinal and cross sectional analysis	Plasma levels of βDG was associated with plasma viral load, I-FABP, LPS, markers of IDO-1 metabolism, and frequency of Tregs. Expression of βDG-specific receptors, Dectin-1 and NKp30, was inversely correlated with plasma levels of βDG but not LPS. PLWH who initiated ART early had lower levels of plasma βDG and elevated βDG did not normalize despite long-term ART.

PLWH, People living with HIV; ART, Antiretroviral Therapy; βDG, (1→3)-β-D-Glucan; LPS, Lipopolysaccharide; LBP, LPS Binding Protein; I-FABP, Intestinal Fatty Acid Binding Protein (marker of epithelial gut damage).

MICROBIAL TRANSLOCATION, INFLAMMATION, AND NON-AIDS EVENTS

Despite the significant success of ART, PLWH still present with high rates of non-AIDS events that includes HIV-associated neurocognitive disorders (HANDs), cardiovascular diseases, renal failure, liver steatosis, and cancer (81, 82). Such non-AIDS events have been associated with epithelial gut damage, microbial translocation, and systemic immune activation (50). Hoenigl et al. have observed in a large cohort of ART-treated PLWH that in addition to soluble urokinase-type plasminogen receptor, plasma levels of βDG, and LBP represent two of the best predictors of increased risk of non-AIDS events (18).

Microbial Translocation and HAND

PLWH present with HANDs including asymptomatic neurocognitive impairment, mild neurocognitive disorder, and dementia (83, 84). Previous studies have found strong associations between plasma levels of sCD14, LPS, and βDG with neurocognitive dysfunction (16, 85). Moreover, ART-treated PLWH with severe neurocognitive dysfunction also presented with elevated sCD14 and βDG in their cerebrospinal fluid (CSF) (16). Supporting the concept of the gut-brain axis, increased microbial translocation likely plays a crucial role in the development of HANDs.

Microbial Translocation and Cardiovascular Diseases

A study with more than 27,000 participants showed that PLWH had a two-fold increased risk of developing acute myocardial infarction in every age group compared to matched control participants (86, 87). Elevated circulation of microbial products and resultant inflammation are associated with increased risk of heart disease (88). Plasma levels of LPS have been associated with known risk factors for cardiovascular diseases such as decreased insulin sensitivity and higher total cholesterol (11). Similarly, elevated plasma levels of βDG have also been associated with cardiopulmonary dysfunction (15).

CONCLUSIONS AND FUTURE DIRECTIONS

Due to the success of ART, the life expectancy and quality of life of PLWH has dramatically improved over the course of the last decade. While early initiation of ART is associated with lower reservoir size and reduced immune activation, PLWH on ART still suffer from unrecovered epithelial gut damage and chronic immune activation (89). It has been recently reported that epithelial gut damage precedes systemic immune activation in a SIV-infected rhesus macaque model (7). Like epithelial gut damage and systemic immune activation, markers of microbial translocation do not normalize despite long-term ART (20). Thus, understanding the mechanisms via which epithelial gut damage and resultant microbial translocation contribute to chronic immune activation is essential toward improving the prognosis of PLWH.

Circulating microbial polysaccharides LPS and βDG are elevated in PLWH (9, 15). Previous research on microbial translocation in PLWH and SIV-infected rhesus macaques has been primarily measured by plasma levels of LPS using the LAL assay. Of note, it has been initially found that LPS measured by the LAL assay also measures βDG (90). While it has been shown that increased plasma levels of LPS are a result of microbial translocation in PLWH, the source of circulating βDG remains to be clarified. Consumption of certain mushrooms, oat fiber, and seaweed can also increase circulating levels of βDG (91). We and others have shown that plasma levels of βDG are positively associated with marker of epithelial gut damage I-FABP and inversely associated with the abundance of protective bacteria, *Lactobacillales*, in the distal gut (19, 20). Furthermore, murine models have shown that mice fed with heat-killed or live *Candida* have increased levels of circulating βDG after cecal ligation and puncture (55). Similarly, people with intestine disorders have increased plasma levels of βDG (56, 92, 93). Hence, there is converging evidence suggesting that elevated plasma levels of βDG in PLWH are a result of increased *Candida* or other fungal colonization, epithelial gut damage, and subsequent microbial translocation.

Both LPS and βDG have been associated with markers of systemic immune activation, inflammation, and the development of non-AIDS events. As such, the individual and potentially synergistic consequences of elevated plasma levels of LPS and βDG on systemic immune activation must be urgently addressed.

Understanding the respective mechanisms by which these two microbial polysaccharides contribute to chronic immune activation may lead to the development of novel therapeutic strategies against inflammation and the development of non-AIDS events in PLWH. Moreover, genetic factors may play a key role in determining the influence of these PAMPs on systemic immune activation. For example, people with CARD9 deficiencies have been shown to have increased susceptibility to fungal infections (94). Furthermore, Palesch et al. demonstrated that sooty mangabeys, a natural host of SIV, had a frameshift mutation in their TLR4 gene that was associated with a blunted response to TLR4 ligands *in vitro* (95). Thus, regular genetic variations in receptors for LPS and βDG may also play a pivotal role in determining the consequences of microbial translocation in PLWH.

In 2014, Kristoff et al. gave Sevelamer, a drug known to decrease circulating LPS (96), to SIV-infected pigtailed macaques. A single dose administration led to partially decreased HIV viral replication, decreased circulation of coagulation markers, and decreased immune activation/inflammation (52). However, when Sandler et al. gave Sevelamer to 36 ART-naïve PLWH, they did not observe a decrease in plasma levels of LPS (measured by LAL assay) nor markers of immune activation/inflammation (97). Future clinical trials should aim to reduce the burden of elevated circulation of products of both bacterial and fungal translocation. While therapeutic strategies targeting elevated circulation of PAMPs should be investigated, future studies should also look to target immune signaling molecules (such as TLR4 and Dectin-1) to reduce LPS and βDG induced systemic immune activation.

Overall, elevated plasma levels of LPS and βDG both play an important role in chronic immune activation in PLWH on long-term ART and may represent a "folie à deux" contributing to the development of non-AIDS events. To this end, gaining a comprehensive understanding of the origin and consequences of these circulating microbial polysaccharides is of critical importance to finding therapeutic strategies to restore mucosal homeostasis, and gut dysbiosis in PLWH.

AUTHOR CONTRIBUTIONS

RR made the first draft, constructed the figure and table, and made revisions to the final draft of the manuscript. RR and SI contributed significantly to conducting the literature review. VM, JC, YZ, and MF critically read and revised the manuscript. J-PR designed the review and critically revised the manuscript.

FUNDING

This study was supported by the Fonds de recherche du Québec—Santé (FRQ-S): Réseau SIDA/Maladies infectieuses and Thérapie cellulaire, the Canadian Institute of Health Research (CIHR grants MOP 103230 and 154051), the Vaccines & Immunotherapies Core of the CIHR Canadian HIV Trials Network (CTN): grant CTN 257, the Canadian Foundation for AIDS Research (CANFAR) grant 02-512, and the Canadian HIV Cure Enterprise Team Grant (HIG-133050) awarded by the CIHR in partnership with CANFAR. RR is an undergraduate student supported by the H. Grenville Smith Studentship, SI is a post-doctoral fellow supported by the William Turner research fellowship, J-PR is the holder of the Louis Lowenstein Chair in Hematology and Oncology at McGill University.

ACKNOWLEDGMENTS

The authors are grateful to study participants for their contribution. We thank Angie Massicotte and Josée Girouard for administrative assistance.

REFERENCES

1. Perez-Lopez A, Behnsen J, Nuccio SP, Raffatellu M. Mucosal immunity to pathogenic intestinal bacteria. *Nat Rev Immunol.* (2016) 16:135–48. doi: 10.1038/nri.2015.17
2. Ouellette AJ. Paneth cells and innate mucosal immunity. *Curr Opin Gastroenterol.* (2010) 26:547–53. doi: 10.1097/MOG.0b013e32833dccde
3. Bry L, Falk P, Huttner K, Ouellette A, Midtvedt T, Gordon JI. Paneth cell differentiation in the developing intestine of normal and transgenic mice. *Proc Natl Acad Sci USA.* (1994) 91:10335–9. doi: 10.1073/pnas.91.22.10335
4. Birchenough GM, Johansson ME, Gustafsson JK, Bergstrom JH, Hansson GC. New developments in goblet cell mucus secretion and function. *Mucosal Immunol.* (2015) 8:712–9. doi: 10.1038/mi.2015.32
5. Luissint AC, Parkos CA, Nusrat A. Inflammation and the intestinal barrier: leukocyte-epithelial cell interactions, cell junction remodeling, and mucosal repair. *Gastroenterology.* (2016) 151:616–32. doi: 10.1053/j.gastro.2016.07.008
6. Ghosn J, Taiwo B, Seedat S, Autran B, Katlama C. HIV. *Lancet.* (2018) 392:685–97. doi: 10.1016/S0140-6736(18)31311-4
7. Hensley-McBain T, Berard AR, Manuzak JA, Miller CJ, Zevin AS, Polacino P, et al. Intestinal damage precedes mucosal immune dysfunction in SIV infection. *Mucosal Immunol.* (2018) 11:1429–40. doi: 10.1038/s41385-018-0032-5
8. Brenchley JM, Douek DC. Microbial translocation across the GI tract. *Annu Rev Immunol.* (2012) 30:149–73. doi: 10.1146/annurev-immunol-020711-075001

9. Brenchley JM, Price DA, Schacker TW, Asher TE, Silvestri G, Rao S, et al. Microbial translocation is a cause of systemic immune activation in chronic HIV infection. *Nat Med.* (2006) 12:1365–71. doi: 10.1038/nm1511
10. Estes JD, Harris LD, Klatt NR, Tabb B, Pittaluga S, Paiardini M, et al. Damaged intestinal epithelial integrity linked to microbial translocation in pathogenic simian immunodeficiency virus infections. *PLoS Pathog.* (2010) 6:e1001052. doi: 10.1371/journal.ppat.1001052
11. Cani PD, Amar J, Iglesias MA, Poggi M, Knauf C, Bastelica D, et al. Metabolic endotoxemia initiates obesity and insulin resistance. *Diabetes.* (2007) 56:1761–72. doi: 10.2337/db06-1491
12. Baker JV, Peng G, Rapkin J, Abrams DI, Silverberg MJ, MacArthur RD, et al. Community programs for clinical research on, CD4+ count and risk of non-AIDS diseases following initial treatment for HIV infection. *AIDS.* (2008) 22:841–8. doi: 10.1097/QAD.0b013e3282f7cb76
13. Mirzaei MK, Maurice CF. Menage a trois in the human gut: interactions between host, bacteria and phages. *Nat Rev Microbiol.* (2017) 15:397–408. doi: 10.1038/nrmicro.2017.30
14. Farhour Z, Mehraj V, Chen J, Ramendra R, Lu H, Routy JP. Use of (1->3)-beta-D-Glucan for diagnosis and management of invasive mycoses in HIV-infected patients. *Mycoses.* (2018) 61:718–22. doi: 10.1111/myc.12797
15. Morris A, Hillenbrand M, Finkelman M, George MP, Singh V, Kessinger C, et al. Serum (1->3)-beta-D-glucan levels in HIV-infected individuals are associated with immunosuppression, inflammation, and cardiopulmonary function. *J Acquir Immune Defic Syndr.* (2012) 61:462–8. doi: 10.1097/QAI.0b013e318271799b
16. Hoenigl M, de Oliveira MF, Perez-Santiago J, Zhang Y, Morris S, McCutchan AJ, et al. (1->3)-beta-D-glucan levels correlate with neurocognitive functioning in HIV-infected persons on suppressive antiretroviral therapy: a cohort study. *Medicine.* (2016) 95:e3162. doi: 10.1097/MD.0000000000003162
17. Hoenigl M, de Oliveira MF, Perez-Santiago J, Zhang Y, Woods SP, Finkelman M, et al. Correlation of (1->3)-beta-D-glucan with other inflammation markers in chronically HIV infected persons on suppressive antiretroviral therapy. *GMS Infect Dis.* (2015) 3:Doc3. doi: 10.3205/id000018
18. Hoenigl M, Moser C, Funderburg N, Bosch R, Kantor A, Zhang Y, et al. Soluble urokinase plasminogen activator receptor (suPAR) is predictive of non-AIDS events during antiretroviral therapy-mediated viral suppression. *Clin Infect Dis.* (2018). doi: 10.1093/cid/ciy966. [Epub ahead of print].
19. Hoenigl M, Perez-Santiago J, Nakazawa M, de Oliveira MF, Zhang Y, Finkelman MA, et al. (1->3)-beta-d-Glucan: a biomarker for microbial translocation in individuals with acute or early HIV infection? *Front Immunol.* (2016) 7:404. doi: 10.3389/fimmu.2016.00404
20. Mehraj V, Ramendra R, Isnard S, Dupuy FP, Ponte R, Chen J, et al. Circulating (1→3)-β-D-Glucan is associated with immune activation during HIV infection. *Clin Infect Dis.*
21. Deeks SG, Tracy R, Douek DC. Systemic effects of inflammation on health during chronic HIV infection. *Immunity.* (2013) 39:633–45. doi: 10.1016/j.immuni.2013.10.001
22. Nash AK, Auchtung TA, Wong MC, Smith DP, Gesell JR, Ross MC, et al. The gut mycobiome of the Human Microbiome Project healthy cohort. *Microbiome.* (2017) 5:15. doi: 10.1186/s40168-017-0373-4
23. Waldman AJ, Balskus EP. The human microbiota, infectious disease, and global health: challenges and opportunities. *ACS Infect Dis.* (2018) 4:14–26. doi: 10.1021/acsinfecdis.7b00232
24. Sheridan BS, Lefrancois L. Intraepithelial lymphocytes: to serve and protect. *Curr Gastroenterol Rep.* (2010) 12:513–21. doi: 10.1007/s11894-010-0148-6
25. Groschwitz KR, Hogan SP. Intestinal barrier function: molecular regulation and disease pathogenesis. *J Allergy Clin Immunol.* (2009) 124:3–20; quiz 21–2. doi: 10.1016/j.jaci.2009.05.038
26. Batman PA, Miller AR, Forster SM, Harris JR, Pinching AJ, Griffin GE. Jejunal enteropathy associated with human immunodeficiency virus infection: quantitative histology. *J Clin Pathol.* (1989) 42:275–81. doi: 10.1136/jcp.42.3.275
27. Batman PA, Kotler DP, Kapembwa MS, Booth D, Potten CS, Orenstein JM, et al. HIV enteropathy: crypt stem and transit cell hyperproliferation induces villous atrophy in HIV/Microsporidia-infected jejunal mucosa. *AIDS.* (2007) 21:433–9. doi: 10.1097/QAD.0b013e3280142ee8
28. Heise C, Dandekar S, Kumar P, Duplantier R, Donovan RM, Halsted CH. Human immunodeficiency virus infection of enterocytes and mononuclear cells in human jejunal mucosa. *Gastroenterology.* (1991) 100:1521–7. doi: 10.1016/0016-5085(91)90648-5
29. Klatt NR, Harris LD, Vinton CL, Sung H, Briant JA, Tabb B, et al. Compromised gastrointestinal integrity in pigtail macaques is associated with increased microbial translocation, immune activation, and IL-17 production in the absence of SIV infection. *Mucosal Immunol.* (2010) 3:387–98. doi: 10.1038/mi.2010.14
30. Milush JM, Mir KD, Sundaravaradan V, Gordon SN, Engram J, Cano CA, et al. Lack of clinical AIDS in SIV-infected sooty mangabeys with significant CD4+ T cell loss is associated with double-negative T cells. *J Clin Invest.* (2011) 121:1102–10. doi: 10.1172/JCI44876
31. Gordon SN, Klatt NR, Bosinger SE, Brenchley JM, Milush JM, Engram JC, et al. Severe depletion of mucosal CD4+ T cells in AIDS-free simian immunodeficiency virus-infected sooty mangabeys. *J Immunol.* (2007) 179:3026–34. doi: 10.4049/jimmunol.179.5.3026
32. Buccigrossi V, Laudiero G, Nicastro E, Miele E, Esposito F, Guarino A. The HIV-1 transactivator factor (Tat) induces enterocyte apoptosis through a redox-mediated mechanism. *PLoS ONE.* (2011) 6:e29436. doi: 10.1371/journal.pone.0029436
33. Canani RB, De Marco G, Passariello A, Buccigrossi V, Ruotolo S, Bracale I, et al. Inhibitory effect of HIV-1 Tat protein on the sodium-D-glucose symporter of human intestinal epithelial cells. *AIDS.* (2006) 20:5–10. doi: 10.1097/01.aids.0000198088.85572.68
34. Planes R, Ben Haij N, Leghmari K, Serrero M, BenMohamed L, Bahraoui E. HIV-1 Tat protein activates both the MyD88 and TRIF pathways to induce tumor necrosis factor alpha and interleukin-10 in human monocytes. *J Virol.* (2016) 90:5886–98. doi: 10.1128/JVI.00262-16
35. Maresca M, Mahfoud R, Garmy N, Kotler DP, Fantini J, Clayton F. The virotoxin model of HIV-1 enteropathy: involvement of GPR15/Bob and galactosylceramide in the cytopathic effects induced by HIV-1 gp120 in the HT-29-D4 intestinal cell line. *J Biomed Sci.* (2003) 10:156–66. doi: 10.1007/BF02256007
36. Clayton F, Kotler DP, Kuwada SK, Morgan T, Stepan C, Kuang J, et al. Gp120-induced Bob/GPR15 activation: a possible cause of human immunodeficiency virus enteropathy. *Am J Pathol.* (2001) 159:1933–9. doi: 10.1016/S0002-9440(10)63040-4
37. Allam O, Samarani S, Mehraj V, Jenabian MA, Tremblay C, Routy JP, et al. HIV induces production of IL-18 from intestinal epithelial cells that increases intestinal permeability and microbial translocation. *PLoS ONE.* (2018) 13:e0194185. doi: 10.1371/journal.pone.0194185
38. Nowarski R, Jackson R, Gagliani N, de Zoete MR, Palm NW, Bailis W, et al. Epithelial IL-18 equilibrium controls barrier function in colitis. *Cell.* (2015) 163:1444–56. doi: 10.1016/j.cell.2015.10.072
39. Mehraj V, Jenabian MA, Ponte R, Lebouche B, Costiniuk C, Thomas R, et al. Montreal primary Hiv infection, the plasma levels of soluble ST2 as a marker of gut mucosal damage in early HIV infection. *AIDS.* (2016) 30:1617–27. doi: 10.1097/QAD.0000000000001105
40. Ponte R, Mehraj V, Ghali P, Couedel-Courteille A, Cheynier R, Routy JP. Reversing gut damage in HIV infection: using non-human primate models to instruct clinical research. *EBioMedicine.* (2016) 4:40–9. doi: 10.1016/j.ebiom.2016.01.028
41. Mehraj V, Ponte R, Routy JP. The dynamic role of the IL-33/ST2 axis in chronic viral-infections: alarming and adjuvanting the immune response. *EBioMedicine.* (2016) 9:37–44. doi: 10.1016/j.ebiom.2016.06.047
42. Derikx JP, Luyer MD, Heineman E, Buurman WA. Non-invasive markers of gut wall integrity in health and disease. *World J Gastroenterol.* (2010) 16:5272–9. doi: 10.3748/wjg.v16.i42.5272
43. Brenchley JM, Schacker TW, Ruff LE, Price DA, Taylor JH, Beilman GJ, et al. CD4+ T cell depletion during all stages of HIV disease occurs predominantly in the gastrointestinal tract. *J Exp Med.* (2004) 200:749–59. doi: 10.1084/jem.20040874
44. Mehandru S, Poles MA, Tenner-Racz K, Horowitz A, Hurley A, Hogan C, et al. Primary HIV-1 infection is associated with preferential depletion of CD4+ T lymphocytes from effector sites in the gastrointestinal tract. *J Exp Med.* (2004) 200:761–70. doi: 10.1084/jem.20041196
45. Lim SG, Condez A, Lee CA, Johnson MA, Elia C, Poulter LW. Loss of mucosal CD4 lymphocytes is an early feature of HIV infection. *Clin Exp Immunol.* (1993) 92:448–54. doi: 10.1111/j.1365-2249.1993.tb03419.x

46. Jenabian MA, El-Far M, Vyboh K, Kema I, Costiniuk CT, Thomas R, et al. Montreal primary, and G slow progressor study, immunosuppressive tryptophan catabolism and gut mucosal dysfunction following early HIV infection. *J Infect Dis.* (2015) 212:355–66. doi: 10.1093/infdis/jiv037
47. Klatt NR, Estes JD, Sun X, Ortiz AM, Barber JS, Harris LD, et al. Loss of mucosal CD103+ DCs and IL-17+ and IL-22+ lymphocytes is associated with mucosal damage in SIV infection. *Mucosal Immunol.* (2012) 5:646–57. doi: 10.1038/mi.2012.38
48. Macpherson AJ, Smith K. Mesenteric lymph nodes at the center of immune anatomy. *J Exp Med.* (2006) 203:497–500. doi: 10.1084/jem.20060227
49. Brenchley JM, Douek DC. HIV infection and the gastrointestinal immune system. *Mucosal Immunol.* (2008) 1:23–30. doi: 10.1038/mi.2007.1
50. Marchetti G, Tincati C, Silvestri G. Microbial translocation in the pathogenesis of HIV infection and AIDS. *Clin Microbiol Rev.* (2013) 26:2–18. doi: 10.1128/CMR.00050-12
51. Pandrea I, Gaufin T, Brenchley JM, Gautam R, Monjure C, Gautam A, et al. Cutting edge: experimentally induced immune activation in natural hosts of simian immunodeficiency virus induces significant increases in viral replication and CD4+ T cell depletion. *J Immunol.* (2008) 181:6687–91. doi: 10.4049/jimmunol.181.10.6687
52. Kristoff J, Haret-Richter G, Ma D, Ribeiro RM, Xu C, Cornell E, et al. Early microbial translocation blockade reduces SIV-mediated inflammation and viral replication. *J Clin Invest.* (2014) 124:2802–6. doi: 10.1172/JCI75090
53. Triantafilou M, Triantafilou K. Lipopolysaccharide recognition: CD14, TLRs and the LPS-activation cluster. *Trends Immunol.* (2002) 23:301–4. doi: 10.1016/S1471-4906(02)02233-0
54. Barclay GR. Endogenous endotoxin-core antibody (EndoCAb) as a marker of endotoxin exposure and a prognostic indicator: a review. *Prog Clin Biol Res.* (1995) 392:263–72.
55. Panpetch W, Somboonna N, Bulan DE, Issara-Amphorn J, Finkelman M, Worasilchai N, et al. Oral administration of live- or heat-killed *Candida albicans* worsened cecal ligation and puncture sepsis in a murine model possibly due to an increased serum (1->3)-beta-D-glucan. *PLoS ONE.* (2017) 12:e0181439. doi: 10.1371/journal.pone.0181439
56. Issara-Amphorn J, Surawut S, Worasilchai N, Thim-Uam A, Finkelman M, Chindamporn A, et al. The synergy of endotoxin and (1->3)-beta-D-glucan, from gut translocation, worsens sepsis severity in a lupus model of Fc gamma receptor IIb-deficient mice. *J Innate Immun.* (2018) 10:189–201. doi: 10.1159/000486321
57. Leelahavanichkul A, Worasilchai N, Wannalerdsakun S, Jutivorakool K, Somparn P, Issara-Amphorn J, et al. Gastrointestinal leakage detected by serum (1->3)-beta-D-glucan in mouse models and a pilot study in patients with sepsis. *Shock.* (2016) 46:506–18. doi: 10.1097/SHK.0000000000000645
58. Opal SM. Endotoxins and other sepsis triggers. *Contrib Nephrol.* (2010) 167:14–24. doi: 10.1159/000315915
59. Caradonna L, Amati L, Magrone T, Pellegrino NM, Jirillo E, Caccavo D. Enteric bacteria, lipopolysaccharides and related cytokines in inflammatory bowel disease: biological and clinical significance. *J Endotoxin Res.* (2000) 6:205–14. doi: 10.1177/09680519000060030101
60. Vaure C, Liu Y. A comparative review of toll-like receptor 4 expression and functionality in different animal species. *Front Immunol.* (2014) 5:316. doi: 10.3389/fimmu.2014.00316
61. Freudenberg MA, Tchaptchet S, Keck S, Fejer G, Huber M, Schutze N, et al. Lipopolysaccharide sensing an important factor in the innate immune response to Gram-negative bacterial infections: benefits and hazards of LPS hypersensitivity. *Immunobiology.* (2008) 213:193–203. doi: 10.1016/j.imbio.2007.11.008
62. Sandler NG, Wand H, Roque A, Law M, Nason MC, Nixon DE, et al. Plasma levels of soluble CD14 independently predict mortality in HIV infection. *J Infect Dis.* (2011) 203:780–90. doi: 10.1093/infdis/jiq118
63. Brown GD, Taylor PR, Reid DM, Willment JA, Williams DL, Martinez-Pomares L, et al. Dectin-1 is a major β-glucan receptor on macrophages. *J Exp Med.* (2002) 196:407–12. doi: 10.1084/jem.20020470
64. McDonald JU, Rosas M, Brown GD, Jones SA, Taylor PR. Differential dependencies of monocytes and neutrophils on dectin-1, dectin-2 and complement for the recognition of fungal particles in inflammation. *PLoS ONE.* (2012) 7:e45781. doi: 10.1371/journal.pone.0045781
65. Taylor PR, Brown GD, Reid DM, Willment JA, Martinez-Pomares L, Gordon S, et al. The B-glucan receptor, dectin-1, is predominantly expressed on the surface of cells of the monocyte/macrophage and neutrophil lineages. *J Immunol.* (2002) 169:3876–82. doi: 10.4049/jimmunol.169.7.3876
66. Elder MJ, Webster SJ, Chee R, Williams DL, Hill Gaston JS, Goodall JC. beta-glucan size controls dectin-1-mediated immune responses in human dendritic cells by regulating IL-1beta production. *Front Immunol.* (2017) 8:791. doi: 10.3389/fimmu.2017.00791
67. Hefter M, Lother J, Weiss E, Schmitt AL, Fliesser M, Einsele H, et al. Human primary myeloid dendritic cells interact with the opportunistic fungal pathogen *Aspergillus fumigatus* via the C-type lectin receptor Dectin-1. *Med Mycol.* (2017) 55:573–8. doi: 10.1093/mmy/myw105
68. Li SS, Kyei SK, Timm-McCann M, Ogbomo H, Jones GJ, Shi M, et al. The NK receptor NKp30 mediates direct fungal recognition and killing and is diminished in NK cells from HIV-infected patients. *Cell Host Microbe.* (2013) 14:387–97. doi: 10.1016/j.chom.2013.09.007
69. Tremblay-McLean A, Bruneau J, Lebouche B, Lisovsky I, Song R, Bernard NF. Expression profiles of ligands for activating natural killer cell receptors on HIV infected and uninfected CD4(+) T cells. *Viruses.* (2017) 9:295. doi: 10.3390/v9100295
70. Pandey R, DeStephan CM, Madge LA, May MJ, Orange JS. NKp30 ligation induces rapid activation of the canonical NF-kappaB pathway in NK cells. *J Immunol.* (2007) 179:7385–96. doi: 10.4049/jimmunol.179.11.7385
71. Lawrence T. The nuclear factor NF-kappaB pathway in inflammation. *Cold Spring Harb Perspect Biol.* (2009) 1:a001651. doi: 10.1101/cshperspect.a001651
72. Swidergall M, Solis NV, Lionakis MS, Filler SG. EphA2 is an epithelial cell pattern recognition receptor for fungal beta-glucans. *Nat Microbiol.* (2018) 3:53–61. doi: 10.1038/s41564-017-0059-5
73. Hahn AS, Desrosiers RC. Binding of the Kaposi's sarcoma-associated herpesvirus to the ephrin binding surface of the EphA2 receptor and its inhibition by a small molecule. *J Virol.* (2014) 88:8724–34. doi: 10.1128/JVI.01392-14
74. Legentil L, Paris F, Ballet C, Trouvelot S, Daire X, Vetvicka V, et al. Molecular interactions of beta-(1->3)-glucans with their receptors. *Molecules.* (2015) 20:9745–66. doi: 10.3390/molecules20069745
75. Noss I, Doekes G, Thorne PS, Heederik DJ, Wouters IM. Comparison of the potency of a variety of beta-glucans to induce cytokine production in human whole blood. *Innate Immun.* (2013) 19:10–9. doi: 10.1177/1753425912447129
76. Sonnier DI, Bailey SR, Schuster RM, Gangidine MM, Lentsch AB, Pritts TA. Proinflammatory chemokines in the intestinal lumen contribute to intestinal dysfunction during endotoxemia. *Shock.* (2012) 37:63–9. doi: 10.1097/SHK.0b013e31823cbff1
77. Vujkovic-Cvijin I, Dunham RM, Iwai S, Maher MC, Albright RG, Broadhurst MJ, et al. Dysbiosis of the gut microbiota is associated with HIV disease progression and tryptophan catabolism. *Sci Transl Med.* (2013) 5:193ra91. doi: 10.1126/scitranslmed.3006438
78. Favre D, Mold J, Hunt PW, Kanwar B, Loke P, Seu L, et al. Tryptophan catabolism by indoleamine 2,3-dioxygenase 1 alters the balance of TH17 to regulatory T cells in HIV disease. *Sci Transl Med.* (2010) 2:32ra36. doi: 10.1126/scitranslmed.3000632
79. Jenabian MA, Patel M, Kema I, Kanagaratham C, Radzioch D, Thebault P, et al. Distinct tryptophan catabolism and Th17/Treg balance in HIV progressors and elite controllers. *PLoS ONE.* (2013) 8:e78146. doi: 10.1371/journal.pone.0078146
80. Chen J, Xun J, Yang J, Ji Y, Liu L, Qi T, et al. Plasma indoleamine 2,3-dioxygenase activity is associated with the size of HIV reservoir in patients receiving antiretroviral therapy. *Clin Infect Dis.* (2018) 10:676. doi: 10.1093/cid/ciy676
81. Kenneth Castro MDJ, Laurence Slutsker WWG, James Buehler PH, Harold Jaffe W, Ruth Berkelman MD. *1993 Revised Classification System 638 for HIV Infection and Expanded Surveillance Case Definition for AIDS Among Adolescents 639 and Adults.* Centre For Disease Control (1992).
82. Hsu DC, Sereti I, Ananworanich J. Serious Non-AIDS events: immunopathogenesis and interventional strategies. *AIDS Res Ther.* (2013) 10:29. doi: 10.1186/1742-6405-10-29
83. Clifford DB, Ances BM. HIV-associated neurocognitive disorder. *Lancet Infect Dis.* (2013) 13:976–86. doi: 10.1016/S1473-3099(13)70269-X

84. Ancuta P, Kamat A, Kunstman KJ, Kim EY, Autissier P, Wurcel A, et al. Microbial translocation is associated with increased monocyte activation and dementia in AIDS patients. *PLoS ONE.* (2008) 3:e2516. doi: 10.1371/journal.pone.0002516
85. Lyons JL, Uno H, Ancuta P, Kamat A, Moore DJ, Singer EJ, et al. Plasma sCD14 is a biomarker associated with impaired neurocognitive test performance in attention and learning domains in HIV infection. *J Acquir Immune Defic Syndr.* (2011) 57:371–9. doi: 10.1097/QAI.0b013e3182237e54
86. Justice AC, Dombrowski E, Conigliaro J, Fultz SL, Gibson D, Madenwald T, et al. Veterans aging cohort study (VACS): overview and description. *Med Care.* (2006) 44:S13–24. doi: 10.1097/01.mlr.0000223741.02074.66
87. Marconi VC, Duncan MS, So-Armah K, Re VL III, Lim JK, Butt AA, et al. Bilirubin is inversely associated with cardiovascular disease among HIV-positive and HIV-negative individuals in VACS (Veterans aging cohort study). *J Am Heart Assoc.* (2018) 7:7792. doi: 10.1161/JAHA.117.007792
88. Drosatos K, Lymperopoulos A, Kennel PJ, Pollak N, Schulze PC, Goldberg IJ. Pathophysiology of sepsis-related cardiac dysfunction: driven by inflammation, energy mismanagement, or both? *Curr Heart Fail Rep.* (2015) 12:130–40. doi: 10.1007/s11897-014-0247-z
89. Chen RRJ, Lu H, Routy JP. The early bird gets the worm: benefits and future directions with early antiretroviral therapy initiation in primary HIV infection. *Future Virol.* (2018) 13:11. doi: 10.2217/fvl-2018-0110
90. Wong J, Zhang Y, Patidar A, Vilar E, Finkelman M, Farrington K. Is endotoxemia in stable hemodialysis patients an artefact? Limitations of the limulus amebocyte lysate assay and role of (1->3)-beta-D glucan. *PLoS ONE.* (2016) 11:e0164978. doi: 10.1371/journal.pone.0164978
91. Hashimoto N, Mori T, Hashida R, Sakurai M, Koda Y, Toyama T, et al. False-positive serum (1, 3)-beta-D-glucan elevation due to intake of seaweed in a hematopoietic stem cell transplant recipient. *Transpl Infect Dis.* (2017) 19. doi: 10.1111/tid.12653
92. Zainab Shahid NSK, Restrepo A, Haider S, Muzaffar J, Grazziutti M, Nucci M, et al. Elevated serum beta-D-glucan (BDG) as a marker for chemotherapy-induced mucosal barrier injury (MBI) in adults with hematologic malignancies: a retrospective analysis. In: *IDSA Annual Meeting.* Boston, MA (2011).
93. Ellis M, Al-Ramadi B, Finkelman M, Hedstrom U, Kristensen J, Ali-Zadeh H, et al. Assessment of the clinical utility of serial beta-D-glucan concentrations in patients with persistent neutropenic fever. *J Med Microbiol.* (2008) 57:287–95. doi: 10.1099/jmm.0.47479-0
94. Gavino C, Cotter A, Lichtenstein D, Lejtenyi D, Fortin C, Legault C, et al. CARD9 deficiency and spontaneous central nervous system candidiasis: complete clinical remission with GM-CSF therapy. *Clin Infect Dis.* (2014) 59:81–4. doi: 10.1093/cid/ciu215
95. Palesch D, Bosinger SE, Tharp GK, Vanderford TH, Paiardini M, Chahroudi A, et al. Sooty mangabey genome sequence provides insight into AIDS resistance in a natural SIV host. *Nature.* (2018) 553:77–81. doi: 10.1038/nature25140
96. Stinghen AE, Goncalves SM, Bucharles S, Branco FS, Gruber B, Hauser AB, et al. Sevelamer decreases systemic inflammation in parallel to a reduction in endotoxemia. *Blood Purif.* (2010) 29:352–6. doi: 10.1159/000302723
97. Sandler NG, Zhang X, Bosch RJ, Funderburg NT, Choi AI, Robinson JK, et al. Sevelamer does not decrease lipopolysaccharide or soluble CD14 levels but decreases soluble tissue factor, low-density lipoprotein (LDL) cholesterol, and oxidized LDL cholesterol levels in individuals with untreated HIV infection. *J Infect Dis.* (2014) 210:1549–54. doi: 10.1093/infdis/jiu305

19

Measuring the Inducible, Replication-Competent HIV Reservoir Using an Ultra-Sensitive p24 Readout, the Digital ELISA Viral Outgrowth Assay

*Erin L. Stuelke[1], Katherine S. James[1], Jennifer L. Kirchherr[1], Brigitte Allard[1], Caroline Baker[1], Joann D. Kuruc[1,2], Cindy L. Gay[1,2], David M. Margolis[1,2,3,4] and Nancie M. Archin[1,2]**

[1] University of North Carolina HIV Cure Center, UNC Institute for Global Health and Infectious Diseases, Chapel Hill, NC, United States, [2] Department of Medicine, UNC Chapel Hill School of Medicine, Chapel Hill, NC, United States, [3] Department of Microbiology and Immunology, UNC Chapel Hill School of Medicine, Chapel Hill, NC, United States, [4] Department of Epidemiology, UNC Chapel Hill School of Public Health, The University of North Carolina at Chapel Hill, Chapel Hill, NC, United States

***Correspondence:**
Nancie M. Archin
nancie_archin@med.unc.edu

Quantifying the inducible HIV reservoir provides an estimate of the frequency of quiescent HIV-infected cells in humans as well as in animal models, and can help ascertain the efficacy of latency reversing agents (LRAs). The quantitative viral outgrowth assay (QVOA) is used to measure inducible, replication competent HIV and generate estimations of reservoir size. However, traditional QVOA is time and labor intensive and requires large amounts of lymphocytes. Given the importance of reproducible and accurate assessment of both reservoir size and LRA activity in cure strategies, efforts to streamline the QVOA are of high priority. We developed a modified QVOA, the Digital ELISA Viral Outgrowth or DEVO assay, with ultra-sensitive p24 readout, capable of femtogram detection of HIV p24 protein in contrast to the picogram limitations of traditional ELISA. For each DEVO assay, 8–12 $\times$ 10^6 resting CD4 + T cells from aviremic, ART-treated HIV + participants are plated in limiting dilution and maximally stimulated with PHA, IL-2 and uninfected allogeneic irradiated PBMC. CD8-depleted PHA blasts from an uninfected donor or HIV-permissive cells (e.g., Molt4/CCR5) are added to the cultures and virus allowed to amplify for 8–12 days. HIV p24 from culture supernatant is measured at day 8 by Simoa (single molecule array, ultra-sensitive p24 assay) confirmed at day 12, and infectious units per million CD4 + T cells (IUPM) are calculated using the maximum likelihood method. In all DEVO assays performed, HIV p24 was detected in the supernatant of cultures as early as 8 days post stimulation. Importantly, DEVO IUPM values at day 8 were comparable or higher than traditional QVOA IUPM values obtained at day 15. Interestingly, DEVO IUPM values were similar with or without the addition of allogeneic CD8-depleted target PHA blasts or HIV permissive cells traditionally used to expand virus. The DEVO assay uses fewer resting CD4 + T cells and provides an assessment of reservoir size in less time than standard QVOA. This assay offers a new platform to quantify replication competent HIV during limited cell availability. Other potential applications include evaluating LRA activity, and measuring clearance of infected cells during latency clearance assays.

Keywords: QVOA, DEVO, HIV, outgrowth, IUPM

INTRODUCTION

With an estimated 40 million people living with HIV (PLWH), and given the health, stigma, and financial burden associated with chronic HIV infection, eliminating the HIV pandemic remains a priority both from a public health and societal perspective. While successful antiretroviral therapy (ART) has significantly reduced the mortality and morbidity associated with HIV infection, the existence of long-lived viral reservoirs capable of reigniting fulminant infection in the absence of ART remains one of the major barriers toward achieving an HIV cure. With two documented functional cures, first the Berlin Patient (1) and more recently the London Patient (2), there is renewed hope and interest in the quest to eliminate persistent HIV infection. Modalities to target HIV persistence are being tested in the clinic. A large proportion of persistent HIV is defective and unable to replicate (3–5). Clinical interventions targeting the HIV reservoir would benefit greatly from assays that can rapidly and precisely quantitate the replication competent HIV reservoir in order to assess the efficacy of therapeutic interventions aimed at depleting the reservoir. Standard PCR-based assays offer a relatively rapid and sensitive method to quantitate persistent HIV infection. However, as most of these assays amplify one conserved genomic region, they do not distinguish between replication-competent and defective provirus (3–5). The recently reported Intact Proviral DNA Assay (IPDA) has the added advantage over standard PCR assays in that by using two sets of primer probes targeting an intact packaging signal (PS) and the Rev-responsive element within *Env*, it increases the probability of amplifying mostly intact proviral genome (6). Although relatively streamlined and amenable to high throughput, 30–40% of virus amplified by this method is likely to be defective, and sequence polymorphism may limit the ability of primers and probes to amplify intact provirus (6, 7). The QVOA is considered the gold standard to measure replication-competent, inducible provirus. The QVOA provides a minimal, but definitive estimate of the inducible HIV reservoir (8–10). However, this assay can be costly and labor intensive. Additionally, as latently infected CD4 + T cells are present at low frequency, large numbers of cells are often required to increase sensitivity. Furthermore for some participants, the QVOA may under-represent the true frequency of latent but replication-competent proviruses due in part to the presence of "non-induced" proviruses unresponsive to a single round of cell stimulation (4, 11). Despite its limitations, the QVOA remains the most reliable method to measure replication competent HIV (12). Thus several modifications of this assay have been made to improve throughput, sensitivity and increased its dynamic range [reviewed in Falcinelli et al. (13)]. We report here a modified QVOA, the Digital ELISA Viral Outgrowth or DEVO assay which takes advantage of the Simoa platform (Quanterix Inc., Billerica, MA, United States) (14, 15). The Simoa or single molecule array is an ultrasensitive, fully automated immune assay platform capable of femtogram detection of HIV p24 protein in contrast to the picogram limitations of traditional ELISA (15–17). During the DEVO assay 8–12 × 10^6 purified resting CD4 + T cells from aviremic, ART-treated HIV + participants are PHA stimulated in limiting dilution in a 96 well-format and HIV p24 measured by Simoa.

To reduce non-specific signal, we use an optimized Simoa p24 protocol (16) in our assay. We found that virus can be expanded using either the CD4 T cell input alone (i.e., addition of exogenous donor cells is not necessary), PHA blasts from an uninfected donor, or HIV permissive cell lines such as the MOLT4/CCR5. Furthermore, with the DEVO assay, we obtained IUPM comparable or higher than the traditional QVOA at an earlier time point, thus reducing the overall length of the assay (18). While there have been other reports using the Simoa as a p24 readout for other QVOA modifications (19–21), to our knowledge, this is the first study describing a specific Simoa HIV outgrowth assay that has been meticulously and carefully evaluated for demonstrable accuracy and reproducibility.

RESULTS

Participant Characteristics

To develop the DEVO assay we used resting CD4 + T cells isolated from 12 PLWH, stably suppressed (<50 copies of HIV-1 RNA/ml on ART). Participants were 75% male and 25% female, had a mean age of 43.5 years with an average CD4 count of 740 cells/μl, and on ART for an average of 7.3 years, with a mean duration of suppression of 4.9 years (**Supplementary Table S1**). Leukapheresis or whole blood samples were obtained from participants through an ongoing longitudinal collection protocol approved by the University of North Carolina (UNC) biomedical institutional review board. All samples were collected in accordance with UNC guidelines and all participants provided informed consent prior to sample donation.

Simoa Detects HIV *gag* p24 Earlier Than Standard p24 ELISA During QVOA

Our primary goal for developing the DEVO assay was to investigate whether or not using ultra-sensitive p24 measurements by Simoa would shorten the duration of standard QVOA by detecting HIV p24 positive wells earlier than traditional ELISA methods. To that end, we harvested

TABLE 1 | HIV antigen is detected earlier using Simoa compared to standard ELISA in the traditional QVOA$^{\Psi}$.

	Number of HIV p24 positive wells/total wells cultured		
	Day 8		Day 15
Resting CD4 + T cells (×10^6)	Simoa	Standard ELISA	Standard ELISA
2.5	18/18	2/18	18/18
0.5	4/6	2/6	5/6
0.1	0/6	0/6	0/6
IUPM	1.927	0.088	2.49

$^{\Psi}$ *Representative QVOA experiment.*

supernatant from a standard QVOA assay on days 8, 15, and 19 post-stimulation and measured HIV p24 by both Simoa (day 8) and standard HIV *gag* p24 ELISA (days 8, 15, and 19). Seventy three percent of the wells were p24 positive by Simoa at day 8 compared to 13% of the wells by standard ELISA (**Table 1**). Importantly, 95% of the wells slated to become positive at day 15 during the traditional QVOA assay were already positive at day 8 by Simoa and the IUPM at day 8 were comparable to the day 15 traditional QVOA IUPM (**Table 1**).

We next performed a pilot experiment to determine whether the sensitivity of the Simoa would be maintained when fewer cells are used for the viral outgrowth assay. We stimulated approximately 8 million resting CD4 + T cells in limiting dilution as described under methods. Culture wells were then targeted with PHA blasts to amplify virus. We subsequently assessed p24 production from culture supernatant at day 8 post-stimulation. We observed that detection of p24 positive wells by Simoa was more sensitive with 10 positive wells detected, as compared to 3 wells by standard ELISA (**Supplementary Figure S1**).

Determination of the Lower Limit of Quantitation of the DEVO Assay

During the development of the DEVO assay, we initially used the lower limit of quantitation (LLOQ) generated from the Simoa assay standard curve, which is approximately 12 fg/ml and 3 times the median absolute deviation (MAD) as the cut off value from which to assign a well as positive. Additionally, to reduce non-specific noise in the assay, we employed an optimized Simoa p24 protocol developed by our colleagues at Merck Pharmaceuticals (16). However, despite these careful approaches, we observed that in some cases, wells that were low-positive for HIV p24 would become negative if cultured for additional days, suggesting further modification of the DEVO assay was necessary to capture true replication competent-HIV and avoid recording poorly adapted virus that are incapable of spreading in culture. To better understand the level of background noise in the assay, we performed a mock viral outgrowth assay using PBMC isolated from an uninfected donor. Approximately 2–6 million PBMC were maximally stimulated in limiting dilution with PHA/IL-2/irradiated PBMC or with survival amount of IL-2 (10–20 U/ml) and cultured over 8 days. Cultures were targeted with PHA-blasts or no targets were added. Supernatant from cultures were harvested on day 8 and assayed by Simoa, using the optimized HIV p24 protocol referenced. Although false p24 signal was detectable in most of the wells, the values were below the limit of quantitation of the assay except for two wells in the PHA-stimulated, no target added culture conditions where values above the LLOQ were registered (**Figure 1**).

To eliminate the influence of low-level false p24 positive signal in the assay, we next employed the methods standardized by The Clinical and Laboratory Standards Institute (CLSI) to determine a new limit of quantitation based on total error of the assay (22). Resting CD4 + T cells were isolated from a normal donor and stimulated with PHA/IL-2/irradiated PBMC for 24 h. Cultures were washed to remove the PHA and targeted with PHA-blasts from an uninfected donor twice over the course of 19 days. On three separate days, supernatant harvested on days 8 and 12 post-stimulation were spiked with different concentrations of HIV p24 (Quanterix, Inc.) and assayed by Simoa. Values obtained were used to calculate assay bias, total error and percent total error as described under methods. The concentration at which there was <20% of total error was found to be approximately 50 fg/ml and this value was used as the DEVO assay LLOQ onward (**Figure 2**). In addition, for added rigor and to eliminate recording cryptic p24 signal from wells containing only defective provirus, only wells exhibiting sustained or increase in p24 production over the 2 days of the assay are scored as positive (**Supplementary Tables S2, S3**).

Comparison of the DEVO Assay to the Traditional QVOA

Using the optimizations defined above, we next compared the performance of the DEVO assay to the traditional QVOA in measuring the replication competent HIV reservoir of stably suppressed, ART-treated PLWH. Both assays were set-up in parallel using resting CD4 + T cells isolated from HIV + ART-suppressed donors. The QVOA was performed as described elsewhere (12, 23) using 34–50 million resting CD4 + T cells that are maximally stimulated with PHA/IL2/irradiated PBMC in limiting dilution. PHA-blasts from an uninfected CCR5 high donor are added to the cultures twice to expand virus and supernatant harvested on days 15 and 19 and assayed for HIV p24 by ELISA. For the DEVO assay 8–12 million resting CD4 + T cells are stimulated in limiting dilution as done for QVOA. Wells were either targeted with PHA blasts or in corresponding experiments received no blasts in order to assess whether virus can be expanded without the addition of exogenous cells. Culture supernatant were initially harvested on days 8, 12, 15, and 19 and p24 measured by Simoa. For both assays, the maximum likelihood method (24, 25) was used to calculate IUPM values. At day 8 post-stimulation, the DEVO assay generated IUPM values that were comparable to or in some assays higher than QVOA IUPM obtained at day 15 post-stimulation (**Figure 3A** and **Supplementary Figure S2**). However, the overall difference in IUPM between the DEVO at day 8 and the QVOA at day 15 were not statistically significant. Importantly, IUPM values for the two assays highly correlated (**Figure 3B**). Interestingly,

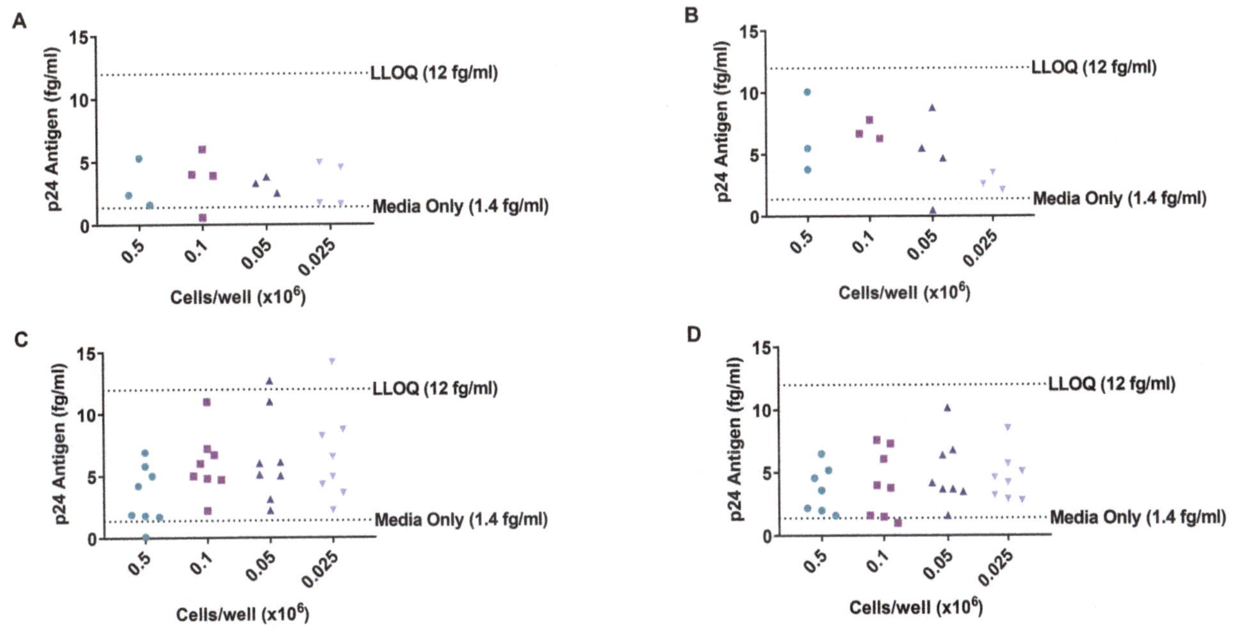

FIGURE 1 | Limiting dilution culture of uninfected donor PBMC reveals background noise of Simoa. PBMC from an uninfected donor were stimulated in limiting dilution with PHA/IL-2 and irradiated PBMC or treated with low amount of IL-2 only. Cultures were either targeted with PHA blasts or no targets were added. Supernatant were harvested at day 8 and HIV p24 assayed by Simoa. **(A)** Low IL-2 treated/no targets added. **(B)** Low IL-2 treated/cultures targeted with PHA blasts. **(C)** PHA stimulated/no targets added. **(D)** PHA stimulated/cultures targeted with PHA blasts. Each dot represents a well at the indicated cell dilution. LLOQ, lower limit of quantitation.

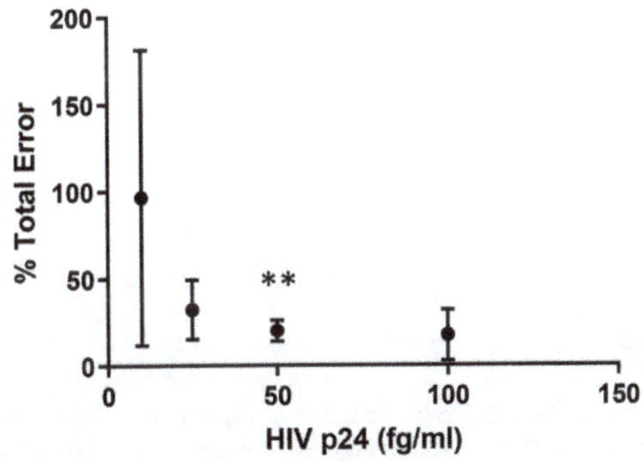

FIGURE 2 | The lower limit of quantitation for the DEVO assay. Freshly isolated resting CD4 + T cells from an uninfected donor were stimulated with PHA and irradiated PBMC, then co-cultured with PHA blasts over the course of 19 days. On three separate, but not consecutive days, supernatant from day 8 and 12 were spiked with HIV p24 protein at different dilutions and assayed by Simoa. Bias, total error and % total error was calculated from replicate well values using the following formula: Bias = Average − Actual Value; Total Error = |Bias| + 2 × Standard Deviation; % Total Error = Total Error Actual Value × 100. The concentration with <20% total error was determined to be 49.21fg/ml**. This value was used as the DEVO lower limit of quantitation.

similar IUPM values were obtained in the DEVO assay whether or not exogenous cells were added to expand virus, suggesting that the assay can be performed without the addition of target cells (**Figure 4A**). Additional days in culture beyond day 12 post-stimulation increased the number of positive wells in some, but not all assays (**Figure 4B**; not shown). This is similar to the standard QVOA where in most assays, all wells containing HIV outgrowth are p24 positive by day 15 with very few or no additional wells turning positive with longer culture. As one of the goals of the DEVO was to reduce the length of the QVOA assay, and given that by day 8, IUPM values were comparable or higher than the traditional QVOA assay, day 8 p24 assessment with a day 12 confirmation were subsequently selected as the assay endpoint (**Supplementary Tables S2, S3**).

The use of HIV permissive cell lines such as Molt4/CCR5 instead of PHA-blasts to amplify virus outgrowth in co-culture assays could diminish the cost associated with PHA-blast production and eliminate donor-to-donor variability in longitudinal studies (26). We therefore compared the ability of Molt4/CCR5 cells to expand virus in the DEVO assay as compared to PHA blasts. We observed no significant difference in IUPM values whether Molt4/CCR5 or PHA blasts were used in the assay (**Figure 4C**).

Longitudinal Variation of the DEVO Assay

Longitudinal reservoir measurements are important metrics to evaluate the efficacy of therapeutic interventions and therefore depend on reliable and reproducible assays for accurate assessment. We previously reported on the longitudinal reproducibility of the traditional QVOA (12) and therefore, we compared the reproducibility of the DEVO assay with the QVOA. In two participants, the DEVO assay was run in parallel with the QVOA using resting CD4 + T cells collected longitudinally, spanning 6–14 months. In one participant, we compared the

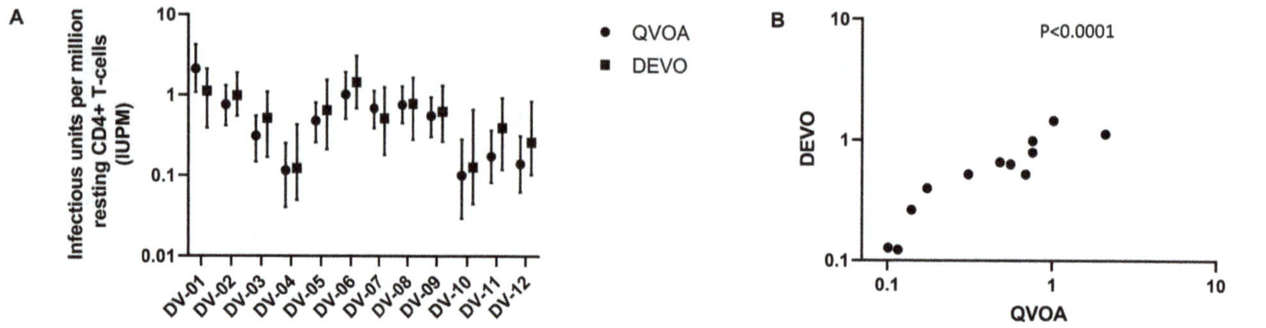

FIGURE 3 | Comparison of IUPM values obtained in the DEVO assay at day 8 post-stimulation versus IUPM values obtained from the QVOA at day 15 post-stimulation. **(A)** The DEVO assay generated IUPM values that were either comparable or in some cases higher than values obtained with the traditional QVOA. However, overall, there was no significant difference in IUPM values between the two assays. $P = 0.1294$, Wilcoxon matched-pairs signed rank test. Twelve independent, paired assays from 12 distinct participants is shown. IUPM + 95% CI (upper and lower limits) is shown. **(B)** Correlation of the DEVO assay at day 8 post-stimulation with the QVOA at day 15 post-stimulation. Spearman $r = 0.9282$.

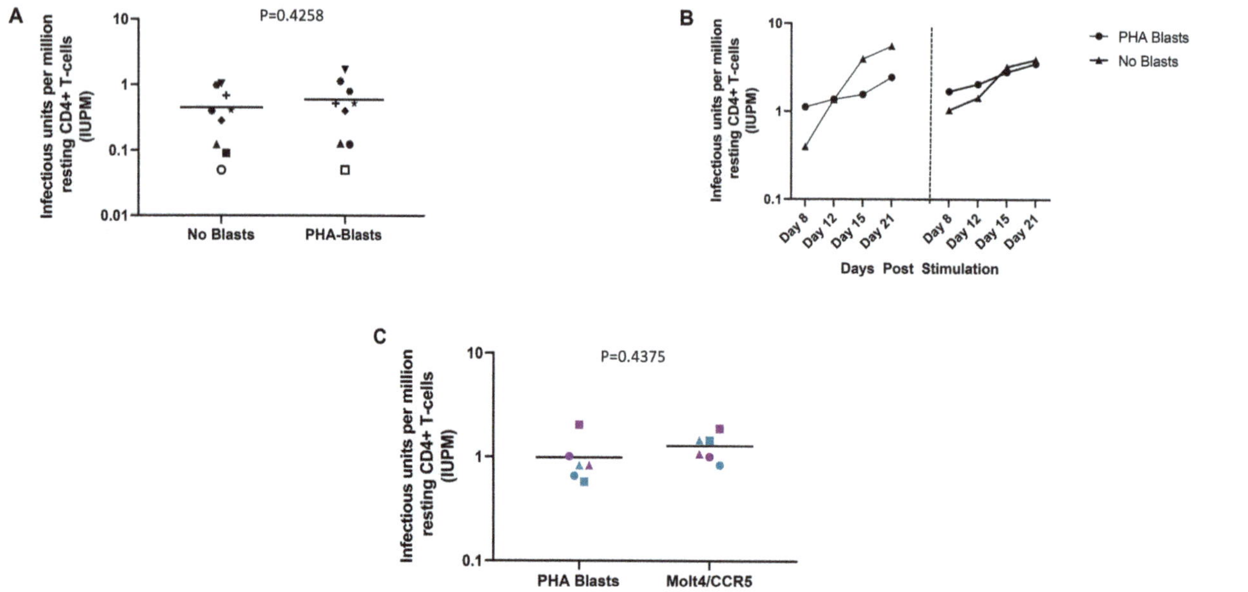

FIGURE 4 | DEVO assay outcome using either no blasts, or PHA blasts or the HIV permissive cell line, Molt4/CCR5 to expand virus. **(A)** Increase in IUPM values over time in cultures receiving either PHA blasts or no exogenous targets (no blasts). Two independent assays using cells from two participants are shown (left and right panel, DV-01 and DV-02). **(B)** Similar IUPM values are obtained in the DEVO assay whether or not exogenous targets to expand virus are used. Each symbol represents an independent assay performed with cells from distinct participants. **(C)** The HIV permissible cell line Molt4/CCR5 expands virus as well as PHA blasts in the DEVO assay. Results from independent assays performed with cells from three different participants (DV-01, DV-05 and DV-06) at day 8 (green) and day 12 (purple) are shown. For each experiment, cultures either received Molt4/CCR5 or PHA blasts to expand virus. Each symbol represents a participant. Open symbols indicate values below the limit of detection. Wilcoxon matched-pairs signed rank test was used to compare statistical differences.

DEVO assay performed using whole blood resting CD4 T cells collected longitudinally (17.5 months between donations), with the QVOA performed using leukapheresis-derived resting CD4 T cells acquired within 3 months of the blood cells (15.2 months between donations). We observed that the DEVO assay tracked with the QVOA within a given participant and across participants over time (**Figure 5**).

The ability to perform the DEVO assay using whole blood-derived instead of leukapheresis-derived resting CD4 + T cells would be beneficial for several reasons. It could reduce the costs associated with obtaining leukapheresis product and the time a participant spends in the clinic. Removing the need for leukapheresis procedures would also allow for the inclusion of additional time points to measure the replication competent reservoir during clinical trials. We therefore compared the performance of the DEVO assay on resting CD4 + T cells isolated from peripheral blood versus cells donated at leukapheresis in three different donors. We observed no significant difference in IUPMs obtained from the DEVO assay performed with the two different sources of resting CD4 T cells suggesting that the DEVO assay could be incorporated as an important tool in clinical trials seeking to deplete the HIV reservoir (**Figure 6**).

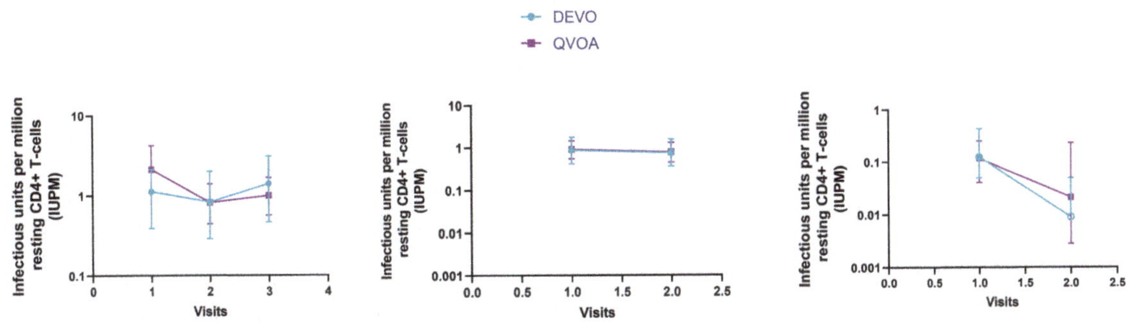

FIGURE 5 | The DEVO assay tracked similarly overtime as the traditional QVOA. The DEVO assay and QVOA were performed with resting CD4 + T cells collected at multiple time points from 3 participants, DV-01 (first panel), DV-09 (second panel), and DV-04 (third panel). All assays were performed using cells from the same leukapheresis donation, except for VV-09 where the DEVO was performed using cells from whole blood donated within 3 months of leukapheresis donations used for the QVOA. The time elapsed between visits 1 and 2, 1 and 3, and 2 and 3 for DV-01 is 7.9, 14.1, and 6.2 months respectively; for DV-09 the time elapsed between visit 1 and 2 is 17.9 months (DEVO) and 14.9 months (QVOA); For DV-04, the time between the first and second donation is 15. 9 months. IUPM + 95% CI (upper and lower limits) is shown.

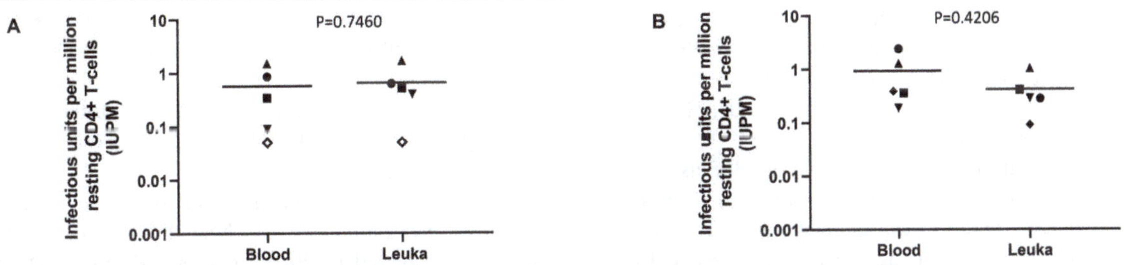

FIGURE 6 | Comparison of the DEVO assay using resting CD4 + T cells isolated from whole blood vs leukapheresis product (Leuka). **(A)** Targets (either PHA blasts or MOLT4/CCR5) added to expand virus. **(B)** No targets added. Whole blood was collected 6–17 months from leukapheresis donation time. Each symbol represents an independent assay performed using cells from 4 distinct participants (DV-02, DV-03, DV-04, DV-09 and DV-11). For each experiment, cultures either received exogenous targets to expand virus or no targets. Open symbols indicate values below the limit of detection. The Mann–Whitney *U* test was used to compare statistical differences.

DISCUSSION

Interventions to deplete the HIV reservoir are being explored in the clinic and would greatly benefit from endpoint assays that can rapidly and reliably measure the replication competent HIV reservoir. While PCR assays to measure DNA and RNA are high-throughput, rapid and relatively streamlined, they do not distinguish between defective proviruses and replication competent virus (3–5). The newly described IPDA offers a significant advantage over traditional PCR methods targeting only a single genomic region of the virus as the IPDA uses primer/probe sets simultaneously targeting multiple conserved regions of the HIV genome to more accurately detect intact provirus. However, the IPDA still over-estimates the frequency of true intact proviruses (6, 7). Near full-length or full genome sequencing may provide better assessment of intact proviruses than standard DNA PCR, however, the inefficiency associated with long distance PCR for DNA sequencing, and the extreme costs and labor involved makes them difficult to apply on a large scale [reviewed in Falcinelli et al. (13)]. The QVOA, though labor intensive, provides a minimal estimate of the frequency of latent HIV infection, and is still the gold standard for measuring true replication competent HIV. We report here a validated, modified version of the QVOA which incorporates a digital p24 ELISA as a readout for sensitive and accelerated detection of HIV. We showed that the DEVO assay can be performed in less time and with fewer cells than the traditional QVOA. Importantly, IUPM values obtained from the DEVO assay were comparable or in some cases higher than the values from the traditional QVOA. Finally, we also show that the assay varies minimally longitudinally and can be performed using resting CD4 + T cells isolated from either whole blood or leukapheresis product. An optimized HIV p24 protocol is used in the DEVO assay to improve sensitivity (16). Additionally, to improve accurate measurement of replication competent virus, we meticulously defined a limit of quantitation for the assay and included an additional day of culture to confirm positive wells. While others have reported using the Simoa to quantitate the inducible reservoir, to our knowledge this the first report with detailed description of the steps taken to validate the assay and demonstrate longitudinal reproducibility and accuracy.

Given the importance of the QVOA in assessing replication competent HIV, it is no surprise that efforts have been devoted to streamlining the assay (13). Increasing sensitivity to detect viral outgrowth while minimizing cell input has been a common goal in the field. Other laboratories have also reported modifications of the assay to use fewer than 10 million cells while maximizing the ability to record the frequency of latently infected cells (19, 27, 28). One of the challenges of all viral outgrowth assays is the phenomenon of non-induced, replication competent virus (4, 11). Capturing cell free RNA from the supernatant of outgrowth wells using magnetic beads before assaying for HIV gag by PCR, was shown to increase sensitivity to detect inducible HIV (19, 28). However, while RNA measurements may provide more sensitivity, the detection of RNA may not represent a replication-competent viral particle. Further, false positive detection because of PCR contaminants could be a disadvantage. In a more recent report, effector memory T cells were found to contain a higher frequency of inducible HIV, leading to the suggestion that the effector memory state was overall more conducive to HIV latency reversal than other T cell differentiation states (29). This lead to the development of a modified QVOA termed the dQVOA, during which resting CD4 + T cells are first differentiated into effector memory T cells using a cocktail of cytokines before the stimulation and viral outgrowth steps (27). The differentiation step resulted in significantly higher frequencies of reactivated HIV compared to the traditional QVOA (27). Whether or not including this differentiation-to-effector-memory step in the DEVO assay would further increase the frequency of virus detected remains to be determined.

There are some limitations to our assay. Because we are interrogating fewer cells, the confidence interval around our point estimate (IUPM) is wide, especially when the frequency of latently infected cells is low. Thus in stably suppressed PLWH with extremely small inducible reservoirs, or if someday anti-latency interventions are able to significantly deplete the reservoir to very low levels, the applicability of the DEVO assay as described, in such situations will be limited as large numbers of cells will have to be interrogated to make an accurate assessment of the frequency of replication competent HIV. In such cases, either a modified DEVO assay or standard QVOA using large numbers of cells might be preferred. As an alternative, murine viral outgrowth models (mVOA or hmVOA) may provide an attractive, *in vivo* approach to record difficult to detect replication competent virus [(30, 31) reviewed in Schmitt and Akkina (32)]. Another limitation of our assay relates to selecting day 8 as the assay end point. As mentioned previously, in some assays, additional days of culture produce additional p24 positive wells. Thus wells that were p24 negative at day 8 may become positive at a later day but would not be considered positive, and result in a lower IUPM estimate than if the assay was extended to a later timepoint. However, there are obvious costs to extending times in culture, and a negative result (no positive cultures at the end of an assay) simply defines a limit of detection under the conditions employed. Increased sensitivity, at the burden of increased cost, may be obtained by extending time in culture.

In summary, the DEVO assay represents an advance to the available validated toolkit to measure replication competent HIV. The DEVO assay offers a new platform to quantify replication competent HIV for a variety of applications, such as measuring the frequency of infection in situations where the number of cells available may be limited, evaluating LRA activity, and measuring clearance of infected cells following the addition of autologous immune effectors.

MATERIALS AND METHODS

Cell Culture

MOLT4/CCR5 cells were acquired from the NIH AIDS Reagent Bank. Cells were maintained in culture in RPMI supplemented with 1% penicillin/streptomycin (Gibco, ThermoFisher), 10% FBS (Gibco, ThermoFisher) and 1 mg/mL G418 until use.

PHA-blasts were prepared from PBMC obtained from selected HIV seronegative donors screened for adequate CCR5 expression (33). PBMC were CD8-depleted and maintained in culture in IMDM supplemented with 1% penicillin/streptomycin, 10% FBS and 20 U/ml IL-2. Cells were stimulated for 2–3 days with 2 μg/ml PHA prior to usage.

Isolation of Resting CD4 + T Cells

HIV+ participants underwent continuous flow leukapheresis to obtain large amount of white blood cells or 150 ml of whole blood was obtained by venipuncture at a different time point from the leukapheresis from selected participants. PBMCs were isolated by Ficoll-gradient. Resting CD4 + T cells were isolated from PBMC by negative selection as previously described (34). Resting CD4 + T cells were maintained in culture for 1–2 days in the presence of ARV, without IL-2 prior to performing outgrowth assays.

Buffy coats from HIV seronegative donors were obtained from the New York Blood Center (New York, NY, United States) and PBMC isolated by Ficoll-gradient. Resting CD4 + T cells were isolated using the EasySep™ Human Resting CD4 + T Cell Isolation Kit (StemCell Technologies, Vancouver, BC, United States). Cells were cultured overnight in media containing 20 U/ml IL-2 prior to assay set-up.

Traditional QVOA

The QVOA assay was performed as previously described (12, 23). Briefly, 34–50 million resting CD4 + T cells were plated in replicate limiting dilutions of 2.5 million (12–18 cultures), 0.5 million (6 cultures) and 0.1 million (6 cultures) cells per well, activated with PHA (Remel, ThermoFisher) and a fivefold excess of allogeneic irradiated PBMCs from a seronegative donor, and 60 U/ml IL-2 for 24 h. Cultures were washed and co-cultivated with CD8-depleted PHA-blasts. Culture supernatants were harvested on days 15 and 19 and assayed for virus production by p24 antigen capture ELISA (ABL, Rockville, MD, United States). Cultures were scored as positive if p24 was detected at day 15 and was increased in concentration at day 19. A maximum likelihood method was used to estimate the frequency of resting cell infection, reported as infectious units per million CD4 + T cells (24, 25). Unless otherwise indicated, IUPM from day 15 post-stimulation of the QVOA is reported.

DEVO Assay

Resting CD4 + T cells were plated in limiting dilution of a combination of 0.5×10^6, 0.25×10^6, 0.1×10^6, 0.05×10^6 and 0.025×10^6 cells per well at 12 replicates each. Cells were stimulated with 2 μg/mL PHA, 60 U/mL Interleukin-2 (IL-2), and irradiated PBMCs from an HIV-seronegative donor.

After 24 h, the cells were washed to remove the PHA, and MOLT-CCR5 or PHA-blasts were added at 0.05 × 10^6 or 0.2 × 10^6 per well respectively to amplify outgrowth of the virus. For experiments testing whether virus outgrowth would occur without the addition of exogenous feeder cells, no targets were added to the wells. Fresh media was added to cultures every 3–4 days. On day 8, the wells were split and targeted with another round of MOLT-CCR5 or PHA blasts. Supernatants were harvested on days 8, 12, 15, and 19 or just days 8 and 12. An optimized protocol was used to quantify HIV p24 antigen in culture supernatant by the Simoa HD-1 Analyzer (Quanterix, Billerica, MA, United States). Only wells exhibiting sustained or increase in p24 expression over the multiple days of harvest were scored as positive. A maximum likelihood method was used to estimate the frequency of resting cell infection, reported as infectious units per million CD4 + T cells (24, 25). Unless otherwise indicated, all DEVO assays were performed with the addition of exogenous targets (PHA blasts or Molt4/CCR5) to amplify virus and IUPM from day 8 post-stimulation is reported.

Determination of DEVO LLOQ

Sero-negative donor resting CD4 + T cells were cultured in triplicate at 1 × 10^6 cells/ml in cIMDM with 0.2 × 10^6 irradiated normal donor PBMCs/ml, 3 μg/ml PHA and 100 units/ml IL-2. After 1 day, cells were washed one time to remove PHA. Cells were then co-cultured with target cells with wells receiving 0.4 × 10^6 normal donor PHA-stimulated, CD8-depleted PBMCs per million resting cells. On day 5, a half of media was removed and replaced with an equivalent volume of media containing IL-2. On day 8, supernatant was collected, aliquoted and stored at −80°C. An equivalent volume of media containing IL-2 and the appropriate number of targets cells were added back to each culture. Half volume of supernatant was collected from each well on days 8,12, 15, and 19, aliquoted and stored at −80°C for later processing.

On three separate, but not consecutive days, Using Calibrator I from Quanterix Simoa HIV p24 kit, day 8 and day 12 supernatants were spiked in triplicate at 100, 50, 25, 10, and 0 fg/ml of p24 and assayed on the Simoa on. For each concentration, supernatant day and assay day, the average and standard deviation of the three replicates were used to determine the bias, total error and% total error using the following formula: Bias = Average − Actual Value; Total Error = |Bias| + 2 × Standard Deviation; % Total Error = Total Error Actual Value × 100 (22). Percent total error versus concentration was plotted and fit using a 4-pl curve fit. From this fit, the concentration at which there is <20% total error was interpolated and found to be approximately 50 fg/ml. This value is used as the DEVO assay lower limit of quantitation.

Statistical Analyses

All statistical analyses were performed using GraphPad Prism version 8.0.0. Wilcoxon matched-pairs signed rank or Mann-Whitney *U* Test were used as appropriated to compare differences between groups. For IUPM below the limit of detection, resting cell infection was estimated assuming that 1 culture at the highest input cells was positive, and one-half of this value was used for the statistical analyses (12). Correlations between the DEVO and QVOA were assessed using the Spearman correlation coefficient. A *p* value of less or equal to 0.05 was considered to be significant in all analyses performed.

ETHICS STATEMENT

Samples were obtained from participants through an ongoing longitudinal collection protocol approved by the University of North Carolina (UNC) biomedical institutional review board. All samples were collected in accordance with UNC guidelines and all participants provided written informed consent prior to sample donation.

AUTHOR CONTRIBUTIONS

NA and ES conceptually designed the study. ES, KJ, JLK, and BA performed the experiments. NA, ES, and KJ performed the data analysis. NA wrote the manuscript. JDK, CB, DM, and CG provided clinical coordination and support. All authors edited and approved the final version.

ACKNOWLEDGMENTS

The authors would like to thank all the HIV seronegative and positive participants who made the study possible. The authors also would like to thank Nancie Hergert and Simon Ghofrani for technical support; Mary Napier for operational support; Katie Mollan and Jake Mathura for statistical support; Francesca Prince, Y. Park and the staff of the UNC Blood Bank and the UNC CTRC for clinical support.

REFERENCES

1. Hutter G, Nowak D, Mossner M, Ganepola S, Mussig A, Allers K, et al. Long-term control of HIV by CCR5 Delta32/Delta32 stem-cell transplantation. *N Engl J Med.* (2009) 360:692–8. doi: 10.1056/NEJMoa0802905
2. Gupta RK, Abdul-Jawad S, McCoy LE, Mok HP, Peppa D, Salgado M, et al. HIV-1 remission following CCR5Delta32/Delta32 haematopoietic stem-cell transplantation. *Nature.* (2019) 568:244–8. doi: 10.1038/s41586-019-1027-4
3. Eriksson S, Graf EH, Dahl V, Strain MC, Yukl SA, Lysenko ES, et al. Comparative analysis of measures of viral reservoirs in HIV-1 eradication studies. *PLoS Pathog.* (2013) 9:e1003174. doi: 10.1371/journal.ppat.1003174
4. Ho YC, Shan L, Hosmane NN, Wang J, Laskey SB, Rosenbloom DI, et al. Replication-competent noninduced proviruses in the latent reservoir increase barrier to HIV-1 cure. *Cell.* (2013) 155:540–51. doi: 10.1016/j.cell.2013.09.020
5. Bruner KM, Murray AJ, Pollack RA, Soliman MG, Laskey SB, Capoferri AA, et al. Defective proviruses rapidly accumulate during acute HIV-1 infection. *Nat Med.* (2016) 22:1043–9. doi: 10.1038/nm.4156

6. Bruner KM, Wang Z, Simonetti FR, Bender AM, Kwon KJ, Sengupta S, et al. A quantitative approach for measuring the reservoir of latent HIV-1 proviruses. *Nature.* (2019) 566:120–5. doi: 10.1038/s41586-019-0898-8
7. Gaebler C, Lorenzi JCC, Oliveira TY, Nogueira L, Ramos V, Lu CL, et al. Combination of quadruplex qPCR and next-generation sequencing for qualitative and quantitative analysis of the HIV-1 latent reservoir. *J Exp Med.* (2019) 216:2253–64. doi: 10.1084/jem.20190896
8. Finzi D, Hermankova M, Pierson T, Carruth LM, Buck C, Chaisson RE, et al. Identification of a reservoir for HIV-1 in patients on highly active antiretroviral therapy. *Science.* (1997) 278:1295–300. doi: 10.1126/science.278.5341.1295
9. Chun TW, Carruth L, Finzi D, Shen X, DiGiuseppe JA, Taylor H, et al. Quantification of latent tissue reservoirs and total body viral load in HIV-1 infection. *Nature.* (1997) 387:183–8. doi: 10.1038/387183a0
10. Siliciano JD, Siliciano RF. Enhanced culture assay for detection and quantitation of latently infected, resting CD4+ T-cells carrying replication-competent virus in HIV-1-infected individuals. *Methods Mol Biol.* (2005) 304:3–15.
11. Hosmane NN, Kwon KJ, Bruner KM, Capoferri AA, Beg S, Rosenbloom DI, et al. Proliferation of latently infected CD4(+) T cells carrying replication-competent HIV-1: Potential role in latent reservoir dynamics. *J Exp Med.* (2017) 214:959–72. doi: 10.1084/jem.20170193
12. Crooks AM, Bateson R, Cope AB, Dahl NP, Griggs MK, Kuruc JD, et al. Precise quantitation of the latent HIV-1 reservoir: implications for eradication strategies. *J Infect Dis.* (2015) 212:1361–5. doi: 10.1093/infdis/jiv218
13. Falcinelli SD, Ceriani C, Margolis DM, Archin NM. New frontiers in measuring and characterizing the HIV reservoir. *Front Microbiol.* (2019) 10:2878. doi: 10.3389/fmicb.2019.02878
14. Rissin DM, Kan CW, Campbell TG, Howes SC, Fournier DR, Song L, et al. Single-molecule enzyme-linked immunosorbent assay detects serum proteins at subfemtomolar concentrations. *Nat Biotechnol.* (2010) 28:595–9. doi: 10.1038/nbt.1641
15. Wilson DH, Rissin DM, Kan CW, Fournier DR, Piech T, Campbell TG, et al. The simoa HD-1 analyzer: a novel fully automated digital immunoassay analyzer with single-molecule sensitivity and multiplexing. *J Lab Autom.* (2016) 21:533–47. doi: 10.1177/2211068215589580
16. Wu G, Swanson M, Talla A, Graham D, Strizki J, Gorman D, et al. HDAC inhibition induces HIV-1 protein and enables immune-based clearance following latency reversal. *JCI insight.* (2017) 2:e92901. doi: 10.1172/jci.insight.92901
17. Chang L, Song L, Fournier DR, Kan CW, Patel PP, Ferrell EP, et al. Simple diffusion-constrained immunoassay for p24 protein with the sensitivity of nucleic acid amplification for detecting acute HIV infection. *J Virol Methods.* (2013) 188:153–60. doi: 10.1016/j.jviromet.2012.08.017
18. Stuelke ELSK, Kirchherr JL, Allard B, Margolis DM, Archin NM, *Abstracts of the Eighth International Workshop on HIV Persistence During Therapy 12–15 December 2017.* Miami, FL: Elsevier. (2017). Available online at: https://www.sciencedirect.com/journal/journal-of-virus-eradication/vol/3/suppl/S5
19. Rosenbloom DIS, Bacchetti P, Stone M, Deng X, Bosch RJ, Richman DD, et al. Assessing intra-lab precision and inter-lab repeatability of outgrowth assays of HIV-1 latent reservoir size. *PLoS Comput Biol.* (2019) 15:e1006849. doi: 10.1371/journal.pcbi.1006849
20. Descours B, Petitjean G, Lopez-Zaragoza JL, Bruel T, Raffel R, Psomas C, et al. CD32a is a marker of a CD4 T-cell HIV reservoir harbouring replication-competent proviruses. *Nature.* (2017) 543:564–7. doi: 10.1038/nature21710
21. Passaes CP, Bruel T, Decalf J, David A, Angin M, Monceaux V, et al. Ultrasensitive HIV-1 p24 assay detects single infected cells and differences in reservoir induction by latency reversal agents. *J Virol.* (2017) 91:e02296-16. doi: 10.1128/JVI.02296-16
22. CLSI. *Evaluation of Detection Capability for Clinical Laboratory Measurement Procedures; Approved Guidline.* 2nd ed. Wayne, PA: Clinical and Laboratory Standards Institute (2012).
23. Archin NM, Kirchherr JL, Sung JA, Clutton G, Sholtis K, Xu Y, et al. Interval dosing with the HDAC inhibitor vorinostat effectively reverses HIV latency. *J Clin Invest.* (2017) 127:3126–35. doi: 10.1172/JCI92684
24. Myers LE, McQuay LJ, Hollinger FB. Dilution assay statistics. *J Clin Microbiol.* (1994) 32:732–9. doi: 10.1128/JCM.32.3.732-739.1994
25. Trumble IM, Allmon AG, Archin NM, Rigdon J, Francis O, Baldoni PL, et al. SLDAssay: a software package and web tool for analyzing limiting dilution assays. *J Immunol Methods.* (2017) 450:10–6. doi: 10.1016/j.jim.2017.07.004
26. Laird GM, Eisele EE, Rabi SA, Lai J, Chioma S, Blankson JN, et al. Rapid quantification of the latent reservoir for HIV-1 using a viral outgrowth assay. *PLoS Pathog.* (2013) 9:30. doi: 10.1371/journal.ppat.1003398
27. Wonderlich ER, Subramanian K, Cox B, Wiegand A, Lackman-Smith C, Bale MJ, et al. Effector memory differentiation increases detection of replication-competent HIV-l in resting CD4+ T cells from virally suppressed individuals. *PLoS Pathog.* (2019) 15:e1008074. doi: 10.1371/journal.ppat.1008074
28. Massanella M, Yek C, Lada SM, Nakazawa M, Shefa N, Huang K, et al. Improved assays to measure and characterize the inducible HIV reservoir. *EBioMedicine.* (2018) 36:113–21. doi: 10.1016/j.ebiom.2018.09.036
29. Kulpa DA, Talla A, Brehm JH, Ribeiro SP, Yuan S, Bebin-Blackwell AG, et al. Differentiation into an effector memory phenotype potentiates HIV-1 latency reversal in CD4(+) T Cells. *J Virol.* (2019) 93:e00969-19. doi: 10.1128/JVI.00969-19
30. Charlins P, Schmitt K, Remling-Mulder L, Hogan LE, Hanhauser E, Hobbs KS, et al. A humanized mouse-based HIV-1 viral outgrowth assay with higher sensitivity than in vitro qVOA in detecting latently infected cells from individuals on ART with undetectable viral loads. *Virology.* (2017) 507:135–9. doi: 10.1016/j.virol.2017.04.011
31. Metcalf Pate KA, Pohlmeyer CW, Walker-Sperling VE, Foote JB, Najarro KM, Cryer CG, et al. A murine viral outgrowth assay to detect residual HIV type 1 in patients with undetectable viral loads. *J Infect Dis.* (2015) 212:1387–96. doi: 10.1093/infdis/jiv230
32. Schmitt K, Akkina R. Ultra-sensitive HIV-1 latency viral outgrowth assays using humanized mice. *Front Immunol.* (2018) 9:344. doi: 10.3389/fimmu.2018.00344
33. Archin NM, Liberty AL, Kashuba AD, Choudhary SK, Kuruc JD, Crooks AM, et al. Administration of vorinostat disrupts HIV-1 latency in patients on antiretroviral therapy. *Nature.* (2012) 487:482–5. doi: 10.1038/nature11286
34. Keedy KS, Archin NM, Gates AT, Espeseth A, Hazuda DJ, Margolis DM. A limited group of class I histone deacetylases acts to repress human immunodeficiency virus type 1 expression. *J Virol.* (2009) 83:4749–56. doi: 10.1128/JVI.02585-08

Permissions

All chapters in this book were first published by Frontiers; hereby published with permission under the Creative Commons Attribution License or equivalent. Every chapter published in this book has been scrutinized by our experts. Their significance has been extensively debated. The topics covered herein carry significant findings which will fuel the growth of the discipline. They may even be implemented as practical applications or may be referred to as a beginning point for another development.

The contributors of this book come from diverse backgrounds, making this book a truly international effort. This book will bring forth new frontiers with its revolutionizing research information and detailed analysis of the nascent developments around the world.

We would like to thank all the contributing authors for lending their expertise to make the book truly unique. They have played a crucial role in the development of this book. Without their invaluable contributions this book wouldn't have been possible. They have made vital efforts to compile up to date information on the varied aspects of this subject to make this book a valuable addition to the collection of many professionals and students.

This book was conceptualized with the vision of imparting up-to-date information and advanced data in this field. To ensure the same, a matchless editorial board was set up. Every individual on the board went through rigorous rounds of assessment to prove their worth. After which they invested a large part of their time researching and compiling the most relevant data for our readers.

The editorial board has been involved in producing this book since its inception. They have spent rigorous hours researching and exploring the diverse topics which have resulted in the successful publishing of this book. They have passed on their knowledge of decades through this book. To expedite this challenging task, the publisher supported the team at every step. A small team of assistant editors was also appointed to further simplify the editing procedure and attain best results for the readers.

Apart from the editorial board, the designing team has also invested a significant amount of their time in understanding the subject and creating the most relevant covers. They scrutinized every image to scout for the most suitable representation of the subject and create an appropriate cover for the book.

The publishing team has been an ardent support to the editorial, designing and production team. Their endless efforts to recruit the best for this project, has resulted in the accomplishment of this book. They are a veteran in the field of academics and their pool of knowledge is as vast as their experience in printing. Their expertise and guidance has proved useful at every step. Their uncompromising quality standards have made this book an exceptional effort. Their encouragement from time to time has been an inspiration for everyone.

The publisher and the editorial board hope that this book will prove to be a valuable piece of knowledge for researchers, students, practitioners and scholars across the globe.

List of Contributors

Vikram Mehraj
Chronic Viral Illness Service, McGill University Health Centre, Montreal, QC, Canada
Infectious Diseases and Immunity in Global Health Program, Research Institute, McGill University Health Centre, Montreal, QC, Canada
University of Montreal Hospital Health Centre (CRCHUM), Montreal, QC, Canada
Centre de Recherche du Centre Hospitalier de l'Université de Montréal, Montreal, QC, Canada

Stéphane Isnard, Jun Chen, Franck P. Dupuy and Cecilia Costiniuk
Chronic Viral Illness Service, McGill University Health Centre, Montreal, QC, Canada
Infectious Diseases and Immunity in Global Health Program, Research Institute, McGill University Health Centre, Montreal, QC, Canada

Madéleine Durand and Carl Chartrand-Lefebvre
University of Montreal Hospital Health Centre (CRCHUM), Montreal, QC, Canada

Rayoun Ramendra
Chronic Viral Illness Service, McGill University Health Centre, Montreal, QC, Canada
Infectious Diseases and Immunity in Global Health Program, Research Institute, McGill University Health Centre, Montreal, QC, Canada
Department of Microbiology and Immunology, McGill University, Montreal, QC, Canada

Bertrand Lebouché
Chronic Viral Illness Service, McGill University Health Centre, Montreal, QC, Canada
Infectious Diseases and Immunity in Global Health Program, Research Institute, McGill University Health Centre, Montreal, QC, Canada
Department of Family Medicine, McGill University, Montreal, QC, Canada

Réjean Thomas
Clinique Médicale l'Actuel, Montreal, QC, Canada

Jason Szabo
Chronic Viral Illness Service, McGill University Health Centre, Montreal, QC, Canada
Clinique Médicale Quartier Latin, Montreal, QC, Canada

Jean-Guy Baril, Benoit Trottier and Pierre Coté
Clinique Médicale Quartier Latin, Montreal, QC, Canada

Roger LeBlanc
Clinique Médicale OPUS, Montreal, QC, Canada

Ido Kema
Department of Laboratory Medicine, University Medical Center, University of Groningen, Groningen, Netherlands

Yonglong Zhang and Malcolm Finkelman
Associates of CapeCod Inc., Falmouth, MA, United States

Cécile Tremblay
University of Montreal Hospital Health Centre (CRCHUM), Montreal, QC, Canada
Département de Microbiologie, Infectiologie et Immunologie, Université de Montréal, Montreal, QC, Canada

Jean-Pierre Routy
Chronic Viral Illness Service, McGill University Health Centre, Montreal, QC, Canada
Infectious Diseases and Immunity in Global Health Program, Research Institute, McGill University Health Centre, Montreal, QC, Canada
Hematology Clinic, McGill University Health Centre, Montreal, QC, Canada

Hok Yee Chan, Jiajia Zhang and Kellie N. Smith
Bloomberg-Kimmel Institute for Cancer Immunotherapy, Johns Hopkins School of Medicine, Baltimore, MD, United States
Sidney Kimmel Comprehensive Cancer Center, Johns Hopkins School of Medicine, Baltimore, MD, United States

Caroline C. Garliss and Abena K. Kwaa
Department of Medicine, Johns Hopkins School of Medicine, Baltimore, MD, United States

Joel N. Blankson
Department of Medicine, Johns Hopkins School of Medicine, Baltimore, MD, United States
Department of Molecular and Comparative Pathobiology, Johns Hopkins School of Medicine, Baltimore, MD, United States

Tori Huffman and Joy A. Pickeral
Department of Surgery, Duke University School of Medicine, Durham, NC, United States

Justin Pollara, Shalini Jha and Guido Ferrari
Department of Surgery, Duke University School of Medicine, Durham, NC, United States
Human Vaccine Institute, Duke University School of Medicine, Durham, NC, United States

R. Whitney Edwards and Thomas N. Denny
Human Vaccine Institute, Duke University School of Medicine, Durham, NC, United States

Chia-Ying Kao Lam, Liqin Liu, Gundo Diedrich and Jeffrey L. Nordstrom
Macrogenics, Inc., Rockville, MD, United States

Sallie R. Permar
Human Vaccine Institute, Duke University School of Medicine, Durham, NC, United States
Department of Pediatrics, Duke University School of Medicine, Durham, NC, United States

Lin-Bo Yin, Cheng-Bo Song, Jie-Fu Zheng, Ya-Jing Fu, Shi Qian, Yong-Jun Jiang, Jun-Jie Xu, Hai-Bo Ding, Hong Shang and Zi-Ning Zhang
NHC Key Laboratory of AIDS Immunology (China Medical University), Department of Laboratory Medicine, The First Affiliated Hospital of China Medical University, Shenyang, China
Key Laboratory of AIDS Immunology of Liaoning Province, The First Affiliated Hospital of China Medical University, Shenyang, China
Key Laboratory of AIDS Immunology, Chinese Academy of Medical Sciences, Shenyang, China
Collaborative Innovation Center for Diagnosis and Treatment of Infectious Diseases, Hangzhou, China

Allan Bowen and Elizabeth E. Sweeney
The George Washington Cancer Center, The George Washington University, Washington, DC, United States

Rohan Fernandes
The George Washington Cancer Center, The George Washington University, Washington, DC, United States
Department of Medicine, The George Washington University, Washington, DC, United States

Ryan Tjitro, Jessica Johnson and Julia A. Najera
Department of Neurosciences, The Scripps Research Institute, La Jolla, CA, United States

Lee A. Campbell
LAC Intramural Research Program, National Institute on Drug Abuse, Baltimore, MD, United States

Liana Basova and Maria Cecilia Garibaldi Marcondes
Department of Neurosciences, The Scripps Research Institute, La Jolla, CA, United States
San Diego Biomedical Research Institute, San Diego, CA, United States

Alexander Lindsey
San Diego Biomedical Research Institute, San Diego, CA, United States

José M. Martinez-Navio, Sebastian P. Fuchs, Desiree E. Mendes and Ronald C. Desrosiers
Department of Pathology, Miller School of Medicine, University of Miami, Miami, FL, United States

Eva G. Rakasz
Wisconsin National Primate Research Center, University of Wisconsin, Madison, WI, United States

Guangping Gao
Gene Therapy Center, University of Massachusetts Medical School, Worcester, MA, United States

Jeffrey D. Lifson
AIDS and Cancer Virus Program, Frederick National Laboratory for Cancer Research, Frederick, MD, United States

Xiao Yu, Lei Gao, Haha Wang, Zhuang Yin, Jian Fang and Haibo Xu
Department of Radiology, Zhongnan Hospital of Wuhan University, Wuhan University, Wuhan, China

Jing Chen
Publicity Department, Zhongnan Hospital of Wuhan University, Wuhan University, Wuhan, China

Qiang Li and Xien Gui
Training Centre of AIDS Prevention and Cure of Hubei Province, Zhongnan Hospital of Wuhan University, Wuhan University, Wuhan, China

Pep Coll, Maria C. Puertas, Sara Morón-López, Marta Ruiz-Riol, Marta Marszalek, Anuska Llano and Samandhy Cedeño
IrsiCaixa AIDS Research Institute-HIVACAT, Badalona, Spain

Miriam López, Jessica Toro and Cristina Miranda
Fundació Lluita contra la Sida, Infectious Diseases Department, Hospital Universitari Germans Trias i Pujol, Badalona, Spain

Beatriz Mothe
IrsiCaixa AIDS Research Institute-HIVACAT, Badalona, Spain
Fundació Lluita contra la Sida, Infectious Diseases Department, Hospital Universitari Germans Trias i Pujol, Badalona, Spain
Faculty of Medicine, Universitat de Vic-Central de Catalunya (UVic-UCC), Vic, Spain
Centre for Health and Social Care Research (CESS), Faculty of Medicine, University of Vic - Central University of Catalonia (UVic - UCC), Vic, Spain

Miriam Rosás-Umbert
IrsiCaixa AIDS Research Institute-HIVACAT, Badalona, Spain
Department of Cellular Biology, Physiology and Immunology, Universitat Autonoma de Barcelona (UAB), Barcelona, Spain

Bonaventura Clotet
IrsiCaixa AIDS Research Institute-HIVACAT, Badalona, Spain
Fundació Lluita contra la Sida, Infectious Diseases Department, Hospital Universitari Germans Trias i Pujol, Badalona, Spain
Faculty of Medicine, Universitat de Vic-Central de Catalunya (UVic-UCC), Vic, Spain
Department of Cellular Biology, Physiology and Immunology, Universitat Autonoma de Barcelona (UAB), Barcelona, Spain
Department of Infectious Diseases, Hospital Germans Trias i Pujol, Badalona, Spain
Centre for Health and Social Care Research (CESS), Faculty of Medicine, University of Vic - Central University of Catalonia (UVic - UCC), Vic, Spain

Christian Manzardo, Irene Ruiz, Cristina Rovira and Jose M. Miró
Hospital Clinic- IDIBAPS, University of Barcelona, Barcelona, Spain

Yovaninna Alarcón-Soto, Guadalupe Gómez Melis and Klaus Langohr
Departament d'Estadística i Investigació Operativa, Universitat Politècnica de Catalunya/ BARCELONATECH, Barcelona, Spain

Ana M. Barriocanal
Department of Cellular Biology, Physiology and Immunology, Universitat Autonoma de Barcelona (UAB), Barcelona, Spain
Department of Infectious Diseases, Germans Trias i Pujol Research Institute, Badalona, Spain

Antonio Carrillo
Department of Infectious Diseases, Germans Trias i Pujol Research Institute, Badalona, Spain

José Moltó
Fundació Lluita contra la Sida, Infectious Diseases Department, Hospital Universitari Germans Trias i Pujol, Badalona, Spain
Department of Infectious Diseases, Germans Trias i Pujol Research Institute, Badalona, Spain

Michael Meulbroek
Projecte dels NOMS-Hispanosida, BCN Checkpoint, Barcelona, Spain

Alison Crook and Edmund G. Wee
The Jenner Institute, University of Oxford, Oxford, United Kingdom

Marta Valle
Department of Cellular Biology, Physiology and Immunology, Universitat Autonoma de Barcelona (UAB), Barcelona, Spain
Pharmacokinetic/Pharmacodynamic Modeling and Simultation, Institut de Recerca de l'Hospital de la Santa Creu i Sant Pau-IIB Sant Pau, Barcelona, Spain

Javier Martinez-Picado and Christian Brander
IrsiCaixa AIDS Research Institute-HIVACAT, Badalona, Spain
Faculty of Medicine, Universitat de Vic-Central de Catalunya (UVic-UCC), Vic, Spain
ICREA, Pg. Lluis Companys, Barcelona, Spain
Centre for Health and Social Care Research (CESS), Faculty of Medicine, University of Vic - Central University of Catalonia (UVic - UCC), Vic, Spain

Marco A. Fernández
Flow Cytometry Facility, Health Sciences Research Institute Germans Triasi Pujol, Badalona, Spain

Tomáš Hanke
The Jenner Institute, University of Oxford, Oxford, United Kingdom
Joint Research Center for Human Retrovirus Infection, Kumamoto University, Kumamoto, Japan

Riley M. F. Pihl
Flow Cytometry Core Facility, Boston University School of Medicine, Boston, MA, United States

Anna C. Belkina
Flow Cytometry Core Facility, Boston University School of Medicine, Boston, MA, United States
Department of Pathology and Laboratory Medicine, Boston University School of Medicine, Boston, MA, United States

Alina Starchenko, Elizabeth A. Proctor and Douglas A. Lauffenburger
Department of Biological Engineering, Massachusetts Institute of Technology, Cambridge, MA, United States

Katherine A. Drake
Cytobank, Inc., Santa Clara, CA, United States

Alex Olson and Nina Lin
Department of Medicine, Boston University School of Medicine, Boston, MA, United States

Jennifer E. Snyder-Cappione
Flow Cytometry Core Facility, Boston University School of Medicine, Boston, MA, United States
Department of Microbiology, Boston University School of Medicine, Boston, MA, United States

Florent Colomb, Leila B. Giron, Emmanouil Papasavvas, Luis J. Montaner and Mohamed Abdel Mohsen
Vaccine and Immunotherapy Center, The Wistar Institute, Philadelphia, PA, United States

Thomas A. Premeaux, Brooks I. Mitchell and Lishomwa C. Ndhlovu
Department of Tropical Medicine, Hawaii Center for AIDS, John A. Burns School of Medicine, University of Hawaii, Honolulu, HI, United States

Toshiro Niki
GalPharma Co., Ltd., Takamatsu-shi, Takamatsu, Japan
Department of Immunology and Immunopathology, Kagawa University, Takamatsu, Japan

Janne Tegder Martinsen, Jesper Damsgaard Gunst, Jesper Falkesgaard Højen, Martin Tolstrup and Ole Schmeltz Søgaard
Department of Infectious Diseases, Aarhus University Hospital, Aarhus, Denmark

Nicholas Rhoades, Norma Mendoza, Allen Jankeel, Suhas Sureshchandra, Alexander D. Alvarez, Brianna Doratt and Ilhem Messaoudi
Molecular Biology and Biochemistry, University of California Irvine, Irvine, CA, United States

Omeid Heidari
School of Nursing, John Hopkins University, Baltimore, MD, United States

Rod Hagan, Steven Scheibel and Theodore Marbley
Stonewall Medical Center, Borrego Health, Cathedral City, CA, United States

Brandon Brown
School of Medicine, University of California, Riverside, Riverside, CA, United States

Jeff Taylor
HIV+ Aging-Palm Springs, Palm Springs, CA, United States

Maria Pino, Colin King, Kevin Nguyen and Inbo Shim
Division of Microbiology and Immunology, Yerkes National Primate Research Center, Emory University, Atlanta, GA, United States

Srijayaprakash Babu Uppada and Kabita Pandey
Department of Pharmacology and Experimental Neuroscience, University of Nebraska Medical Center, Omaha, NE, United States

Kenneth Rogers and Francois Villinger
New Iberia Research Center, University of Louisiana at Lafayette, New Iberia, LA, United States

Mirko Paiardini
Division of Microbiology and Immunology, Yerkes National Primate Research Center, Emory University, Atlanta, GA, United States
Department of Pathology and Laboratory Medicine, Emory University School of Medicine, Atlanta, GA, United States

Siddappa N. Byrareddy
Department of Pharmacology and Experimental Neuroscience, University of Nebraska Medical Center, Omaha, NE, United States
Department of Genetics, Cell Biology and Anatomy, University of Nebraska Medical Center, Omaha, NE, United States
Department of Biochemistry and Molecular Biology, University of Nebraska Medical Center, Omaha, NE, United States

Bethany M. Henrick
Evolve Biosystems, Davis, CA, United States
Department of Food Science and Technology, University of Nebraska, Lincoln, NE, United States

Xiao-Dan Yao, Muhammad Atif Zahoor and Kenneth L. Rosenthal
Department of Pathology and Molecular Medicine, McMaster University, Hamilton, ON, Canada

Alash'le Abimiku and Sophia Osawe
Institue of Human Virology-Nigeria, Abuja, Nigeria

Mansi Saxena, Rachel L. Sabado, Hanqing Dong and Nina Bhardwaj
Icahn School of Medicine at Mount Sinai, New York, NY, United States

Elizabeth Miller
Icahn School of Medicine at Mount Sinai, New York, NY, United States
Laboratory of Investigative Dermatology, The Rockefeller University, New York, NY, United States

Melissa La Mar, Hiroshi Mohri and Martin Markowitz
Aaron Diamond AIDS Research Center, Rockefeller University, New York, NY, United States

Andres M. Salazar
Oncovir, Inc., Washington, DC, United States

Joel Correa Da Rosa
Laboratory of Investigative Dermatology, The Rockefeller University, New York, NY, United States

Erin L. Stuelke, Katherine S. James, Jennifer L. Kirchherr, Brigitte Allard and Caroline Baker
University of North Carolina HIV Cure Center, UNC Institute for Global Health and Infectious Diseases, Chapel Hill, NC, United States

Joann D. Kuruc, Cindy L. Gay and Nancie M. Archin
University of North Carolina HIV Cure Center, UNC Institute for Global Health and Infectious Diseases, Chapel Hill, NC, United States
Department of Medicine, UNC Chapel Hill School of Medicine, Chapel Hill, NC, United States

David M. Margolis
University of North Carolina HIV Cure Center, UNC Institute for Global Health and Infectious Diseases, Chapel Hill, NC, United States
Department of Medicine, UNC Chapel Hill School of Medicine, Chapel Hill, NC, United States
Department of Microbiology and Immunology, UNC Chapel Hill School of Medicine, Chapel Hill, NC, United States
Department of Epidemiology, UNC Chapel Hill School of Public Health, The University of North Carolina at Chapel Hill, Chapel Hill, NC, United States

Francesco Indiveri
Centre of Excellence for Biomedical Research and Department of Internal Medicine, University of Genoa, Genoa, Italy

Index